# MEDICAL RADIOLOGY

Diagnostic Imaging and Radiation Oncology – Softcover Edition

Springer
*Berlin*
*Heidelberg*
*New York*
*Barcelona*
*Hong Kong*
*London*
*Milan*
*Paris*
*Singapore*
*Tokyo*

S. K. Mukherji · J. A. Castelijns (Eds.)

# Modern Head and Neck Imaging

With Contributions by

B. Biswal · V. Carrasco · J. A. Castelijns · M. Castillo · V. Chong · D. L. Daniels
R. De Bree · J. L. Duerk · M. Gapany · F. M. Grund · B. M. Hemminger · R. Hermans
L. Jäger · A. G. Janssen · M. Lapela · S. Leskinen · J. S. Lewin · P. Lindholm
M. G. Mack · L. P. Mark · E. M. Merkle · H. Minn · K. Mosier · S. K. Mukherji · J. J. Quak
J. C. Roos · G. B Snow · J. L. Ulmer M. W. M. Van Den Brekel · G. A. M. S. Van Dongen
T. J. Vogl · D. M. Yousem

Series Editor's Foreword by

J. E. Youker

Forewords by

H.C. Pillsbury and G.B. Snow

With 166 Figures in 318 Separate Illustrations, 51 in Color

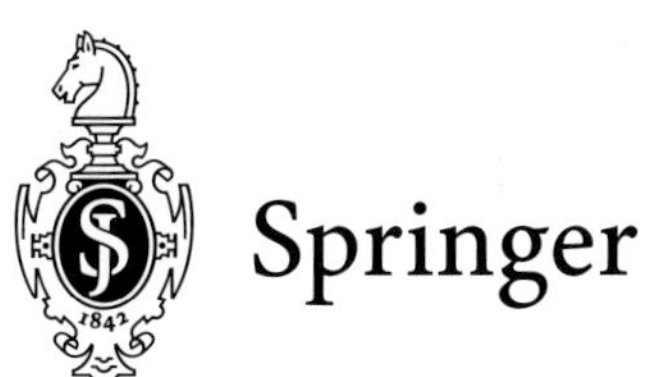


Springer

Suresh K. Mukherji, MD
Department of Radiology
The School of Medicine
University of North Carolina at Chapel Hill
Chapel Hill, NC 27599-7510
USA

J.A. Castelijns, MD
Academisch Ziekenhuis Vrije Universiteit
Department of Radiology
P.O.Box 7057
1007 MB Amsterdam
The Netherlands

MEDICAL RADIOLOGY · Diagnostic Imaging and Radiation Oncology

Continuation of
Handbuch der medizinischen Radiologie
Encyclopedia of Medical Radiology

ISSN 0942-5373
ISBN 3-540-66344-4 Springer-Verlag Berlin Heidelberg New York

Library of Congress Cataloging-in-Publication Data applied for

Die Deutsche Bibliothek – CIP-Einheitsaufnahme. Modern head and neck imaging / S. K. Mukherji; J. A. Castelijns (ed.). With contributions by B. Biswal ... Ser. ed. foreword by J. E. Youker. Forewords by H. C. Pillsbury and G. B. Snow. – Berlin; Heidelberg; New York; Barcelona; Hong Kong; London; Milan; Paris; Singapore; Tokyo: Springer, 2000 (Medical radiology). ISBN 3-540-66344-4. Radiology Trauma. – 2000.



Printed in Germany



Cover design: Joan Greenfield, New York

Typesetting: Best-set Typesetter Ltd., Hong Kong

SPIN: 10741894 21/3135 – 5 4 3 2 1 – Printed on acid-free paper

*To my wife Rita, for her love and understanding*

*To my mother, Chandra Mukherji, MD*
*for her undying love and encouragement*

*In loving memory of my father,*
*Phatick Mukherji, MD*

*To my daughter Anika,*
*who represents the future generations that we, as academicians*
*and researchers, hope will benefit from our work*

SURESH K. MUKHERJI

*To my dear parents for their support and stimulation*

*To my beloved wife Brigitte*
*for understanding my continuing dedication*

*and to my two young heroes, Brent and Luc,*
*for giving me immediate relaxation*

JONAS A. CASTELIJNS

# Foreword

Historically, the diagnosis of clinical problems in the head and neck has relied on a combination of physical examination and plain film radiography. Although Ziedses des Plantes' invention of tomography had a major impact on head and neck diagnosis, it remained for the development of CT, MR and modern nuclear medicine to truly revolutionize the specialty. Not only have these new techniques provided better definition of osseous structures and soft tissues but adaptations of these techniques have allowed us to study function as well as anatomy. Utilization of the modern imaging techniques has also provided a springboard for new interventional techniques which promise to redefine the treatment of head and neck problems.

As a consequence there are now many highly specific diagnostic and therapeutic applications of these new technologies that are not familiar to the average practicing radiologist or otolaryngologist. Drs. Mukherji and Castelijns have made an important contribution by bringing together a group of outstanding authors from around the world who explain in detail how these new techniques can be applied and what their impact is on patient care. Included among the authors are both radiologists and otolaryngologists. The volume will serve as a practical, easy reference guide to physicians when unusual problems are encountered in this somewhat unfamiliar area of patient care. The volume should be of particular value to the radiologist who deals with these new modalities on a day-to-day basis.

Milwaukee James E. Youker

# Foreword

The role of the neuroradiologist with a special interest in head and neck imaging has become essential for those of us who deal with complex cases from a diagnostic and therapeutic point of view. The editors and authors in this book have done a superb job of bringing together the critical issues in head and neck imaging that impact on neuroradiologists, surgeons and those interested in arriving at an accurate diagnosis when there are problems in the head and neck region for which they have to plan therapy. The techniques described and discussed in this text are state of the art, and the expertise of the contributors is beyond question.

Having worked with Dr. Suresh Mukherji for several years, I have found him personally to be a tremendous asset to our service and a valued member of our team. I have grown to respect his expertise as well as enjoy his friendship. I think all who read this book will be impressed with its content and learn a great deal from it.

Chapel Hill HAROLD C. PILLSBURY

# Foreword

Imaging of the head and neck has made great progress during the last 25 years. Superb anatomical CT and MR Images are now routinely available, allowing for improved delineation of lesions in the head and neck, particularly of their deeper extension. These advances in imaging have helped clinicians considerably in the selection and the planning of treatment of patients with diseases of the head and neck. However, many diagnostic problems in the head and neck remain to be solved and these are strong motive for imaging technology to continue to develop.

This book comprehensively reviews the latest developments of head and neck imaging in the 1990s. It is a multi-authored book written by well-known American and European experts who are acknowledged leaders in imaging modalities in the head and neck. To complete a book with a distinguished group of specialists on such a broad range of modalities is in itself an admirable achievement by the editors Dr. S. K. Mukherji and Dr. J. A. Castelijns. Ten chapters deal with application of special MR techniques, such as magnetisation transfer, T2 gradient echo imaging, functional MRI and MR spectroscopy. The value of nuclear medicine techniques like PET, SPECT and immunoscintigraphy is discussed extensively in three chapters. Two chapters discuss the role of 3D-CT in the extracranial head and neck. Comparison between various techniques has been made for the larynx and the neck. Finally, interventional procedures, using MR guidance and balloon dilatation, are dealt with in three chapters. The great majority of the chapters address important topics in head and neck oncology, such as the assessment of "occult" lymph node metastasis in the neck, detection of "unknown" primary tumours, the evaluation of the response to treatment and the differential diagnosis between "early" recurrence and post-treatment changes. Other chapters concentrate on pathology in the temporal bone, the skull base and the lacrimal duct system. Two chapters address functional MR imaging respectively of hearing and swallowing.

The strength of this book is the extensive and in-depth coverage of advanced imaging modalities in the head and neck, providing unique information that is a welcome supplement to the already existing literature. The book deserves a prominent position in the library of readers who seek information on the newer fields of application in radiology and nuclear medicine. Many of these imaging techniques hold great promise and their potential clinical relevance is highlighted.

Modern Head and Neck Imaging brings the reader up to date about what is going on and about what lies ahead in this fascinating field. This book is warmly recommended to both radiologists, nuclear medicine physicians and otolaryngologists/head and neck surgeons who want to familiarize themselves with advanced imaging techniques in the head and neck.

Amsterdam G. B. Snow

# Preface

The past 15 years have seen dramatic changes in imaging of the head and neck. Technical advances in computed tomography and magnetic resonance imaging, coupled with their widespread availability, have made cross-sectional imaging an important adjunct to the evaluation of patients with disease of the extracranial head and neck. At the majority of institutions, cross-sectional imaging is now a routine part of the initial evaluation of these patients. The most recent advances in head and neck imaging are those developed from new metabolic and functional imaging techniques.

We have attempted to make Modern Head and Neck Imaging a clear and concise text reviewing the recent advances in the field of head and neck imaging. We have especially emphasized the clinical applications of these techniques. In fact, many chapter authors are otolaryngologists, and their perspectives on these techniques is especially welcome. The clinical topics that are addressed include: (1) techniques that are useful in improving the ability to distinguish between tumor and post-treatment changes; (2) new techniques that add new information for evaluating patients with sensorineural hearing loss; (3) advances that can help in differentiation between metastatic and normal cervical lymph nodes; (4) new minimally invasive procedures that may be performed for diagnosis and treatment that can avoid an open intraoperative procedure; and (5) clinical applications of three-dimensional imaging.

Despite these advances, the primary goal of head and neck imaging has not changed. As this is one of the few radiological subspecialties where the referring clinician can directly identify the pathology on physical examination, the challenge is to continue to provide clinically relevant information that cannot be ascertained by the referring physician. It is important that radiologists understand the clinical utility of these new imaging techniques and emphasize the "added value" of performing these studies for the overall care of the patient. Otherwise, we, as radiologists, run the risk of having our clinical colleagues consider these new modalities as "radiological curiosities" rather than important adjuncts to the treatment and management of patients with various head and neck disorders. We must always remember that the field of head and neck imaging will only continue to advance if the new imaging techniques can provide information that cannot be determined on examination and will directly alter outcome. We hope our text will provide the basis for future investigations, which will further demonstrate the benefits of these important advances in patient care.

Chapel Hill
Amsterdam

Suresh K. Mukherji
Jonas A. Castelijns

**Acknowledgements**

I would like to acknowledge my colleagues in the sections of Neuroradiology and Otolaryngology, Head and Neck Surgery and Joseph K.T. Lee, MD, for providing an environment that fosters creativity; my parents for instilling in me the belief that no hard work goes unrewarded.

SURESH K. MUKHERJI

I would like to thank my colleagues who graciously gave me the opportunity to complete this work, to my fellow neuroradiologists for stimulating a climate of high creativity, and my secretary, Helma Drukker, for her untiring support.

JONAS A. CASTELIJNS

We both would like to acknowledge Ursula Davis, at Springer-Verlag, for her continuing support, understanding and enthusiasm for our ideas. Many individuals have contributed to the preparation of this text and we apologize for any unintended omissions.

SURESH K. MUKHERJI and JONAS A. CASTELIJNS

# Contents

# 1 Magnetization Transfer Imaging of the Extracranial Head and Neck

D.M. Yousem

CONTENTS



## 1.1 Introduction

Magnetization transfer imaging (MTI) of head and neck lesions is a fertile area of research that has yet to see its potential fulfilled. While a few promising articles on the uses of this technique for evaluating masses in the cervical region have been published, magnetization transfer imaging has not been accepted as a routine methodology for head and neck MR imaging. Part of the reason widespread use has not gained favor is that the emphasis in the literature has centered around predicting the histology of lesions and, in the feeling of many, no imaging study is going to obviate the need for histologic sampling of most head and neck masses. In the opinion of this author, MTI research must shift from predicting histology to defining tumor margins and distinguishing "reactive, edematous change" from neoplastic infiltration. Only then will the technique make significant clinical inroads.

D.M. Yousem, MD, Departments of Radiology and Otorhinolaryngology: Head and Neck Surgery, University of Pennsylvania Medical Center, 3400 Spruce Street, Philadelphia, PA 19104, USA

## 1.2 The Concept of Magnetization Transfer

Currently MR imaging focuses on the contribution of freely mobile water protons because of their great abundance and their sharp resonance frequency. Protons in macromolecules such as complex proteins and cellular membranes induce relaxation of these mobile water protons, thereby contributing to the signal derived in routine MR imaging. These protons in the macromolecular proteins have restricted motion and hence very short T2 relaxation values, so short, in fact, that they are invisible to routine imaging (Eng et al. 1991; Balaban and Ceckler 1992). These macromolecules subsequently restrict the motion of the nearby water molecules through dipolar coupling, cross-relaxation, and chemical exchange (Eng et al. 1991; Balaban and Ceckler 1992; Wolff and Balaban 1989; Wolff et al. 1991b). In so doing, they tend to shorten both the T1 and the T2 relaxation time of the free protons, but the major effect is that of T2 shortening. The rate of magnetization transfer to the free water pool is influenced by several factors, including the macromolecule composition (Grossman et al. 1994; Fralix et al. 1991), the macromolecule's concentration (Balaban and Ceckler 1992), the presence of nearby paramagnetic compounds, the T1 of the water (Yang and Schleich 1994; Morris and Freemont 1992), and the degree of mobility of the macromolecules (Morris and Freemont 1992). Thus, complex and highly concentrated immobile protons such as those in cerebral white matter, hypercellular tissues, and muscular proteins have the greatest degree of magnetization transfer.

The macromolecular proton pool appears as a very broad peak in the MR spectrum, extending over many KHz. By placing a radiofrequency suppressor pulse far away from the resonant frequency of water into this broad macromolecular pool, one can assess the contribution of the macromolecular protons to the MR signal. This is done most easily by comparing scans with and without the suppressor pulse applied and/or by performing subtraction imaging of the two sequences. The difference in intensity between the two scans reflects the degree to which magnetization has been transferred from the macromolecular pool to the free proton pool. The term "magnetization transfer ratio" (MTR) has been coined for the ratio of Ms/Mo (intensity with the MT suppressor pulse over the intensity without the MT pulse applied) (GROSSMAN et al. 1994; GROSSMAN 1994). Defining the magnetization transfer rate as such means that the higher the value the greater the degree of transfer of relaxation.

T1 and T2 relaxation rates are increased by magnetization transfer interactions. The degree of T1 relaxation of free water depends on the magnetization transfer rates and on the ability of the immobile protons to transfer that magnetization (ENG et al. 1991). In the evaluation of absolute MTR values, the T1 of a lesion should be considered as a potential confounding factor. T1 and MTR are related by the equation:

$$MTR = K_a \times T1_a,$$

where $K_a$ is the rate of magnetization transfer from water to macromolecules and $T1_a$ is the apparent T1 of the bulk water pool measured after irradiation (ENG et al. 1991). To acknowledge the issue of the T1 effects many researchers use the term "apparent MTR" (MITTL et al. 1993; BOORSTEIN et al. 1994a,b; DOUSSET et al. 1992; DOUSSET 1993; LOEVNER et al. 1995a,b; GROSSMAN 1994; GROSSMAN et al. 1994; GOMORI et al. 1993; HIEHLE et al. 1995) rather than "MTR," since T1 values are not kept constant.

In the past, researchers have assumed, based on previous studies, that there is relatively little variation in T1s of most cancers or nodes (DOOMS et al. 1984, 1985; DOOMS and HRICAK 1986). Qualitatively there has been little variation in the signal intensity of the masses on T1-weighted scans. Certainly in cases of melanoma, colloid-containing papillary carcinomas, or calcified lesions the T1 values may vary considerably. MTRs should be viewed with caution when these lesions are evaluated.

## 1.3 The Concept of Spin Lock Imaging

Spin lock imaging is closely related to MTI. At low field strengths, the spin lock technique has been employed to study similar off-resonance effects. With this technique, a radiofrequency pulse is applied to "lock" the relaxation of the spins in the low frequency range. This allows greater sensitivity to macromolecular concentration, mobility, and spin interactions at low field strength (ULMER et al. 1996). The spin lock technique requires a preparation pulse that is applied at the resonance frequency, and the length of the locking pulse is designated by the term TL (typically 10–100 ms). A saturation pulse is also applied. In the head and neck, spin lock (SL) effects parallel those of MT; however, fat has intermediate SL values (reported to be due to "thermal vibrations"), whereas it has a very low MTR (MARKKOLA et al. 1996). The spin lock technique can generate MT-like contrast in normal and pathologic conditions.

ULMER et al. (1996) have studied the spin lock effect at high field strength. These authors have shown that, at frequency offsets from water in the 100 to 1000 Hertz range, saturation effects can be seen that appear to be independent of MT even at high-Tesla imaging. Manganese chloride, which is devoid of macromolecules, should have no MT effect. However, when a saturation pulse was applied at less than 2000 Hz from water resonance, ULMER et al. saw diminution in the signal intensity of a vial of manganese chloride. The authors attributed the effect to the spin lock mechanism. The effect is optimized in tissues with high T1/T2 ratios (brain, fat).

While MTI has been employed in research institutions to evaluate lesions of the brain (LUNDBOM et al. 1990, 1995; LUNDBOM 1992; MITTL et al. 1993; BOORSTEIN et al. 1994a,b; DOUSSET et al. 1992; DOUSSET 1993; LOEVNER et al. 1995a,b; GROSSMAN 1994; GROSSMAN et al. 1994; GOMORI et al. 1993; HIEHLE et al. 1995), liver (OUTWATER et al. 1992; KAHN et al. 1993; MORRISON and HENKELMAN 1995; KOMU and ALANEN 1994; LOESBERG et al. 1993), knee (FLAMIG et al. 1992; BALABAN and CECKLER 1992; FELLNER et al. 1995; OUTWATER et al. 1992; WOLFF et al. 1991a,b) and heart (BALABAN and CECKLER 1992; BALABAN et al. 1991; KOBAYASHI et al. 1993; PRASAD et al. 1993), the head and neck region has only recently been evaluated with this new contrast technique. Because the head and neck contain structures that have a wide range of protein, fat, and water content, the implementation of MTI in the head and neck appears to have great potential. Additionally, since one of the drawbacks of spin echo MR scanning of the head and neck is the inability to distinguish tumoral edema from tumor cells, MTI may ultimately be useful in defining boundaries of rapidly proliferating cancers. Presumably the differentiation of freely mobile edema protons from the more restricted tumor cell membrane proton pool will be possible.

## 1.4 History of MTI

The earliest publications on the implementation of magnetization transfer techniques centered on the alteration in contrast of gradient echo images. With MT applied, it is possible to produce a more T2-weighted scan without the need for longer repetition times or shorter flip angles (Balaban and Ceckler 1992; Balaban et al. 1991; Kobayashi et al. 1993; Prasad et al. 1993; Wolff and Balaban 1989; Wolff et al. 1991a,b; Lipton et al. 1991; Jones and Southon 1991; Ordidge et al. 1991; Dixon 1991; Outwater et al. 1992). Alternatively, scans in which MT contrast was maximized could be used to provide gray scale differentiation that is distinct from T1 and T2 contrast. The MT technique ultimately became linked to magnetic resonance angiography, where background suppression is critical to the visualization of smaller blood vessels, particularly with the time-of-flight (TOF) technique (Atkinson et al. 1994; Edelman et al. 1992; Pike et al. 1992; Li et al. 1995; Tkach et al. 1993). At this time, most intracranial TOF sequences have MT-based background suppression. While the suppression of flowing blood also occurs with MTI, the background suppression that occurs is far greater than the suppression of the blood flow, giving improved visibility of vessels.

MR scanner manufacturers have capitalized on the background suppression quality of MTI to combine the technique with postcontrast T1-weighted imaging. Investigators have promoted the use of a single-dose contrast-enhanced, MT-suppressed T1-weighted scan as an effective (and more economical) alternative to high-dose (double- and triple-dose) gadolinium techniques (Elster et al. 1994). Since so many studies have suggested that enhancing intracranial lesions are more conspicuous with MT suppressor pulses applied (Elster et al. 1994; Mehta et al. 1995; Kurki et al. 1992, 1994; Finelli et al. 1994; Mathews et al. 1995, 1997; Burke et al. 1996; Gillams et al. 1995), this begs a more vexing question. Can reduced dose rates (below manufacturers' recommendations) of contrast agents be used if MT suppression is employed? The economic ramifications of this question for the health care industry, pharmaceutical companies, and hospitals have not yet been addressed. While these studies have focused on the brain, at least one study has also shown that the use of MTI with contrast administration can improve visualization of head and neck neoplasms (Gillams et al. 1996).

## 1.5 MTI in the Head and Neck: Normative Data (Figs. 1.1, 1.2)

In an attempt to determine the feasibility of MTI in the head and neck, the normal anatomy of 32 subjects was studied with a standard MTI technique. Normative data for head and neck structures, and intersubject and intrasubject variability of magnetization transfer ratios were provided (Yousem et al. 1994b).

The MTI scanning protocol employed a repetition trone (TR) of 500 ms, a time to echo (TE) of 12 ms, and a flip angle of 20° using a multiplanar gradient echo pulse sequence in a 2D mode. Scanning was performed with and without the magnetization transfer pulse employed, using the same scanning, receive attenuation, and transmit attenuation parameters. The magnetization transfer pulse had a duration of 19 ms, was offset from the resonance frequency of water by 2000 Hz, and employed an area of wave form approximately 10 times that of the 90° spin echo pulse. The technique employed a single cycle sinc pulse (typical slice selection pulses are four cycles) to induce a broad homogeneous suppression of the macromolecular pool. This suppression pulse was applied approximately 1 ms before routine imaging pulses. Previous studies using this technique had demonstrated specific absorption rates ranging from 1.16 to 2.89 W/kg for patients weighing between 45 and 136 kg, which was within acceptable FDA limits (Outwater et al. 1992). The average B1 intensity was $3.67 \times 10^{-6}$ T.

Regions of interest for signal intensity measurements were sampled at the exact same locations for the scans before and after the magnetization transfer pulse was applied. This was achieved by keeping the position, shape, and volume of the cursor for the region of interest constant between measurements of the pre- and post-MTI sequence. This allowed calculation of the apparent MTR for various structures in the head and neck (masseter muscles, pterygoid muscles, tongue intrinsic muscles, submandibular glands, parotid glands, thyroid glands, tonsils, cerebrospinal fluid within the cervical spinal canal, and subcutaneous fat). Right and left asymmetry between the same structures within an individual subject provided intrasubject variability. Intersubject variability was reflected by standard deviations of MTR means for the 32 individuals. The data were analyzed using Student's two-tailed *t*-test for unpaired samples.

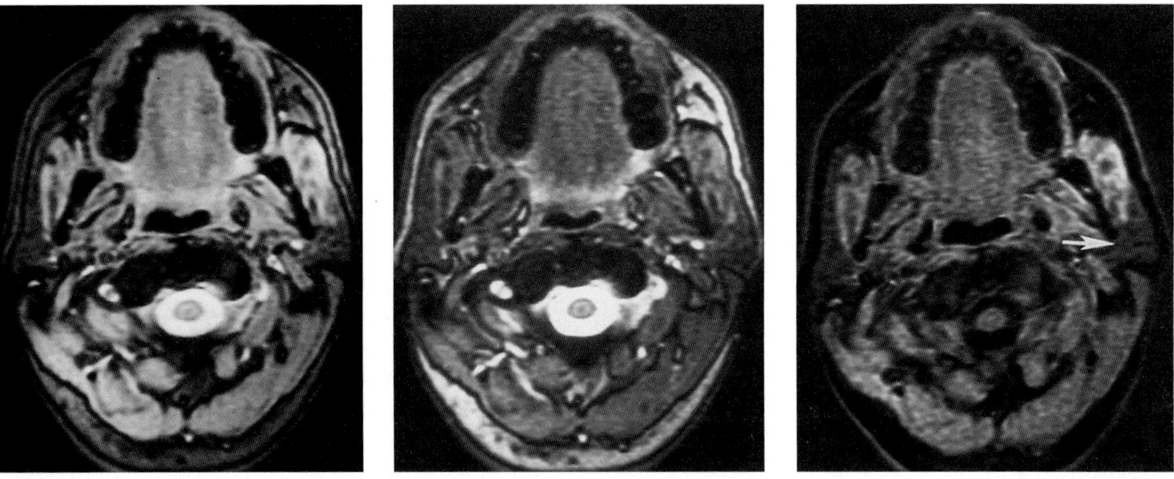


**Fig. 1.1 a–c.** Normal anatomy. **a** Initial gradient echo scan without magnetization transfer pulses (pre-MT) applied shows the normal head and neck anatomy at the level of the retromolar trigone. **b** With magnetization transfer applied (post-MT), note a diminution in the signal intensity of the muscles with relative preservation of the signal intensity of the cerebrospinal fluid (CSF). In the sites with the greatest difference in intensity between the scans, a greater amount of transfer of magnetization (saturation) has occurred. **c** In this subtraction image, the higher the signal intensity the greater the degree of transfer of saturation and, hence, the higher the apparent magnetization transfer ratio. One can see that muscles (note in particular the paraspinal, tongue, and masseter muscles) have the highest signal intensity, whereas CSF and fat have the lowest signal intensity. The parotid gland (*arrow*) has intermediate signal intensity and therefore intermediate MTR values

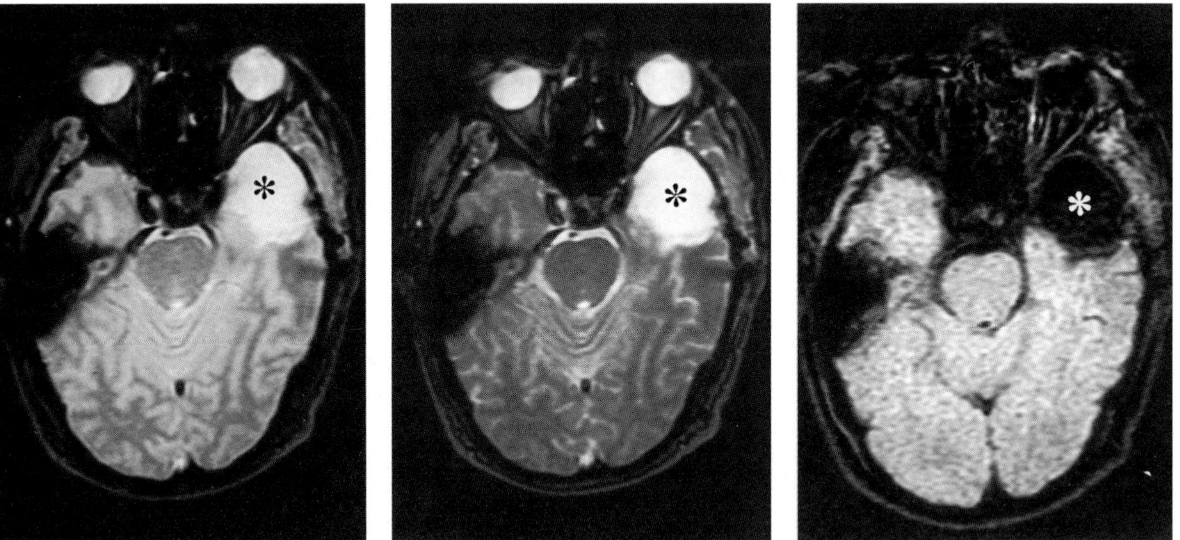


**Fig. 1.2 a–c.** Arachnoid cyst. **a** Pre-MT saturation pulse, **b** post-MT saturation pulse, and **c** subtraction image demonstrate the absence of transfer in the vitreous humor of the orbit, the orbital fat, and in the arachnoid cyst (*) in the left middle cranial fossa. An epidermoid tumor was considered in the differential diagnosis of this case; however with the black signal intensity on the subtraction image, only CSF and fat would appear this way

The magnetization transfer ratios of the masseter, pterygoid, and tongue muscles were similar, and were grouped together for the determination of muscle MTRs. Table 1.1 shows the MTRs of normal structures of the head and neck (Yousem et al. 1994b).

As expected, cerebrospinal fluid and fat, with a predominance of mobile protons and fewer macromolecular proteins, had the lowest magnetization transfer ratios. Muscle, on the other hand, had the highest MTRs, reflecting the greater number of restricted macromolecular protein protons. Glandular

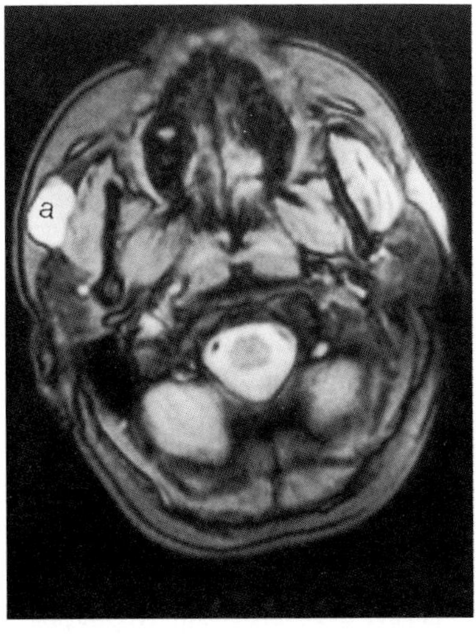

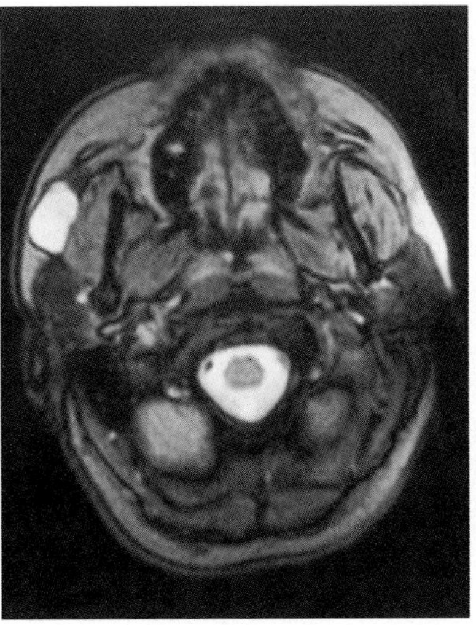
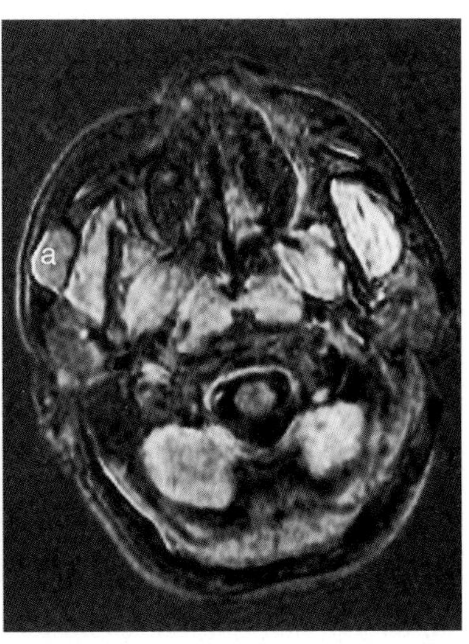


a,b c

**Fig. 1.3 A–C.** Pleomorphic adenoma. **a** This lesion (*a*) is bright on the pre-MT image and is located in the parotid tissue superficial to the masseter muscle. **b** On the post-MT scan, very little change in signal intensity in the lesion is noted and it remains quite bright. **c** The subtraction image demonstrates lower signal intensity in the lesion (*a*) than in muscle, but higher intensity than in normal parotid glandular tissue. The MTR value was 0.24, within the range of a benign neoplasm, whereas the masseter muscular intensity was 0.50

**Table 1.1.** Normal structures and magnetization transfer ratios (*MTRs*)

| Structure | Number of measurements | Mean MTR | SD |
|---|---|---|---|
| Muscle (pterygoid, masseter, tongue) | 100 | 0.54 | 0.09 |
| Submandibular gland | 41 | 0.41 | 0.09 |
| Parotid gland | 50 | 0.39 | 0.09 |
| CSF | 46 | 0.05 | 0.03 |
| Fat | 32 | 0.07 | 0.04 |
| Thyroid | 17 | 0.41 | 0.15 |
| Tonsil | 37 | 0.44 | 0.09 |

tissue (salivary and thyroid glands) had intermediate values. Of note was the fairly wide range of standard deviations in the values of the MTRs. These wide standard deviations proved to be a problem once MTI was applied to pathology in the head and neck.

## 1.6 MTI and Head and Neck Tumors (Figs. 1.3–1.8)

In a separate study, patients with head and neck neoplasms were examined with the same MTI sequences and protocol (Yousem et al. 1994a). The rationale for performing studies in patients with neoplasms was spurred by work in the brain. Lundbom had analyzed the role of MTI in determining the histologic grade of brain tumors (Lundbom 1992). The mean MTR of high-grade astrocytomas was greater than that of low-grade astrocytomas ($P = 0.0005$), presumably due to a difference in cellularity and nuclear material. The MTRs of astrocytomas were significantly lower than those of meningiomas and pituitary adenomas (Lundbom 1992). The issue arose as to whether MTI would be useful in the analysis of head and neck carcinomas where the hypercellular neoplasm often replaces adjacent fat.

Fifty-one patients with head and neck neoplasms were examined with MTI. Using the technique described in the normal control study, MTR values were derived for the neoplasms, CSF, fat, and muscle in every patient, in order to ensure that the MT pulse sequence was applied correctly and to provide an internal control (muscle). The muscle used was the masseter, pterygoid, or sternocleidomastoid muscle. For each squamous cell carcinoma, two to four values were obtained in nonoverlapping regions of the tumor to assess intratumoral variation in MTRs. Because some lesions were very small and could not support more than one nonoverlapping region of interest, intratumoral variation was available for only 20 of 33 squamous cell carcinomas.

After the MTR values had been determined for all neoplasms, a head and neck pathologist without any knowledge of the MTR data retrospectively reviewed the pathological slides on all cases (Table 1.2). The

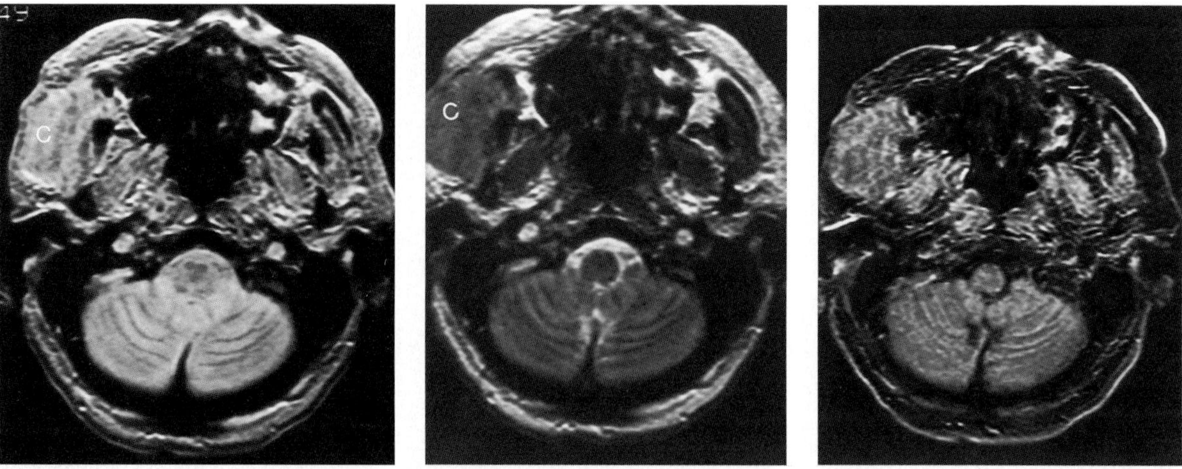


a,b c

**Fig. 1.4 a–c.** Mucoepidermoid carcinoma Contrast the difference in signal intensity on **a** the pre-MTI sequence and **b** the post-MTI sequence in this mucoepidermoid carcinoma (*C*) of the parotid tissue over the masseter muscle with the relative absence of intensity change in the pleomorphic adenoma in Fig. 1.3. **c** On the subtraction image the signal intensity of the mass is similar to that of the pterygoid musculature and one cannot distinguish tumor from masseter muscle. The MTR (magnetization transfer ratio) was 0.37, and the MTR of the unaffected (masseter) muscle was 0.46

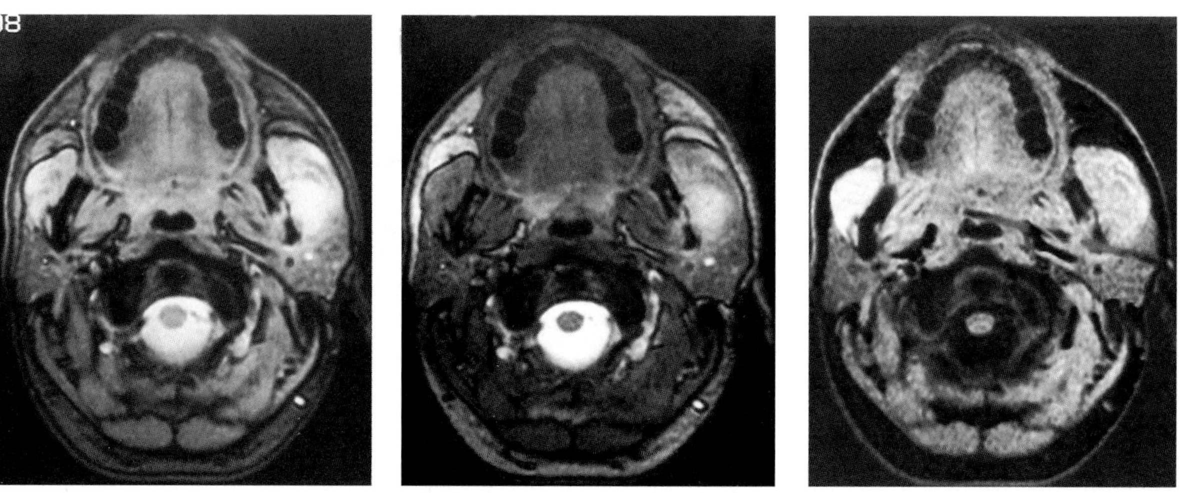

a,b c

**Fig. 1.5 a–c.** Lymphoma. **a** Pre-MT saturation pulse, **b** post-MT saturation pulse, and **c** subtraction image of this mandibular lesion, which had grown into the masseter muscle, demonstrates absence of contrast between the lesion and the masseter muscle on the subtraction image. The borders of the lesion with the masseter muscle are best seen on the pre-MT saturated image (**a**). The MTR of the tumor was 0.42. Because of edema, the ipsilateral masseter muscle had a MTR similar to that of the lesion. The contralateral masseter muscle had an MTR of 0.61 (note the difference in signal intensity in **c**)

pathologist graded all squamous cell carcinomas for (1) the degree of differentiation of the squamous cell carcinomas, (2) the amount of keratin, and (3) the cellular density as measured by the number of cells per high-power field, derived from a mean of 5 fields per patient, and (4) mitoses per square millimeter, derived from a mean of 5 fields per patient (Yousem et al. 1994a).

Data analysis was performed for three approaches and hypotheses: (1) Paired *t*-tests were used to assess whether MTRs of squamous cell carcinomas were different than MTRs of muscle, CSF, and fat, (2) Pearson correlation coefficients were used to assess whether there was a correlation between neoplasms' MTRs and degree of differentiation, cell counts per microscopic high-power field, number of mitoses per square millimeter, and keratin formation, and (3) unpaired T-tests. Since the data did not fit a normal distribution, the Mann–Whitney test was used to assess for differences in MTRs of squamous cell car-

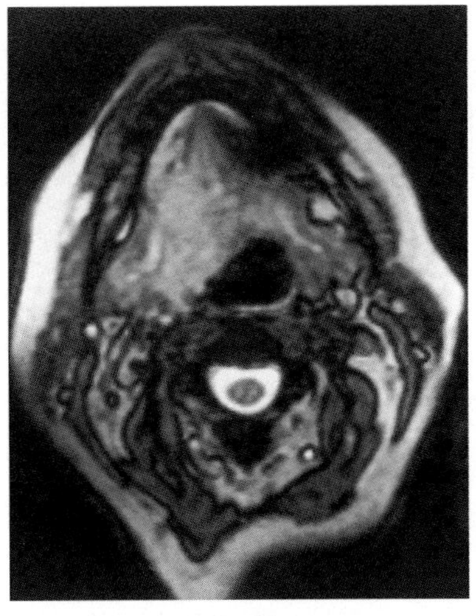
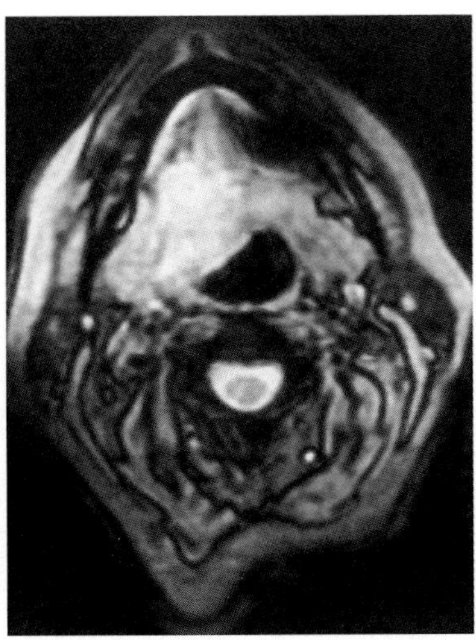
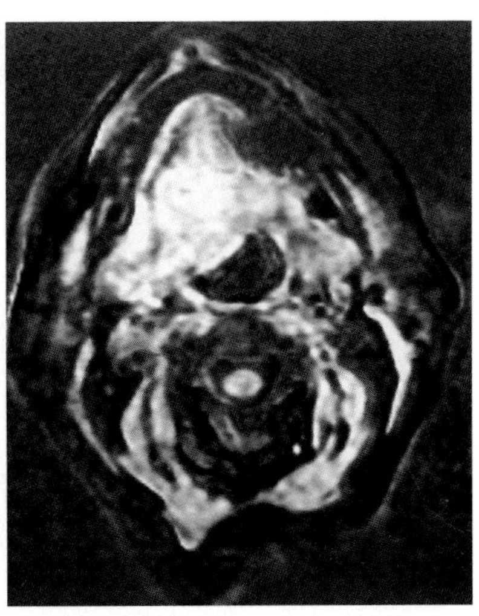

a,b c

**Fig. 1.6 a–c.** Poorly differentiated squamous cell carcinoma. **a** Pre-MT saturation pulse, **b** post-MT saturation pulse, and **C** subtraction images demonstrate a great degree of magnetization transfer in this lesion affecting base of tongue and floor of mouth. Note how high the signal intensity is in the carcinoma of the tongue base on the right side on the subtraction image (**c**)

**Table 1.2.** Pathological data from 33 squamous cell carcinomas

| Pathological factor | Number |
|---|---|
| Degree of differentiation | |
| Well | 5 |
| Well to moderate | 4 |
| Moderate | 9 |
| Moderate to poor | 2 |
| Poor | 13 |
| Keratin formation | |
| Minimal | 13 |
| Moderate | 8 |
| Extensive | 7 |
| Cells per high-power field | |
| 0–250 | 8 |
| 250-1000 | 15 |
| >1000 | 5 |
| Mitotic rate | |
| 0–4 | 13 |
| 5–10 | 5 |
| 10–20 | 6 |
| >20 | 4 |

**Table 1.3.** Histologies of benign neoplasms and non-squamous cell carcinomas

| Histology of tumor | Number |
|---|---|
| Benign | |
| Castleman's disease | 1 |
| Hemangioma | 1 |
| Hemangiopericytoma | 2 |
| Inverted papilloma | 2 |
| Lipoma | 1 |
| Condyloma | 1 |
| Pleomorphic adenoma | 2 |
| Non-squamous cell malignancy | |
| Adenoid cystic carcinoma | 3 |
| Leukemia, lymphoma | 2 |
| Malignant hemangiopericytoma | 1 |
| Melanoma | 2 |
| Mucoepidermoid carcinoma | 1 |
| Papillary carcinoma | 1 |
| Sarcoma | 1 |

cinomas, non-squamous cell malignancies, and benign tumors.

The histologies of the benign tumors and the non-squamous cell carcinomas are found in Table 1.3 and the mean values and standard deviations for MTRs are reported in Table 1.4 (Yousem et al. 1994a).

There was a statistically significant difference in MTRs of neoplasms and muscle ($P < 0.01$), CSF ($P < 0.001$), and fat ($P < 0.001$). In every case except

**Table 1.4.** MTR values of tumors and normal tissue

| Measured tissue (no.) | MTR of lesion (mean, SD) |
|---|---|
| Squamous cell carcinoma (33) | 0.394, 0.097 |
| Non-squamous cell carcinomas (10) | 0.370, 0.104 |
| Benign neoplasms (10) | 0.255, 0.146 |
| Muscle (44) | 0.563, 0.097 |
| CSF (44) | 0.046, 0.034 |
| Fat (44) | 0.066, 0.049 |

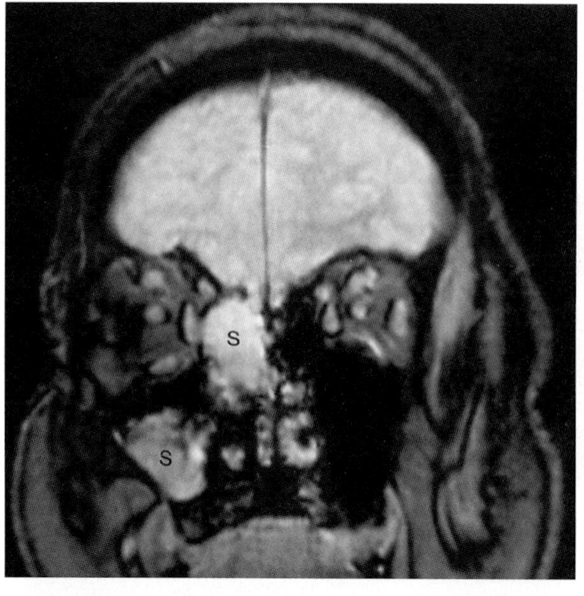

a

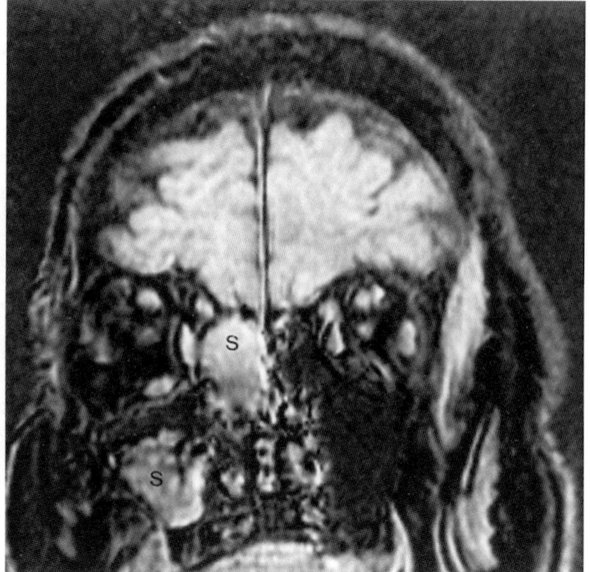

c

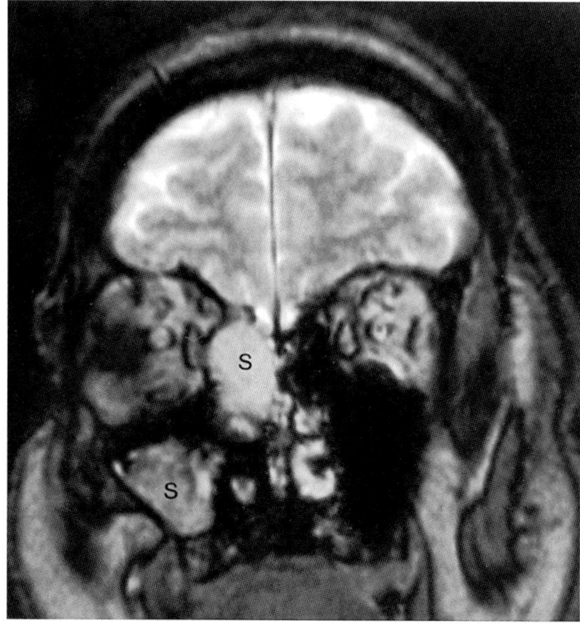

b

**Fig. 1.7 a–c.** Multifocal small cell carcinoma. On routine spin echo imaging it was thought that this patient had retained secretions in the right maxillary antrum. **a** Pre-MT, **b** post-MT, and **c** subtraction images suggested that the lesions (*s*) were similar in magnetization transfer character, and in fact, multifocal small cell carcinoma of the sinonasal cavity was detected. Contrast this case with those of sinusitis (Figs. 1.10, 1.11)

one, the MTR of muscle exceeded the MTR of squamous cell carcinoma, which in turn exceeded the MTRs of fat or CSF.

No correlations were identified between MTRs of squamous cell carcinomas and degree of differentiation ($P = 0.369$), keratin formation ($P = 0.485$), cells per high-power field ($P = 0.304$), and mitoses per square millimeter ($P = 0.663$). To correct for the variation in MT across the entire image due to field inhomogeneity, we also performed the data analyses using lesion MTR/ muscle versus degree of differentiation, keratin formation, cells per high-power field, and mitoses per square millimeter for squamous cell carcinomas. Again no correlations were found.

Statistically significant differences between the MTRs of squamous cell carcinomas and benign tumors ($P < 0.01$), non-squamous cell carcinomas and benign tumors ($P < 0.03$) and all malignant tumors versus benign tumors ($P < 0.01$) were found (using Mann-Whitney tests). No differences were noted between the MTRs of squamous cell carcinomas and non-squamous cell carcinomas ($P$-value 0.73 for Mann-Whitney).

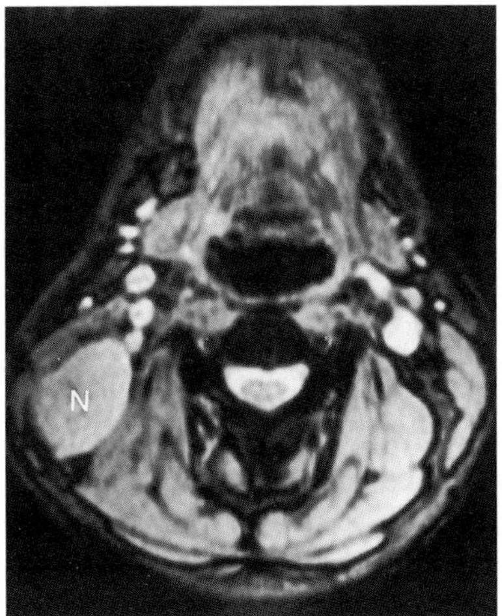

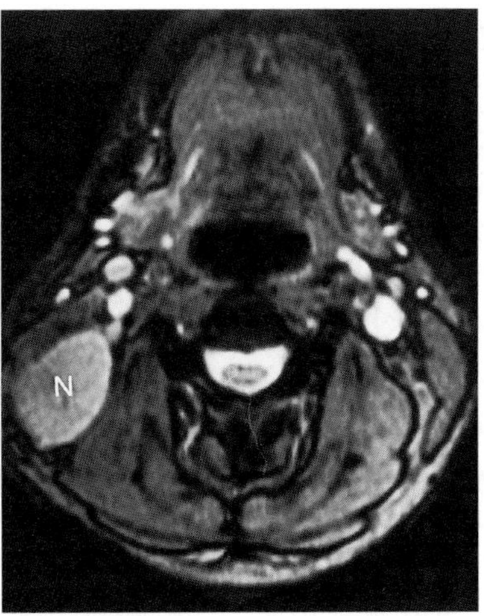

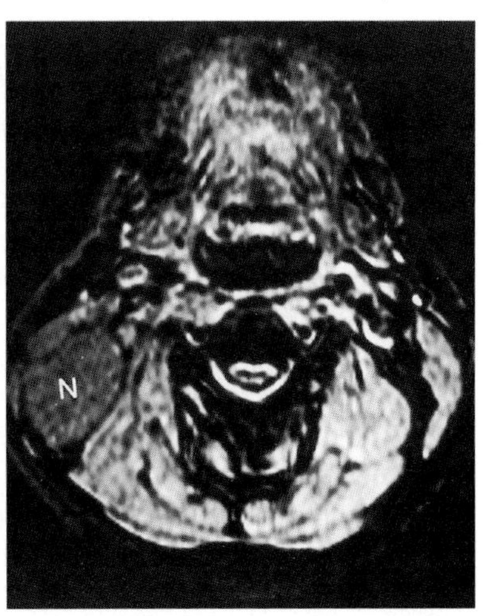


a,b c

**Fig. 1.8 a–c.** Benign adenopathy. There is relatively little change in signal intensity between the pre-MT (**a**) and post-MT (**b**) images of the large right posterior triangle lymph node (*N*). **c** The subtraction image (c) shows no intensity to the mass, suggesting a small amount of magnetization transfer and thus a low MTR. The MTR value was 0.24, and aspiration cytology revealed Castleman's disease

The assessment of intratumoral variation in MTRs was quantified using the mean MTR of the multiple MTR values within a tumor as the denominator and the maximum deviation from that mean as the numerator. For 20 squamous cell carcinomas the mean maximum intratumoral variation was 10.2% (standard deviation 8.7%).

From these data, it was concluded that MTI provided a unique, quantitative means of evaluating head and neck neoplasms. While there was some overlap of MTR values, one could readily assign maximum and minimum MTR limits that could be used to separate benign from malignant primary tumors of the head and neck. The wide standard deviations were accounted for by the presence of "premalignant" masses, such as inverted papillomas and condylomata, which had higher MTRs than typical benign masses, and necrotic primary tumors, which had lower MTRs (since most fluids have lower MTRs than solid masses).

Subsequently, Markkola et al. (1996) examined 40 consecutive patients with histologically verified head and neck tumors (20 malignant and 20 benign) using MTI and spin lock (SL) imaging. These authors computed MTRs and SL ratios for benign versus malignant lesions. When the authors set a magnetization transfer ratio of 0.32 as their threshold, the sensitivity for detecting malignancies (excluding major salivary gland tumors) was 100% with a specificity of 83%, leading to an accuracy of 95%. They found that analyzing signal intensity, borders, and size of the masses was not as accurate a method as utilizing the MTRs and SLRs. In fact, there was only one squamous cell carcinoma that was falsely negative (had a low MTR), and this was a tumor that showed necrosis (a known cause for a low MTR). It should also be noted that in Markkola et al.'s work, the standard deviation for the MTRs of squamous cell carcinomas was only 0.04, with a mean value of 0.40 (Table 1.5). The mean results for benign (0.25 ± 0.13) and malignant masses (0.36 ± 0.10) published in Markkola et al.'s article closely approximate the results found in Tables 1.3 and 1.4 (Yousem et al. 1994a). If the threshold suggested by Markkola was applied to Yousem et al.'s data (Yousem et al. 1994a), the accuracy of predicting benign versus malignant would reach Markkola's value of 78% for all lesions. If the threshold was reduced to 0.30, 9 of 11 benign lesions and 29 of 33 squamous cell carcinomas would have been correctly reported in Yousem's series of primary tumors (Yousem et al. 1994a). This would lead to an accuracy rate of 86.4% (sensitivity 87.9% and specificity, 81.8%). If, on the other hand, a maximum value of 0.32 were set for the MTR, the

**Table 1.5.** MTR values reported by Markkola et al. (1996)

| Measured tissue (no.) | MTR of lesion (mean, SD) |
|---|---|
| Squamous cell carcinoma (9) | 0.40, 0.04 |
| Non-squamous cell carcinomas (10) | 0.36, 0.03 |
| Malignant neoplasms (20) | 0.36, 0.10 |
| Benign neoplasms (20) | 0.25, 0.13 |

only benign lesions that would fall into this category would be the inverted papillomas. Similarly, if a minimal value of 0.24 were set, only 1 of 33 squamous cell carcinomas would fall below this value. These findings suggest that, though there may be a middle territory where there is some overlap in values, one can set high and low thresholds for MTRs which are highly accurate for predicting benignity or malignancy.

While many head and neck studies are ordered purely to stage a cancer where the diagnosis (squamous cell carcinoma) has already been obtained or can be surmised based on risk factors, Markkola and associates provided data from lesions where the histology is unlikely to be known prior to surgery or biopsy. The teaching has been that hypointense lesions on T2 weighting are malignant, whereas those that are bright on T2 scans are benign (Som et al. 1988a–d, 1989; Som and Biller 1989; Zagdanski et al. 1994; Kaneda et al. 1994; Hebert et al. 1993; Sigal et al. 1992a,b, 1996; Grevers et al. 1994; Yousem et al. 1990, 1992). Lesions with irregular margins are more likely to be malignant, and well-defined lesions are most often benign (Zagdanski et al. 1994; Hebert et al. 1993; Sigal et al. 1992b). Too often, however, the head and neck radiologist has found that the exceptions overwhelm the rule (i.e. dark lesions such as inverted papillomas, Warthin's tumors, radiation sialadenitis, odontogenic masses, oncocytomas that are benign, and malignant lesions such as low-grade mucoepidermoid carcinomas, adenoid cystic carcinomas, sarcomas, adenocarcinomas, malignant neurofibrosarcomas, and lymphomas that are bright on T2-weighted scanning) (Schlakman and Yousem 1993; Sigal et al. 1992b; Yousem et al. 1990). Markkola et al.'s results reinforce the notion that observing T2-weighted signal intensity is not an infallible way of predicting histology. When T2-weighted signal intensity alone (hyperintense benign and hypo/isointense malignant) was used, the T2-weighted studies were accurate in distinguishing benign from malignant salivary gland masses in 9 (64%) of 14 cases and in only 10 (48%) of 21 nonsalivary gland lesions, giving an overall ability of 54%. However, when SLR and MTR thresholds from their data were used in addition, the accuracy rose to 78–80% for all masses and 92–95% for non-salivary gland lesions. Then again, fine needle aspiration and/or biopsy provide greater assurance to the head and neck surgeon.

## 1.7 MTI of Adenopathy (Figs. 1.9, 1.10)

Curtin et al. (1998) have found that, for the same size criteria, CT is slightly more accurate than MRI in detecting lymph node metastases. However, the positive predictive value of CT using the standard

a,b

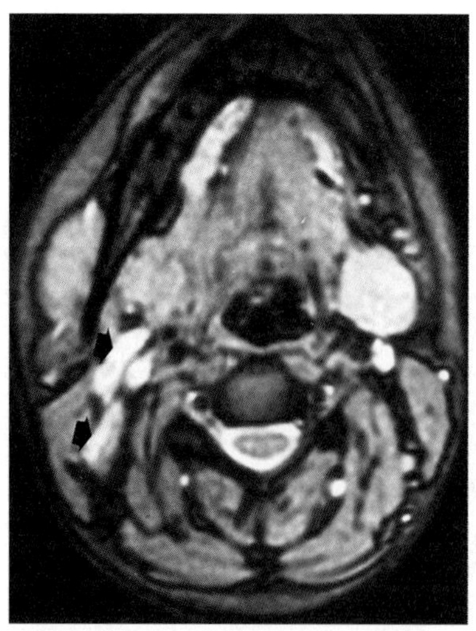

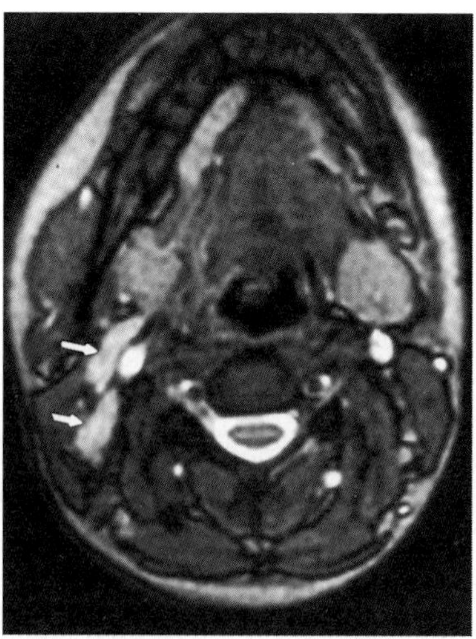

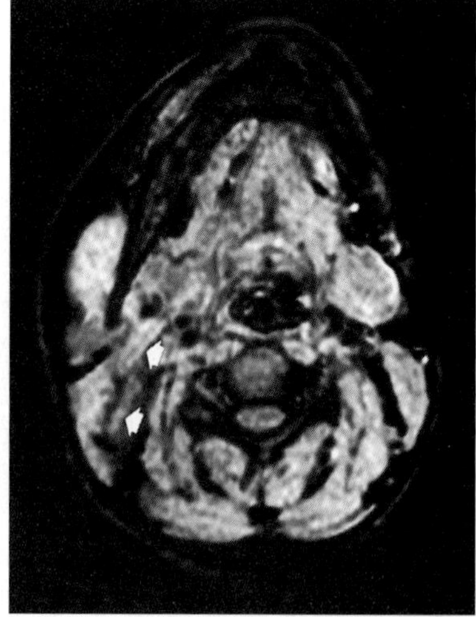

c

**Fig. 1.9 a–c.** Malignant adenopathy. **a** Pre-MT, **b** post-MT, and **C** subtraction images demonstrate lymph nodes (*arrows*) on the right side behind the mandible and deep sternocleidomastoid muscle. These lymph nodes have signal intensity approximating that of the muscle, and the MTR value (0.36) was within a range characteristic of neoplastic infiltration. These were lymph node metastases from papillary carcinoma of the thyroid gland

1.0 cm size criterion was only 50%, while that of MR was 52%. The negative predictive values were 84% and 79% for CT and MR, respectively (Curtin et al. 1998). To achieve negative predictive values of 90% or greater, a 5-mm size criterion had to be used. The failure of CT, MR and, for that matter ultrasound (US), is that radiologists are still bound by size criteria and macroscopic nodal morphology to decide whether nodes have tumor infiltration (Van Den Brekel et al. 1994). This raises the issue as to whether MTI can play a part in evaluating lymph nodes.

In a study reported at the ASNR in 1994 (Sheppard and Yousem 1994), 21 lymph nodes (8 malignant and 13 reactive) were examined and correlated with histology. The mean MTR of malignant adenopathy (mean 0.375 with standard deviation of 0.07) was statistically different ($P < 0.02$ on Mann-Whitney) from that of benign adenopathy (mean 0.253 with standard deviation of 0.12). The intranodal variation in MTRs within the nodes was less than 15% (Table 1.6). These data are in keeping with the previously reported findings from primary tumors showing statistically significant differences between squamous cell carcinomas and benign neoplasms (Yousem et al. 1994a; Markkola et al. 1996). Once again the outliers accounting for the wide standard deviation in the malignant nodes were caused by the inclusion of nodes with necrosis (which brings the MTR value down). From these initial data it was stressed that, when using MTI for cervical adenopathy, one can only sample the non-necrotic portions of the lymph nodes. The study, though promising, did not compare MTR values versus size criteria in these same nodes.

Gillams et al. (1996) also examined MTRs in benign and malignant nodes. They noted that the range of values for benign nodes (0.72–0.77) only modestly overlapped the values for malignant adenopathy (0.76–0.88). These authors employed a 0.1 T magnet, where the MT effect can be optimized without running into specific absorption rate (SAR) limitations (Gillams et al. 1996). They also found that MTI enhanced the contrast between most head and neck lesions and non-fatty background tissue before and after administration of contrast material.

**Table 1.6.** MTRs of cervical adenopathy: raw data (*MTI* magnetic transfer imaging)

| Malignant node MTI value | Benign node MTI value |
|---|---|
| 0.34 | 0.145 |
| 0.48 | 0.375 |
| 0.44 | 0.27 |
| 0.30 | 0.41 |
| 0.40 | 0.48 |
| 0.40 | 0.19 |
| 0.36 | 0.12 |
| 0.28 (necrotic) | 0.12 |
| | 0.26 |
| | 0.21 |
| | 0.14 |
| | 0.23 |
| | 0.25 |

a,b 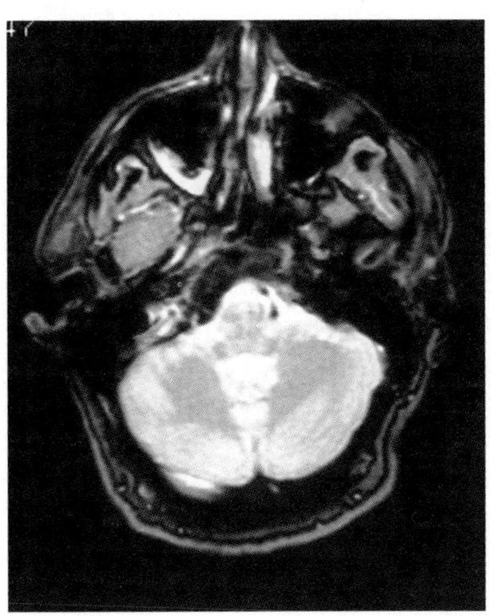 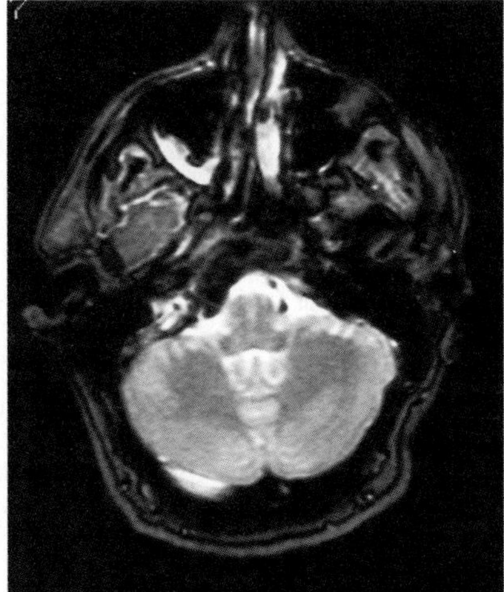 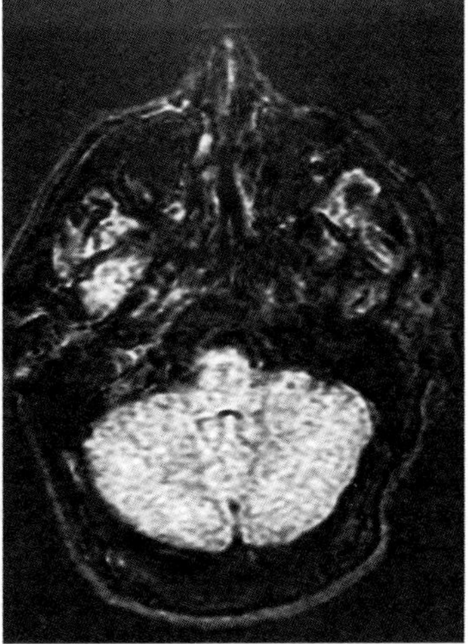 c

**Fig. 1.10 a–c.** Sinus secretions. **a** Pre-MT and **b** post-MT (B) images demonstrate no loss of signal intensity of the secretions in the right maxillary sinus. **C** On the subtraction image, absence of signal suggests that the sinus is filled with secretions rather than a solid neoplasm. Contrast this case with that of small cell carcinoma (Fig. 1.7)

## 1.8 MTI and Optic Neuritis

Boorstein et al. (1997) have recently published an article describing the usefulness of MTRs in assessing the optic nerves for changes suggestive of optic neuritis. These authors measured the MTRs of one optic nerve and compared it with the contralateral nerve using a 3D gradient echo MTI pulse sequence with a TR of 106 and TE of 5 ms and a 12° flip angle. The MT saturation pulse had similar parameters to that applied in the 2D MTI sequence applied above; however, because they used a 3D pulse sequence, the authors were able to employ 3-mm contiguous sections.

The mean MTR for asymptomatic optic nerves was 41.1 ± 1.9, which is similar to MTRs found in the normal white matter of healthy subjects (Boorstein et al. 1994b; Loevner et al. 1995a). In 21 symptomatic optic nerves that were abnormal on T2-weighted scans the MTRs were decreased to 30.6 ± 2.4. In 12 of 18 optic nerves that were symptomatic, but normal on routine spin echo scanning, the MTRs were also depressed (mean 36.3 ± 1.6). This suggests that calculating MTRs would provided a greater sensitivity (84.6%) for detecting optic neuritis than standard MR imaging with and without contrast enhancement (53.8%). At the same time, the specificity of MTI was 100% (Boorstein et al. 1997).

Based on these results, one might predict that MTI might prove useful in the characterization of benign nerve sheath lesions of the head and neck, since they would have high MTR values expected for myelinated fibers. The differentiation of schwannomas from paragangliomas in the carotid space might be a potential avenue of research for the "MT-minded" head and neck radiologist.

## 1.9 The Future of MTI

The most intriguing question about MTI in the head and neck concerns the underlying biochemistry behind the MT phenomenon. What are we looking at when we compare MTRs of benign and malignant tumors and why are they different? Previous reports of intracranial neoplasms have noted that MTRs increase with a brain tumor's cellularity, nuclear pleomorphism and amount of nuclear material, but not with its dried weight (Lundbom 1992; Lundbom et al. 1995). Collagen content in meningiomas correlated with the observed MTR (as collagen content went up, MTRs went up, presumably because collagen has high crosslinking leading to greater bound water interaction) (Lundbom 1992; Lundbom et al. 1995). In the head and neck, no relationships between MTRs and degree of neoplastic differentiation, cells per high-power field, mitotic rate or keratin formation have been noted (Yousem et al. 1994a). Markkola et al. (1996) refer to "high molecular-weight proteins," "degree of macromolecular cell wall protein interactions," "cytoplasmic interfilament proteins," and "cytokeratins" as possible sources of MT in head and neck masses. They also refer to the presence of serous and mucous spaces to explain low MTRs in pleomorphic adenomas, but high-molecular-weight macromolecules which exhibit cross-linking to account for high MTRs in mucoceles. The correlation of MTRs with protein levels in the paranasal sinuses has been suggested also in abstract form, but without extensive biochemical analysis (Yousem et al. 1993; Fig. 1.11). Since there is incomplete understanding of the pathophysiology of MTR variation in head and neck lesions, further investigation is required. It is only by understanding the underlying mechanisms that we can hope to identify the potential pitfalls and/or benefits of the technique.

Because of the known inaccuracy associated with fine needle aspiration cytology of the parotid and thyroid glands (plus the relatively high rate of lesion occurrence there), MTI studies of lesions in these sites may be fruitful. Reliable preoperative information could impact substantially on clinical management.

Continued MTI work on cervical lymphadenopathy is warranted. Radiologists would have a huge impact on patient management if a more reliable method than simple size criteria could be used to detect neoplastic infiltration.

Most importantly, MTI should be evaluated for its potential for more accurate staging and mapping of squamous cell carcinomas of the head and neck. Currently, MRI suffers from a relatively high rate of false-positive studies in the evaluation of the laryngeal cartilages (Zbaren et al. 1996, 1997; Becker et al. 1995), the bone marrow (Chung et al. 1994), the pre-epiglottic fat (Zbaren et al. 1996; Loevner et al. 1997), the dura (Eisen et al. 1996), and the prevertebral muscles (Ott et al. 1996). Since MTI has the potential for separating the effects of free water (edema or inflammation) from highly cellular tissue with a large concentration of cell membranes (squamous cell carcinoma), one would hope that this tech-

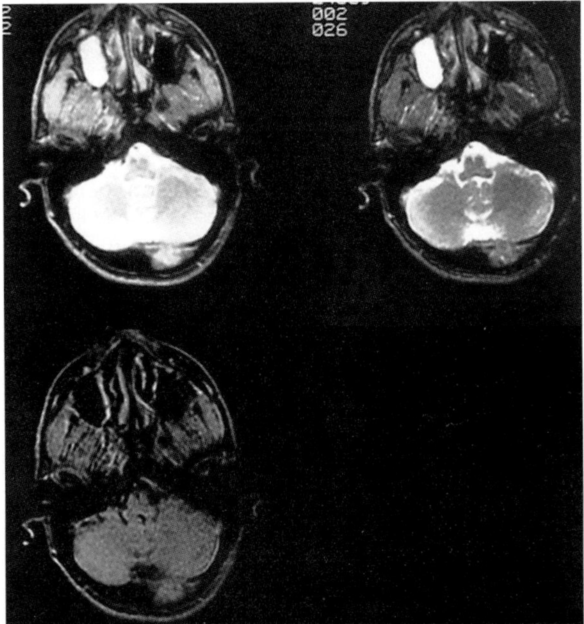

a

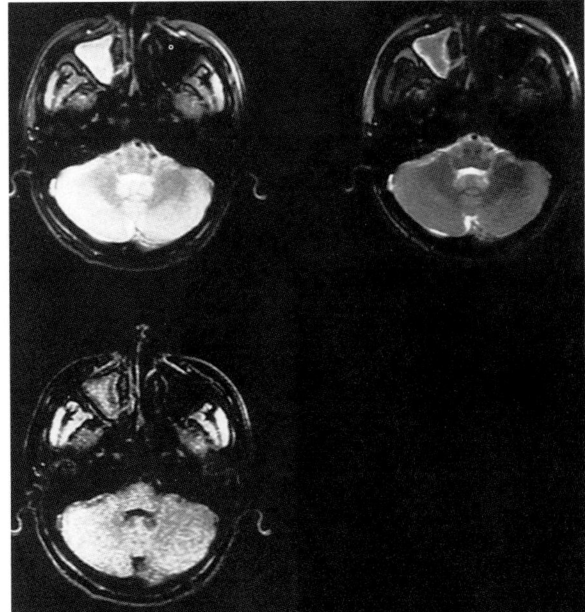

c

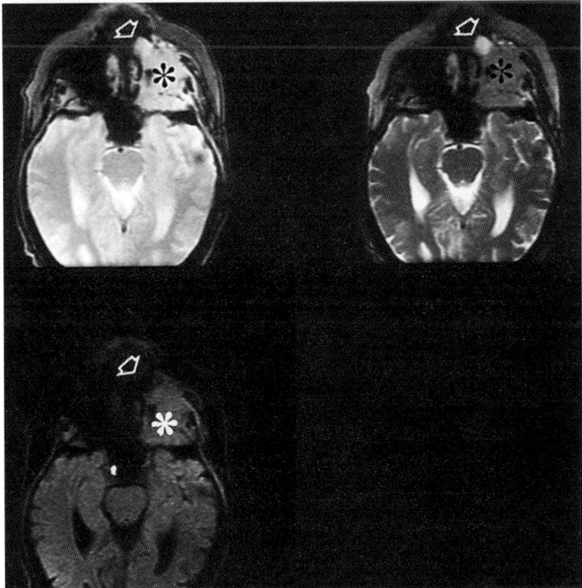

b

**Fig. 1.11 a–c.** Evaluation of paranasal sinus pathology with MTI. **a** Mucous retention cyst. Pre-MT (*top left*), post-MT (*top right*), and subtraction image (*bottom left*) demonstrate complete opacification of the right maxillary antrum on the top images, with contents that show no magnetization transfer on subtraction images. This is indicative of low-protein serous fluid, and not of neoplastic tissue. **b** Squamous cell carcinoma. Note that the retained secretions in the anteromedial aspect of the maxillary antrum (*arrow*) on the *left* demonstrates suppression on the subtraction image (*bottom left*), whereas the moderately differentiated squamous cell carcinoma (*asterisk*) transfers a relatively high degree of saturation, accounting for its higher signal intensity on the subtraction image. **c** Chronic sinusitis. A problem arises in this case of a patient with high-protein secretions in the center of the right maxillary antrum. In this case, the central secretions have a higher MTR, and therefore a higher signal intensity on the subtraction image (*bottom left*). This may simulate a neoplasm

nique could help improve the accuracy of MR in detecting tumor.

In summary, measuring MTRs has been shown to achieve accuracy rates in the 80–90% range for predicting whether a primary tumor is benign or malignant. Data on differentiating reactive vs malignant adenopathy are scant, but also suggest that MTI may provide additional data to size criteria. MTR values can help detect optic neuritis in otherwise apparently normal optic nerves. The application of MTI to distinguishing peritumoral edema, while conceptually promising, has not been investigated thus far. We have only scratched the surface of the value of MTI. The future looks bright.

## References

Atkinson D, Brant-Zawadzki M, Gillan G, Purdy D, Laub G (1994) Improved MR angiography: magnetization transfer suppression with variable flip angle excitation and increased resolution. Radiology 190:890–894

Balaban RS, Ceckler TL (1992) Magnetization transfer contrast in magnetic resonance imaging. Magn Reson Quart 8:116–137

Balaban RS, Chesnick S, Hedges K, Samaha F, Heineman FW (1991) Magnetization transfer contrast in MR imaging of the heart. Radiology 180:671–675

Becker M, Zbaren P, Laeng H, Stoupis C, Porcellini B, Vock P (1995) Neoplastic invasion of the laryngeal cartilage: comparison of MR imaging and CT with histopathologic correlation (see comments). Radiology 194:661–669

Boorstein JM, Grossman RI, Bolinger L (1994a) Magnetization transfer imaging in metatastic disease to the brain. Radiology 191:799–803

Boorstein JM, Wong KT, Grossman RI, Bolinger L, McGowan JC (1994b) Metastatic lesions of the brain: imaging with magnetization transfer. Radiology 191:799–803

Boorstein JM, Moonis G, Boorstein SM, Patel YP, Culler AS (1997) Optic neuritis: imaging with magnetization transfer. Am J Roentgenol 169:1709–1712

Burke JW, Mathews VP, Elster AD, Ulmer JL, McLean FM, Davis SB (1996) Contrast-enhanced magnetization transfer saturation imaging improves MR detection of herpes simplex encephalitis. AJNR Am J Neuroradiol 17:773–776

Chung TS, Yousem DM, Seigerman HM, Schlakman BN, Weinstein GS, Hayden RE (1994) MR of mandibular invasion in patients with oral and oropharyngeal malignant neoplasms. AJNR Am J Neuroradiol 15:1949–1955

Curtin HD, Ishwaran H, Mancuso AA, Dalley RW, Caudry DJ, McNeil BJ Comparison of CT and MRI in staging of neck metastases. Radiology 1998 207:123-130

Dixon WT (1991) Use of magnetization transfer contrast in gradient-recalled echo images (editorial; comment). Radiology 179:15–16

Dooms GC, Hricak H (1986) Radiologic imaging modalities, including magnetic resonance, for evaluating lymph nodes. West J Med 144:49–57

Dooms GC, Hricak H, Crooks LE et al (1984) Magnetic resonance imaging of the lymph nodes: comparison with CT. Radiology 153:719–724

Dooms GC, Hricak H, Moseley ME, Bottles K, Fisher MR, Higgins CB (1985) Characterization of lymphadenopathy by magnetic relaxation times: preliminary results. Radiology 155:691–697

Dousset V (1993) Magnetization transfer imaging in vivo study of normal brain tissues and characterization of multiple sclerosis and experimental allergic encephalomyelitis lesions (letter). J Neuroradiol 20:297

Dousset V, Grossman RI, Ramer KN, Schnall MD, Young LH, Gonzalez-Scarano F, Lavi E, Cohen JA (1992) Experimental allergic encephalomyelitis and multiple sclerosis: lesion characterization with magnetization transfer imaging [published erratum appears in Radiology 1992, 183(3):878]. Radiology 182:483–491

Edelman RR, Ahn SS, Chien D et al (1992) Improved time-of-flight MR angiography of the brain with magnetization transfer contrast. Radiology 26:S255–S256

Eisen MD, Yousem DM, Montone KT, Kotapka MJ, Bigelow DC, Bilker WB, Loevner LA (1996) Use of preoperative MR to predict dural, perineural, and venous sinus invasion of skull base tumors. AJNR Am J Neuroradiol 17:1937–1945

Elster AD, Mathews VP, King JC, Hamilton CA (1994) Improved detection of gadolinium enhancement using magnetization transfer imaging. Neuroimaging Clin North Am 4:185–192

Eng J, Ceckler TL, Balaban RS (1991) Quantitative 1H magnetization transfer imaging in vivo. Magn Reson Med 17:304–314

Fellner C, Geissler A, Held P, Strotzer M, Treibel W, Fellner F (1995) Signal, contrast, and resolution in optimized PD- and T2-weighted turbo SE images of the knee. J Comput Assist Tomogr 19:96–105

Finelli DA, Hurst GC, Gullapali RP, Bellon EM (1994) Improved contrast of enhancing brain lesions on postgadolinium, T1-weighted spin-echo images with use of magnetization transfer. Radiology 190:553–559

Flamig DP, Pierce WB, Harms SE, Griffey RH (1992) Magnetization transfer contrast in fat-suppressed steady-state three-dimensional MR images. Magn Reson Med 26:122–131

Fralix TA, Ceckler TL, Wolff SD, Simon SA, Balaban RS (1991) Lipid bilayer and water proton magnetization transfer: effect of cholesterol. Magn Reson Med 18:214–223

Gillams AR, Silver MS, Carter AP (1995) Clinical utility of a new contrast option from magnetization transfer contrast. J Magn Reson Imaging 5:545–550

Gillams AR, Fuleihan N, Grillone G, Carter AP (1996) Magnetization transfer contrast MR in lesions of the head and neck. AJNR Am J Neuroradiol 17:355–360

Gomori JM, Grossman RI, Asakura T, Schnall MD, Atlas S, Holland G, Mittl RL Jr (1993) An in vitro study of magnetization transfer and relaxation rates of hematoma. AJNR Am J Neuroradiol 14:871–880

Grevers G, Ihrler S, Vogl TJ, Weiss M (1994) A comparison of clinical, pathological and radiological findings with magnetic resonance imaging studies of lymphomas in patients with Sjogren's syndrome. Eur Arch Otorhinolaryngol 251:214–217

Grossman RI (1994) Magnetization transfer in multiple sclerosis. Ann Neurol 36:S97–99

Grossman RI, Gomori JM, Ramer KN, Lexa FJ, Schnall MD (1994) Magnetization transfer: theory and clinical applications in neuroradiology. Radiographics 14:279–290

Hebert G, Ouimet-Oliva D, Nicolet V, Bourdon F (1993) Imaging of the salivary glands. Can Assoc Radiol J 44:342–349

Hiehle JF Jr, Grossman RI, Ramer KN, Gonzalez-Scarano F, Cohen JA (1995) Magnetization transfer effects in MR-detected multiple sclerosis lesions: comparison with gadolinium-enhanced spin-echo images and nonenhanced T1-weighted images. AJNR Am J Neuroradiol 16:69–77

Jones RA, Southon TE (1991) A magnetization transfer preparation scheme for snapshot FLASH imaging. Magn Reson Med 19:483–488

Kahn CE Jr, Perera SD, Sepponen RE, Tanttu JI, Tierala EK, Lipton MJ (1993) Magnetization transfer imaging of the abdomen at 0.1 T: detection of hepatic neoplasms. Magn Reson Imaging 11:67–71

Kaneda T, Minami M, Ozawa K, Akimoto Y, Okada M, Yamamoto H, Suzuki H, Sasaki Y (1994) Imaging tumors of the minor salivary glands. Oral Surg Oral Med Oral Pathol 78:385–390

Kobayashi A, Okayama Y, Yamazaki N (1993) 31P-NMR magnetization transfer study of reperfused rat heart. Mol Cell Biochem 119:121–127

Komu M, Alanen A (1994) Magnetization transfer in fatty and low-fat livers. Physiol Measurement 15:243–250

Kurki TJ, Niemi PT, Lundbom N (1992) Gadolinium-enhanced magnetization transfer contrast imaging of intracranial tumors. J Magn Reson Imaging 2:401–406

Kurki TJ, Niemi P, Valtonen S (1994) MR of intracranial tumors: combined use of gadolinium and magnetization transfer. AJNR Am J Neuroradiol 15:1727–1736

Li KC, Hopkins KL, Moore SG, Loh NN, Bergman G, Pike GB, Glover GH (1995) Magnetization transfer contrast MRI of musculoskeletal neoplasms. Skeletal Radiol 24:21–25

Lipton MJ, Sepponen RE, Tanttu JI, Kuusela T (1991) Magnetization transfer technique for improved magnetic resonance imaging contrast enhancement in whole body imaging. Invest Radiol 26:S255–256 (discussion S263–255)

Loesberg AC, Kormano M, Lipton MJ (1993) Magnetization transfer imaging of normal and abnormal liver at 0.1 T. Invest Radiol 28:726–731

Loevner LA, Grossman RI, Cohen JA, Lexa FJ, Kessler D, Kolson DL (1995a) Microscopic disease in normal-appearing white matter on conventional MR images in patients with multiple sclerosis: assessment with magnetization-transfer measurements. Radiology 196:511–515

Loevner LA, Grossman RI, McGowan JC, Ramer KN, Cohen JA (1995b) Characterization of multiple sclerosis plaques with T1-weighted MR and quantitative magnetization transfer. AJNR Am J Neuroradiol 16:1473–1479

Loevner LA, Ott IL, Yousem DM, Montone KT, Thaler ER, Chalian AA, Weinstein GS, Weber RS. Neoplastic fixation to the pervertebral compartment by squamous cell carcinoma of the head and neck. Am J Roentgenol 1988 170:1389-1394

Loevner LA, Yousem DM, Montone KT, Weber R, Chalian AA, Weinstein GS ( 1997) Can radiologists accurately predict preepiglottic space invasion with MR imaging? Am J Roentgenol 169:1681–1688

Lundbom N (1992) Determination of magnetization transfer contrast in tissue: an MR imaging study of brain tumors. AJR Am J Roentgenol 159:1279–1285

Lundbom N, Brown RD III, Koenig SH et al (1990) Magnetic field dependence of 1/T1 of human brain tumors: correlation with histology. Invest Radiol 25:1197–1205

Lundbom N, Kurki T, Komu M, Kormano M (1995) Magnetization transfer contrast imaging of brain tumors. Rontgenpraxis 48:42–44

Markkola AT, Aronen HJ, Paavonen T, Hopsu E, Sipila LM, Tanttu JI, Sepponen RE (1996) Spin lock and magnetization transfer imaging of head and neck tumors. Radiology 200:369–375

Mathews VP, Elster AD, King JC, Ulmer JL, Hamilton CA, Strottmann JM (1995) Combined effects of magnetization transfer and gadolinium in cranial MR imaging and MR angiography. AJR Am J Roentgenol 164:169–172

Mathews VP, Caldemeyer KS, Ulmer JL, Nguyen H, Yuh WT (1997) Effects of contrast dose, delayed imaging, and magnetization transfer saturation on gadolinium-enhanced MR imaging of brain lesions. J Magn Reson Imaging 7:14–22

Mehta RC, Pike GB, Haros SP, Enzmann DR (1995) Central nervous system tumor, infection, and infarction: detection with gadolinium-enhanced magnetization transfer MR imaging. Radiology 195:41–46

Mittl RL Jr, Gomori JM, Schnall MD, Holland GA, Grossman RI, Atlas SW (1993) Magnetization transfer effects in MR imaging of in vivo intracranial hemorrhage. AJNR Am J Neuroradiol 14:881–891

Morris GA, Freemont AJ (1992) Direct observation of the magnetization exchange dynamics responsible for magnetization transfer contrast in human cartilage in vitro. Magn Reson Med 28:97–104

Morrison C, Henkelman RM (1995) A model for magnetization transfer in tissues. Magn Reson Med 33:475–482

Ordidge RJ, Knight RA, Helpern JA (1991) Magnetization transfer contrast (MTC) in flash MR imaging. Magn Reson Imaging 9:889–893

Ott IL, Loevner LA, Yousem DM, Montone KT, Chalian AA, Hayden RE, Weinstein GS (1996) Prevertebral muscular invasion in patients with squamous cell carcinoma of the head and neck: assessment with MR. American Society of Head and Neck Radiology, 30th annual meeting, Los Angeles, 26 Apr 1996, paper no 005

Outwater E, Schnall MD, Braitman LE, Dinsmore BJ, Kressel HY (1992) Magnetization transfer of hepatic lesions: evaluation of a novel contrast technique in the abdomen. Radiology 182:535–540

Pike GB, Hu BS, Glover GH, Enzmann DR (1992) Magnetization transfer time-of-flight magnetic resonance angiography. Magn Reson Med 25:372–379

Prasad PV, Burstein D, Edelman RR (1993) MRI evaluation of myocardial perfusion without a contrast agent using magnetization transfer. Magn Reson Med 30:267–270

Schlakman BS, Yousem DM (1993) Magnetic resonance imaging of intra-parotid masses. AJNR Am J Neuroradiol 14:1173–1180

Sheppard LM, Yousem DM (1994) MT1 of cervical adenopathy. ASNR, paper 130

Sigal R, Chancelier MD, Luboinski B, Shapeero LG, Bosq J, Vanel D (1992a) Synovial sarcomas of the head and neck: CT and MR findings. AJNR Am J Neuroradiol 13:1459–1462

Sigal R, Monnet O, de Baere T, Micheau C, Shapeero LG, Julieron M, Bosq J, Vanel D, Piekarski JD, Luboinski B et al (1992b) Adenoid cystic carcinoma of the head and neck: evaluation with MR imaging and clinical-pathologic correlation in 27 patients. Radiology 184:95–101

Sigal R, Zagdanski AM, Schwaab G, Bosq J, Auperin A, Laplanche A, Francke JP, Eschwege F, Luboinski B, Vanel D (1996) CT and MR imaging of squamous cell carcinoma of the tongue and floor of the mouth. Radiographics 16:787–810

Som PM, Biller HF (1989) High-grade malignancies of the parotid gland: identification with MR imaging. Radiology 173:823–826

Som PM, Sacher M, Stollman AL et al (1988a) Common tumors of the parapharyngeal space: refined imaging diagnosis. Radiology 169:81–86

Som PM, Shapiro MD, Biller HF, Sasaki C, Lawson W (1988b) Sinonasal tumors and inflammatory tissues: differentiation with MR imaging. Radiology 167:803–808

Som PM, Shugar JM, Sacher M, Stollman AL, Biller HF (1988c) Benign and malignant parotid pleomorphic adenomas: CT and MR studies. J Comput Assist Tomogr 12:65–69

Som PM, Shugar JM, Troy KM, Sacher M, Stollman AL (1988d) The use of magnetic resonance and computed tomography in the management of a patient with intrasinus hemorrhage. Arch Otolaryngol Head Neck Surg 114:200–202

Som PM, Dillon WP, Sze G et al (1989) Benign and malignant sinonasal lesions with intracranial extension: differentiation with MR imaging. Radiology 172:763–766

Tkach JA, Ruggieri PM, Ross JS, Modic MT, Dillinger JJ, Masaryk TJ (1993) Pulse sequence strategies for vascular contrast in time-of-flight carotid MR angiography. J Magn Reson Imaging 3:811–820

Ulmer JL, Mathews VP, Hamilton CA, Elster AD, Moran PR (1996) Magnetization transfer or spin-lock? An investigation of off-resonance saturation pulse imaging with varying frequency offsets. AJNR Am J Neuroradiol 17:805–819

van den Brekel MW, Castelijns JA, Snow GB (1994) Detection of lymph node metastases in the neck: radiologic criteria (editorial; comment). Radiology 192:617–618

Wolff SD, Balaban RS (1989) Magnetization transfer contrast (MTC) and tissue water proton relaxation in vivo. Magn Reson Med 10:135–144

Wolff SD, Chesnick S, Frank JA, Lim KO, Balaban RS (1991a) Magnetization transfer contrast: MR imaging of the knee. Radiology 179:623–628

Wolff SD, Eng J, Balaban RS (1991b) Magnetization transfer contrast: method for improving contrast in gradient-recalled-echo images (see comments). Radiology 179:133–137

Yang H, Schleich T (1994) T1 discrimination contributions to proton magnetization transfer in heterogeneous biological systems. Magn Reson Med 32:16–22

Yousem DM, Lexa FJ, Bilaniuk LT, Zimmerman RI (1990) Rhabdomyosarcomas in the head and neck: MR imaging evaluation. Radiology 177:683–686

Yousem DM, Fellows DW, Kennedy DW, Bolger WE, Kashima H, Zinreich SJ (1992) Inverted papilloma: evaluation with MR imaging. Radiology 185:501–505

Yousem DM, Jarvik J, Chung TS (1993) Magnetization transfer imaging of sinonasal secretions and neoplasms. ASHNR, Vancouver, paper no 054

Yousem DM, Montone KT, Sheppard LM, Rao VM, Weinstein GS, Hayden RE (1994a) Head and neck neoplasms: magnetization transfer analysis. Radiology 192:703–707

Yousem DM, Schnall MD, Dougherty L, Weinstein GS, Hayden RE (1994b) Magnetization transfer imaging of the head and neck: normative data. AJNR Am J Neuroradiol 15:1117–1121

Zagdanski AM, Sigal R, Bosq J, Bazin JP, Vanel D, Di Paola R (1994) Factor analysis of medical image sequences in MR of head and neck tumors. AJNR Am J Neuroradiol 15:1359–1368

Zbaren P, Becker M, Lang H (1996) Pretherapeutic staging of laryngeal carcinoma. Clinical findings, computed tomography, and magnetic resonance imaging compared with histopathology. Cancer 77:1263–1273

Zbaren P, Becker M, Lang H (1997) Staging of laryngeal cancer: endoscopy, computed tomography and magnetic resonance versus histopathology. Eur Arch Otorhinolaryngol [Suppl] 1:S117–122

# 2 Magnetic Resonance Imaging-Guided Intervention in the Head and Neck

E.M. Merkle, J.S. Lewin, and J.L. Duerk

CONTENTS



## 2.1 Introduction

Interventional magnetic resonance imaging (I-MRI) is the use of MR images for biopsy and drainage, and for both guidance and monitoring of minimally invasive therapy (including thermal destruction of tumors). As a result, MRI is rapidly becoming an important tool in the performance of interventional procedures; the medical use of MRI may be expanded from diagnosis only to treatment. However, MRI pulse sequences must be adapted to meet the requirements for: (a) high temporal resolution during biopsy needle insertion, (b) high spatial resolution for accurate needle tip localization, (c) rapid reconstruction/display to achieve near-real-time guidance, and (d) contrast between normal and pathologic tissue and the interventional devices.

This chapter first discusses passive visualization of MR-compatible needles and the effects of field strength, sequence design, and orientation of the needle relative to the static magnetic field of the scanner. In the second section, guidelines for patient preparation, antisepsis and detailed descriptions of the interventional procedures are delineated. The final portion of this chapter will be a report of the current status of I-MRI in the head and neck.

## 2.2 Passive Visualization of MR-Compatible Needles

Unlike ultrasound and CT, MR is beset by the problem that many factors can influence passive visualization of MR-compatible needles, which results from magnetic polarization of the needle causing local disruption of $B_0$. This is a "susceptibility artifact," which depends on field strength, orientation of the needle relative to the static magnetic field ($B_0$), sequence design, needle orientation to frequency-encoding axis, and instrument alloy. It is important that radiologists understand these factors, to ensure correct device selection and to maximize the safety and accuracy of the method.

### 2.2.1 Field Strength

At a given angle $\beta$ (needle orientation to the static magnetic field of the scanner), both apparent needle width and absolute error in tip position depend on field strength (Frahm et al. 1996; Lewin et al. 1996). Artifactual widening of the needle is much more apparent at 1.5 T than at 0.2 T (Frahm et al. 1996; Lewin et al. 1996), as is any error in accurate localization of the needle tip position (Table 2.1). Artifac-

E.M. Merkle, M.D., Department of Radiology, University Hospitals of Cleveland / Case Western Reserve University, 11100 Euclid Avenue, Cleveland, OH 44106, USA
J.S. Lewin, M.D., Department of Radiology, University Hospitals of Cleveland / Case Western Reserve University, 11100 Euclid Avenue, Cleveland, OH 44106, USA
J.L. Duerk, Ph.D., Department of Radiology, University Hospitals of Cleveland / Case Western Reserve University, 11100 Euclid Avenue, Cleveland, OH 44106, USA

**Table 2.1.** Average values on imaging for all needles with shafts perpendicular to static magnetic field (*FISP* fast imaging with steady state free precession, *SE* spin-echo, *FLASH* fast low-angle shot, *TSE* turbo spin-echo). Reproduced with permission from LEWIN et al. (1996)

| Imaging sequence (relationship of needle shaft to frequency-encoded axis) | Width (mm) | | Absolute error in tip position (mm) | |
|---|---|---|---|---|
| | 0.2 T | 1.5 T | 0.2 T | 1.5 T |
| FISP (parallel) | 7.0 | 13.9 | 0.9 | 3.1 |
| FISP (perpendicular) | 6.8 | 13.0 | 1.1 | 3.1 |
| FLASH (parallel) | 6.3 | 12.6 | 1.0 | 3.3 |
| FLASH (perpendicular) | 6.3 | 12.6 | 1.4 | 2.9 |
| SE (parallel) | 1.9 | 4.0 | 1.3 | 2.3 |
| SE (perpendicular) | 3.8 | 7.1 | 0.9 | 1.1 |
| TSE (parallel) | 2.1 | 4.4 | 0.8 | 1.4 |
| TSE (perpendicular) | 4.1 | 6.6 | 0.5 | 1.1 |

**Table 2.2.** Average values on imaging for all needles with shafts parallel to static magnetic field. Reproduced with permission from LEWIN et al. (1996)

| Imaging sequence (relationship of needle shaft to frequency-encoded axis) | Width (mm) | | Absolute error in tip position (mm) | |
|---|---|---|---|---|
| | 0.2 T | 1.5 T | 0.2 T | 1.5 T |
| FISP (parallel) | 2.0 | 1.6 | 2.0 | 4.0 |
| FISP (perpendicular) | 2.0 | 1.6 | 2.0 | 4.1 |
| FLASH (parallel) | 1.5 | 1.5 | 1.9 | 4.5 |
| FLASH (perpendicular) | 1.8 | 1.5 | 1.5 | 4.0 |
| SE (parallel) | 1.8 | 1.6 | 1.6 | 3.8 |
| SE (perpendicular) | 1.8 | 1.6 | 2.4 | 3.4 |
| TSE (parallel) | 1.9 | 1.6 | 1.5 | 3.5 |
| TSE (perpendicular) | 1.9 | 1.8 | 2.1 | 2.5 |

tual widening of the needle is also increased, but tip localization is improved when the needle shaft is perpendicular to the static magnetic field ($\beta = 90°$) (Table 2.1). On the other hand, artifactual widening is much less apparent when the needle shaft is parallel ($\beta = 0°$) to the static magnetic field (FRAHM et al. 1996; LEWIN et al. 1996; MUELLER et al. 1986). Regardless of orientation, the error in tip position is still larger at 1.5 T than at 0.2 T (Table 2.2).

### 2.2.2 Orientation of the Needle Relative to the Static Magnetic Field ($B_0$)

Apparent width and absolute error in needle tip position obviously depend on the needle orientation relative to $B_0$. In general, a larger angle $\beta$ relative to $B_0$ (up to 90°) causes larger artifacts (Tables 2.1, 2.2) (FRAHM et al. 1996; LEWIN et al. 1996; MUELLER et al. 1986). At both 0.2 T and 1.5 T, there is a marked increase (factor 3–4 at 0.2 T; factor 6–7 at 1.5 T) in the apparent needle width on gradient echo sequences (fast imaging with steady state free precession, FISP; fast low-angle shot, FLASH) in comparison with the apparent width at $\beta = 0°$. This increase is especially significant in the range of $0° < \beta < 60°$. In the range of $60° < \beta < 90°$, only a small further increase of the apparent needle width is seen (LEWIN et al. 1996). For SE and turbo spin echo (TSE) sequences, there is no definite artifactual needle widening at 0.2 T with the frequency-encoding axis parallel to the needle shaft; however, a small but definite dependence on orientation is seen at 0.2 T, with the frequency-encoding axis perpendicular to needle shaft in SE and TSE sequences (twofold increase). At 1.5 T, a small trend toward reduction in apparent width is also observed with SE and TSE sequences (factor 2–3), though the dependence of the apparent width is more pronounced when the orientation of the frequency-encoding axis is perpendicular to the needle (Tables 2.1, 2.2).

With regard to the error that will be observed in visualization of needle tip position, a larger angle $\beta$ relative to $B_0$ (up to 90°) causes smaller errors with all pulse sequences for 0.2 T and 1.5 T. The error in tip position is larger at higher field strengths, and also when imaging is performed with gradient echo sequences (Tables 2.1, 2.2).

### 2.2.3 Sequence Design

In general, gradient echo sequences are more sensitive to spin dephasing promoted by the local field inhomogeneities occurring around the needle, because of the lack of a 180° refocusing pulse (LUFKIN et al. 1987). For this reason, gradient echo sequences (FISP, FLASH) cause both larger artifacts and larger absolute errors in tip position than do SE and TSE sequences. These effects are more obvious at higher field strength and when the needle shaft is perpendicular to the main magnetic field (LEWIN et al. 1996). SE and TSE sequences do not differ significantly in apparent needle width or absolute error in tip position (FRAHM et al. 1996; LEWIN et al. 1996).

a,b
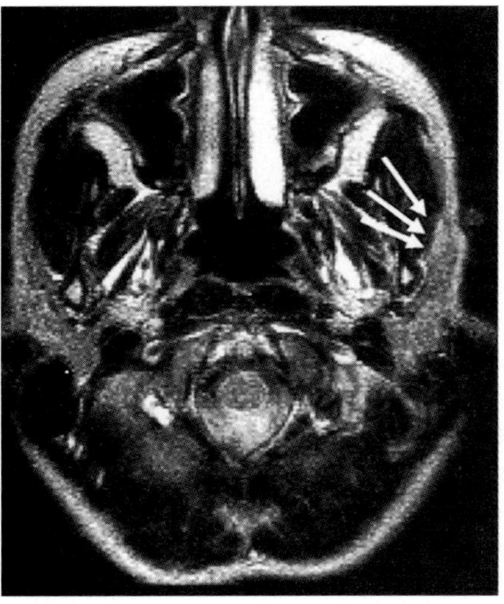
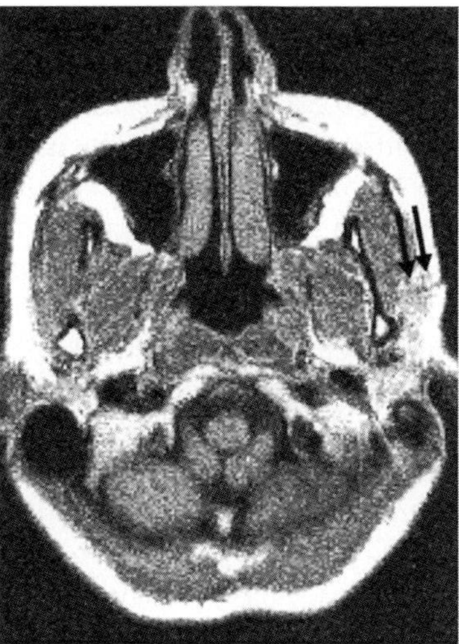
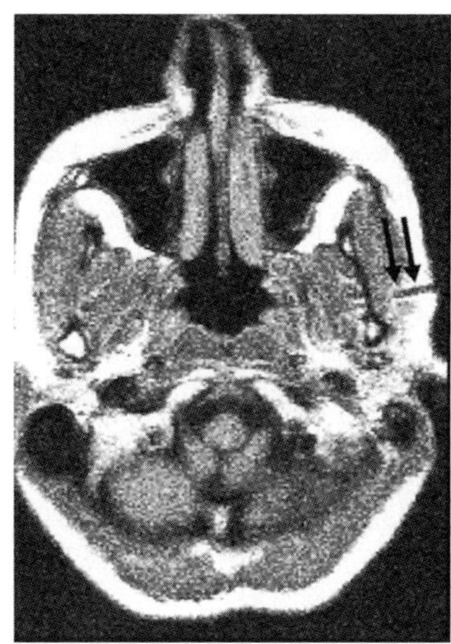
c

**Fig. 2.1 a–c.** Influence of swapping phase-encoding and frequency-encoding axes using TSE sequences. **a** Axial T2-weighted image: 40-year-old patient with history of non-Hodgkin lymphoma and new 1-cm mass in the left parotid space (*arrows*). **b** Axial image for needle position confirmation using a turbo spin echo (TSE) sequence (TR/TE/NEX 2000/105/1). Artifactual widening from the needle (22G) is difficult to see (*solid arrows*), because the frequency-encoding axis is almost parallel to the needle shaft. **c** Using the same sequence, but swapping phase-encoding and frequency-encoding axes, artifactual widening from the needle (22G) is seen much better (*solid arrows*), because needle angulation relative to frequency-encoding axis is almost perpendicular. The cytology sample was negative for malignancy

### 2.2.4 Needle Orientation to Frequency-Encoding Axis

Using SE and TSE sequences, the apparent needle width at $\beta = 90°$ is diminished by a factor of approximately 0.3–0.5 if the read-out gradient is applied parallel to the needle shaft (Frahm et al. 1996; Lewin et al. 1996; Sinha et al. 1989) (Fig. 2.1). The error in needle tip position, however, is decreased by a factor of 0.2–0.5 if the frequency-encoding axis is perpendicular to the needle shaft, because the needle is more conspicuous. When SE and TSE sequences are applied at $\beta = 0°$ this rotation of the image plane has no influence on apparent needle width.

On gradient echo sequences, swapping the phase-encoding and frequency-encoding axes has no observable effect on apparent needle width or on absolute error in tip position, regardless of the field strength (Frahm et al. 1996; Lewin et al. 1996).

### 2.2.5 Alloy

As one would expect, larger diameter (lower gauge) MR-compatible needles cause larger artifacts. But there are also differences of up to a factor of 1.4 in apparent needle width with the same needle size from different manufacturers, depending on the metallurgical compositions (Frahm et al. 1996; Lewin et al. 1996); this effect is especially dependent on the nickel content. Nickel reduces the ferromagnetic properties of iron in alloys and generally decreases magnetic susceptibility differences between the alloy and the surrounding tissues. Nickel works by changing the highly susceptible form of $\alpha$-iron into less susceptible $\gamma$-iron (Lufkin et al. 1987).

## 2.3 Issues and Recommendations for Low- and High- Field Scanners

### 2.3.1 Low-Field

The primary issue at 0.2 T results from too little artifactual widening rather than too much. Insufficient artifactual widening with SE and TSE sequences makes the positions of smaller needles difficult to determine. Gradient echo pulse sequences reveal an increase in apparent needle diameter that is sufficient to facilitate needle visualization but not so large as to preclude accurate needle tip localization. It is also fortunate that the rapid scan times provided by gradient echo pulse sequences are well suited to near-real-time feedback during device placement. Gradient echo pulse sequences are the sequences of choice for monitoring needle insertion at 0.2 T.

After needle insertion, accurate confirmation of trajectory and tip position is necessary before extraction of the specimen, particularly with cutting needles. Both TSE and SE sequences provide accurate localization of tip position, with little problem of artifactual needle widening that can obscure adjacent structures. Unfortunately, the small degree of artifactual widening also makes needle visualization in tissue difficult. Selection of a frequency-encoding axis perpendicular to the needle shaft results in only slight artifactual widening, thereby increasing visibility and facilitating assessment of the accuracy of tip placement.

The orientation of the needle relative to the static magnetic field also has practical implications for MR-guided interventional procedures, because the degree of artifactual widening decreases as the needle shaft approaches the axis of the static magnetic field. With an anterior approach in MR-guided biopsies (in an open C-arm scanner with vertically oriented main magnetic field), the needle shaft would be parallel to $B_0$. This would result in artifactual widening insufficient for visualization during needle placement using gradient echo pulse sequences. Therefore, the direct anterior approach has to be modified to create a visible needle artifact.

### 2.3.2 High Field

Unlike 0.2 T MRI, imaging at 1.5 T requires that ferromagnetic artifacts be reduced as much as possible. Gradient echo pulse sequences yield artifacts that render images suboptimal for accurate needle tip localization. Therefore, despite scan times that are longer than desirable, monitoring of needle insertion may be best performed at 1.5 T with TSE and SE sequences (Lewin et al. 1996). As an alternative, gradient echo pulse sequences with a very short TE can be used, because artifactual widening increases directly with increasing echo time (Frahm et al. 1996; Mahfouz et al. 1996).

For confirmation of needle tip position before tissue sampling, the frequency-encoding axis should be perpendicular to the needle shaft to decrease distortion along the needle while also increasing the accuracy of tip localization. This approach will produce greater apparent widening of the needle tip and may obscure structures adjacent to the needle shaft. Thus, supplemental images obtained with the frequency-encoding axis parallel to the needle shaft also may be necessary.

The use of needles manufactured from less ferromagnetic materials (increased content of nickel, or titanium alloys) is essential for scanning at 1.5 T. Removal of the needle stylet before imaging may also be useful in reducing artifacts.

The orientation of the needle relative to the static magnetic field also has practical implications for MR-guided interventional procedures at 1.5 T. Here, in the opposite situation to a low-field scanner, an approach closer to the axis of the static magnetic field may be helpful. This approach will reduce artifactual widening of the needle, at the expense of an increase in error in determining needle tip position. This might be of importance for MR-guided biopsies of supraclavicular masses, where, in general, an approach closer to the axis of the main magnetic field is possible.

## 2.4 Patient Preparation and Description of Interventional Procedures

The following discussion describing the technique for head and neck biopsies is geared toward those performed on open scanner systems. These techniques may also be applicable, in part, to biopsies that are performed on conventional "closed" MR imaging systems. However, the obligate delay resulting from table repositioning and coil tuning may make performance of head and neck biopsies a long and tedious procedure in a "closed" system, and may negate many of the advantages that MR has to offer.

On our open imaging system, which is based on a C-shaped vertical field scanner with an in-room high-resolution liquid crystal display monitor, most lesions of the head and suprahyoid neck are best approached with the patient in a supine position using a conventional head coil with open sides. Infrahyoid or supraclavicular lesions require a solenoidal coil, either positioned next to the neck with the needle passing through the center of the coil, or placed around the neck with the needle passing just above or below the coil. For open scanners that allow an approach from only one side, such as ours, the patient must be positioned either "head right" or "head left" in the scanner to allow access to the lesion from the open side of the scanner. Next, routine images of the region of interest are typically performed immediately before the procedure, using "conventional" T1-weighted and TSE T2-weighted spin echo sequences. After selection of the safest biopsy needle trajectory from the preprocedure images and selection of an appropriate biopsy device, a fast gradient echo sequence (e.g. FISP) is chosen and the in-room monitor is set up with an automatic display of all acquired images. Using the fast GRE sequence, a near-real-time "MR fluoroscopy" is achieved (3 images every 6–9 s).

The localization of the needle insertion point (on the skin) is the next step. This can be done most simply using a fluid-filled pointer and a fast T2-weighted biopsy sequence. (Note: Instead of expensive fluid-filled pointers, a water-filled 3-cc or 5-cc syringe can also be used. Although the radiologist can also simply use his or her finger on the MR fluoroscopic images, the thickness of the finger means less accurate slice localization.) A four-segment window display is chosen on the in-room monitor, and the most appropriate target slice (from the preprocedure scan) is placed in the left bottom segment of the display. The biopsy is set up with three contiguous parallel slices of 5 mm each filling the three remaining segments of the screen (e.g. positions –5 mm, 0 mm, and +5 mm) (Fig. 2.2). Each of these three images is automatically updated every 2–3 s, allowing continual comparison with the target slice. The water-filled pointer is positioned on the skin, and under MR guidance the needle insertion point is depicted and marked using a water-resistant marker.

The skin is then scrubbed with disinfectant and the biopsy area is covered with sterile towels and drapes. After local anesthesia of the skin, an MR-

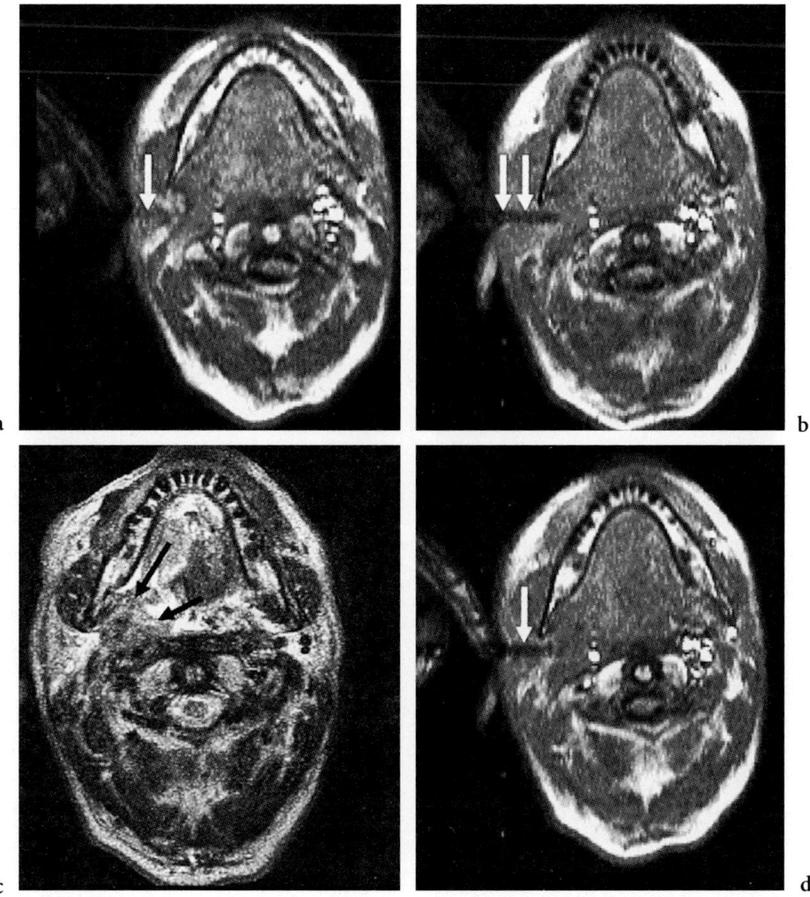

**Fig. 2.2 a–d.** Display illustration of the in-room monitor as used during MR-guided interventional procedures (55-year-old patient with history of laryngectomy and recent oropharyngeal hemorrhage). **a**, **b**, **d** Three parallel fast GRE axial slices, located A 5 mm cranial to **b** at the same position as, and **d** 5 mm caudad to the previously chosen reference slice (**c**). Slices shown in **a**, **b**, and **d** are updated every 3 s and displayed automatically, whereas C remains unchanged in the display. Of note is the high vascular conspicuity, which demonstrates bright signal on fast 2D GRE sequences. Cytology revealed recurrence of an oropharyngeal carcinoma (*white arrows* 22G MR-compatible needle, *black arrows* suspect lesion)

compatible needle is inserted using continuous visual control with fast GRE sequences. An important factor of these sequences is the excellent visualization of the blood vessels as bright structures (Fig. 2.3). After the needle tip has reached the target, a higher spatial resolution spin echo or turbo spin echo sequence is obtained in order to confirm accurate tip position (Fig. 2.1).

The following are our standard approaches to different locations in the head and neck; they are, in part, identical to those previously described (LUFKIN et al. 1997):

1. The subzygomatic/infratemporal approach can be used to access lesions in the skull base, parapharyngeal space, and infratemporal fossa.
2. The retromandibular approach is useful for accessing the paraoropharyngeal, parotid and the lower masticator spaces. The needle is placed just posterior to the angle of the mandible and no less than 1 cm inferior to the tragus, to avoid damaging the facial nerve.
3. The submastoid approach can be used to sample lesions in the skull base. The needle is inserted 1 cm below the mastoid tip along the anterior aspect of the sternocleidomastoid muscle.
4. An anterior paramaxillary approach (Fig. 2.3) can be used to reach the buccal space or anterior parapharyngeal or masticator spaces. This is best performed with the head partially turned to place the needle nearer perpendicular to the vertical static magnetic field of our system. This greatly improves the visibility of the needle, as discussed above.
5. Infrahyoid and cervical spine lesions can be approached from a direct or oblique lateral direction, but care must be taken to choose a trajectory that will avoid puncture of the carotid or vertebral

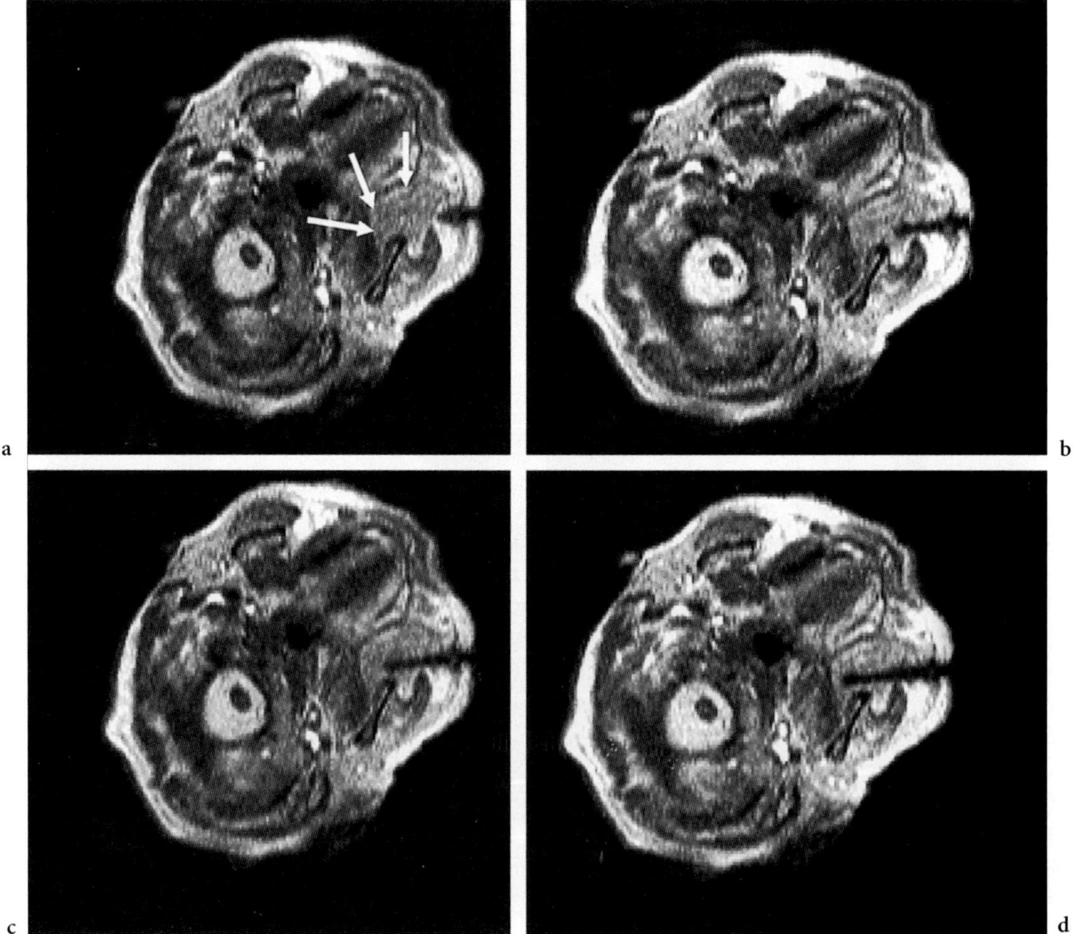


**Fig. 2.3.** Insertion of an 18G MR-compatible needle under permanent visual control within 1 min. Histology revealed a meningioma in the left masticator space (*arrows*)

arteries or entry of the spinal canal if the needle passes through or deflects off the lesion being sampled.

6. Supraclavicular lesions are often easier to target when a coronal or oblique imaging plane and a superolateral approach are used in preference to direct axial imaging. This allows simultaneous visualization of the lesion, the lung apex, and often the brachial plexus, so that pneumothorax and inadvertent neural injury are avoided.

## 2.5 Current Status of I-MRI in the Head and Neck

Although MR-guided aspiration cytology for deep-seated head and neck lesions has been performed over the last 10 years (Duckwiler et al. 1989; Lufkin and Layfield 1989; Lufkin et al. 1987, 1988; Trapp et al. 1989), it has become a standard procedure at only a few institutions. For example:

1. The group in Stanford reported their experience of four patients in 1997 using an open 0.5 T system (Norbash et al. 1997). Their patients included: a 39-year-old woman with suspected recurrent papillary thyroid carcinoma with cystic jugulodigastric lymphadenopathy; a second biopsy of abnormal paratracheal solid enhancing soft tissue was performed in the same patient. Abnormally enhancing sphenoid sinus fullness was sampled in a patient with a history of multiple myeloma, bone marrow transplant, and aspergillosis. Soft palate asymmetry and thickening in a 39-year-old female patient with documented recurrent nasopharyngeal carcinoma was also sampled. In a fourth patient, access to the stellate ganglion anterior to the transverse process of C6 was secured for stellate ganglion blockade with local anesthesia. No complications occurred in these four procedures.
2. The group at UCLA (Borges et al. 1997) reported their experience in 36 cases. Thirteen biopsies were done using a closed 1.5 T scanner. The remaining 23 procedures were performed in an open 0.2 T scanner. No differences in lesion depiction or accuracy of fine needle aspiration diagnosis were detected between the open and closed systems. No complications were observed for either group. It was not possible in this study to obtain data on the duration of all the procedures. However, there was a general belief that biopsies were much faster and required fewer image acquisitions when performed in the open magnet.
3. At the same scientific meeting, the group from Zurich (Kacl et al. 1997) reported MR-guided fine needle aspirations of the maxilla and the skull base in 10 patients using a 0.5 T open scanner. All patients were biopsied successfully without complications. Instrument time averaged under 30 min in all cases.
4. During a 3-year period, at University Hospitals/Case Western Reserve University in Cleveland, a total of 50 MR-guided procedures have been performed in 37 patients (age 6 months to 88 years) in the head and neck, including the mucosal, masticator and parapharyngeal spaces ($n$ = 17), parotid space ($n$ = 6), submandibular space ($n$ = 2), cervical vertebral column/paraspinal tissues ($n$ = 8), skull base ($n$ = 1), larynx or hypopharynx ($n$ = 3), and infrahyoid nodal chains and surrounding tissues ($n$ = 13) (Lewin et al. 1998). A clinical 0.2 T C-arm imaging system was used, supplemented with an in-room radiofrequency-shielded liquid crystal monitor, rapid gradient echo sequences for needle guidance, and MR-compatible anesthesia, monitoring, and surgical lighting equipment. Tissue sampling included fine needle aspiration ($n$ = 49) and cutting needle core biopsy ($n$ = 24), with 23 patients undergoing both procedures. Successful needle placement was accomplished in all cases without complication, with tissue sufficient for pathological diagnosis obtained for all but 5 patients with an average of 2.1 passes per patient. For fine needle aspiration, instrument time averaged 7.8 min per pass, while cutting needle core biopsy averaged 9.2 min.

In conclusion, MR-guided biopsies in the head and neck area are not only safe and feasible, but also reasonable in terms of time considering the available options. Currently, most patients scheduled for MR-guided biopsy at our institution have lesions that are not easily amenable to guidance under other imaging methods (i.e. ultrasound, CT). In many of these patients, the only alternative is an open biopsy in the operation room under general anesthesia.

## 2.6 Future Directions

Few would have predicted the rapid evolution of interventional MRI over the past 5 years, and it is equally challenging to predict what will evolve in the next 5. A few changes are certain. Interventional MRI hardware will almost certainly evolve to include new magnet geometry, higher field strength, and greater integration of intraoperative and interventional tools, including display and localization systems and RF-laser-focused ultrasound ablation systems. Other hardware on the clinical horizon that will support interventional MRI is at the forefront of scientific development today. This includes devices for active tip-tracking, which will be used for automated scan plane definition.

From a clinical perspective, such minimal invasive therapy modalities as interstitial thermotherapy modalities (laser-induced, radiofrequency-induced, high-intensity-focused ultrasound, and cryotherapy) might be included in the treatment of lesions of the head, neck, and skull base. These lesions often have close proximity to major vessels and cranial nerves, and wide local resection may result in both cosmetic and functional deformities. Preliminary clinical trials of laser-induced interstitial thermotherapy have been reported by the groups in Los Angeles and Berlin (Castro et al. 1992; Vogl et al. 1995). These techniques may offer an alternative treatment option for patients with recurrence of cancer in the head and neck area.

*Acknowledgements.* The authors would like to thank the rest of the Interventional MRI Research Team at University Hospitals of Cleveland/Case Western Reserve University. The University Hospitals of Cleveland/Case Western Reserve University Interventional MR Program is supported in part through research collaborations with Siemens Medical Systems and Radionics, and through grants from the Whitaker Foundation, the American Cancer Society, the Mary Ann S. Swetland Fund, and the M.E. and F.J. Callahan Foundation.

## References

Borges A, Villablanca JP, Lufkin RB (1997) MR imaging-guided biopsies in the head and neck region: a comparative evaluation of low field open and high field closed MR systems. Radiology 205 (P):531(abstract)

Castro DJ, Lufkin RB, Saxton RE, Nyerges A, Soudant J, Layfield LJ, Jabour BA, Ward PH, Kangarloo H (1992) Metastatic head and neck malignancy treated using MRI guided interstitial laser phototherapy: an initial case report. Laryngoscope 102:26–32

Duckwiler G, Lufkin RB, Teresi L, Spickler E, Dion J, Vinuela F, Bentson J, Hanafee W (1989) Head and neck lesions: MR-guided aspiration biopsy. Radiology 170: 519–522

Frahm C, Gehl HB, Melchert UH, Weiss HD (1996) Visualization of magnetic resonance-compatible needles at 1.5 and 0.2 Tesla. Cardiovasc Intervent Radiol 19:335–340

Kacl GM, Carls FP, Sailer HF et al (1997) Interactive MR-guided biopsies of the maxilla and the skull base. Radiology 205 (P):531(abstract)

Lewin JS, Duerk JL, Jain VR, Petersilge CA, Chao CP, Haaga JR (1996) Needle localization in MR-guided biopsy and aspiration: effects of field strength, sequence design, and magnetic field orientation. Am J Roentgenol 166: 1337–1345

Lewin JS, Petersilge CA, Hatem SF et al (1998) Interactive MR imaging-guided biopsy and aspiration with a modified clinical C-arm system. Am J Roentgenol 170:1593–1601

Lufkin R, Layfield L (1989) Coaxial needle system of MR- and CT-guided aspiration cytology. J Comput Assist Tomogr 13:1105–1107

Lufkin R, Teresi L, Hanafee W (1987) New needle for MR-guided aspiration cytology of the head and neck. Am J Roentgenol 149:380–382

Lufkin R, Teresi L, Chiu L, Hanafee W (1988) A technique for MR-guided needle placement. Am J Roentgenol 151: 193–196

Lufkin RB, Gronemeyer DW, Seibel RM (1997) Interventional MRI: update. Eur Radiol 7:187–200

Mahfouz AE, Rahmouni A, Zylbersztejn C, Mathieu D (1996) MR-guided biopsy using ultrafast T1- and T2-weighted reordered turbo fast low-angle shot sequences: feasibility and preliminary clinical applications. Am J Roentgenol 167:167–169

Mueller PR, Stark DD, Simeone JF, Saini S, Butch RJ, Edelman RR, Wittenberg J, Ferrucci JTJ (1986) MR-guided aspiration biopsy: needle design and clinical trials. Radiology 161:605–609

Norbash AM, Daniel BL, Butts K et al (1997) Magnetic Resonance Therapy (MRT) guided biopsies in the skull base, suprahyoid neck, and infrahyoid neck. Proceedings of the SMR meeting 1997, p 530 (abstract)

Sinha S, Sinha U, Lufkin R, Hanafee W (1989) Pulse sequence optimization for use with a biopsy needle in MRI. Magn Reson Imaging 7:575–579

Trapp T, Lufkin R, Abemayor E, Layfield L, Hanafee W, Ward P (1989) A new needle and technique for MRI-guided aspiration cytology of the head and neck. Laryngoscope 99: 105–108

Vogl TJ, Mack MG, Muller P, Phillip C, Bottcher H, Roggan A, Juergens M, Deimling M, Knobber D, Wust P (1995) Recurrent nasopharyngeal tumors: preliminary clinical results with interventional MR imaging-controlled laser-induced thermotherapy. Radiology 196:725–733

# 3 MR-Guided Therapy of Head and Neck Cancers

T.J. Vogl and M.G. Mack

CONTENTS



## 3.1 Introduction

The head and neck area includes a multitude of small, complexly arranged anatomical structures; intimate knowledge of normal spatial relationships and variations is necessary to plan and implement appropriate therapy. Lesions often lie near vital structures, complicating diagnostic and therapeutic procedures. Improved visualization during such procedures can therefore provide the physician with critical information, permitting innovative procedures. The first treatment choice for head and neck cancer is surgery, often followed by radiation therapy. If surgery is not possible because of extensive tumor infiltration or general contraindications for surgery the treatment of first choice is radiation therapy or chemotherapy or a combination of both. So far there are no accepted indications for MR-guided therapy modalities, such as MR-guided laser-induced thermotherapy, in the primary treatment of head and neck cancer.

However, palliative treatment options for recurrent head and neck cancer are limited by the proximity of vital vascular and neural structures and the aggressive nature of these tumors. Depending on the localization of the recurrent tumor a minimally invasive treatment modality such as interventional MR-guided laser-induced thermotherapy (LITT) offers a number of potential treatment benefits. First, MR imaging provides unparalleled topographic accuracy owing to its excellent soft-tissue contrast and high spatial resolution. Secondly, the temperature sensitivity of especially designed MR sequences can be used to monitor the temperature elevation in the tumor and surrounding normal tissues (Batnar et al. 1997; Bleier et al. 1991; Delannoy et al. 1991; Dickinson et al. 1986; Jolese et al. 1988; Vogl et al. 1997a), thus increasing safety. On-line MR imaging during LITT therefore allows early detection of local complications and treatment effects, such as bleeding, hemorrhage, or necrosis. Thirdly, recovery time, length of hospital stay, and the risk of infection and other complications can be reduced compared with those attendant on conventional palliative surgery. Finally, successful implementation of such minimal invasive procedures would allow significantly reduced costs compared with those of surgical procedures. A further, indirect, advantage is the psychological effect that would arise from the avoidance of cosmetic deformities that can result from major reconstructive surgery.

Interstitial LITT is a minimally invasive technique for local tumor destruction within solid organs. Interventionally applied Nd:YAG laser applicators with a diffusor tip result in a well-defined area of coagulative necrosis. Thus, the laser can destroy tumor by direct heating, while greatly limiting damage to surrounding structures. Experimental work has shown that a well-defined area of coagulative necrosis is obtained around the fibre tip, with minimal damage to surrounding structures. Pilot clinical studies have demonstrated that this technique is practical for the palliation of hepatic tumors. The success of LITT is dependent on delivering the optical fibers to the target area, real-time monitoring of the effects of the treatment, and

T.J. Vogl, M.D., Virchow-Klinikum, Humboldt University of Berlin, Strahlenklinik und Poliklinik, Augustenburger Platz 1, D-13353 Berlin, Germany
M.G. Mack, M.D., Virchow-Klinikum, Humboldt University of Berlin, Strahlenklinik und Poliklinik, Augustenburger Platz, 1, D-13353 Berlin, Germany

subsequent evaluation of the extent of thermal damage. The key to achieving these objectives is the selection of imaging methods. The magnetic resonance (MR) findings of LITT in the experimental setting have been described, but the clinical role of MRI during and after LITT has been described only in a small series of patients (VOGL et al. 1995; CASTRO et al. 1992a,b).

## 3.2 Technique

### 3.2.1 Laser System and Application Set

Laser coagulation was performed using a Neodymium-YAG laser (Dornier MediLas 5060, Martin MY 30, Zeiss Opmilas) with a specially developed scattering dome light emitter. For an effective LITT procedure, a special diffusing applicator and an application kit for percutaneous treatment were developed and optimized for our purposes.

Laser light with a wavelength of 1046 nm was transmitted to tissue with a diffusing applicator. On a 400-μm silica fiber core a protective glass dome 1.4 mm in diameter was mounted, also frosted on its inner surface, which emittes laser light to an effective distance of 12–15 mm. Laser light of this wavelength penetrates deeply into biological tissue, where photon absorption and heat conduction lead to coagulative and hyperthermic effects. The tissue destruction may be immediate or delayed.

The laser application kit (SOMATEX, Berlin, Germany) consists of a cannulation needle with a tetragonally sharpened tip and the guidewire, a sheath system with mandrin (length 20 cm, 7 Ch), and a special protective catheter (length 43 cm, 4 Ch) which is closed at the distal end. The protective catheter prevents direct contact of the laser applicator with the patient and allows complete removal of the applicator even in the unlikely event of any damage to it. This increases patients' safety and simplifies the procedure. The catheter is transparent for laser radiation, and heat resistant (up to 400°C) (MACK et al. 1997). Marks on the sheath and the protective catheter allow exact positioning of both in the lesion. This system without water cooling can be used with a laser power of a maximum of 6 W over 20 min.

In addition, a water-cooled power laser application system (Fig. 3.1) was developed to increase the volume of coagulative necrosis. The maximum laser power for this system is 30 W over a period of 25 min. The internal cooling of the laser applicator prevents carbonization at the tip of the laser applicator (VOGL et al. 1997b).

Both systems are fully compatible with MR imaging systems. Magnetite markers on the laser applicator or specially designed localization fibers allow an easier visualizing and positioning procedure.

The laser itself is installed outside the examination unit, the light being transmitted via a 10-m-long optical fiber.

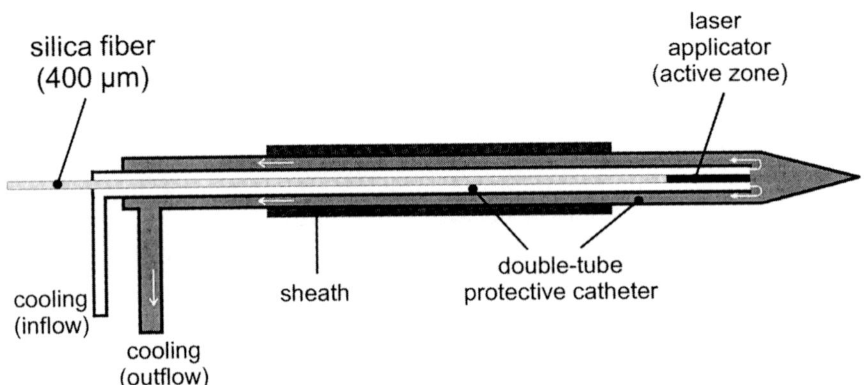


**Fig. 3.1.** The internally cooled power laser system

### 3.2.2 MR-guided LITT

Before LITT treatment all patients undergo a contrast-enhanced MRI study at least 2 days prior to the intervention, and informed consent is obtained from each. Immediately before the procedure and during the procedure patients receive pethidine (25–100 mg) intravenously. After localization of the tumor with CT, 20 ml of 1% lidocaine is infiltrated.

A 7-F catheter is then inserted via a percutaneous approach under CT guidance, and subsequently a special thermostable plastic catheter is introduced. In a third step a software program calculates the parameters for the laser treatment, such as energy and total application time. Once the patient is positioned at the MR table, the laser catheter is inserted into the guide catheter and the patient is asked to stay calm.

### 3.2.3 MR Thermometry

A variety of different sequences has been described and evaluated for MR thermometry (Batnar et al. 1997; Bleier et al. 1991; Delannoy et al. 1991; Vogl et al. 1997a; Castren Person et al. 1992; Castro et al. 1990; Cline et al. 1994; Matsumoto et al. 1992; Panych et al. 1992). However for our clinical applications the T1 method has proven the most adequate, because these sequences still work if there is slight patient movement during the treatment. Therefore, for our purposes we performed MR thermometry by the use of a turbo-FLASH (fast low-angle shot) sequence (TR/TE/TI = 7/3/400) and a thermo-FLASH-2D sequence (TR/TE/flip angle = 102/8/15), which is more sensitive for the detection of thermally induced changes in signal and morphology.

Before and after LITT treatment T1-weighted (SE, GE), and T2-weighted (SE) images are obtained at 1.5 T magnet. Of special importance is a dynamic Turbo-FLASH sequence protocol, which is started precontrast and with a short delay (6 s) post-contrast over a total duration of 180 s. Nonenhanced and contrast-enhanced imaging studies are also performed 1 week, 4 weeks, 3, and 6 months after therapy. Qualitative and quantitative parameters are evaluated, including size, morphology and contrast enhancement pattern at early and late follow-up.

## 3.3 Results

### 3.3.1 MR Thermometry

The in vitro study using muscle tissue demonstrated reproducible loss of signal intensity corresponding to increasing tissue temperatures. With an energy of 5 W and an application time of 12 min, the maximum diameter of the region with signal loss was 25 mm. This effect was best monitored using the thermo-turboFLASH sequence at repetition times (TR) of 300–400 ms, providing a nearly linear, inverse correlation between signal intensity and temperature. By comparison, this correlation was somewhat less linear with the FLASH-2D sequence; this sequence did, however, provide higher spatial resolution and clearer delineation of topographical structures.

### 3.3.2 In Vivo Study

In a prospective study, 13 patients underwent LITT of the head and neck under MRI guidance via an interventional subzygomatic approach for recurrent tumors of the nasopharynx and parapharyngeal space. Lesions of the floor of the mouth and the larynx were directly punctured. Pretherapeutic MR scans revealed tumor recurrence in all patients. All patients had already surgery and/or chemotherypy before the LITT intervention.

All patients but 1 tolerated the procedure well. One patient with a recurrent squamous cell carcinoma and infiltration of the sublingual gland developed pain 5 min after the laser was started. No long-term side effects related to treatment were observed. The 4-year MR control study of the patients with the pleomorphic adenoma showed no recurrent tumor (Fig. 3.2).

MR thermometry enabled on-line display of the hyperthermic effects, seen as progressively decreased signal from spaces surrounding tumor. Criteria for evaluating the success of treatment included clinical data, such as pain or other local symptoms, and pre- and posttherapeutic changes in signal and tumor morphology. We were able to induce coagulative necrosis in all patients (volume range: 3 $cm^3$ to 25 $cm^3$) and to reduce clinical symptoms in 9 patients.

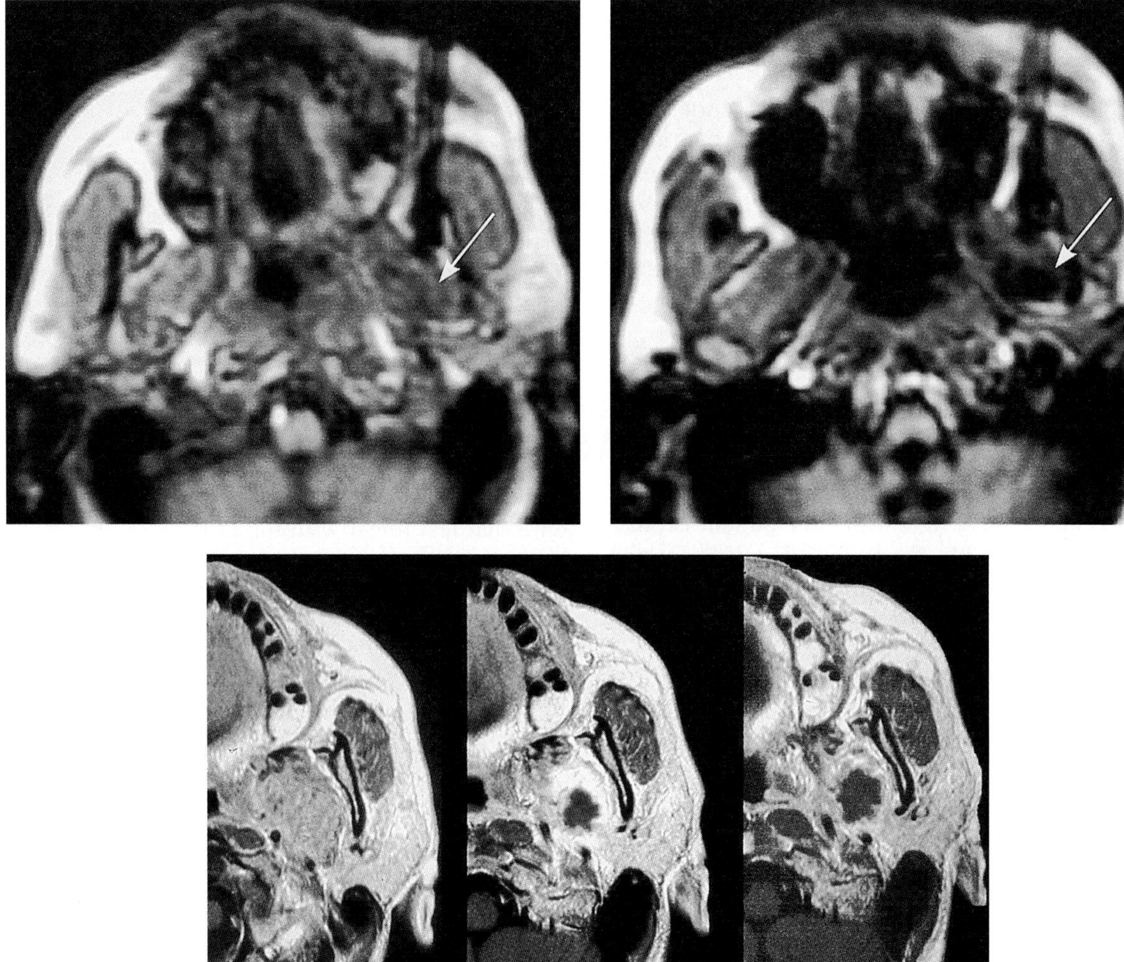


**Fig. 3.2 a–f.** Laser-induced thermotherapy (LITT) of pleomorphic adenoma. **a** Thermo-turboFLASH (fast low-angle shot) image (TR/TE/TI/flip angle = 7/3/400/8°) demonstrates recurrence (*arrow*) of the pleomorphic adenoma in the prestyloid compartment of the right parapharyngeal space, nearly isointense with muscle tissue. A subzygomatic approach was used for positioning of the laser applicator. Note the signal loss of the laser applicator due to the magnetite marker. The active zone (length 2 cm) of the laser applicator starts 1 cm in front of the end of the magnetite marker. **b** Thermo-turboFLASH image obtained 12 min after starting the laser shows a signal loss around the active zone of the laser applicator owing to an increase in tissue temperature caused by prolongation of T1 relaxation time. **c** *Left image* The contrast-enhanced (0.1 mmol/kg b.w. Gd-DTPA) T1-weighted spin echo (SE) image (TR/TE = 700/15) before LITT demonstrates the recurrent pleomorphic adenoma in the prestyloid compartment of the left parapharyngeal space with strong contrast-enhancement, displacing the internal carotid artery on the left side posteriorly. *Middle image* The contrast-enhanced image 2 days after LITT with 5.8 W over 20 min demonstrates the induced coagulative necrosis with strong enhancement in the border of the lesion, most probably representing postinterventional reactive changes. *Right image* The contrast-enhanced image 1 week after LITT shows decreasing postinterventional reactive changes and an increase in volume of coagulative necrosis obtained. **d** *Left image* The contrast-enhanced (0.1 mmol/kg b.w. Gd-DTPA) T1-weighted SE image (TR/TE = 700/15) 4 weeks after LITT demonstrates a further decrease in the reactive changes in the border of the treated recurrent tumor. However, in the anterior portion of the tumor pathologic contrast enhancement could still be visualized. Therefore, a second LITT treatment was performed to treat this part of the recurrent tumor also. *Middle image* The contrast-enhanced image 3 months after LITT demonstrates the coagulative necrosis induced, with some residual reactive changes in the border of the lesion. *Right image* The contrastenhanced image 2 years after LITT shows decreasing postinterventional reactive changes. **e** The plain T1-weighted SE-image (TR/TE = 700/15) obtained 4 years after laser treatment demonstrates mainly residual scar tissue in the prestyloid compartment of the left parapharyngeal space. **f** The contrast-enhanced (0.1 mmol/kg b.w. Gd-DTPA) T1-weighted SE-image (TR/TE = 700/15) no longer demonstrates any pathologic contrast enhancement in the prestyloid compartment of the left parapharyngeal space

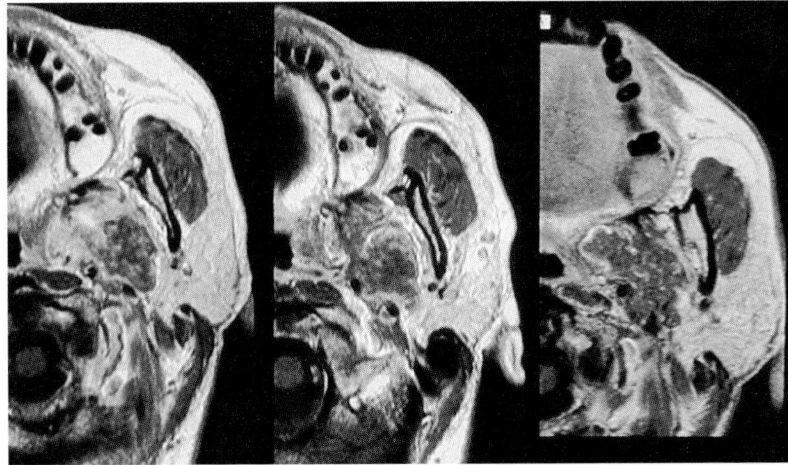


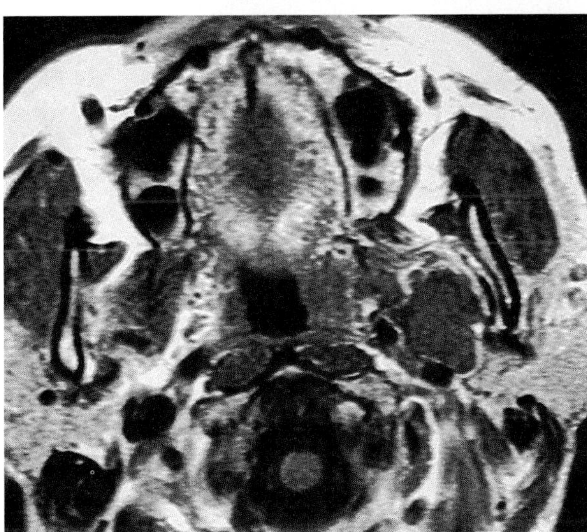


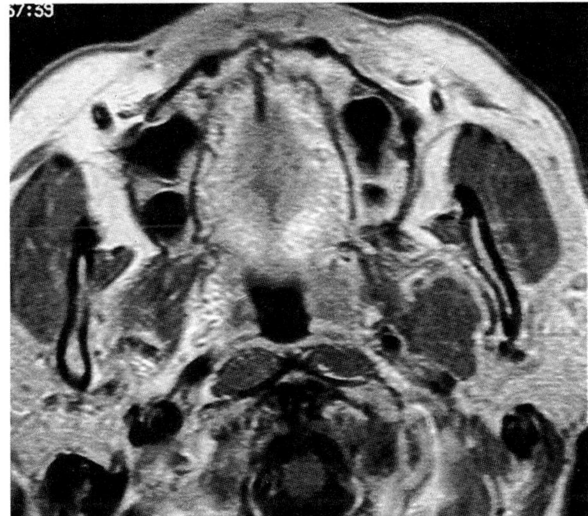


**Fig. 3.2.** *Continued*

## 3.4 Conclusion

MR-guided LITT allows accurate on-line thermometry during the interventional procedure. Dynamic gadolinium-enhanced MRI is suitable for early and late follow-up studies on lesions treated with LITT. Follow-up studies indicate that the laser-induced effects lead to reliable palliation in recurrent head and neck tumors.

## References


Batnar R, Steiner P, Erhart P, Debatin J, von Schulthess GK (1997) Absolute temperature quantification in near real-time with an open 0.5 Tesla interventional MR-scanner. Proc Int Soc Magn Reson Med 3:1957

Bleier AR, Jolesz FA, Cohen MS et al (1991) Real-time magnetic resonance imaging of laser heat deposition in tissue. Magn Reson Med 21:132–137

Castren Persons M, Lipasti J, Puolakkainen P, Schroder T (1992) Laser-induced hyperthermia: comparison of two different methods. Lasers Surg Med 12:665–668

Castro DJ, Saxton RE, Layfield LJ et al (1990) Interstitial laser phototherapy assisted by magnetic resonance imaging: a new technique for monitoring laser-tissue interaction. Laryngoscope 100:541–547

Castro DJ, Lufkin RB, Saxton RE et al (1992a) Metastatic head and neck malignancy treated using MRI guided interstitial laser phototherapy: an initial case report. Laryngoscope 102:26–32

Castro DJ, Saxton RE, Lufkin RB (1992b) Interstitial photoablative laser therapy guided by magnetic resonance imaging for the treatment of deep tumors. Semin Surg Oncol 8:233–241

Cline HE, Hynynen K, Hardy CJ, Watkins RD, Schenck JF, Jolesz FA (1994) MR temperature mapping of focused ultrasound surgery. Magn Reson Med 31: 628–636

Delannoy J, Chen CN, Turner R, Levin RL, Le Bihan D (1991) Noninvasive temperature imaging using diffusion MRI. Magn Reson Med 19:333–339

Dickinson RJ, Hall AS, Hind AJ, Young IR (1986) Measurement of changes in tissue temperature using MR imaging. J Comput Assist Tomogr 10:468–472

Jolesz FA, Bleier AR, Jakab P, Ruenzel PW, Huttl K, Jako GJ (1988) MR imaging of laser-tissue interactions. Radiology 168:249–253

Mack MG, Vogl TJ, Roggan A et al (1997) Design of a percutaneous application set for MR-controlled laser induced thermotherapy. ISMRM abstracts, 1951

Matsumoto R, Oshio K, Jolesz FA (1992) Monitoring of laser and freezing-induced ablation in the liver with T1-weighted MR imaging. J Magn Reson Imaging 2:555–562

Panych LP, Hrovat MI, Bleier AR, Jolesz FA (1992) Effects related to temperature changes during MR imaging. J Magn Reson Imaging 2:69–74

Vogl TJ, Mack MG, Muller P et al (1995) Recurrent nasopharyngeal tumors: preliminary clinical results with interven-tional MR imaging controlled laser-induced thermotherapy. Radiology 196:725–733

Vogl TJ, Mack MG, Hirsch HH et al (1997a) In-vitro evaluation of MR-thermometry for laser-induced thermotherapy. Fortschr Rontgenstr 167:638–644

Vogl TJ, Mack MG, Staub R, Roggan A, Knappe V, Felix R (1997b) Internally cooled laser applicator system for MR-guided laser induced thermotherapy. Radiology 205(P):177

# 4 Magnetic Resonance Spectroscopy of the Extracranial Head and Neck

S.K. Mukherji, V. Chong, M. Castillo

**Contents**



## 4.1 Introduction

The majority of clinical applications for MR spectroscopy (MRS) have centered on the evaluation of intracranial disease processes. Recent investigations have been focused on the use of MRS for evaluating diseases of the extracranial head and neck (Mukherji et al. 1996, 1997, 1998; Schiro et al. 1998; Mafee et al. 1989). This chapter will summarize the recent investigations that have been performed to evaluate the MRS findings in a variety of pathologic processes involving the upper aerodigestive tract. We will also comment on the potential clinical role of MRS in the extracranial head and neck. The primary focus will be on 1dimensional (1D) 1H-MRS; however, the results of P-31 MRS and two-dimensional correlated spectroscopy analysis will also be presented when available.

S.K. Mukherji, MD, Departments of Radiology and Surgery, The School of Medicine, and Department of Diagnostic Sciences, The School of Dentistry, University of North Carolina at Chapel Hill, Chapel Hill, NC 27599-7510, USA
V. Chong, MD, Department of Diagnostic Radiology, Singapore General Hospital, Outsam Road, Singapore
M. Castillo, MD, Department of Radiology, The School of Medicine, University of North Carolina at Chapel Hill, Chapel Hill, NC 27599-7510, USA

## 4.2 Imaging Strategies

The upper aerodigestive tract is an inherently difficult area for performance of MRS. In order to obtain highly resolved spectra, a very homogeneous magnetic field is required in the area to be examined (i.e. $\leq$ 0.1 parts per million deviation in the magnetic field). Numerous structural interfaces exist in this region that result in large magnetic field inhomogeneities. In many cases, these large field inhomogeneities cannot be corrected by the use of magnetic field shim. Susceptibility artifact from the paranasal sinuses and pharyngeal airway often prohibits analysis of low-volume tumors located adjacent to these structures. Susceptibility artifact from bone prevents spectral analysis of small to moderate size tumors that directly abut on the skull base or mandible. Pulsations from the carotid artery result in rhythmical field inhomogeneities and may prevent spectral analysis of lesions that involve the poststyloid parapharyngeal space (Mukherji et al. 1998).

Motion artifact is much more problematic in the upper aerodigestive tract than in the brain or extremities. Normal respiration usually will not interfere with primary parapharyngeal, nasopharyngeal, tonsillar, or masticator space masses. However, masses that arise in the visceral space and partially obstruct the airway often cause dyspnea. The resultant increase in respiratory motion will prevent adequate shimming prior to spectral analysis. Thus, the role of 1H-MRS in evaluating advanced laryngeal or hypopharyngeal carcinomas is very limited, especially if the patient is tracheostomy dependent (Mukherji et al. 1998).

Fat contamination of proton spectra is often a major problem when 1D 1H-MRS is performed in the extracranial head and neck. The fat planes surrounding the various muscle groups are very helpful in identifying deep extension of tumor on CT or noncontrast T1-weighted MR imaging. However, these fat planes can result in contamination of proton spectra by a dominant lipid peak that prevents identification of the choline or creatine peak (Mukherji et al. 1998). When lesions that abut on fat are evaluated, every attempt should be made to center the voxel directly over the lesion. It is especially important in these cases to minimize the voxel size without excessively increasing the acquisition time. Our experience has shown that, despite proper placement of the acquisition voxel over a malignant tumor, the intrinsically high fat content of the tongue and tonsil may result in fat contamination of the choline and creatine resonances (Mukherji et al. 1998).

Currently, a single-voxel technique is the method of choice for 1H-MRS. Two-dimensional chemical shift imaging in not suitable in this region owing to the impossibility of obtaining an adequate shim from the numerous susceptibility artifacts located in this region. One of the drawbacks of single volume 1D 1H-MRS is the relatively large voxel size necessary for *in vivo* studies. Although the voxel size for 1H-MRS is typically smaller than that required for P-31 MRS, it is still significantly larger than that required for high-field (11 T) spectroscopy of tissue specimens. At the present time, a 2x2x2 cm voxel (8 cc) is the smallest volume we can define using the PRESS sequence. However, head and neck studies of 1 $cm^3$ have been performed (Van Zijl et al. 1990).

In our experience, 1H-MRS can be performed for patients with non-obstructing lesions. Because voxel size and acquisition time tend to be competing factors, the study parameters should be individualized depending on the patient status and location of the lesion in question. A smaller voxel size with longer spectral acquisition time could be used in cooperative patients with a masticator space mass. However, a larger voxel size that allows a reduction in acquisition time may be a better strategy in patients with masses that extend into the airway and result in mild to moderate dyspnea. In the future, the best results will likely be obtained by using dedicated spectroscopy coils developed solely for use in the extracranial head and neck.

## 4.3 Pathology

### 4.3.1 Squamous Cell Carcinoma

Squamous cell carcinoma (SCCA) is the most common malignancy of the upper aerodigestive tract, with approximately 500,000 new cases diagnosed annually worldwide (Million 1994; American Cancer Society). This tumor accounts for more than 90% of all malignancies and can be found in all areas of the upper aerodigestive tract. SCCA has been analyzed with both P-31 MRS and 1H-MRS.

#### 4.3.1.1 P-31 MR Spectrosopy

Initial P-31 analysis of tumors has demonstrated increased concentrations of phosphomonoester (PME), phosphodiester (PDE), and inorganic phosphate (Pi) relative to normal muscle (Mukherji et al.1998; McKenna et al.1989; Fig. 4.1). These elevated resonances are believed to be composed, in part, of phosphocholine and/or phosphoserine. It is thought that the increase in phosphocholine levels may reflect increased membrane turnover and be analo-

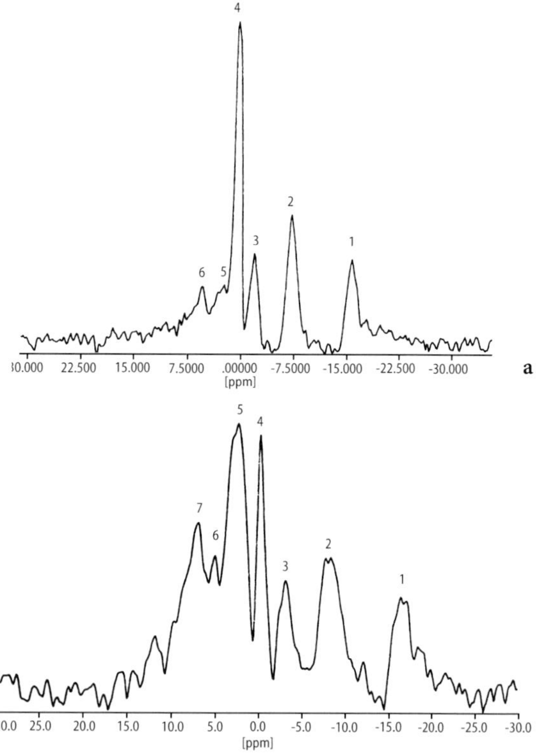


**Fig. 4.1 a, b.** P-31 spectra (frequency 25.93 MHz 1.5 T). (Reprinted with permission from Mukherji et al. 1998.) **A** Normal muscle. P-31 spectra of normal calf muscle demonstrate the following spectral peaks: *1* beta phosphate of ATP, *2* alpha phosphate group of ATP, *3* gamma phosphate group of ATP, *4* phosphocreatine, *5* phosphodiesters, *6* inorganic phosphate. **b** Tumor. P-31 spectra show elevation of spectral peaks of phosphodiester, inorganic phosphate, and phosphomonoester, and a reduction in the level of phosphocreatine compared with the P-31 spectra of normal muscle shown in Fig. 6A. *1* beta phosphate of ATP, *2* alpha phosphate group of ATP, *3* gamma phosphate group of ATP, *4* phosphocreatine, *5* phosphodiesters, *6* inorganic phosphate, *7* phosphomonoester

gous to the elevated choline levels that have been identified in various malignancies analyzed with $^{1}$H-MRS. The concentration of phosphocreatine (PCr) within tumor appears to be markedly reduced compared with that in normal muscle. The levels of the alpha, beta, and gamma – nucleoside phosphates (NTP) peaks are variable in SCCA and do not exhibit a definite trend. Areas of necrosis are associated with increased levels of Pi (VOGL et al. 1989; HENDRIK et al. 1990)

### 4.3.1.2 1H-MR Spectroscopy

Recent *in vitro* investigations have suggested that the most reliable 1H-MRS markers, which can distinguish SCCA from normal muscle of the extracranial head and neck, are the relative levels of choline (Cho) and creatine (Cr) (MUKHERJI et al. 1996,1997; Figs.4.2-4.4). Elevation of the Cho/Cr ratio appears

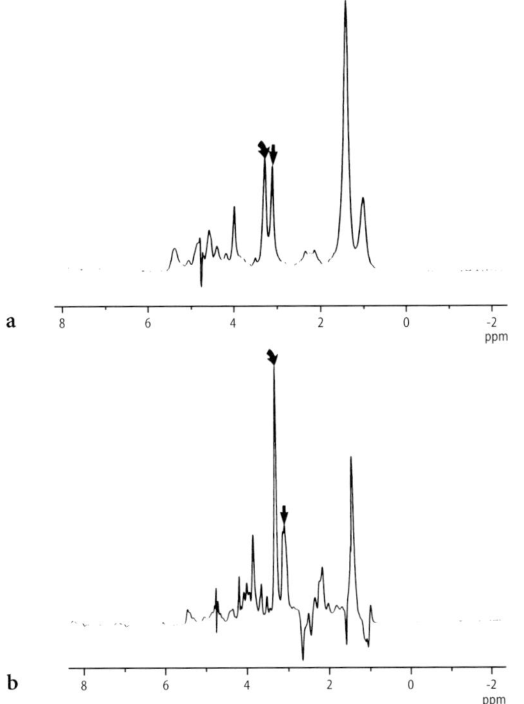


**Fig. 4.2 a, b.** In vitro 1H-MRS magnetic resonancespectroscopy: (TR, repetition time = 2000 ms / TE, time to echo = 136 ms). (Reprinted with permission from MUKHERJI et al. 1997.) **a** 1H MRS of normal tissue sample obtained from strap muscle shows similar areas of the choline (*curved arrow*) and creatine (*straight arrow*) resonances. The choline to creatine (Cho/Cr) ratio is 1.06. **b** 1H MRS of epiglottic SCCA tissue sample obtained from the same patient as illustrated in Fig. 4.1A shows elevation of the choline resonance (*curved arrow*) with respect of the creatine resonance (*straight arrow*). The Cho/Cr ratio is 1.92

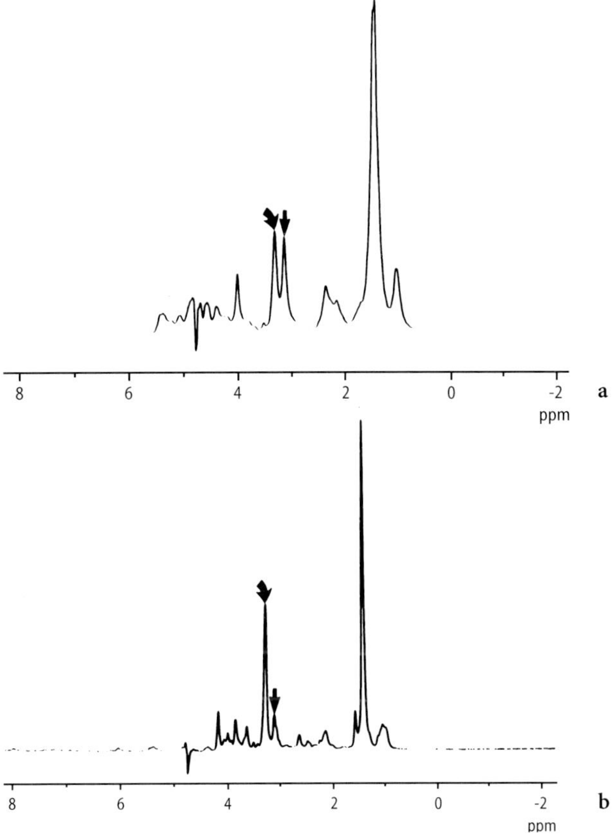


**Fig. 4.3a, b.** In vitro 1H-MRS (TR = 2000 ms / TE = 272 ms). (Reprinted with permission from MUKHERJI et al. 1997). **a** 1H MRS of the same normal tissue sample as shown in Fig. 4.2A, performed with a TE = 272 ms shows a similar appearance of the Cho (*curved arrow*) and Cr (straight arrow) resonances to that seen in Fig. 4.1A. The Cho/Cr ratio is 1.06. **b** 1H MRS of the same SCCA tissue sample as seen in Fig. 4.2B. Spectra demonstrate elevation of the Cho/Cr ratio obtained at TE = 272 ms (4.4) relative to the spectra obtained at TE = 136 msec (1.92). Also note the marked difference in Cho/Cr ratio when compared to the spectra of the normal tissue sample obtained from the same patient. (cf. Fig. 4.2A)

to be a consistent finding in SCCA and has also been identified in analyses of various SCCA cell cultures and SCCA-containing cervical metastatic lymph nodes (MUKHERJI et al. 1997; Figs. 4.5,4.6).

Choline, a nutrient that is present in most foods, is absorbed from the diet and is ubiquitous throughout the body, serving as a precursor of two important molecules: acetylcholine and phosphatidylcholine (MILLER 1991). Choline is believed to be an important constituent in the phospholipid metabolism of all cell membranes (KINOSHITA et al. 1994). The Cho molecule is transported intracellularly by a low-affinity system with its mechanism coupled to the synthesis of phosphatidylcholine (THOMPSON 1973). Once intracellular, Cho is initially phosphorylated by

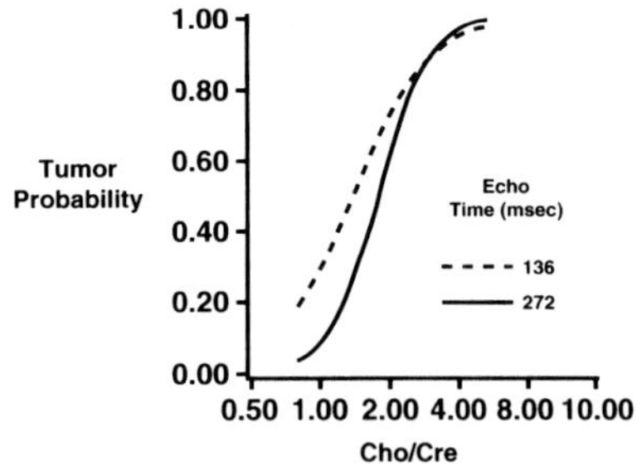


**Fig. 4.4.** Plot of the tumor probabilities based on the Cho/Cr ratio. The curves have an S-shaped configuration (ogive) and support the contention that the Cho/Cr ratio is an important metabolic marker that differentiates tumor and normal tissue. The greater slope of the 272 curve than to the 136 curve between the 20th and 80th percentiles suggests that longer TEs may provide better discrimination between tumor and normal tissue. (Reprinted with permission from MUKHERJI et al.1997)

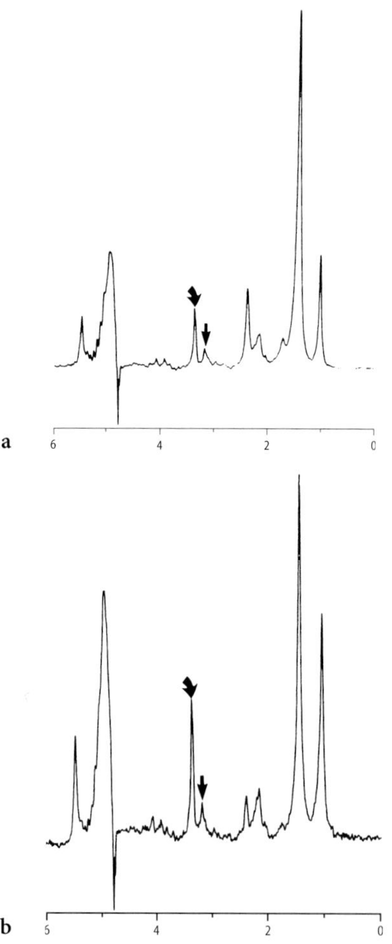


**Fig. 4.5a,b.** In Vitro [1]H-MRS of SCCA cell line (TR = 2000 ms/ TE = 136 ms). (Reprinted with permission from MUKHERJI et al.1997). **a** 1D 1H-MRS of SCCA cell culture shows elevation of Cho/Cr ratio which measures 4.5 (choline *curved arrow*, creatine *straight arrow*). **a** 1D 1H-MRS performed on the same sample as in **a** with a TE = 272 ms demonstrates elevation of the Cho/Cr ratio (5.7) relative to that seen at TE = 136 ms (see **a**). This increase in Cho/Cr ratio is similar to that demonstrated in the SCCA tissue samples (choline *curved arrow*, creatine *straight arrow*)

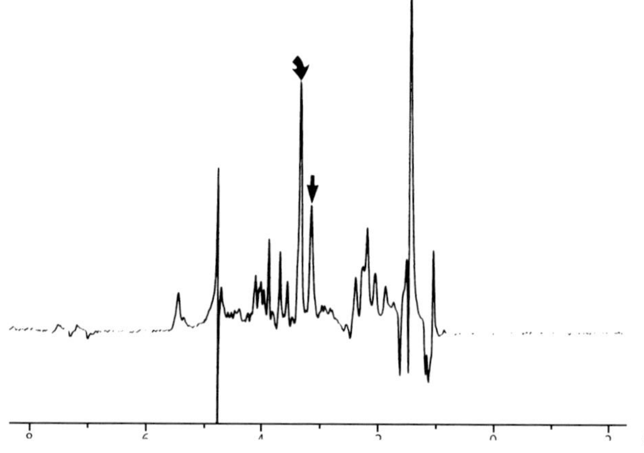


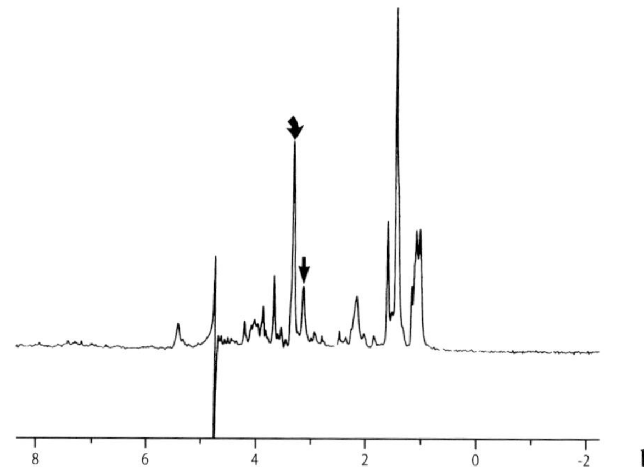


**Fig. 4.6a, b.** In Vitro 1D 1H-MRS of a metastatic cervical lymph node (TR = 2000 ms/TE = 136 ms). (Reprinted with permission from MUKHERJI et al.1997). **a** 1D 1H-MRS demonstrates elevation of Cho/Cr ratio, which is 1.98 (cholin *curved arrow*, creatine *straight arrow*). **b** 1D 1H-MRS performed on the same sample as shown in **a** demonstrates elevation of the Cho/Cr ratio (3.36) relative to that seen at TE = 136 ms. The progressive increase in Cho/Cr ratio is similar to that was previously illustrated in SCCA tissue samples and SCCA cell culture. (Cho *curved arrow*, Cr *straight arrow*)

Cho phosphotransferase to form phosphocholine. This latter molecule is the precursor of phosphatidylcholine, which is formed by the Kennedy pathway (WURTMAN 1979).

The n-methyl [$^{+}N(CH_3)_3$] group of Cho and Cho-based metabolites is detected at 3.2 ppm (MOUNTFORD et al.1984a). The total Cho resonance peak is believed to be composed of Cho, phosphocholine, phosphatidylcholine, and glycerophosphocholine. Elevation of this peak is not specific for SCCA and has been demonstrated in several tumors. Increased levels of Cho are thought to be related to increased cellular membrane phospholipid biosynthesis and raised Cho is, therefore, felt to be an active marker for cellular proliferation (LEAN et al. 1992; RUIZ-CABELLO and COHEN 1992; NEGENDAK et al. 1992; MOUNTFORD et al. 1993; KUESEL et al. 1990; DE CESTAINES et al. 1993).

Creatine (Cr) plays a part in the maintenance of energy metabolism. It may be obtained from the diet or synthesized *de novo* within the liver, kidneys, and pancreas by precursor molecules, which include arginine, glycine, and s-adenosylmethionine (Miller 1991; DE CESTAINES et al. 1993). Cr is converted to phosphocreatine by the enzyme creatine kinase. Phosphocreatine acts as a store for high-energy phosphates in the cytosol of muscles and neurons and is also believed to buffer cellular adenosine triphosphate and adenosine diphosphate (MILLER 1991; KINOSHITA et al.1994). Because phosphocreatine is a high-energy phosphate compound, it has been postulated that it may help sustain levels of adenosine triphosphate in energy-demanding tissues such as actively proliferating tumors. The Cr resonance observed at 3.02 ppm is felt to be comprised of both phosphocreatine and Cr (ROSS 1992). Currently, exact concentrations of total Cr, as measured by 1H-MRS in normal and diseased tissue (i.e. tumor or inflammation), and its clinical significance are unknown (MILLER 1991; KINOSHITA et al. 1994)

These *in vitro* findings have been demonstrated in *in vivo* studies performed in patients with SCCA of the extracranial head and neck. 1H-MRS analysis of SCCA performed at 1.5 T has demonstrated significant elevation of the Cho/Cr ratio in patients with tumors compared with normal tongue muscle. The spectrum for normal tongue muscle is dominated by a broad lipid peak centered at 1.3–0.9 ppm (Mukherji et al. 1997). The Cho and Cr peaks are typically not detected in *in vivo* normal muscle by the single-voxel technique (MUKHERJI et al. 1997,1998).

Elevation of the Cho/Cr ratio has also been demonstrated in a variety of other malignant neoplasms, including various brain tumors, gynecological tumors, and lymphomas (GILL et al. 1990; DELIKATNY et al. 1993; NEGENDAK et al. 1996; Wang et al.1995; CASTILLO et al. 1996). These findings suggest that the Cho/Cr ratio is a ubiquitous 1H-MRS tumor marker that can be used to clearly identify the presence of a variety of tumors. It should be emphasized that the Cho/Cr ratio is nonspecific and cannot distinguish between tumors; nor can it differentiate between grades of squamous cell carcinoma or metastatic potential. However, this ratio may be used as a spectral tumor marker in an attempt to identify a malignancy or to differentiate recurrent tumor from nonmalignant posttreatment changes in the extracranial head and neck using 1H-MRS.

### 4.3.1.3 Clinical Applications

The clinical applications of MRS are currently under investigation. Initial results suggest there are spectroscopic markers that can identify malignant lesions and differentiate these from normal tissue. (Figs. 4.7, 4.8)

However, it is unlikely that MRS will be able to identify the specific histological type of a tumor. (Figs. 4.9–4.11)

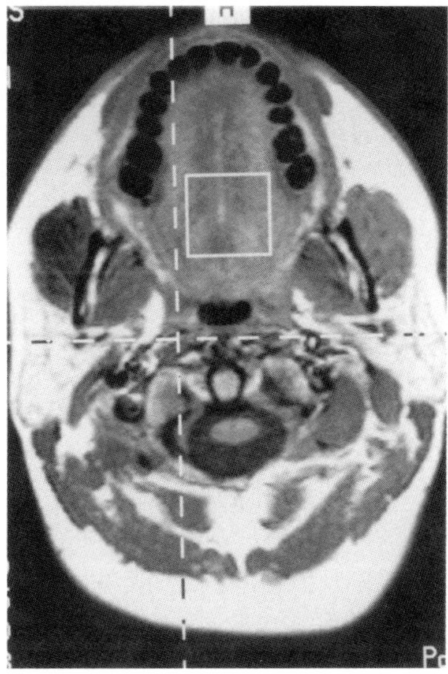

a

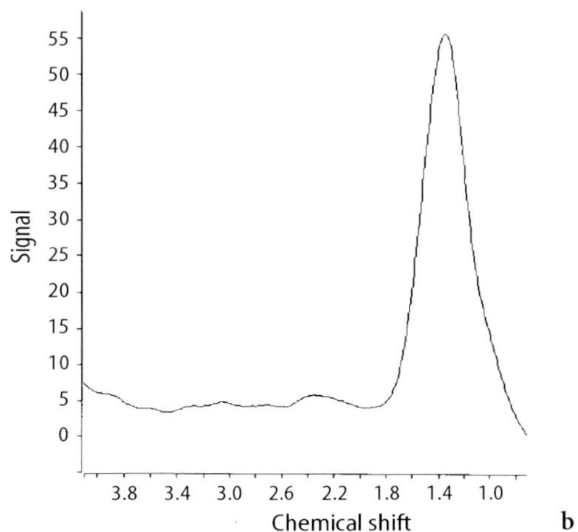


b

**Fig. 4.7a,b.** In Vivo (1.5 T) 1H-MRS of normal tongue base. (TR = 2000ms/ TE = 136 ms). (Reprinted with permission from MUKHERJI et al.1997). **a** Axial T1-weighted image (TR = 3500ms/ TE = 93 ms) illustrates the location of the voxel for **b** In vivo $^{1}$H-MRS demonstrates a very broad lipid peak without detectable levels of Cho or Cr

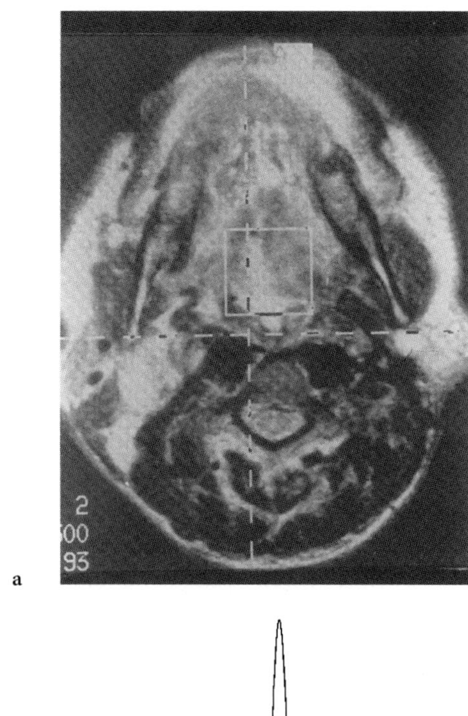


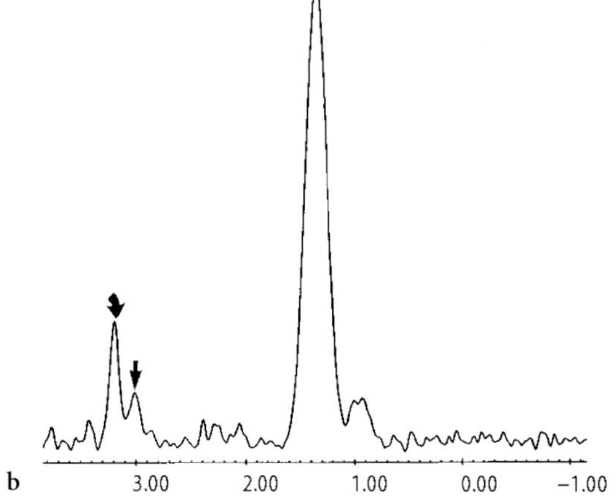


Fig. 4.8a, b. In Vivo (1.5 T) 1H-MRS of SCCA arising from the tongue base. (TR = 2000ms/ TE = 136 ms). (Reprinted with permission from MUKHERJI et al.1997). **a** Axial T2-weighted image (TR = 3500ms/TE = 93 ms) shows location of the voxel for **b**. **b** In vivo 1H-MRS demonstrates elevation of the Cho peak (*curved arrow*) relative to the Cr peak (*straight arrow*). The Cho/Cr ratio was 3.33

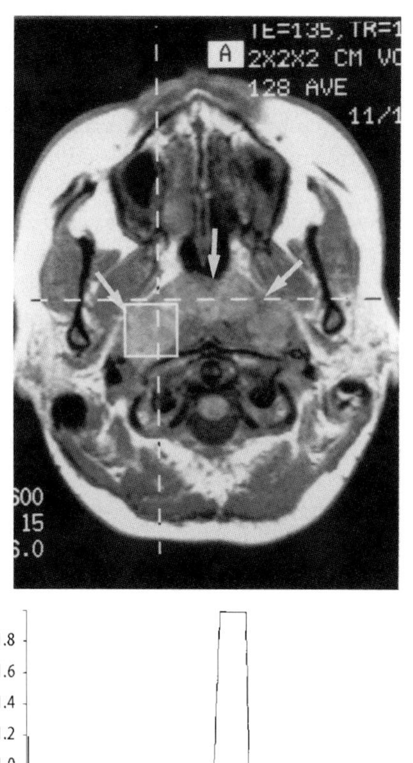


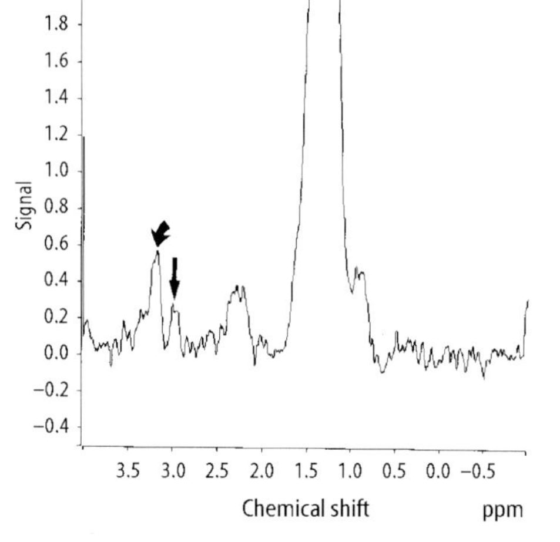


Fig. 4.9a, b. In Vivo (1.5 T) $^{1}$H-MRS of nasopharyngeal carcinoma. (TR = 2000ms/TE = 136 ms). **a** Axial non contrast T1-weighted image demonstrates a nasopharyngeal carcinoma (*arrows*). The voxel demonstrates the location of the acquired spectra. **b** In vivo 1H-MRS demonstrates elevation of the Cho peak (*curved arrow*) relative to the Cr peak (*straight arrow*), similar to that identified in the SCCA of the tongue base (cf. Fig. 4.8B)

Our *in vitro* and *in vivo* investigations have shown that elevation of the Cho/Cr ratio can be seen in a variety of benign neoplasms, including glomus tumors, pleomorphic adenomas, vagal schwannomas, inverting papillomas, and inflammatory polyps (MUKHERJI et al. 1988; Figs.4.12–4.14). These results also suggest that MRS may not be able to separate benign from malignant tumors on the basis of the Cho/Cr ratio alone. (Fig. 4.15) Thus, histological confirmation is necessary for all neoplasms of the upper aerodigestive tract, and initial treatment decisions should not be based on spectroscopic findings alone.

The importance of identifying and isolating consistent and reproducible MRS metabolic markers for malignancies of the upper aerodigestive tract rests not in the ability to initially diagnose a tumor, but in the potential for MRS to identify early recurrent tumors and treatment monitoring (GILL et al. 1990; NEGENDAK et al. 1996). The detection of recurrent

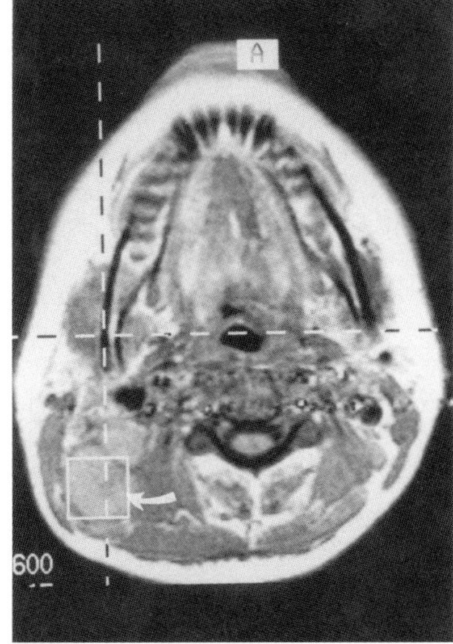


a

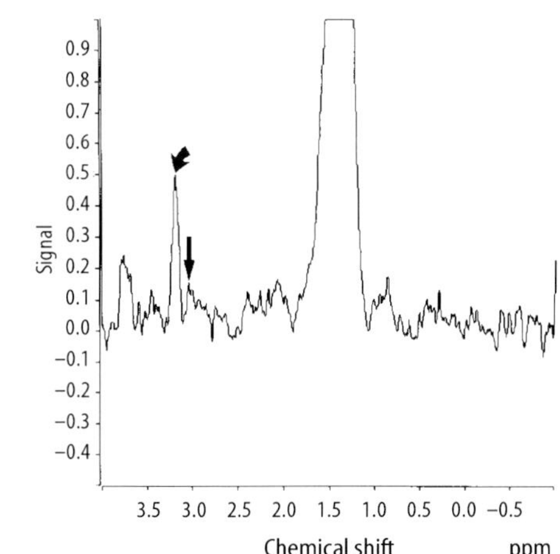


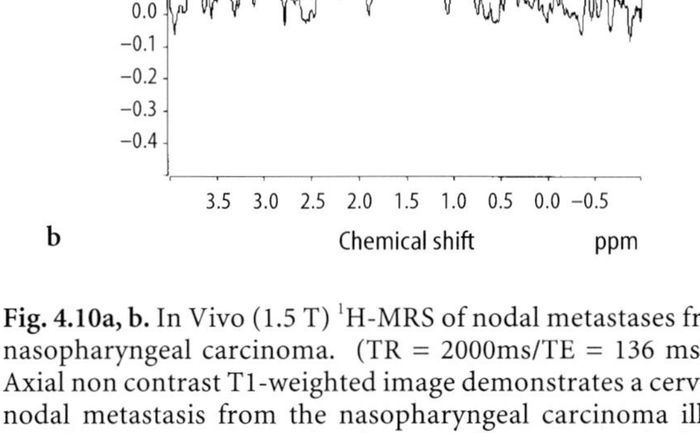


b

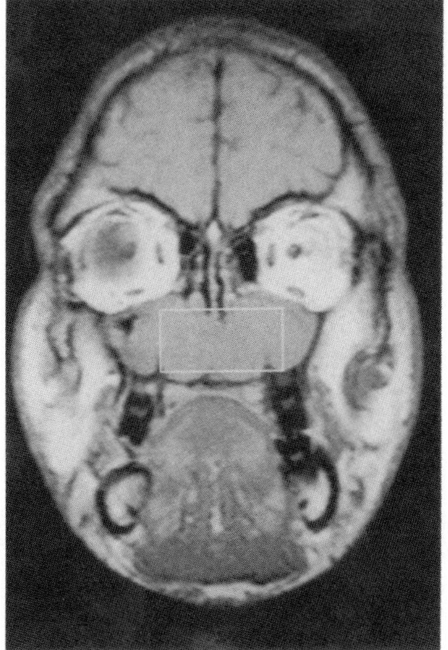

a

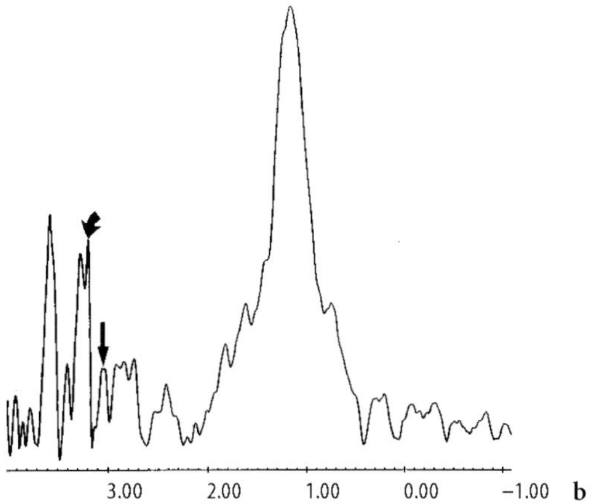


b

**Fig. 4.10a, b.** In Vivo (1.5 T) $^{1}$H-MRS of nodal metastases from nasopharyngeal carcinoma. (TR = 2000ms/TE = 136 ms). **a** Axial non contrast T1-weighted image demonstrates a cervical nodal metastasis from the nasopharyngeal carcinoma illustrated in Fig. 4.9A (*arrow*). The voxel demonstrates the location of the acquired spectra. **b** In vivo 1H-MRS demonstrates elevation of the Cho peak (*curved arrow*) compared to the Cr peak (*straight arrow*) similar to that seen in the primary tumor (cf. Fig. 4.9 B)

**Fig. 4.11a, b.** In Vivo (1.5 T) 1H-MRS of Osteosarcoma of the nasal cavity (TR = 2000ms/TE = 135 ms). (Reprinted with permission from MUKHERJI et al.1997). **a** Coronal T1-weighted image illustrates the location of voxel for b. **b** *In vivo* 1H-MRS shows elevation of the Cho peak (*curved arrow*) with respect to the Cr peak (*straight arrow*)

tumors by physical examination and imaging (CT and MRI) is difficult after treatment, as surgery and radiotherapy result in scarring and fibrosis of underlying tissues, which often preclude adequate physical and radiological examinations. Earlier detection of recurrent tumor after surgery has the potential to increase the likelihood of cure in those patients who fail initial treatment.

Currently, it is difficult to detect early recurrent tumors by physical examination or imaging studies alone. Radiation therapy (RT) causes significant erythema and induration within the treated area. These treatment-associated changes often prevent thorough endoscopic evaluation and reduce the ability to accurately detect persistent tumor that is unresponsive to therapy. This task is made even more difficult by the fact that persistent tumors are often situated below the mucosal surface and are not often directly visible to the examining physician. A technique that could detect chemical alterations and in-

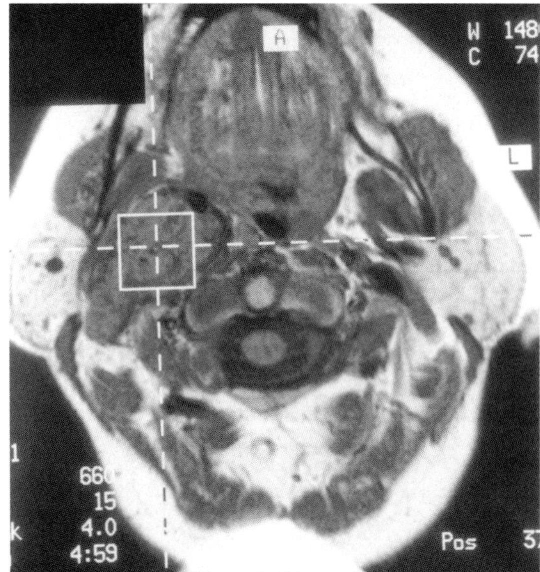


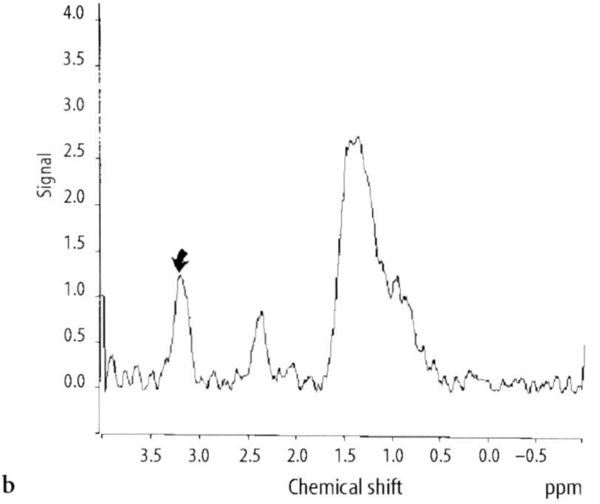


**Fig. 4.12.a, b.** In Vivo (1.5 T) 1H-MRS of glomus vagale tumor. (TR = 1600ms/TE = 135 ms). **a** Axial T1-weighted image illustrates the acquisition voxel overlying a glomus vagale tumor. **b** In vivo 1H-MRS shows elevation of the Cho peak (*curved arrow*) in this benign tumor

dicate whether a tumor is being successfully treated would be very beneficial and potentially life- saving.

Standard imaging modalities, including computed tomography (CT) and magnetic resonance (MR) imaging, can be used as adjuncts to clinical examination following treatment. However, the role of these modalities is restricted owing to the nonspecific radiographic appearance of tumors (Mancuso et al.1998). The posttreatment imaging findings differ with the type of treatment and the location and extent of the primary tumor. RT results in an inflammatory response (granulation tissue) in the tumor bed (Mukherji et al. 1994a,b; Manara 1966). In most sites, this inflammatory response progresses to end-stage fibrosis (scar) within 3–4 months after the completion of RT (Mukherji et al.1994a,b; Manara 1966). Unfortunately, this inflammatory response, which occurs prior to the formation of scar tissue, is indistinguishable from tumor by CT and MR imaging (Mancuso et al. 1998) .

Early results suggest that 1H-MRS may be used to differentiate recurrent tumor from posttreatment changes in patients with a prior malignancy of the upper aerodigestive tract that has been subjected previous treatment (Mukherji et al. 1998). Elevation of the Cho/Cr ratio detected in an indeterminate mass is indicative of recurrent tumor, whereas a low ratio is suggestive of posttreatment changes (Mukherji et al. 1998; Fig.4.16). Despite the encouraging early results of 1H-MRS, it is unlikely that microscopic foci of tumor can be completely excluded by $^{1}$H-MRS alone, regardless of the field strength. Thus, indeterminate masses without the characteristic spectral tumor markers still warrant close clinical and radiographic follow-up, regardless of the MR spectroscopic findings. It should be emphasized that, in any attempt to use 1H-MRS for differentiating recurrent tumor from posttreatment changes, the acquisition voxel should be completely centered over the area of interest to prevent spectral contamination from adjacent tissues.

MRS also may be used for tumor mapping prior to either surgical resection or radiation therapy (Castillo et al. 1996). Because it is dependent on the tissue's metabolic composition rather than anatomical information, MRS may be able to provide information on the extent of disease that cannot be determined by MR or CT (Kuesel et al.1990;Fig. 4.17). This potential future application will be dependent on future advances that permit analysis using smaller voxel sizes than are currently permissible.

One of the most promising clinical applications for MRS is noninvasive treatment monitoring in patients with SCCA of the upper aerodigestive tract who are treated nonsurgically. Accurate assessment of the response of the primary tumor to RT and/or chemotherapy is extremely important in patients treated nonsurgically, since the malignancy is treated *in situ* rather than resected. Early identification of an unresponsive malignancy may indicate the need for additional therapy or may necessitate surgical resection (salvage surgery).

Rapid decrease in tumor volume is a poor measure of ultimate local control. Rather, it is thought to measure the rapidity with which a tumor expresses radiation damage and the ability of the body to remove dead tissue, rather than the degree of tumor is destruction achieved. For this reason, serial CT dur-

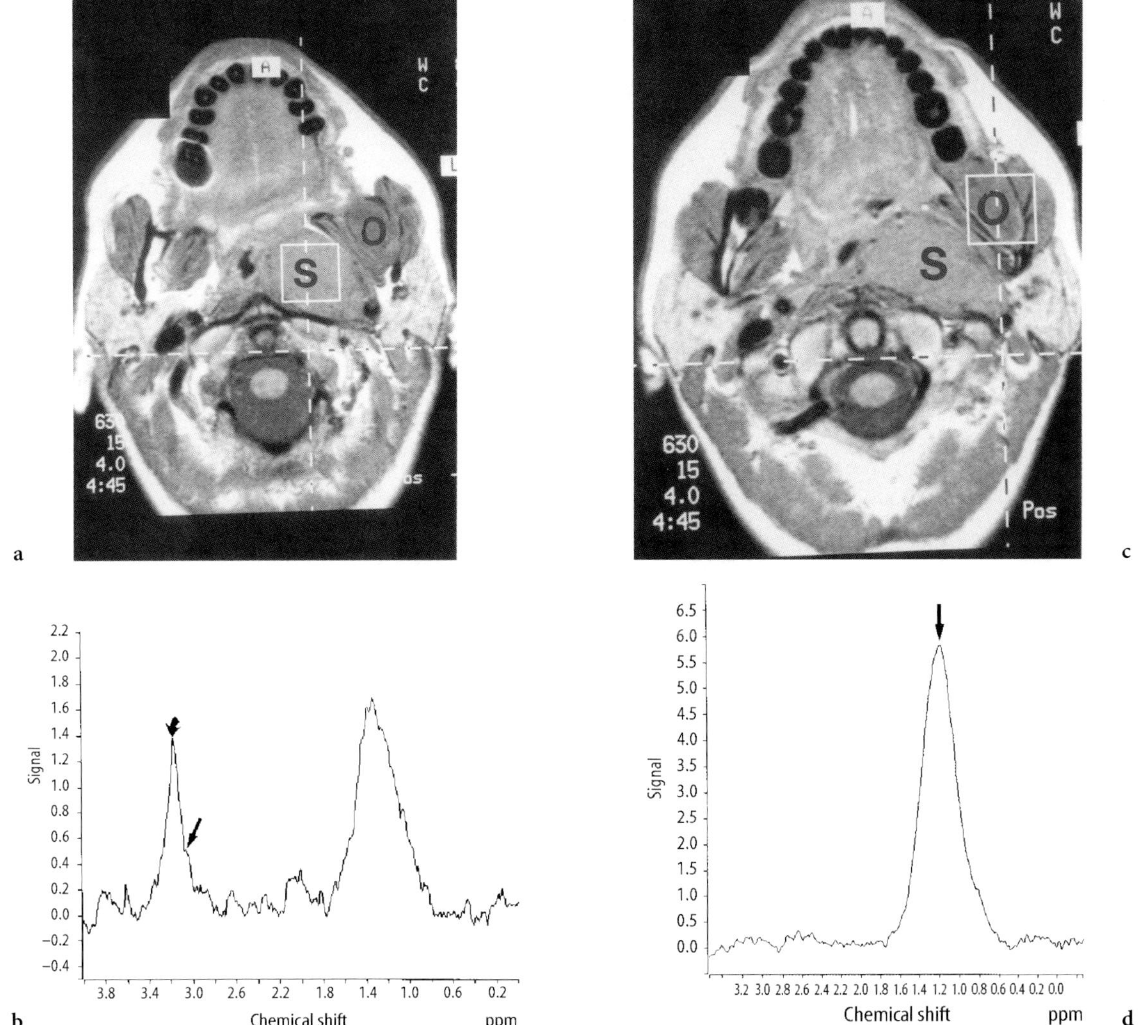


**Fig. 4.13a–d.** In Vivo (1.5 T) 1H-MRS of a Patient with a vagal schwannoma (*S*) and odontogenic keratocyst (*O*) (TR = 1600ms/ TE = 135 ms). **a** Axial non contrast T1-weighted image shows the location of the schwannoma and odontogenic keratocyst. The voxel position for the spectra illustrated in **b** is centered over the schwannoma. **b** 1H-MRS for the vagal schwannoma shows elevation of the Cho peak (*curved arrow*) in this benign tumor. The Cr peak cannot be completely separated from the Cho peak. The small peak denoted by the *straight arrow* probably denotes the Cr peak. **C** Axial non contrast T1-weighted image shows the location of the spectra illustrated in **d** centered over the odontogenic keratocyst. **d** In vivo 1H-MRS for the odontogenic keratocyst shows a broad fluid peak (*arrow*) without detectable Cho or Cr resonances. These findings are indicative of the cystic nature of these benign lesions

ing RT is not used as a measure of tumor response, and it is necessary to wait for at least 4 months after completion of therapy before such volume measurements are useful (Manara et al. 1966). MRS has the potential to be a much earlier indicator of tumor response, not by measuring volumetric changes but by measuring the internal chemistry of the treated tumor cells.

The noninvasive nature of MRS allows frequent interval studies to be performed both during and following treatment. The usefulness of 1H-MRS for prospective treatment monitoring for SCCA is currently being investigated. Based on the early results, reductions in specific resonances associated with tumors during treatment would be expected to indicate a tumor that is successfully responding to ongoing therapy. On the other hand, persistence or elevation of these spectroscopic tumor resonances would indicate a tumor that is not responding to treatment (Cazzaniga et al. 1994; Tzika et al. 1997).

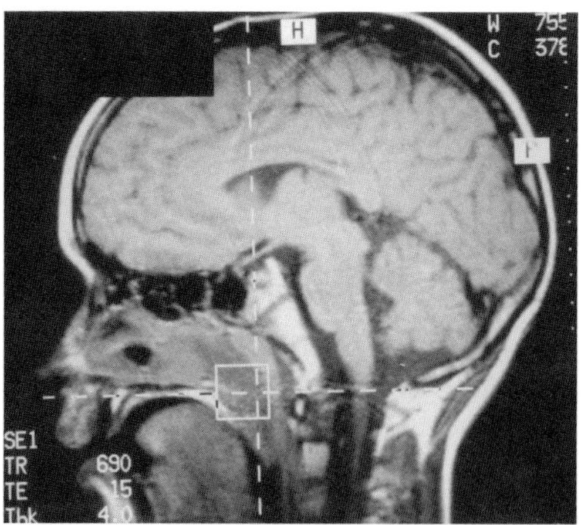


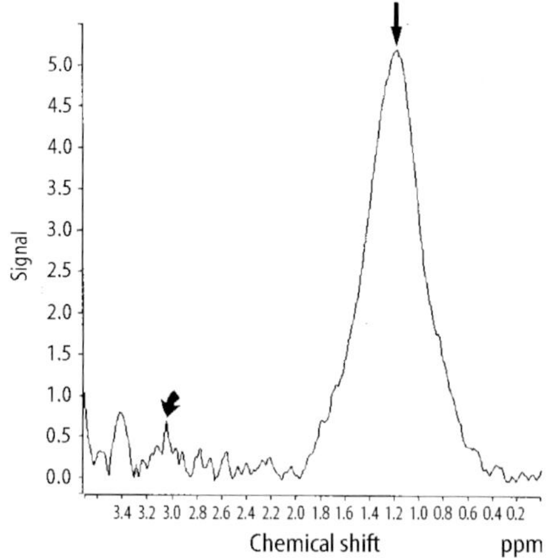


**Fig. 4.14a, b.** In Vivo (1.5 T) 1H-MRS of inflammatory polyp (TR = 2000ms/TE = 135 ms). **a** Sagittal non-contrast T1weighted image shows a mass situated within the nasopharynx. The voxel demonstrates the location of the spectra obtained in **b. b** 1H-MRS for the inflammatory polyp shows mild elevation of the Cho peak (*curved arrow*) and a broad fluid peak (*straight arrow*). The fluid peak is similar to that seen in the case of the odontogenic keratocyst, indicating a large fluid component. The elevation of the Cho peak indicates a proliferating solid component of this benign mass

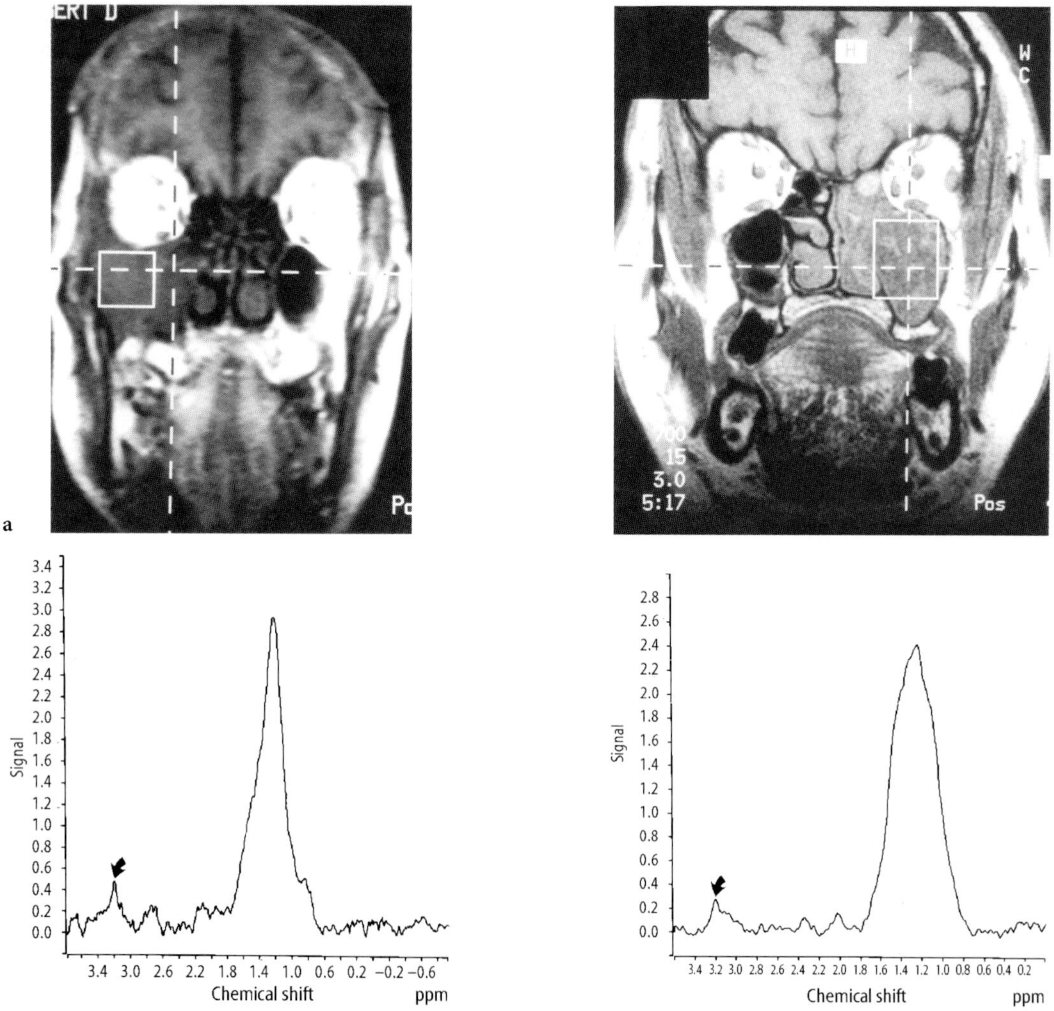

**Fig. 4.15a-d.** Example of the difficulty of using In vivo (1.5 T) 1H-MRS (TR = 2000ms/TE = 135 ms) to distinguish between benign and malignant tumors. **a** Coronal non contrast T1-weighted sequence demonstrates the location of the voxel in a patient with a right maxillary sinus mass. **b** 1H-MRS spectra obtained from **a** show mild elevation of the choline peak (*curved arrow*) in a patient with pathologically proven squamous cell carcinoma. **c** Coronal non contrast T1-weighted sequence demonstrates the location of the voxel in a patient with a left maxillary sinus mass. **d** 1H-MRS spectra obtained from **c** show mild elevation of the Cho peak (*curved arrow*) similar to that seen in **b**. Pathology revealed inverting papilloma.

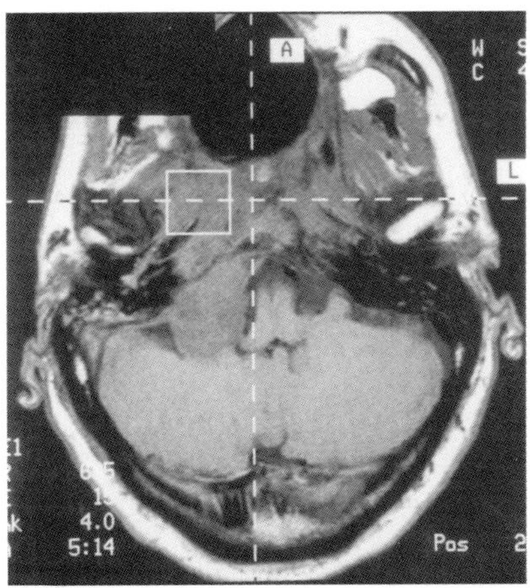


a

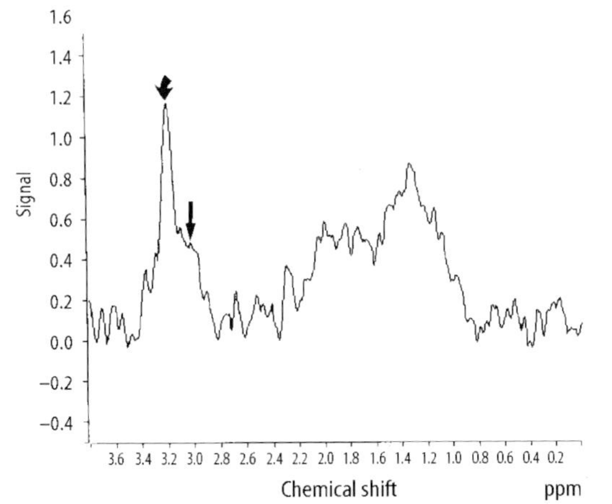


b

**Fig. 4.16a, b.** In Vivo (1.5 T) $^{1}$H-MRS of recurrent adenoid cystic carcinoma of the nasopharynx (TR = 1600ms/TE = 135 ms). (Reprinted with permission from MUKHERJI et al.1998). **a** Axial non contrast T1-weighted image obtained in a patient previously treated for adenoid cystic carcinoma illustrates location of the voxel for **b**. **b** In vivo 1H-MRS shows marked elevation of the Cho peak (*curved arrow*). The Cr peak cannot be completely separated from the Cho peak, but, is probably identified by the *straight arrow*

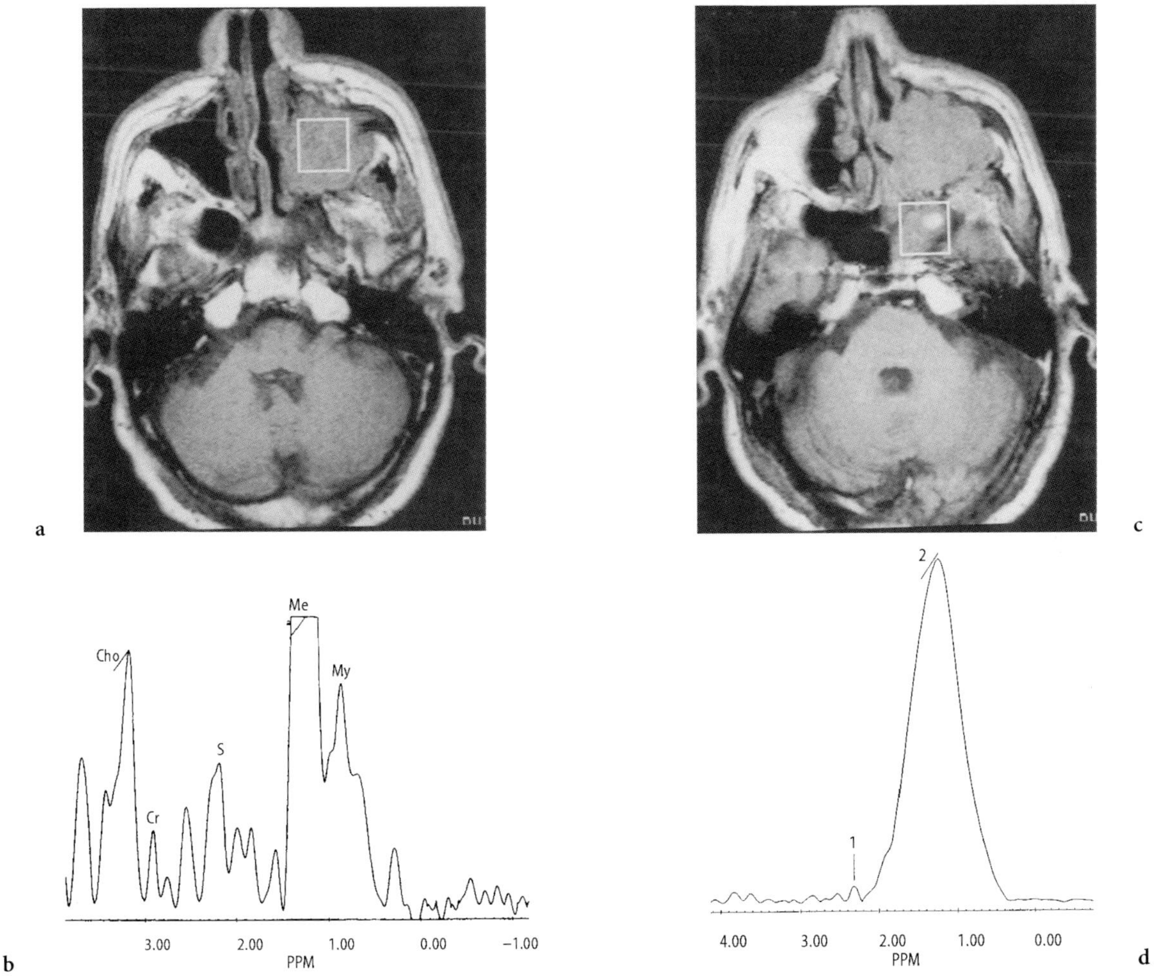

**Fig. 4.17a-d.** Tumor mapping of SCCA of the maxillary sinus. (Reprinted with permission from CASTILLO et al. 1996). **a** Axial T1-weighted MR shows the location of a voxel within a SCCA of the left maxillary sinus. **b**: $^{1}$H-MRS shows elevated Cho relative to Cr. Sialic acid (*S*), methylene groups (*Me*) and methyl groups (*My*), are found in membrane lipids of malignancies. **c** Axial T1-weighted MR shows the voxel encompassing the left sphenoid sinus. It was unclear whether the opacification of the sinus was secondary to postobstructive inflammation or to tumor invasion. **d** 1H-MRS from the sphenoid sinus shows no discernible Cho or Cr resonances. A small peak for sialic acid (*1*) is present. A large peak (*2*) at 1.3 ppm may be related to lipids in inflammatory tissues. At surgery, only inflammatory mucosal changes and retained secretions were found in this region

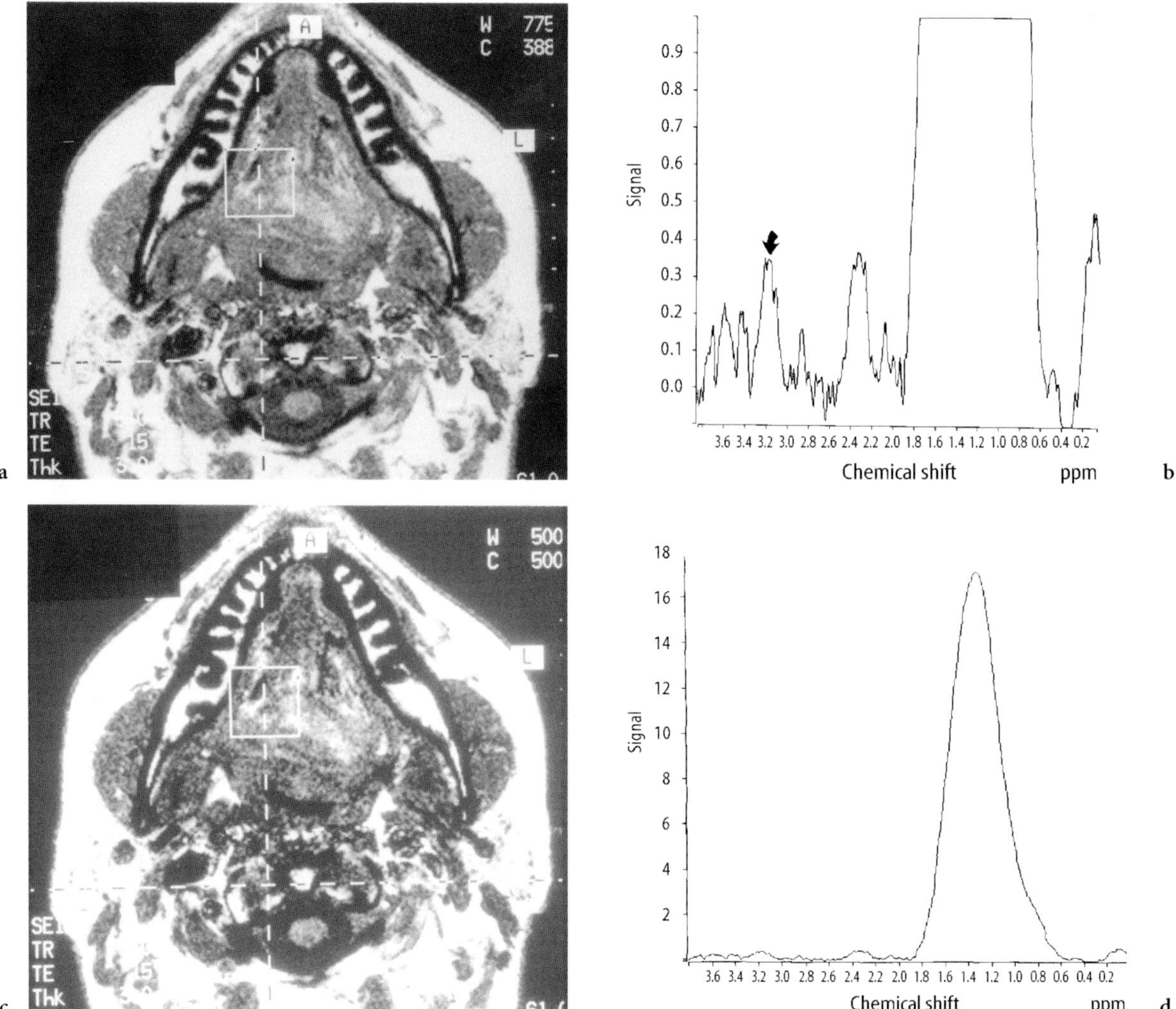


**Fig. 4.18a-d.** Prospective treatment monitoring of SCCA of the tongue base using 1H-MRS. **a** Axial non contrast T1-weighted MR demonstrates the voxel location in a patient with a right tongue base SCCA prior to initiation of combined radiation and chemotherapy. **b** Corresponding spectra prior to treatment show elevation of the Cho resonance (*curved arrow*). **c** Axial non contrast T1-weighted MR demonstrates the voxel location for 1H-MRS performed one week after completion of therapy. **d** Posttreatment proton spectroscopy shows reduction of the Cho and Cr peaks, which is suggestive of a successfully controlled tumor. This patient has no evidence of recurrent disease 2 years after completion of non surgical organ-conservating therapy.

Initial experience with P-31 MRS for treatment monitoring has been disappointing. Early results suggested that levels of PME were a sensitive indicator of tumor regression: progressively decreasing levels of PME were believed to be indicative of tumor regression (McKenna et al. 1989). However, subsequent investigators have demonstrated that the alterations in PME, Pi, and PDE are nonspecific, and that P-31 MRS cannot reliably predict tumor response to therapy, especially in advance of changes in tumor size (Karczmar et al. 1991).

The results obtained with 1H-MRS have been more encouraging. Recent investigations have shown that progressive reduction in Cho concentrations during treatment are indicative of tumor response (Bizzi et al. 1995; Fig. 4.18). Some investigators have suggested that alterations in 1H-MRS can be used to predict response prior to changes in tumor volume (Van Zijl et al. 1990; Bizzi et al. 1995). Persistence of an elevated Cho/Cr ratio suggests tumors that are not responding to treatment. (Fig. 4.19) There is no information currently available on the time interval following the initiation of treatment, when one would expect to see resolution of spectral markers in tumors that are being successfully treated. Large-scale prospective studies will need to be performed

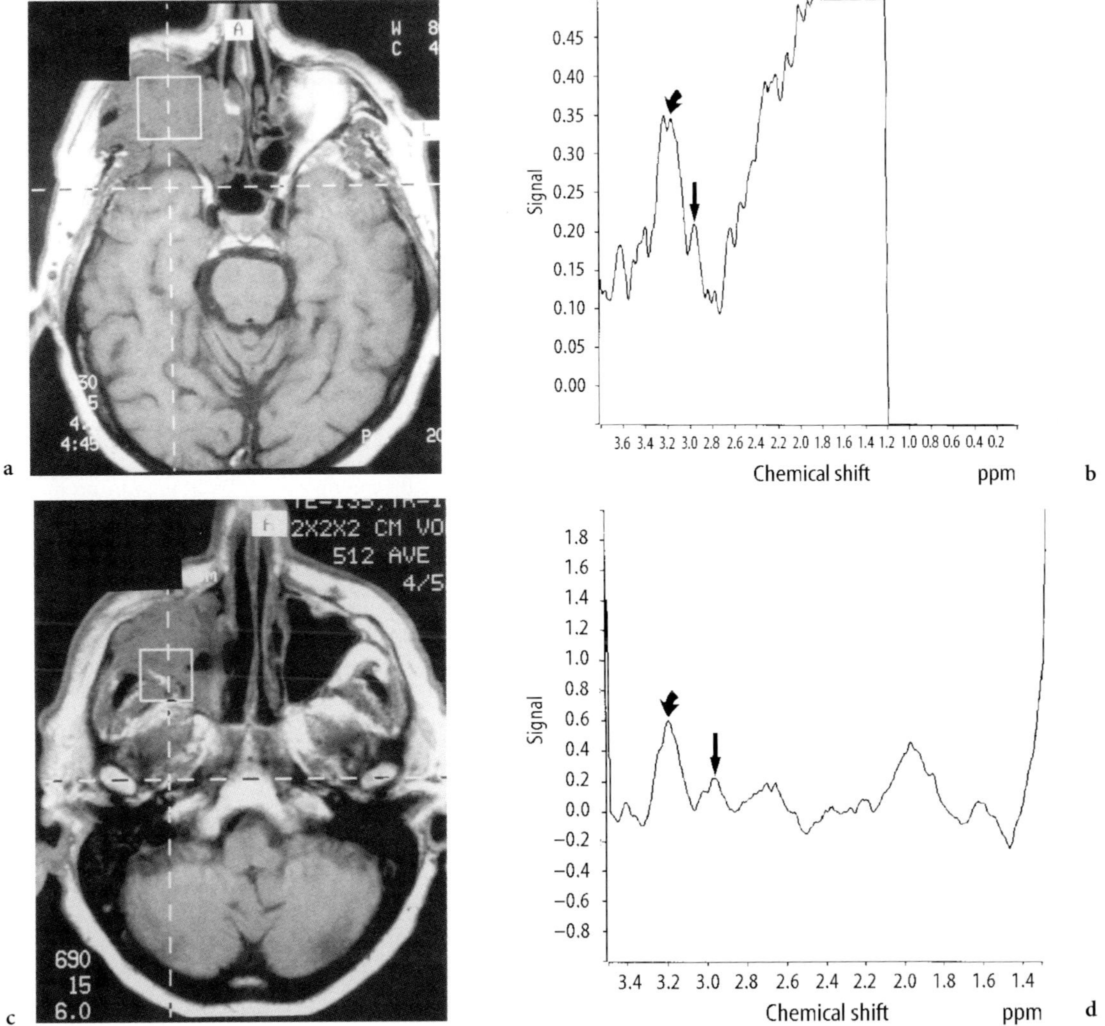


**Fig. 4.19a-d.** Prospective treatment monitoring of SCCA of the maxillary sinus using [1]H-MRS. (Reprinted with permission from MUKHERJI et al.1998). **a** Axial T1-weighted MR demonstrates the location of a voxel situated in a SCCA of the right maxillary sinus prior to initiation of radiation therapy. **b:** Corresponding spectra prior to treatment show marked elevation of the Cho resonance (*curved arrow*) relative to Cr (*straight arrow*). **c** Axial T1-weighted MR performed 4 weeks after initiation of RT demonstrates a large persistent soft tissue mass that has reduced in size compared with the pretreatment study. It is difficult to determine by MR whether this residual mass represents nonresponding tumor or postradiation treatment changes. The voxel indicates the area of acquisition. **d** Posttreatment proton spectroscopy shows persistent elevation of the Cho resonance (*curved arrow*) relative to Cr (*straight arrow*), indicative of residual nonresponding tumor. This patient underwent salvage medial maxillectomy, which confirmed the spectroscopic findings of residual tumor

in order to determine whether 1H-MRS can be reliably used for treatment monitoring in patients with malignancies of the extracranial head and neck.

### 4.3.2 Thyroid Neoplasms

Previous investigations have attempted to determine whether 1H-MRS can distinguish normal thyroid tissue from malignancies, and whether 1H-MRS can distinguish between malignant and benign thyroid nodules (JOHNSON et al. 1989; RUSSELL et al. 1994). These studies have suggested that the ratio between the methyl (0.9 ppm) and methylene (1.3 ppm) is significantly higher than that between normal thyroid tissue and benign thyroid nodules (JOHNSON et al. 1989). This increased ratio is believed to be due to an increase in the amount of low- or very- low-density lipoproteins in the plasma membranes of malignant processes (WILLIAMS et al. 1985). Because these lipoproteins are composed of more unsaturated fats

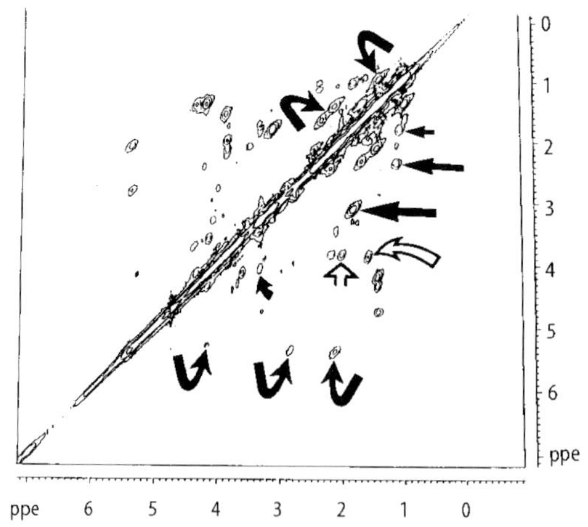


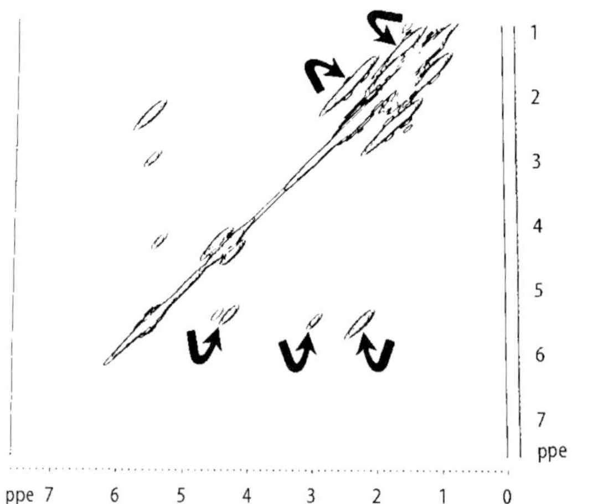


**Fig. 4.20a, b.** 2D Correlated spectroscopy (COSY) of tumor sample illustrates the multiple contours of the various metabolites that had a statistically greater likelihood of being detected in tumors than in normal tissues (**b**). These metabolites include alanine (*curved open arrow*), glutathione (*straight open arrow*), histidine (*curved solid small arrow*), isoleucine (*straight small solid arrow*), valine (*straight medium solid arrow*), and shared cross-peak for polyamine /lysine (*straight large solid arrow*). Note the absence of these metabolites in the 2D COSY spectra of the normal tissue sample (**b**). Note also the difference in the contours of the triglyceride resonances (*large curved solid arrows*). There was no significant difference regarding the presence or absence of the various triglycerides between tumors and normal tissues. However, the contours of the triglyceride peaks are noticeably different. These resonances appear elliptical in normal tissue (**b**: *large curved solid arrows*), whereas in tumor they are narrow and are less elliptical in shape owing decreased chemical shift dispersion (**a**). (Reprinted with permission from MUKHERJI et al.1997)

than lipoproteins in nonmalignant tissue, the number of methylene groups is decreased. The result is a relative increase in the methyl/methylene ratio in malignant tumors compared with normal tissues (JOHNSON et al. 1989).

1H-MRS analysis has demonstrated elevated Cho concentrations to be present in thyroid malignancies compared with normal tissue, benign adenomas, and fibrosis (SOMORJAI et al. 1994). However, a specific analysis attempting to determine whether the Cho/Cr ratio can separate benign from malignant processes has never been performed.(38) Recently, we have demonstrated elevation of the Cho/Cr ratio in a metastatic lymph node containing papillary thyroid carcinoma (unpublished results). These findings suggest that elevation of the Cho/Cr ratio may be able to separate a malignant tumor from normal thyroid tissue.

1H-MRS analysis has also demonstrated elevated Cho concentrations in the thyroid glands of patients with Graves' disease (JOHNSON et al. 1989). Because Cho is thought to be an active marker for cellular proliferation, the elevation of Cho corresponds to a higher rate of tissue cellular replication known to be present within the thyroid glands of patients with Graves' disease. Thus, it seems unlikely that the Cho/Cr ratio alone will be able to differentiate Graves' disease from thyroid carcinoma.

### 4.3.3 Other Neoplasms

The most common type of lymphoma to involve the extracranial head and neck is non-Hodgkin's lymphoma (NHL). The region of Waldeyer's ring is the most common site of NHL of the upper aerodigestive tract. The specific primary sites are the nasopharynx, the tonsil, and the lingual tonsillar tissue situated adjacent to the tongue base. NHL may also present as enlarged cervical lymph nodes. This presentation may be associated with a primary lesion in the oropharynx or nasopharynx, or a more generalized systemic process disease.

P-31 spectroscopy has demonstrated mild elevation of the concentrations of PME and NTP and markedly decreased concentrations of PCr relative to normal muscle. Unlike SCCA, there do not appear to be significant alterations in the concentrations of PDE and Pi compared with normal muscle (VOGL et al. 1989).

*In vitro* and *in vivo* 1D 1H-MRS of lymphoma have shown marked elevation of the Cho/Cr ratio in a pattern similar to that seen in previous studies of SCCA (MUKHERJI et al. 1997, 1998; BIZZI et al. 1995). *In vitro* (11 T) study suggests that the 1D 1H-MRS spectra for lymphoma may be more complex than those for SCCA; however, several of these peaks have not been assigned. Many of these resonances may not be detectable with spectra obtained on current 1.5 T clinical units. Clinical imaging on higher field strength units (3 T or greater) may provide better detection of these other resonances. Thus, it is conceivable that further characterization of these resonances may help distinguish lymphoma from other neoplasms.

On 1H-MRS, lipomas are dominated by a very broad lipid peak centered over 1.3 ppm (Mafee et al. 1989). The imaging findings of lipomas are characteristic on both CT and MR. Occasionally, the imaging appearances of liposarcomas may mimic those of lipomas, making it difficult to differentiate between these entities. It is unlikely that 1H-MRS will be able to distinguish lipomas from low-grade liposarcomas because the very broad lipid resonance may prevent separation of the Cho and Cr resonances. Elevation of the Cho/Cr would be expected in liposarcomas and not in lipomas. However, the broad lipid resonance from the fat would probably prevent adequate analysis of these important resonances.

Other malignant tumors that arise in the extracranial head and neck have demonstrated a similar spectroscopic profile to that seen in SCCA. 1H-MRS of adenoid cystic carcinoma (Fig. 4.16) and osteosarcomas (Fig. 4.11) shows elevation of the Cho/Cr ratio. P-31 MRS of chondrosarcomas and synovial cell sarcomas shows elevation of PME, Pi, and PDE in a manner similar to that described for SCCA (Vogl et al. 1989; Hendrix et al. 1990). 1H-MRS of choroidal melanoma has demonstrated a large resonance at 6.2 ppm, corresponding to melanin (Mafee et al. 1989).

By identifying specific resonances, MRS appears to be able to distinguish tumors of the extracranial head and neck from normal muscle. However, initial experience suggests that MRS may not be able to reliably differentiate benign from malignant tumors. P-31 MRS has shown elevated concentrations of PME, Pi, and PDE in benign tumors, including juvenile angiofibromas (Hendrix et al. 1990). Similarly, *in vivo* 1H-MRS studies have shown elevated Cho levels in paragangliomas, pleomorphic adenomas, schwannomas, inflammatory polyps, and benign inverting papillomas. (Figs. 4.12-4.15). This lack of specificity of MRS is based on the fact that the aforementioned resonances are indicative of cellular proliferation. Therefore, benign processes, which are actively growing, may also demonstrate increased levels of Cho on $^{1}$H-MRS.

### 4.3.4 Infections and Inflammatory Processes

Very little information is currently available on MRS analysis of infectious and inflammatory processes of the extracranial head and neck. $^{1}$H-MRS of benign mucosal thickening is characterized by a very large water peak without elevation of Cho or Cr (Castillo et al. 1996). P-31 MRS of tuberculosis has shown mild elevation of PME, Pi, and PDE (Vogl et al. 1989). Further investigations are needed in order to determine whether 1H-MRS can reliably differentiate infectious or inflammatory processes from malignant tumors.

## 4.4 Two-Dimensional Correlated Spectroscopy

One-dimensional proton magnetic resonance spectroscopy (NMRS) is a relatively sensitive technique that allows detection of numerous metabolites in a variety of tissue samples. However, the chemical shift range of proton spectra is relatively narrow, which leads to overlapping resonances. This overlap may mask important metabolites contained within a single spectral peak. The problem of overlapping resonances becomes more problematic at clinical field strengths (1.5 T) due to spectral broadening caused by lower field strengths and inherent susceptibility artifacts (Schiro et al. 1992; Behar and Ogino 1991).

Two-dimensional correlated spectroscopy (2D COSY) is a technique that can be used to separate the composite 1D spectral MR resonances into their individual resonances by generating a cross-peak in a second dimension. The result of the 2D COSY sequence is a two-dimensional plot that contains a series of cross peaks. These cross-peaks provide information on the presence of additional metabolites that are not visible on the one-dimensional spectrum (Schiro et al. 1998; Mountford et al. 1993; May et al. 1986; Cross et al. 1984). A summary of the assignments is given in Table 4.1. From the numerous metabolites listed in Table 4.1, one can see that 2D COSY provides a more robust technique for spectral analysis than is currently possible with one-dimensional techniques.

**Table 4.1.** Assignments of metabolites to cross-peaks by 2D correlated spectroscopy

| Metabolite | Crosspeak |
|---|---|
| Alanine | 1.49–3.79 |
| Glutathione | 2.21–3.81 |
| Histadine | 3.22–3.95 |
| Isoleucine | 0.97–2.12 |
| Polyamine/lysine | 1.72–3.05 |
| Valine | 1.03–2.34 |
| Choline | 3.50–4.07 |
| Phosphocholine | 3.61–4.25 |
| Glutamic acid | 2.21–2.62 |
| Glycerophosphocholine | 3.69–4.38 |
| Leucine | 0.97–1.78 |
| Fucose/threoni | 1.33–4.27 |
| Inositol | 3.28–3.64 |
| Taurine | 3.28–3.50 |
| Lactate | 1.33–4.12 |
| Triglyceride A | 0.90–1.33 |
| Triglyceride B | 1.33–2.08 |
| Triglyceride C | 2.02–5.38 |
| Triglyceride D | 2.84–5.38 |
| Triglyceride E | 1.33–1.62 |
| Triglyceride F | 1.60–2.30 |
| Triglyceride G1 | 4.12–5.26 |
| Triglyceride G2 | 4.26–5.26 |
| Triglyceride G' | 4.09–4.29 |

Recent *in vitro* investigations have demonstrated that there are a variety of amino acids that have a significantly greater likelihood of being detected in squamous cell carcinoma of the upper aerodigestive than normal muscle. The specific amino acids which were more likely to be detected in tumors are alanine, glutathione, histidine, isoleucine, valine, and the shared cross peak for lysine/polyamine. (2) (Fig. 20) (Mukherji et al. 1997; Fig. 4.20).

The detection of certain amino acids suggests that these compounds are present in higher concentrations in tumors than in normal tissues, which may be due to unregulated protein synthesis in tumors. These metabolites are also likely to be present in normal tissues, but in such small quantities that they are not detected by 2D COSY technique. The amino acids we identified as more prevalent in SCCA than in normal tissues have also been reported to be found in higher concentrations in other tumors. 2D COSY studies performed on colorectal and gynecological carcinomas have demonstrated elevated levels of various metabolites including the aforementioned amino acids (Ruiz-Cabello and Cohen 1992; May et al. 1986; Lean et al. 1992). Delikatny et al. 1993) demonstrated higher levels of alanine, leucine, isoleucine, valine, and lysine in tissue samples of cervical carcinoma. PET studies utilizing C-11 based compounds have also demonstrated an increase in amino acid metabolism in a variety of malignancies, including those arising in the extracranial head and neck (Lapela et al. 1995; Lindholm et al. 1993).

Elevated concentrations of various amino acids may be expected in tumor cells because of their need for more protein synthesis, which is due to rapid cell proliferation. Increased activity of various amino acid transport systems owing to enhanced protein synthesis has been described in tumors (Kinoshita et al. 1994; Starr 1978; Holley 1972). Increased amounts of alanine have been demonstrated in meningiomas and astrocytomas (Kinoshita et al. 1994). Additionally, accessory pathways of protein synthesis may become activated to meet the demands of rapid cell proliferation in tumor (Gill et al. 1990; Yorek et al. 1984).

2D COSY analysis has also identified noticeable differences in the spectral contours of various triglyceride cross-peaks between tumors and normal tissues. The contours of the various triglycerides appeared less elliptical and narrower owing to less chemical shift dispersion in tumors when compared to normal tissues (Figs. 4.6, 4.9). These morphological differences may be due to differences in the fluidity of mobile membrane lipids in tumors versus normal tissues (Wallach 1971; Cherry 1976; Narayana et al. 1988; Meyer 1987). The difference in chemical shift dispersion could also be due to any changes of particular phospholipids which can change the fluidity of the membrane components resulting in alterations in chemical shift dispersion as a result of changes in relaxation times. Prior 1H MRS studies have detected the presence of lipid structures which are highly mobile in the cell membrane of tumors compared to similar membrane lipids analyzed from normal tissue (Ruiz-Cabello and Cohen 1992; Guidoni et al. 1987).

*In vitro* 2D COSY studies of intact cancer cells have suggested metabolic differences that may indicate differences between cells with the capacity to metastasize and those that produce locally invasive tumors (Schiro et al. 1988). Mountford et al. 1984b) used 2D COSY to assess the metastatic potential of primary tumors. They showed that the component resonances in the lipid methylene region at 1.2 ppm could provide information on the biological status of intact cancer cells. They concluded that the ability of cells to metastasize might be attributed to some extent to cell membrane characteristics, which are determined in part by the modulating effects of the plasma membrane lipids. NMR resonances that characterized the metastatic cells were associated with an increased ratio of cholesterol to phospholipid and an increased amount of plasma membrane-bound cholesterol ester (MUKHERJI et al. 1997; SIVARAJA et al. 1994).

2D COSY is primarily an *in vitro* technique. However, recent investigations have shown that this technique can be used *in vivo*. BRERTON et al. (1994) have evaluated the *in vivo* use of 2D COSY of the brain and the tibial marrow. In studies of the brain, peaks seen in 2D, but not in 1D (owing to spectral overlap) included a-CH resonance of NAA, aspartate, and glutamate/glutamine. They also discussed problems that still exist in the application of this method clinically, i.e., the long acquisition times (approximately 2h with setup and spectral acquisition) and large voxel size. THOMAS et al. (1996) also evaluated the use of 3D localized 2D MRS for monitoring metabolites in human brains *in vivo*, specifically to distinguish between lipid and lactate.

Ongoing investigations are evaluating the ability of 2D COSY to evaluate gene function. Owing to the large number of metabolites identified by 2D COSY, it is possible that this technique may be used to identify changes in the 2D COSY metabolic profile caused by altering gene function. 2D COSY has the potential to detect subtle changes in the amino acid profiles that result in selectively activating or deactivating specific oncogenes or tumor suppressor genes. These results could have important implications for gene therapy in those tumors containing known gene mutations (SCHIRO et al. 1998).

## 4.5 Summary

There are specific metabolites that can differentiate tumor from normal tissue of the extracranial head and neck. The early results suggest that MRS has the potential to differentiate recurrent tumor from posttreatment changes in treatment monitoring. These early results indicate that the Cho/Cr ratio is an important spectroscopic marker for differentiating malignant tumors from normal tissue. Further studies need to be performed to evaluate other metabolic peaks in the proton spectra in the hope of identifying global spectral patterns that are specific to certain tumors. The ability of 1H-MRS to differentiate recurrent tumor from posttreatment changes and prospective treatment monitoring are currently being investigated. However, the future role of 1H-MRS will depend directly on advances in coil technology, which will help to facilitate spectroscopic analysis of this difficult region.

## References


American Cancer Society (1990) Cancer facts and figures 1990. Atlanta, American Cancer Society, p 8

Behar KL, Ogino T (1991) Assignment of resonances in the 1H spectrum of rat brain by two-dimensional shift correlated and J-resolved NMR spectroscopy. MRM 17:285-303

Bizzi, A, Movsas B, Tedeschi G et al (1995) Response of non-Hodgkin lymphoma to radiation therapy: early and long term assessment with h-i mr spectroscopic imaging. Radiology 194:271-276

Brerton IM, Galloway GJ, Rose SE, Doddrell DM (1994) Localized two-dimensional shift correlated spectroscopy in humans at 2 tesla. Magn Reson Imaging 32:256-257

Castillo M, Kwock L, Mukherji SK (1996) Clinical applications of proton MR spectroscopy. AJNR 17:1-15

Cazzaniga S, Schold SC, Sostman HD, Charles HC. (1994) Effects of therapy on 1H MRS spectrum of a human glioma line. Magn Reson Med 12:945-950

Cherry R. (1976) Protein and lipid mobility in biologic and model membranes. In: Chapman D, Wallach DFH (eds) Biological membranes. Academic, London, pp 47-97

Cross KJ, Holmes KT, Mountford CE (1984) Assignment of acyl chain resonances from membranes of mammalian cells by two-dimensional NMR methods. Biochemistry 23:5895-5897

De Cestaines JD, Larsen VA, Podo F, Carpinella G, Briot O, Hensiksen O (1993) *In vivo* P-31 MRS of experimental tumors. NMR Biomed 6:345-365

Delikatny EJ, Russell P, Hunter JC et al (1993) Proton MR and human cervical neoplasia: ex vivo spectroscopy allows distinction of invasive carcinoma of the cervix from carcinoma in situ and other preinvasive lesions. Radiology 188:791-796

Gill SG, Thomas DGT, Van Bruggen NV et al (1990) Proton MR spectroscopy of intracranial tumours: *in vivo* and *in vitro* studies. JCAT 14:497-504

Guidoni L, Mariutti G, Rampelli GM, Rosi A, Viti V (1987) Mobile phospholipid signals in NMR spectra of cultured human adenocarcinoma cells. Magn Reson Med 5:578-585

Hendrix RA, Lenkinski RE, Vogele K, Bloch, McKenna WG (1990) 31-P localized magnetic resonance spectroscopy of head and neck tumors-preliminary findings. Otolaryngol Head Neck Surg 103:775

Holley RW (1972) A unifying hypothesis concerning the nature of malignant growth. Proc Natl Acad Sci USA 69:2840-2841

Johnson M, Selinsky B, Davis M et al (1989) *In vitro* nmr evaluation of human thyroid lesions. Invest Radiol 24:666-671

Karczmar GS, Meyerhoff DJ, Boska MD et al P-31 (1991) spectroscopy study of response of superficial human tumors to therapy. Radiology 179:149-153

Kinoshita Y, Kajiwara H, Yokata A, Koga Y (1994) Proton magnetic resonance spectroscopy of brain tumors: an *in vitro* study. Neurosurgery 35:606-614

Kuesel AC, Graschew G, Hull WE, Lorenz W, Thielman HW (1990) $^{31}$P NMR studies of cultured human tumor cells: influences of pH on phospholipid metabolite levels and the detection of CDP-choline. NMR Biomed 3:78-89

Lapela M, Grenman R, Kurki T et al (1995) Head and neck cancer: detection of recurrence with PET and 2-[F-18] fluoro-2-deoxy glucose. Radiology 197:205-211.

Lean CL, MacKinnon WB, Delikatny J, Whitehead RH, Mountford CE (1992) Cell-surface fucosylation and magnetic resonance spectroscopy characterization of human malignant colorectal cells. Biochemistry 31:11092-11105

Lindholm P, Leskinen-Kallio S, Minn H et al (1993) Comparison of fluorine-18-fluoride-oxoglucose and carbon-11-methionine in head and neck cancer. J Nucl Med 186:27-35

Mafee MF, Barany M, Gotsis ED et al (1989) Potential use of *in vivo* proton spectroscopy for head and neck lesions. Radiol Clin North Am 27:243-254

Manara M (1966) Histological changes of the human larynx irradiated with various technical therapeutic methods. Arch Ital Otolaryngol 79:596-635

Mancuso AA, Mukherji SK, Mendenhall WE, Kotzur I, Freeman D (1998) Value of pretreatment CT as a predictor of outcome in supraglottic cancer treated with radiation therapy alone. J Clin Oncol (in press)

May GL, Wright LC, Holmes KT (1986) Assignment of methylene proton resonances in NMR spectra of embryonic and transformed cells to plasma membrane triglycerides. J Biol Chem 261:3048-3053

McKenna WG, Lenkinski RE, Hendrix RA, Vogele K, Bloch P (1989) The use of magnetic resonance imaging and spectroscopy in the assessment of patients with head and neck and other superficial malignancies. Cancer 64:2069-2075

Meyer RA (1987) Echo acquisition during frequency-selective pulse trains for proton spectroscopy of metabolites *in vivo*. Magn Reson Med 4:297-301

Miller BL (1991) A review of chemical issues in 1-H NMR spectroscopy: n-acetyl-L-aspartate, creatine and choline. NMR Biomed 4:47-52

Million RR (1994) Natural history of squamous cell carcinoma. In: Million RR, Cassisi NJ (eds) Management of head and neck cancer: a multidisciplinary approach. Lippincott, Philadelphia, pp 31-33

Mountford CE, Wright LC, Holmes KT, MacKinnon WB, Gregory P, Fox RM (1984a) High resolution nuclear magnetic analysis of metastatic cancer cells. Science 226:1415

Mountford CE, Wright LC, Holmes KT et al (1994b) High-resolution proton nuclear magnetic resonance analysis of metastatic cancer cells. Biochem Biophys Methods 9:323-330

Mountford CE, Lean CL, Hancock R et al (1993) Magnetic resonance spectroscopy detects cancer in draining lymph nodes. Invasion Metast 13:57-51

Mukherji SK, Mancuso AA, Kotzur IM et al (1994a) Radiographic appearance of the irradiated larynx: part I: expected changes. Radiology 193:141-148

Mukherji SK, Mancuso AA, Kotzur IM et al (1994b) Radiographic appearance of the irradiated larynx: part II: primary site response. Radiology 193:149-154

Mukherji SK, Schiro S, Castillo M (1996) Proton MR spectroscopy of squamous cell carcinoma of the upper aerodigestive tract: *in vitro* characteristics. AJNR 17:1485-1490

Mukherji SK, Schiro S, Castillo M, Kwock L, Muller K (1997) MR proton spectroscopy of squamous cell carcinoma of extracranial head and neck: *in vitro* and *in vivo* studies. AJNR 18:1057-1072

Mukherji SK, Kwock L, Schiro S (1998) Magnetic resonance spectroscopy of the extracranial head and neck. In: Mukherji SK (ed) Clinical applications of magnetic resonancce spectroscopy. Wiley, New York (in press)

Narayana PA, Hazle JD, Jackson EF, Fotedar LK, Kulkarni MV (1988) *In vivo* 1H spectroscopic studies of human gastrocnemius muscle at 1.5T. Magn Res Imaging 6:481-485

Negendak WG, Brown TR, Evelhoch JL et al (1992) Proceedings of a national cancer institute workshop: MR spectroscopy and tumor cell biology. Radiology 185:875-883

Negendak WG, Brown TR, Evelhoch JL et al (1996) Proceedings of a national cancer institute workshop: MR spectroscopy and tumor cell biology. Radiology 185:875-883

Ross BD (1992) The biochemistry of living tissues: examination by MRS. NMR Biomed 5:215-219

Ruiz-Cabello J, Cohen JS (1992) Phospholipid metabolites as indicators of cancer cell function. NMR Biomed 5:226-233

Russell P, Lean CL, Delbridge L, May G, Dowd S, Mountford CE (1994) Proton magnetic resonance and human thyroid neoplasia I: discrimination between benign and malignant neoplasms. Am J Med 96:383-388

Schiro S, Blackstock AW, Mukherji SK (1998) New techniques in magnetic resonance spectroscopy: potential clinical applications. In: Mukherji SK (ed) Clinical MR spectroscopy: basic principles and applications. Wiley, New York (in press)

Sivaraja M, Turner C, Souza K, Singer S (1994) Ex vivo two-dimensional proton nuclear magnetic resonance spectroscopy of smooth muscle tumors: advantages of total correlated spectroscopy over homonuclear J-correlated spectroscopy. Cancer Res 54:6037-6041

Somorjai RL, Nikulin AE, Pizzi N, Jackson D et al (1994) Computerized consensus diagnosis: a classification strategy for the robust analysis of MR spectra. MRM 33:257-263

Starr MS (1978) Uptake of taurine by retina in different species. Brain Res 151:604-608

Thomas MA, Ryner LN, Mehta MP et al (1996) Localized 2D J-resolved 1H MR spectroscopy of human brain tumors *in vivo*. J Magn Reson Imaging 1996; 6:453-459

Thompson GA (1973) Phospholipid metabolism in animal tissues. In: Ansell GB, Jawthorne JN, Dawson RMC (eds) Form and function of phospholipids. Elsevier, Amsterdam, pp 67-96

Tzika AA, Vajapeyam S, Barnes PD (1997) Multivoxel proton MR spectroscopy and hemodynamic MR imaging of childhood brain tumors: preliminary observations. AJNR 18:203-218.

Van Zijl PCM, Moonen CTW, Gillen J et al (1990) Proton magnetic resonance spectroscopy of small regions (1 mL) localized inside superficial human tumors. A clinical feasibility study. NMR Biomed 3:227-232

Vogl T, Peer F, Schedel H et al (1989) 31-P Spectroscopy of head and neck tumors-surface coil technique. Magn Reson Imag 7:425-435

Wallach DFH (1971) Cooperativity in Biomembranes. In: Wallach DFH, Fischer H (eds) The dynamic structure of cell membranes. Springer, Berlin Heidelberg New York, pp 181-199

Wang A, Sutton L, Cnann A et al (1995) Proton MR spectroscopy of pediatric cerebellar tumors. AJNR 16:1821-1833

Williams PG, Helmer MA, Wright LC et al (1985) Lipid domain in cancer cell plasma membrane shown by h-1 nmr to be similar to a lipoprotein. FEBS 192:159-164

Wurtman JJ (1979) Sources of choline and lecithin in the diet. Nutr Brain 5:73-81

Yorek MA, Storm DK, Spector AA (1984) Effect of membrane polyunsaturation on carrier-mediated transport in cultured retinoblastoma cells: alterations in taurine uptake. J Neurochem 42:254-261

# 5 Functional MR Imaging and Auditory Activation

J.L. ULMER, L.P. MARK, B.BISWAL and D.L. DANIELS

Contents



J.L. ULMER, MD, Department of Radiology, Medical College of Wisconsin, Froedtert Memorial Lutheran Hospital, 9200 West Wisconsin Avenue, Milwaukee, WI 53226, USA
L.P. MARK, MD, Department of Radiology, Medical College of Wisconsin, Froedtert Memorial Lutheran Hospital, 9200 West Wisconsin Avenue, Milwaukee, WI 53226, USA
B. BISWAL, PhD, Department of Biophysics, Medical College of Wisconsin, Froedtert Memorial Lutheran Hospital, 9200 West Wisconsin Avenue, Milwaukee, WI 53226, USA
D.L. DANIELS, MD, Department of Radiology, Medical College of Wisconsin, Froedtert Memorial Lutheran Hospital, 9200 West Wisconsin Avenue, Milwaukee, WI 53226, USA

## 5.1 Introduction

The processing of sound is one of the most complex sensory functions of the human brain, characterized by extensive modulation of neural signals in the brain stem prior to the ultimate expression of input in the auditory cortex. Processing at the level of the cortex is equally complex, reflecting the capacity of the human animal to decode and encode complex stimuli such as speech. Because of the unique capabilities of the human brain, neurophysiological studies using animals have left us with an incomplete picture of human auditory function. Investigators and clinicians studying hearing are anxious to apply new techniques to the human animal that will allow us to peer even further into the complex workings of the auditory system. Minimally invasive or noninvasive techniques, such as PET, FMRI, and MEG, that allow the study of human auditory function hold great promise and expectations.

Functional magnetic resonance imaging (FMRI) is a recently developed technique capable of detecting regional blood oxygen level changes associated with cortical neuronal activity (BELLIVEAU et al. 1991; BANDETTINI et al. 1992; KWONG et al. 1992; OGAWA et al. 1992), and it has become one of the most useful tools available to study human brain function. Functional MRI has proved capable of investigating cortical activation to a variety of simple and complex auditory stimuli (BINDER et al. 1994a, 1996; MILLEN et al. 1995; ULMER et al. 1996b; TALAVAGE et al. 1996; STRAINER et al. 1997). As a noninvasive technique used to image primary and association auditory cortical activity, FMRI has the potential to improve our understanding of normal auditory function and may ultimately prove useful in evaluating patients with hearing disorders and other auditory processing problems. This chapter focuses on the use of FMRI to image normal primary auditory cortical function, keeping in mind that the understanding of such is still evolving and that FMRI techniques used to study the auditory system have yet to be optimized. Thus, the intended goals of the following discussions on the subject are to introduce the reader to FMRI as a technique, review the functional anatomy of the auditory system, present some preliminary results from recent FMRI investigations, and stimulate further development of this powerful tool for investigating human auditory function and dysfunction.

## 5.2 General Methodology

A variety of FMRI techniques for studying human brain function have been devised, including exogenous diffusible tracers (e.g. $D_2O$, $H_2O^{17}$), spin-labeled ("tagged") $H_2O$ protons, intravascular contrast agents (e.g. Gd, Dy, iron oxide), functional spectroscopy, and BOLD (blood oxygen level-dependent) contrast imaging (DETRE et al. 1991; KWONG et al. 1992; WILLIAMS et al. 1992; CHEN et al. 1993; KWONG et al. 1995; FRAHM et al. 1996). Each of these techniques may ultimately play an important part in FMRI research and clinical applications. However, BOLD contrast imaging is the most readily available and the bulk of FMRI research to date has been carried out using this technique. Additionally, BOLD imaging is the only one of these techniques currently being used with any frequency in clinical practices. Thus, the following sections in this chapter describe BOLD FMRI as a primary technique to study human brain function.

### 5.2.1 BOLD Contrast

BOLD contrast depends upon the shifts in the equilibrium between concentrations of deoxyhemoglobin and oxyhemoglobin in regional microvascular networks of cerebral cortex (Fig. 5.1). Neuronal activity in the cerebral cortex stimulates a vascular response resulting in increased cerebral blood flow, cerebral blood volume, and oxygen concentration, which exceeds the metabolic demands of the activated neurons. This results in an increase in oxyhemoglobin and a decrease in deoxyhemoglobin compared with the nonactivated state (OGAWA et al. 1993). In effect, there is a change in regulatory mechanisms of activated cortex, resulting in the decoupling of oxygen supply and neuronal demand at the regional level (VILLRINGER and DIRNAGL 1995). Because deoxyhemoglobin is paramagnetic, it

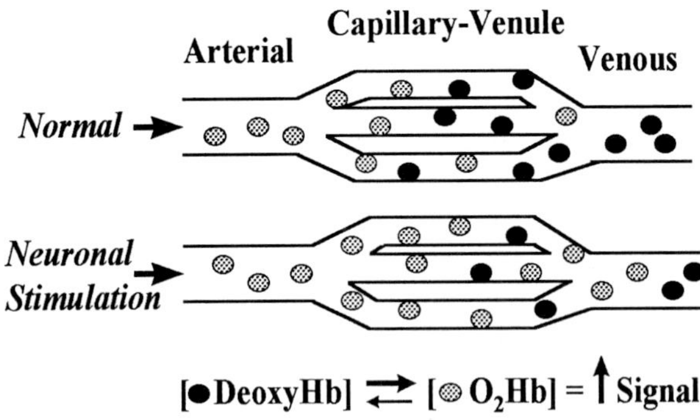


Fig. 5.1. Hyperoxygenation associated with neuronal activity. Neuronal stimulation results in relative shifts in concentrations from deoxyhemoglobin to oxyhemoglobin within the regional microvascular networks of activated cortex, resulting in increased signal on T2*-weighted FAST imaging sequences (cf. Fig. 5.2). In echoplanar imaging, microvascular signal increases by 2–5% owing to regional neuronal activity, while macrovascular (venous) contrast may increase by more than 5% and at sites remote from neuronal activity

produces local susceptibility gradients that can be detected with fast T2*-weighted imaging techniques such as echoplanar imaging. Thus, neuronal activity results in regional decreases in deoxyhemoglobin concentrations and regional increases in BOLD related signal on T2*-weighted sequences. With the echoplanar imaging (EPI) technique, signal changes within the cortical microvasculature related to neuronal activity ranges from 2% to 5% above baseline. However, signal may also increase by considerably more than 5% in the macrovasculature of the region, simulating neuronal activity and providing erroneous maps of cortical function. When analyzing FMRI data sets, is important to avoid this potential pitfall and to differentiate between microvascular and macrovascular contrast (BOXERMAN et al. 1995).

It is equally important for investigators to recognize that the BOLD-related signal is associated with neuronal activity, but does not equal neuronal activity. Rather, the vascular response to regional neuronal activity is mediated by one or more factors, requiring at least 2 s to produce detectable regional changes in deoxyhemoglobin concentrations (BANDETTINI et al. 1992). The vascular response is presumably mediated to some extent by chemical factors, but the exact mechanisms are not entirely clear at this point. A number of chemical mediators have been proposed in the vascular response, including lactate, adenosine, $K^+$, $O_2$, glucose, and NO. Direct neural innervation and mediation at the arteriolar level is also possible. Finally, there could be a cascade of events responsible for mediating the

BOLD effect subsequent to cortical neuronal activity. Thus, BOLD contrast is associated with neuronal activity, but not does necessarily represent a cause-and-effect relationship. It is therefore possible that BOLD contrast does not localize precisely to neuronal activity, but intraoperative mapping studies have confirmed that BOLD activation maps are generally at least accurate to within 1 cm of true activated cortical regions (MALONEK and GRINVOLD 1996; YETKIN et al. 1997).

### 5.2.2 Echoplanar Imaging

The goal of BOLD FMRI techniques is the detection of task-induced signal alterations related to the T2* effects of changing deoxyhemoglobin concentrations (OGAWA et al. 1992). Thus, BOLD pulse sequences are designed to optimize the detection of T2* contrast. A number fast T2*-weighted sequences have been developed, including EPI (BANDETTINI et al. 1992; KWONG et al. 1992), spiral FMRI (NOLL et al. 1995), EPISTAR (EDELMAN et al. 1994), QUIPSS (WONG et al. 1997), FLASH and HASTE (FRANSSON et al. 1997) sequences. Spiral FMRI is a promising new technique that deserves special mention, having the advantage of being able to image the entire brain without the need for additional hardware beyond that on existing MRI systems (NOLL et al. 1995). However, the efficacy of this technique to map cortical function must be confirmed before it will likely replace other techniques. The most widely used FMRI technique to date is single-shot EPI, and the following sections focus on the characteristics and pitfalls of this particular method of cortical activation imaging. EPI, first proposed and implemented by Peter Mansfield (STEHLING et al. 1991), is a T2*-weighted fast image acquisition sequence requiring hardware modifications to that of conventional MRI. In order to image the entire brain with EPI, specialized amplifiers are required to rapidly switch field gradients. Initially, specialized head gradient coils were used exclusively to acquire FMRI data using the EPI technique. However, stronger gradients have recently been designed and incorporated into the body coil of newer MRI systems so that FMRI data can be acquired without the need for these specialized head coils.

In EPI, a series of echoes are generated by rapidly switching the strong phase-encoding gradient during a weaker read gradient. Thus the entire k-space is covered during a single scan; hence the name single-shot EPI. Similar techniques that are derivatives of EPI, such as FLEET and BEST, have also been developed, which cover only a proportion of the k-space. The high speed ability of EPI enables one to acquire an entire image in as little as 50 ms. Up to 20 images covering the entire brain can be obtained every second in a sequential fashion (BISWAL et al. 1997a). Typical EPI parameters at 1.5 T include a 1- to 3-s. repetition time (TR), 40- to 80-ms time to echo (TE), 24 cm field of view (FOV), and a 64×64 imaging matrix.

There is an inverse relationship between the spatial and the temporal resolutions of echoplanar images. For example, 20 images/s can be acquired with EPI on a 1.5 T system, yielding a spatial resolution (pixel) of 3.75 mm using a 64×64 matrix. Alternatively, 10 images/s with a spatial resolution of 1.88 mm can be obtained using a matrix of 128×128, assuming other imaging parameters remain constant. Because the contrast-to-noise ratio of echoplanar BOLD imaging is low (2–5% signal change), alterations in voxel size can dramatically change the apparent cortical activation maps. High-field-strength scanners (i.e. 3 or 4 T) can achieve even higher signal-to-noise ratios in the temporal and spatial domain, but are beset by increased susceptibility artifacts and increased acoustic echoplanar scanner noise. Of course, the 2- to 3-s response time of the BOLD effect and the timing of the task paradigm are generally the limiting factors in the temporal resolution of FMRI data. Multi-shot EPI has the advantage of no special hardware requirements, but acquires fewer images by a factor of 4 than single-shot EPI for any given time frame (TAN et al. 1997).

### 5.2.3 Flow-Related Signal in FMRI

While EPI is able to provide high-resolution T2*-weighted (BOLD) images, the signal changes observed in FMRI using this technique actually arise from a combination of increased cerebral blood flow and from the dominant BOLD effect, and the relative contributions of flow and BOLD contrast cannot be easily distinguished. In the human brain an increase in the metabolic demands of a small region of the cortex can be associated with a substantially larger area of vascular response and change in regional cerebral blood flow. Thus, the BOLD effect related to shifts in the microvascular concentrations of deoxy- and oxyhemoglobin matches the true regions of cortical activity more precisely than do flow-related signal changes. Although most FMRI investigations assume a minor contribution from flow related signal, these effects can be a significant source of error in mapping activated cortex, particularly when larger vessels are near the cortical area of interest. For example, mapping the tonotopic organization of the primary auditory cortex on the superior surface of the superior temporal gyrus (i.e. transverse temporal gyrus) could be problematic if flow-related effects in the macrovasculature within the adjacent sylvian fissure are not considered.

Investigators have recently begun to consider methods of differentiating BOLD from flow-related contrast, which may become critical as FMRI techniques evolve to map cortex with ever increasing spatial resolutions (Kim 1995; Kwong et al. 1995; S.G. Kim et al. 1997). One method proposed uses a pulsed arterial spin labeling modified EPI technique (FAIR) that utilizes endogenous water as a tracer, by alternating between slice-selective and non-slice-selective inversion to differentiate the relative contributions of these two sources of task-activated signal changes. To make this differentiation, resting state and task activation time-courses of FAIR images are acquired with a TI value that suppresses signal from CSF and blood. After the inversion, a time delay before the image is collected allows blood to move into the imaging slice. The blood that moves in during a slice-selective inversion is fresh and enhances the signal, while blood that moves in during a non-slice-selective inversion is inverted and does not change the signal. The even-numbered non-slice-selective images are BOLD-weighted. All odd-numbered images in the image sequence are slice selective BOLD-plus flow-weighted. Subtracting every odd-numbered image from the succeeding even-numbered image results in a time series of images that are flow-weighted. By this simple method, the contribution of flow signal effects can be determined for a given FMRI experiment. However, this single-shot sequence is also a single slice-technique and therefore has limited utility in FMRI experiments of the brain. However, multi-slice techniques using similar methodology are currently under development, which in the future should give researchers the option of differentiating between BOLD- and flow-related signal in FMRI experiments where high spatial resolution is paramount.

### 5.2.4 Experimental Task Design

In FMRI experiments, images are obtained while the subjects are presented with a sensory or cognitive task, and brain function is then determined by comparing signal generated in cortex during an "active" state with signal generated during a "resting" or non-task state. The goal is to design task paradigms to generate predictable "on" and "off" conditions in the cortex, such that signal changes associated with particular brain functions can be referenced to background signal (Fig. 5.2a). This is often the most difficult and important component of an FMRI experimental design. The more complex the cognitive function required of the subject, the harder is it to design paradigms to achieve this goal. In effect, the study must produce temporally discrete brain functions for activated cortex to be detected with FMRI. For example, a simple stimulus such as a pure tone should elicit little in the way secondary cognitive effects and associated cortical activity should reflect the timing of the on-off stimulus. On the other hand, an "on-off" presentation of music or speech may stimulate unintended cognitive effects during the "on" or "off" state of the experiment and therefore alter the cortical activation maps.

In many situations, a separate "control" task during the off state of the experiment is needed to isolate the desired cortical function. Consider, for example, attempts to map receptive (Wernicke's) language areas using a text listening task, to determine the location of eloquent cortex noninvasively. While such tasks will certainly activate receptive language areas associated with language comprehension in alert subjects during the on state of the study, recent investigations have also reported similar distributions of activation throughout the auditory and language system with nonsemantic complex auditory stimuli and no comprehension of content (e.g. unintelligible or backwards language) (Ulmer et al. 1997, 1998a). Thus, FMRI activation maps as determinants of language cortex are not necessarily testing comprehension per se, as is the case with conventional WADA testing in the angiographic suite. The addition of a control task containing nonsemantic complex auditory stimuli during the off state will more accurately delineate the eloquent cortical areas necessary for language comprehension (Ulmer et al. 1997). As FMRI researchers delve into even more complex cognitive functions, effective task designs will likely become some of the more challenging obstacles to

a

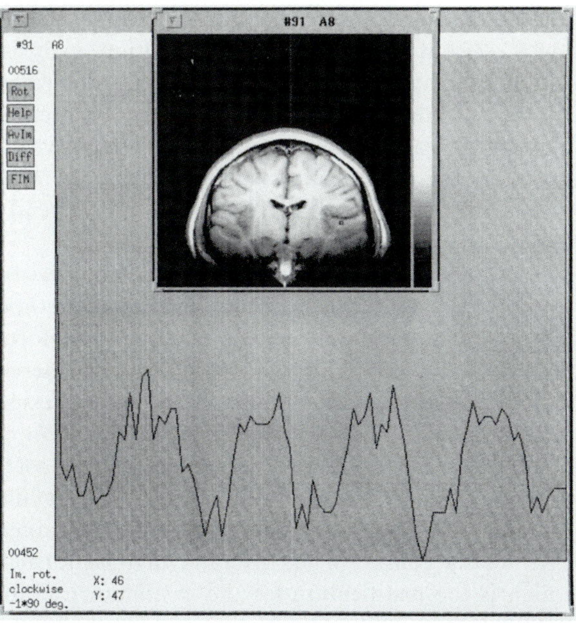


b

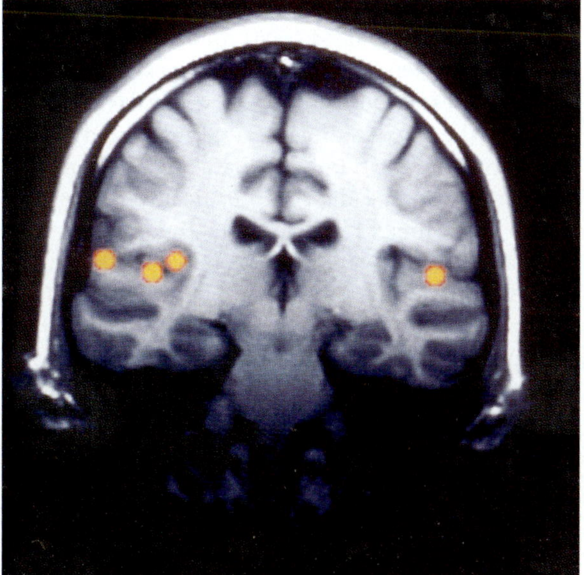


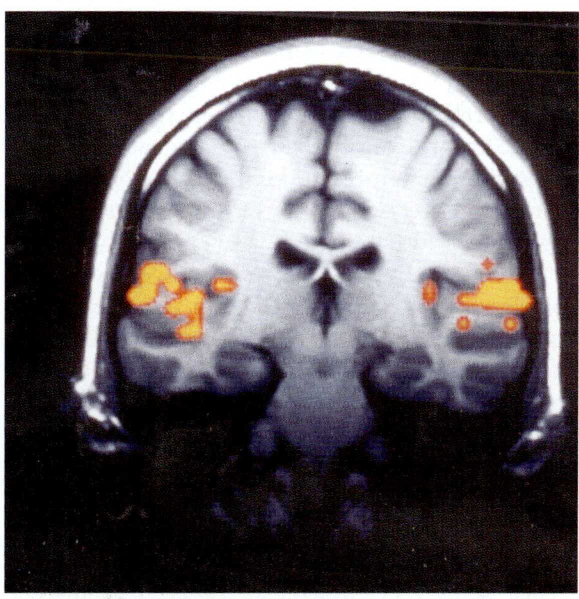


**Fig. 5.2. a** Cortical activity-induced signal changes in a single pixel (voxel) with echoplanar imaging. Pure tones delivered to this normal volunteer in four 20-s "on" intervals results in signal changes within the left transverse temporal gyrus (TTG; *small black box*). The task-induced signal changes correspond to the timing of the task cycle, with five nontask periods interposed by four task (tone) periods. The single pixel shown can be chosen as a reference pixel by which to identify activated regions elsewhere in the brain, using a cross-correlation analysis. **b** Once activated pixels are designated, they are mapped onto high-resolution anatomic images. Pure tone stimuli results in activation in the superior temporal gyri (STG) bilaterally, in the region of the TTG. The more complex stimulus of text listening results in considerably more activity in the TTG and in auditory association cortices surrounding the TTG, including STG, middle temporal gyrus, insular gyrus, and left subcentral gyrus (frontal operculum) regions. (Modified from Strainer et al. 1997)

overcome in using this technique to study higher brain function.

A typical FMRI experiment consists of presenting the subject with a 20- to 30-s stimulus/task alternated with non-task or control periods of equal length for 3-5 cycles during the image acquisitions (Fig. 5.2a). Presenting the stimulus in a simple periodic fashion such as this makes it easy for researchers to analyze task-related signal changes relative to resting background signal of similar periods and to construct maps of activated cortex. An alternative approach is to design a continuously changing task that is in the on state throughout much of the data acquisition period. The stimulus is timed to activate different regions of the cortex during different phases of the stimulus, such that phase-specific analysis of the data allows researchers to determine which portions of the changing stimulus are responsible for activating specific regions of cortex. That is to say that the analysis for this type of paradigm detects activated pixels based on stimuli shifted in time by using corresponding time-shifted reference waveforms. However, this method also requires the paradigm to achieve temporally correlated cortical responses to produce meaningful FMRI result.

### 5.2.5 Analysis of Activation Data

Most FMRI studies are designed such that the time-course of the on-off paradigm is known. When this is the case, a cross-correlation analysis is widely used (Bandettini et al. 1993) to detect and map cortical regions activated by the on-off task. Cross-correlation assumes that neuronal activity and FMRI task-induced signals change proportionally with the stimulus paradigm. With this method, activated pixels are determined by correlating a single reference pixel to all other pixels in the brain region of interest, usually the entire brain. All pixels showing a significant correlation with the selected reference pixel (Fig. 5.2b) are considered to be activated and are mapped onto high-resolution reference images that correspond precisely to the EPI images used to acquire the FMRI data (Fig. 5.3a,b).

A reference waveform to be used for cross-correlation analysis can be chosen in several ways. First, a single pixel from the raw data set with signal changes corresponding to the time frame of the task paradigm can be selected as the reference pixel (Fig. 5.3a). This is the most sensitive method of detecting activated cortex, but probably the least specific in excluding other physiological and technical artifacts, which may simulate cortical activity. This can influence particularly regions of brain with less robust activity (T. Kim et al. 1997). This method requires investigators to use a sufficiently high correlation coefficient to minimize these artifacts in the data analysis. A second method uses a synthesized box-car waveform corresponding to the known time-course of the stimulus presentation which is then cross-correlated with all other pixels on a pixel-by-pixel basis to identify a stimulus-locked response (Fig. 5.3b). This method has high specificity, but may underestimate regions of subtle cortical activity camouflaged by underlying technical or physiologic artifacts. In areas of robust activity, however, these two methods of choosing a reference waveform result in very similar activation distributions (Fig. 5.3c, d) (T. Kim et al. 1997). Many investigators are now using a third method of selecting a reference pixel for cross-correlation analysis, which is a hybrid of the two methods described above. With this method, a synthetic pixel is used to identify activated pixels. A number of the activated pixels are then averaged to cancel out random technical and physiological artifacts, and subsequently used as a reference waveform.

The statistical significance of the cross-correlated pixels is calculated using a semiempirical method (Biswal et al. 1996). If the ideal reference waveform used for cross-correlation FMRI analysis of filtered task-activated pixels is applied to all filtered pixels in the resting state data set, the standard deviation of the distribution of the resting state correlation coefficients is typically somewhat less than 0.1. The histogram of the correlation coefficient values obtained when in this condition has been shown to be normal, which is the justification for the semiempirical approach. Assuming that the resting state data exhibit a normal distribution, five times the standard deviation leads to a typical $P<0.0001$ for activated pixels in FMRI data sets. Because the cross-correlation method uses a point-by-point analysis of signal changes, the $P$-value of correlated (activated) pixels will increase as the number of data points, or images, is increased in the data set. Typically, researchers obtain 70–90 images in a single data set. Thus, a valid comparison of activation between two tasks requires an identical number of images to be collected during the presentation for each task. Also, the sensitivity and specificity of the cortical activation maps can be adjusted by selecting the appropriate correlation coefficient threshold by which a pixel is considered activated (Fig. 5.4a, b). Typical correlation coefficient ($r$) thresholds used by FMRI researchers range from 0.4 (very sensitive) to 0.7 (very specific). In our laboratory, we typically use correlation coefficient thresholds of 0.5 or 0.6.

Although the cross-correlation analysis is the one that is currently most widely used by FMRI investigators, other methods of analysis have been developed (Worsley et al. 1995; Buchel et al. 1996; Brammer et al. 1997). When the on-off cycle is known, a method similar to the cross-correlation method can be used to calculate a Fourier spectrum of each pixel time-course using a fast Fourier transform. Frequency components of the time-course images obtained at the stimulus rate are then obtained to detect activated cortical regions. This method has the advantage of reduced sensitivity to subtle time differences between cortical responses to any given stimulus. In some experiments, the task design does

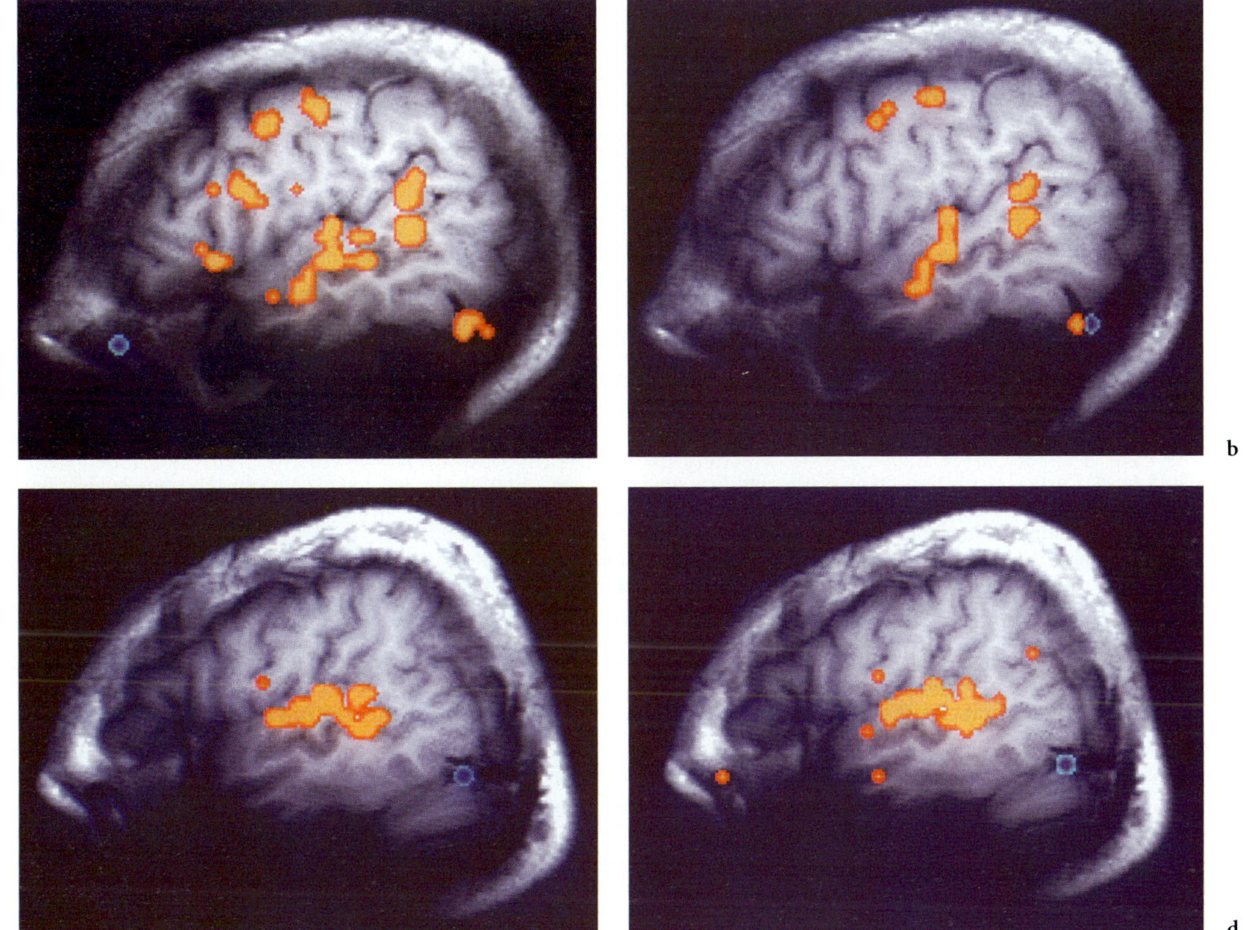


**Fig. 5.3a–d.** For areas of less robust cortical activity, the reference waveform chosen (from the raw data or a synthetic idealized waveform) for the cross-correlation analysis can alter the appearance of the cortical activation maps. Activation maps of auditory and language cortex of the left hemisphere in response to passive text listening, **a, c** using a single pixel from the raw data as a reference waveform and **b, d** using a synthesized square waveform that corresponds precisely to the timing of the task paradigm applied to the same data. In regions of less robust activity (anterior language area), the cross-correlation analysis using a raw data reference waveform (**a**) results in greater apparent activity than is seen when the map is constructed using an idealized square-wave (**b**) as the reference waveform. In regions of robust activity (auditory cortex and posterior language area) activation maps are similar (**c, d**) using the two reference waveforms for the cross-correlation analysis

not lend itself to an on-off cycle or the subjects are not able to respond synchronously to the input of cognitive tasks. In experiments such these, the cross-correlation analysis does not work well. For such conditions, a "resting" state scan can be obtained in addition to the regular stimulus presentation scan, or active state scan. Nonparametric statistics such as the Komogrov-Smirnov test or the Kruskal-Wallis test (Biswal et al. 1994) can then be used to reliably detect regions of activation. Another simple and computationally fast method of detecting activated pixels is to determine the mean and standard deviation of signal change in each FMRI data set and subtract the averaged images obtained during stimulus presentation from the averaged images obtained during rest. This is equivalent to T-test statistics and uses differences between the means to detect regions of activation. Such a method can be employed even if the timing of the on-off cycle is not fully known, but it is especially susceptible to artifacts.

Another approach to FMRI analysis uses statistical clustering techniques (Forman et al. 1995; Baumgartner et al. 1997; Moser et al. 1997). These techniques are not detection analyses, but rather serve to refine existing analysis methods. After all the pixels in the brain that have passed a given activation threshold have been detected, clustering techniques can assess statistically the spatial extent of

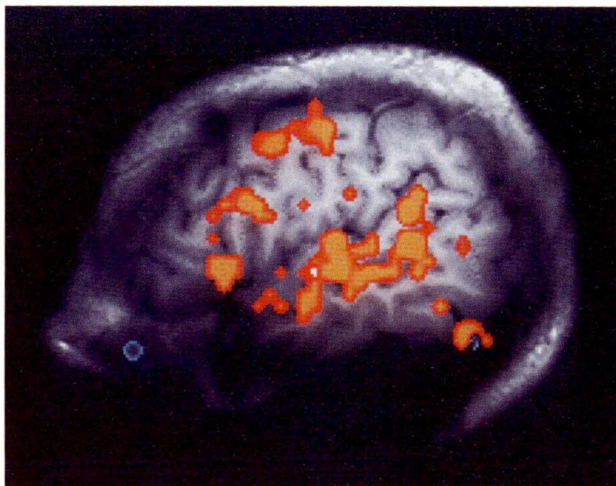
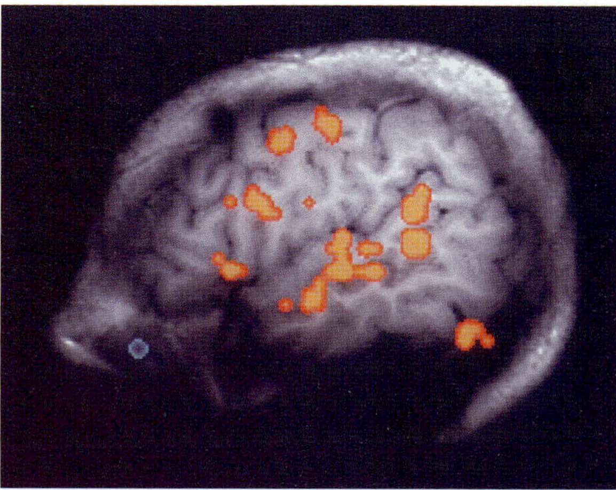

**Fig. 5.4a, b.** Cortical activation maps of the auditory and language cortex of the left hemisphere in the same subject and experiment, generated from a cross-correlation analysis with correlation coefficient thresholds of **a** 0.5 and **b** 0.6. The lower correlation coefficient threshold (**a**) is more sensitive and yields increased areas of activation than the higher threshold (**b**). Increasing the correlation coefficient threshold reduces cortical activation areas, but also reduces apparent activation due to physiological and technical artifacts, and can therefore add specificity to activation maps

activation foci. That is to say, the probability of two or more pixels that have passed the activation threshold being adjacent to one another is computed. Clustering techniques can quantify, for example, the fact that eight neighboring pixels passing a given activation threshold are statistically much less likely to occur by pure chance than two neighboring pixels that have passed the same activation threshold. Thus, clustering methods not only assign a significance value to clusters of activated pixels, but also reject single pixels of activation occurring by chance as a result of technical or physiological artifacts. Several clustering methods of data analysis have been used in FMRI studies, including fuzzy clustering and hierarchical techniques. More research is needed, however, to confirm the utility of this promising refinement of FMRI analysis.

### 5.2.6 Motion Detection and Correction

One experimental condition that all FMRI researchers must face is the exquisite sensitivity of fast T2*-weighted techniques, such as EPI, to subject motion. Even the most subtle head motion can substantially reduce the ability to detect task-induced signal changes. Indeed, even motion of someone other than the study subject in the scanner suite can result in signal changes in FMRI. With task-induced signal changing by only 5% over the mean signal intensity in EPI, changes caused by head motion severely impede detection of cortical activity-induced signal changes. If the motion of a subject or a person delivering a task in the scanner suite corresponds temporally to the task paradigm, the motion-induced signal alterations can be misinterpreted as cortical activation. Head motion can result, not only in translation and rotation, but also in and out of the imaging plane. Images obtained in the presence of head motion exhibit global distortions as well as local signal distortions. In our experience, foam padding considerably reduces head motion while keeping the subject comfortable and relaxed. Bite bars have been used to reduce head motion, but the associated discomfort in relatively lengthy experiments can actually increase head motion.

Because of the potential confounding variables from motion, most FMRI data are generally statistically analyzed for the presence of motion-induced artifacts. Some investigators elect to apply motion correction algorithms to data sets where motion is detected, while others prefer to reject the data altogether. Rejecting the data based on significant motion is feasible in FMRI neuroscience experiments, but may be less than desirable, when FMRI is utilized in the clinical setting where sick patients can have trouble holding still during the examination. While a large number of algorithms exist for the detection (and correction) of misregistered images, image registration using intrinsic properties of the brain can be broadly classified into (a) intensity-based (Woods et al. 1992; Friston et al. 1996) and (b) feature-based (Biswal et al. 1997b) methods. Intensity-based registration techniques maximize (or minimize) intensity of pixels between two or more images according to some predetermined criteria, such as maximizing the correlation coefficients or minimizing the intensity variance. Woods' registration algorithm, a very commonly used algorithm in FMRI and PET, is based on the implicit assumption that when two images are perfectly aligned the variance between the two images is minimized. Similarly, a registration algorithm assumes that the intensity correlation coefficient between the two images would be maximum when they are registered. Intensity-based registration techniques are robust for registering images corrupted with noise or images that have been shifted. If, in addition to the above two contamination sources (noise and shifts), one of the images has local changes in signal intensity, intensity-based registration will not be able to align the images even when the criteria for registration are satisfied. Perfectly aligned images that have local signal variations will be misregistered by an intensity-based registration technique.

Feature-based registration methods match common properties, including geometric and contour properties, present in an image pair. Since head motion can be considered as rigid body motion, any motion occurring in the same imaging plane can be decomposed into translation and/or rotation, both of which preserve features. Thus, a feature-based cross-correlation algorithm using brain contours can detect the presence of - head motion. A contour image of the first image in each data set is used as a reference, and the motion is estimated for every other image in the data set. The contour-based registration can differentiate between task-induced (localized in signal intensity) and motion-induced signal changes. It can improve performance in motion detection in the presence of both task-induced and head motion-induced signal changes. With this method, the estimated motion is tabulated as a function of time for each subject and for each data set. In our laboratory, data sets that exhibit head motion are corrected for motion prior to cross-correlation analysis. Data sets that exhibit head motion by more than two pixels are generally discarded.

### 5.2.7 Filtering Physiological Signal Fluctuations

In FMRI the temporal frequency resolution of the signal change is limited by the choice of TR. Two images (2 TRs) are required to detect a task-induced change in signal. One cannot arbitrarily reduce the value of TR, because such a decrease, when other imaging acquisition parameters are kept the same, leads to a decrease in signal-to-noise ratio. In FMRI the TR is typically between 1000 and 3000 ms, corresponding to a temporal resolution between 0.5 and 0.17 Hz. Since heart rates are in the range of 1-2 Hz, aliasing of flow-related signal changes can result. Respiratory related (BOLD) signal oscillations occur at approximately 0.15 Hz. Thus, physiological artifact frequencies can interfere with the task activation frequency, which typically has a period of 10-20 s. Investigators have found that using physiological filters can increase the number of activated pixels detected for a given threshold (Biswal et al. 1996). Such filters allow additional foci of cortical activation to be mapped and result in an increase in the mean correlation value of activated pixels. The following discussion outlines one reported method for filtering physiological signal artifacts from FMRI data.

To filter physiological oscillations from an FMRI data set, one method proposed uses a pulse oximeter placed on the toe of a subject to obtain a waveform of blood oxygenation during scan acquisition (Biswal et al. 1996). The oximeter is sensitive to the average blood oxygenation of the resting muscle capillary bed. The respiration and heart rates can also be obtained from the pulse oximeter. The analog oximeter output, digitized at a rate of 100 samples/s, provides a frequency resolution of 50 Hz. This is sufficient to record the fundamental frequencies and several harmonics of the heart and respiration rates. To estimate aliased frequencies, the oximeter data is sampled at the same sampling period as that of the FMRI data. In its simplest form, such a resampling can be generated using the formula $y(t1)=x(Nt2)$. The output and input data points at time t are represented by $y(t1)$ and $x(Nt2)$, where $N$ is the decimate factor, $x$ is the original signal sampled very finely, and $y$ is the output signal sampled at a slower rate (aliased signal). Comparison of the Fourier transforms of the resampled data and the experimental FMRI time-course data permits identification of the aliased frequencies.

Once the aliased frequencies in a data set are determined, a finite impulse response (FIR) Gaussian band-reject filter can be used to attenuate the fundamental frequencies and first harmonics of the average aliased heart and respiratory signals. Filter half-widths for heart and respiration are adjusted to accommodate variations in the fundamental frequency during a 4-min scan. The filter parameters are adjusted to minimize side lobes and phase distortion. Typically, the full width at half-maximum of the filters is half the standard deviation of the frequency-domain data obtained during the resting state. A second strategy uses a FIR low-pass filter with a cut-off frequency <0.1 Hz to attenuate the fundamental respiratory and higher frequency noise components for data sets obtained with a TR greater than 2000 ms. Although the respiration frequency can be reliably filtered by this method alone, the heart rate (which is typically in the range of 60–80 cycles/min) remains aliased and buried in the data set.

## 5.3 Auditory System Anatomy

It behooves FMRI investigators of auditory cortical function to recognize the extent of modulation of auditory signals occurring at the level of the cochlea and brain stem. That is to say that cortical activity imaged with FMRI may not only be related to processing within the cortex, but may also be a reflection of extensive upstream auditory processing. Differentiating cortical from brain stem processing is no easy task. A thorough understanding of auditory system functional anatomy is necessary for FMRI investigators to properly analyze and interpret functional imaging data as expressed in the cortex. The understanding of such will become even more important in the near future, as investigators have already begun to image brain stem function using newer FMRI techniques. Also, future FMRI investigations of hearing dysfunction need to appreciate the effects of various pathologic conditions at specific sites along the auditory pathways, from the cochlea to the cortex.

The auditory system consists of multiple components distributed from the auricle to the cerebral cortex and can be conceptualized as having two basic functions: the recognition of sound source and sound patterns. The coding of frequency (FM) and amplitude modulations (AM) and the recognition of complex patterns occurs at many levels in the auditory system, with some stages of sound processing containing independent functions while others are influenced and dependent upon foreign system components. The function and complete elucidation of these complex and interdependent components involved in the processing of auditory stimuli and the experiential phenomenon of hearing, however, still present many unresolved issues and continue to be the focus of intense investigations. The anatomy of the auditory system is also incompletely understood, but some of the defined system components will be the subject of this brief overview section, which will be limited to major landmarks of the cochlea, brain stem auditory pathways, and primary auditory cortex. For further detailed discussion of auditory system functional anatomy, the reader is referred to a recent series of graphically illustrated reviews on the subject (Swartz et al. 1996a, 1996b; Mark et al. 1998), as well as more traditional sources (Celesia 1976; Plomp 1983; Nieuwenhuys 1984; Nieuwenhuys et al. 1988; Lauter et al. 1985; Greenberg 1988; Brugge 1991; Langner 1992; Masterton 1992; Newby and Popelka 1992; Roland 1993; Bannister et al. 1995; Knudsen and Brainard 1995).

### 5.3.1 The Cochlea

The cochlea is an inner ear structure specifically suited to housing the primary auditory sense organ, the organ of Corti. The basic structure of the cochlea is ideally designed to allow the organ of Corti to code a wide range of auditory stimuli, and is therefore worth reviewing here. The snail-shaped cochlea is a helical tubular structure forming about two and one-half turns (Figs. 5.5, 5.6). The wider base of the cochlea is oriented posteromedially, while the smaller apex faces anterolaterally. The modiolus is the bony central axis of the cochlea (Fig. 5.6). The osseous spiral lamina projects from the modiolus toward the cochlea walls, forming a winding shelf-like appearance similar to the flanges of a screw. The space within the cochlea contains perilymph and is divided by the osseous spiral lamina and the endolymph-containing cochlear duct, which extends from the margin of the osseous spiral lamina to the cochlear walls (Figs. 5.6, 5.7). The more anterior (toward the apex) compartment is called the scala vestibuli, while the posterior (toward the base) compartment is labeled the scala tympani. At the cochlear apex, the cochlear duct ends blindly and the two scalae communicate with each other at a point of communication termed the helicotrema (Figs. 5.5, 5.6). In effect, this communication couples the oval and round windows and maintains hemostatic balance during the transmission of sound energy. The posterior wall of the cochlear duct (basilar membrane) is anchored to the bony cochlear walls by an endosteal thickening (spiral ligament) and separates the cochlear duct (scala media) from the scala tympani (Fig. 5.7). The anterior cochlear duct wall (vestibular or Reissner's membrane), which is also attached to the cochlear walls, separates the cochlear duct from scala vestibuli (Fig. 5.7).

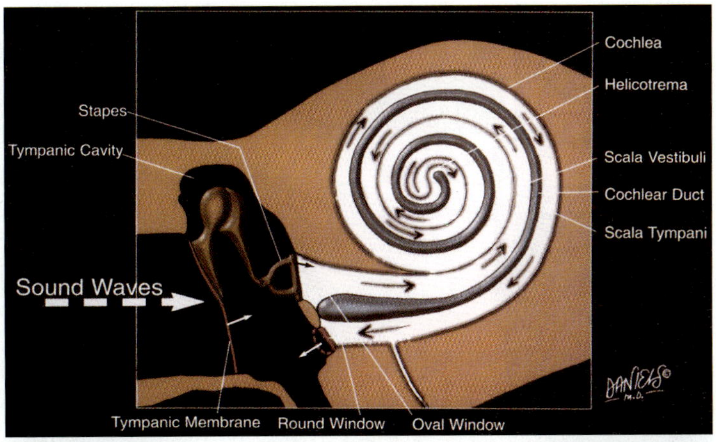

**Fig. 5.5.** Schematic of the tympanic cavity and cochlea. Sound waves causing vibrations in the tympanic membrane are transmitted to the ossicles within the middle ear cavity. Energy transmitted from the stapes to the oval window produces pressure waves that travel in the perilymph from the oval window to the round window, ultimately dissipated into the air containing middle ear cavity. (From SWARTZ et al. 1996a)

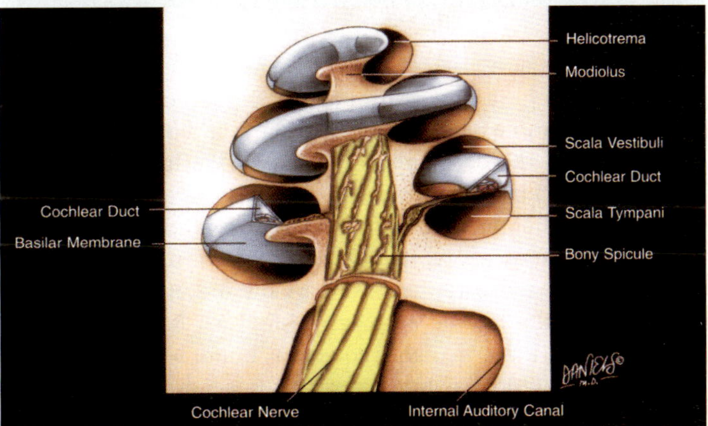


**Fig. 5.6.** Dissected view of the cocheal showing its central osseous axis (modiolus), through which the cochlea nerve reaches the internal auditory canal. Note the spiraling cochlear duct within the turns of the cochlea. (From SWARTZ et al. 1996a)

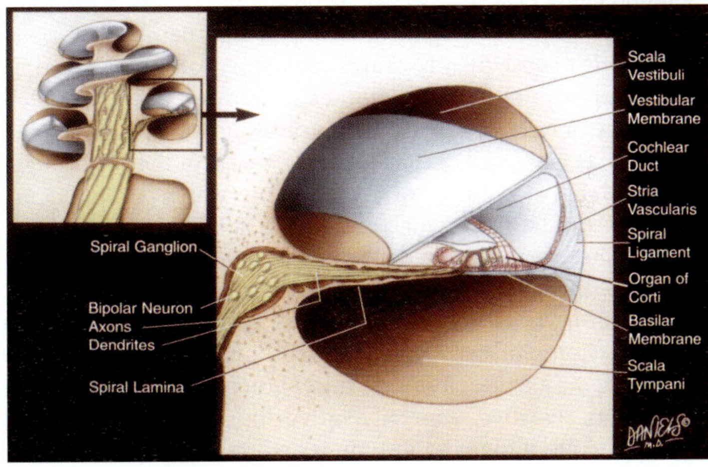


**Fig. 5.7.** Magnified view of the cochlear duct, scala vestibule, and scalal tympani. The organ of Corti is located within the cochlear duct and is positioned on the basilar membrane. The spiral ganglion is formed by bipolar neurons, whose dentrites synapse with hair cells in the organ of Corti and extend through the osseous spiral lamina. Axons of the bipolar neurons form the cochlear nerve. (From SWARTZ et al. 1996a)

## 5.3.2 The Organ of Corti

The organ of Corti is an auditory sense organ designed to convert sound waves into electrical neuronal activity (Fig. 5.8), and it has extraordinary capabilities in deciphering intensity, frequency, and temporal components of sound. The organ of Corti lies on the basilar membrane and contains neuroepithelial hair cells that, when displaced by sound, stimulate the cochlear nerve (Fig. 5.8). The transduction of sound to neural discharges is achieved by a series of steps propagating sound energy through external, middle, and inner ear structures. Sound waves hitting the tympanic membrane (air conduction) are amplified by the ossicles in the middle ear.

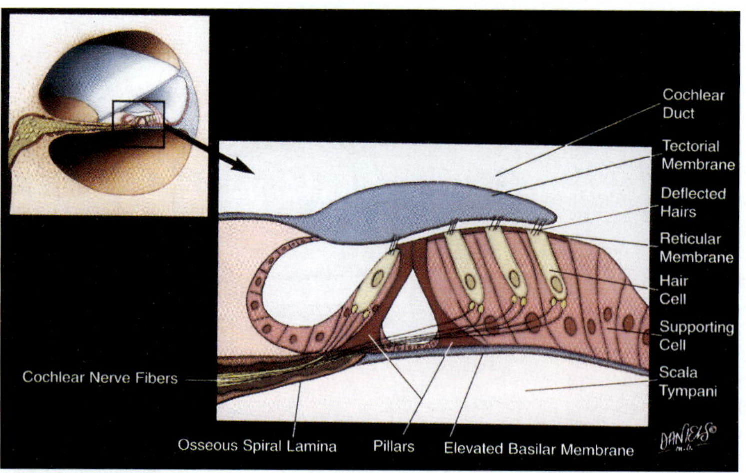


**Fig. 5.8.** Schematic of the organ of Corti. Pressure waves in the perilymph cause the vestibular membrane, cochlear duct, endolymph, and basilar membrane to vibrate. As the basilar membrane is displaced, there is a relative sharing action between basilar and tectorial membranes, resulting in deflection of the hair cell cilia embedded in the tectorial membrane. This sharing motion results in alternating inhibitory and excitatory influences on the hair cells and ultimately in a potential that excites the cochlear nerve fibers. (From Swartz et al. 1996a)

These vibratory waves are propagated to the oval window membrane by the stapes footplate, and then transmitted to the perilymph in the scala vestibuli (Fig. 5.5). Because perilymph is virtually incompressible, the membrane covering the round window at the end of the scala tympani serves to accommodate increased hydrostatic pressure by dissipating it in the air of the middle ear cavity (Fig.5.5). Bone conduction of low- or high-frequency sounds (e.g. <800 and >1500 Hz) also has similar, but less efficient, direct effects on the perilymph.

Sound energy transmitted to the perilymph of the scala vestibuli causes bulging of the vestibular membrane, which subsequently causes movement of the endolymph within the cochlear duct and throws the basilar membrane into a series of traveling waves. These vibratory waves cause a shearing action of the hair cells relative to the tectorial membrane, which is affixed to the hair cell cilia (Fig. 5.8). The sound-induced shearing action of the two membranes relative to one another creates a to-and-fro motion of the cilia, resulting in alternating inhibitory and excitatory effects on hair cell $K^+$ (depolarizing) channels. This produces an alternating electrical potential that is stimulus sensitive, generally mirroring the frequency and amplitude of the auditory stimulus. The hair cells within the organ of Corti are organized into internal and external components. The internal hair cells are innervated primarily by afferent fibers (i.e. cochlea to brain stem) while the external hairs cells are primarily innervated by efferents (brain stem to cochlea), implying that the external cells are under some element of central influence.

### 5.3.3 Cochleotopic Organization

Because of the structural features of the basilar membrane, the magnitude of deflection of the basilar membrane by sound energy is site specific, depending on the frequency of that sound. The basilar membrane is approximately 32 mm long and varies in width from 0.05 mm to 0.5 mm from the cochlear base to the apex. Also, the basement membranes becomes gradually thinner towards the apex. Within the basilar membrane, there are parallel bundles of collagen-like microfibrils measuring 8–10 nm in thickness called auditory strings, which stretch for variable lengths from the cochlear base to its apex. There are approximately 20,000 auditory strings, varying in length from 0.04 mm at the cochlear base to 0.5 mm at the apex. Each sound frequency transmitted to the endolymph causes vibrations in corresponding auditory strings, thus stimulating hair cells at specific locations on the basilar membrane. High-frequency sounds, which have short high-energy traveling waves, are limited to the cochlear base, while lower frequency sounds move farther along the basilar membrane toward the apex. In addition to the frequency specificity of the basilar membrane, selectivity is further enhanced by individual hair cells and cochlear nerve fibers that are tuned to be most sensitive to certain frequencies. This geographic mapping of frequencies along the length of the cochlea is also referred to as a cochleotopic, or tonotopic, organization. Interestingly, the tonotopic distribution of sound frequencies in the cochlea is maintained throughout the complex brain stem pathways and is ultimately expressed in the primary auditory cortex.

Despite the frequency selectivity of the basilar membrane and organ of Corti hair cells, a simple frequency-place model cannot account for the extraordinary capabilities of the auditory system to discrimination pitch. For example, the impulses generated in the auditory nerve of animals is synchronous up to several thousand hertz, but any single nerve fiber is only capable of firing at a rate of a few hundred hertz. Thus, vibrations of the basilar membrane at greater than a few hundred hertz will not be coded as such by any individual auditory unit. Instead, individual fibers respond sequentially and in alternating fashion, such that much higher frequencies can be coded. Exactly how the higher auditory centers process this sort of information is not well known, but the degree of synchrony decreases as the impulses ascend brain stem auditory pathways. The high level of pitch discrimination we enjoy probably involves the processing of both place and impulse frequency information, and undubitably involves considerable modulation of such input by brain stem nuclei. In fact, modulation could even occur at the level of the cochlea, specifically within the organ of Corti. Although the central influence on hair cell activity is not well understood, it is reasonable to suppose that efferent input to the external cells somehow contributes to fine pitch discrimination.

## 5.3.4 The Cochlear Nerve

The fibers that form the cochlear nerve begin in the bipolar neurons forming the spiral ganglion of Corti. This spiral ganglion sits in a bony cavity at the base of the osseous spiral lamina (junction between the spiral lamina and modiolus) (Fig. 5.8). Dendritic fibers of the spiral ganglion course through many fine bony channels in the osseous spiral lamina to synapse with the hair cells of the organ of Corti. Depolarization of the hair cells results in stimulation of the fibers of the cochlear nerve and propagation of the impulses to brain stem nuclei. A spiral chain of axons extends from the spiral ganglion to leave the modiolus via a row of extremely fine spiral bony perforations at the apex of the internal auditory canal. These fibers unite to form the cochlear nerve within the anterior inferior quadrant of the internal auditory canal (Fig. 5.9). The cochlear nerve courses through the internal auditory canal and cerebellar pontine angle cistern to enter the brain stem at the ponto-medullary junction (Fig. 5.9). As discussed above, potentials recorded from the auditory fibers exiting the cochlea are temporally correlated to the frequency of the auditory stimulus. Also, the rate of response and the total number of activated fibers increase with increasing sound intensity, thereby providing a greater neural discharge per unit of time which is apparent in both peripheral and higher auditory centers.

## 5.3.5 The Brain Stem

The anatomy of brain stem auditory pathways is extremely complex and probably reflects the functional complexity of the auditory system. Within the brain stem, the cochlear fibers enter a recondite sophisticated network consisting of fiber tracts and nuclei linking the cochlear nerve with the auditory cortex. While cochlear fibers entering the brain stem arise

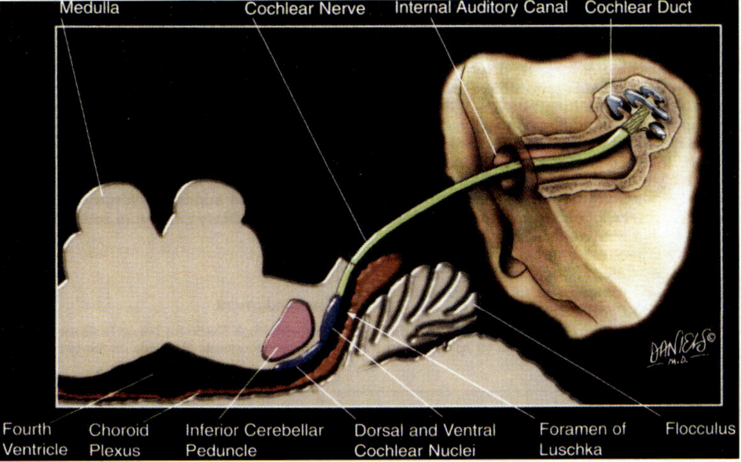


**Fig. 5.9.** Schematic of the cochlear nerve. The cochlear nerve extends through the internal auditory canal and the cerebellopontine angle cistern to synapse with dorsal and ventral cochlear nuclei. These nuclei are located lateral to the inferior cerebellar peduncle and form a slight bulge along the posterior lateral sufrace of the upper medula. (From Swartz et al. 1996b)

from first-order neurons, most neurons reaching the primary auditory cortex are in fact fourth order. The cochlear nuclei contain in the order of 10,000 neurons, but the number of neurons in the ascending auditory nuclei substantially increases, to 35,000–40,000 in the superior olivary and lateral lemniscus nuclei, 350,000–400,000 in the inferior colliculi and medial geniculate bodies, and 10,000,000 in the auditory cortex. Thus, the amplification of neurons in the nuclei of the auditory pathway implies a considerable potential for processing sound stimuli at both the brain stem and cortical levels. In addition, second- and third-order neurons in the brain stem give off collaterals to the reticular formation, providing an indirect sensory pathway to the cortex. Thus, auditory processing in the brain stem may impact arousal and attention functions as well. The conventional description of the brain stem auditory pathways as merely a series of conduits that relay signals from the cochlea to the auditory cortex is probably a specious paradigm, and more recent understanding of brain stem auditory function challenges the persistent notion that the auditory cortex is necessary for the processing of all auditory information.

The anatomic and functional components of the brain stem auditory system are not completely defined at this point, but a framework can be broadly conceptualized as a lattice of fibers and associated nuclei, with main ascending components at the more lateral aspect of the brain stem linked by tracts that cross the midline. The auditory pathways are distributed across many areas: the pontomedullary junction, pons, midbrain, and posterior diencephalon (medial geniculate bodies). A series of nuclei are symmetrically distributed on both sides of the midline as discussed below. Some of the fiber tracts, which interconnect the nuclei, also cross the midline. The majority of the fibers ascend toward the cortex, although a small proportion of fibers form descending pathways from the cortex to the cochlea.

## 5.3.6 The Cochlear Nuclei

The cochlear nerve terminates synapsing with ipsilateral second-order neurons of the cochlear nuclei, which are situated at the lateral aspect of the lower pons and upper medulla near the lateral surface of the inferior cerebellar peduncles (Figs. 5.9, 5.10). The contour of the dorsal cochlear nucleus produces a small protrusion on the farthest lateral aspect of the IV ventricular floor (acoustic tubercle). Because of the purely ipsilateral contribution from the cochlea, lesions near this location can cause unilateral hearing loss. The cochlear nuclei consist of ventral and dorsal components. The ventral cochlear nucleus can be subdivided further into anteroventral and posteroventral nuclei. Auditory units of the cochlear nuclei are sensitive to specific frequencies and are tonotopically organized (Fig. 5.11). Some of the auditory units, however, are inhibitory and serve to filter, or refine, the impulses propagated from the cochlea. Also, the number of discharges in auditory units of the cochlear nuclei is proportional to the intensity of the auditory stimulus. The neurons of

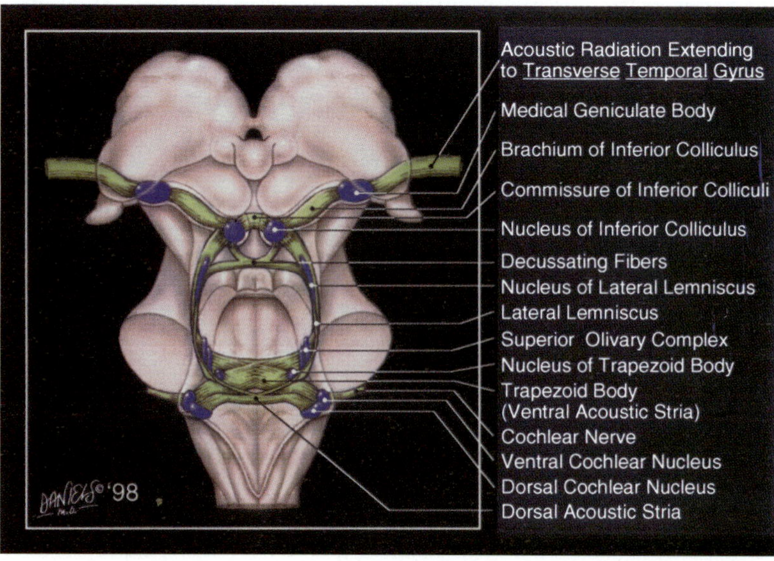


**Fig. 5.10.** Schematic of the nuclei and fiber tracts of the brain stem auditory pathways. Fiber tracts and nuclei are oriented in the lateral aspect of the brain stem, with multiple crossing fibers. Note the extensive interconnections of the brainstem auditory nuclei below the level of the medial geniculate bodies. (From Mark et al. 1998)

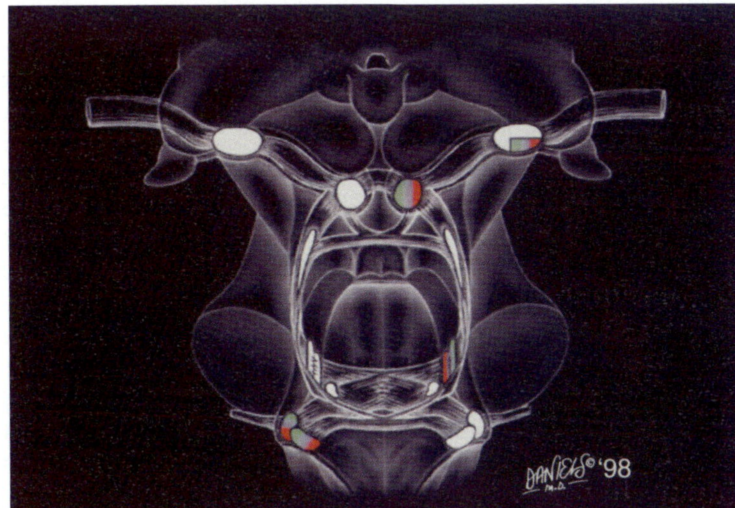


**Fig. 5.11.** Schematic of the tonotopic organization within the brainstem auditory nuclei. The tonotopic orientation within the cochlea is maintained throughout the complex auditory pathways of the brain stem and ultimately expressed in the auditory cortex. (From Mark et al. 1998) Red=low frequency, Green=high frequency

the cochlear nucleus are capable of coding the temporal sound patterns propagated through cochlear nerve discharges. The frequency, amplitude, and temporal features of sound coded in the cochlear nuclei are transmitted throughout ascending auditory nuclei of the brain stem, where considerable modulation of this input takes place.

The second-order neurons of the cochlear nuclei give rise to three major fiber bands that cross the midline: the trapezoid body, dorsal acoustic stria, and intermediate acoustic stria (Fig. 5.10). The trapezoid body, which is the largest of these fiber bands, arises from the ventral cochlear nucleus and courses along the ventral border of the pontine tegmentum. The fibers of the trapezoid body form a gentle arc across the midline, passing through or ventral to the medial lemniscus (ascending sensory fibers from the spinal cord) to reach the contralateral ventrolateral aspect of the pontine tegmentum. Most of the fibers then turn sharply cephalad just dorsolateral to the superior olivary complex to help form the large ascending tract of the lateral lemniscus. The smaller dorsal acoustic strias arise from the dorsal cochlear nucleus and crosses the midline dorsal to the trapezoid body but ventral to the medial longitudinal fasciculus. Most, but not all, of the fiber bundles of the dorsal acoustic stria enter the contralateral lateral lemniscus. The intermediate acoustic stria, which arises from the posteroventral cochlear nucleus, is the smallest of three major fiber groups. The fibers of the intermediate acoustic stria lie dorsal to the trapezoid body in the midline and also contribute to the contralateral lateral lemniscus.

### 5.3.7 The Superior Olivary Complex

Embedded in the trapezoid body is a group of nuclei that form the superior olivary complex (Fig. 5.10). The superior olivary complex consists of the medial and lateral superior olivary nuclei and the nucleus of the trapezoid body. The nucleus of the trapezoid body and the lateral superior olivary nucleus, however, are poorly developed in man. The superior olivary nuclei are the first to receive fiber contributions from both ears, and this region is thought to function in the localization of sound by way of neuronal sensitivities to interaural differences in sound phase and intensity. Surrounding the three cell masses of the superior olivary complex is a zone of varying cell sizes, sometimes collectively designated the periolivary nuclei. The use of the term periolivary nucleus has also been limited to the zone of cells dorsal and medial to the medial superior olivary nucleus. The cells ventral to the superior olivary complex have then been called the preolivary nuclei and the cells dorsal to the complex, the retro-olivary nuclei. The role of the periolivary nuclei is another point of obfuscation, as these nuclei were formerly believed to involve only descending pathways but more current investigations also suggest a role in the ascending fibers. An efferent pathway that crosses the midline in this portion of the brain stem but is not usually discussed with the fibers crossing above is the olivocochlear fascicle or bundle of Rasmussen, which originates in the periolivary nuclei and projects to the cochlea, forming a mechanism for the central nervous system to influence its own sensory input. These fibers provide inhibitory input to the hair cells and the cells of the spiral ganglion, thereby reducing auditory nerve activity to acoustic stimuli.

### 5.3.8 The Nuclei of the Lateral Lemniscus

The lateral lemniscus is the principal ascending auditory pathway of the brain stem (Fig. 5.10). Its fibers are positioned at the dorsolateral aspect of the pontine tegmentum to reach the midbrain, where they terminate at the inferior colliculus. Ventral and dorsal nuclei of the lateral lemniscus are embedded in the fibers of the lateral lemniscus (Fig. 5.10). The dorsal nucleus of the lateral lemniscus, however, is positioned rostral to the ventral component and immediately ventral to the inferior colliculus. The role of the nuclei of the lateral lemniscus in auditory processing in humans is not well known, but it has been suggested that they have a function in echolocation in bats. Neurons in the lateral lemniscus of bats are apparently capable of synchronizing to FM signals with high temporal resolution. These ventral and dorsal nuclei both receive some ascending projections from the lateral lemniscus and contribute fibers to that main ascending pathway. In addition, these nuclei are linked by the commissure or decussation of the lateral lemniscus (Probst's commissure), which contains commissural fibers from the left and right dorsal nuclei of the lateral lemniscus and also fibers passing from those nuclei to the contralateral inferior colliculi.

### 5.3.9 The Nuclei of the Inferior Colliculus and Medial Geniculate Bodies

The midbrain auditory nuclei, as the major relay to the cortex, must be able to code information concerning sound patterns and source propagated from the lower brain stem centers. The inferior colliculus (Fig. 5.10), the lower of the midbrain auditory centers, contains a compact central nucleus and more diffuse lateral zone gray matter, with neurons that respond to ascending AM and FM signals. The inferior colliculus receives both ascending fiber projections from the lateral lemniscus and some descending auditory projections from the cortex. The commissure of the inferior colliculi connects the inferior colliculi. The ascending auditory fibers from the inferior colliculus project to the diencephalic medial geniculate body (Fig. 5.10), which is part of the dorsal thalamus. These fibers from the inferior colliculus to the medial geniculate body form the brachium of the inferior colliculus, which is visible as a surface protuberance on the dorsolateral aspect of the upper brain stem situated between the brachium of the superior colliculus and the cerebral peduncle.

The medial geniculate body is the final relay of auditory information to the auditory cortex (Fig. 5.10). After receiving fibers from the inferior colliculus, the medial geniculate body projects to the ipsilateral auditory cortex via the geniculocortical fibers (auditory radiation), which passes laterally traversing the sublenticular portion of the internal capsule. The medial geniculate body can be subdivided into medial, dorsal, and ventral nuclear divisions. Aside from relaying brain stem signals, the role of these nuclei has been less well studied than the nuclei of the lower auditory centers. Commissural fibers connecting the medial geniculate bodies have yet to be identified, but some auditory cortical regions are linked to the contralateral cortex via the corpus callosum.

The ascending auditory fibers reaching the cortex are also organized by "core" and "belt" projections. Those fiber projections designated as "core" ultimately reach the primary auditory cortex, while the "belt" fibers terminate in the auditory fields that surround the primary auditory cortex (auditory association cortex). At the level of the inferior colliculus, the central nucleus project the core fibers while the lateral zone projects the belt fibers. At higher levels, the ventral nucleus of the medial geniculate body gives rise to the core projections while the remaining nuclear divisions (dorsal and medial) project to the belt area.

### 5.3.10 Tonotopic Organization of the Brain Stem Nuclei

Many anatomic details of the human brainstem auditory system are unresolved, but some organizational patterns can be appreciated. One characteristic feature, for instance, is a tonotopic or cochleotopic organization (Fig. 5.11). At the level of the cochlear nucleus, the apical cochlear fibers (low frequency) project to the ventral portion of the cochlear nuclear complex, while the fibers from the basal turn of the cochlea (high frequency) project to the dorsal aspect of the complex. The full range of frequencies is also distributed in the nucleus of the trapezoid body. The lower frequencies project to the better developed medial nucleus of the superior olivary complex, while the lower frequencies can be found in the less highly developed lateral nucleus. This tonotopic organization can also be found at a more superior level, i.e. that of the inferior colliculus, where the higher frequencies are located at the ventromedial aspect of the central nucleus and the lower frequencies at the dorsolateral aspect of the same nucleus. At the diencephalic level, the ventral nucleus of the medial geniculate body also demonstrates a cochleotopic organization, with the high and low frequencies found at the medial and lateral aspects, respectively. The fact that the frequency representation in the cochlea is maintained throughout the afferent brain stem pathways underlines the importance of the place-frequency phenomenon in the perception of pitch. However, it is important to recognize that central efferent pathways also have important functions that may modulate the perception of pitch. For example, descending fibers from the inferior colliculus, the nuclei of the lateral lemniscus, and superior olivary nuclei inhibit impulses generated by certain frequencies, enhancing other frequencies not subject to central inhibition. These pathways act as a spectral filter of auditory stimuli resulting in a phenomenon known as auditory sharpening.

### 5.3.11 Bilateral Representation of Brain Stem Auditory Nuclei

The anatomy of the fiber tracts and nuclei of the brainstem component of the auditory system does not readily lend itself to a simple schematic model. The various tracts and intercalated nuclei allow for multiple permutations of neuronal activation for any auditory stimulus. Closer evaluation of these brain stem components also reveals an increasing degree of anatomic complexity. Many of the fibers from the cochlear nucleus that form the trapezoid body, for example, extend across the midline to help form the contralateral lateral lemniscus, but some trapezoid fibers terminate in various components of the ipsi- and contralateral superior olivary complexes. Fibers from these complexes can then project to the ipsi- or contralateral lateral lemnisci relative to the side of cochlear stimulation. The dorsal acoustic stria enters the contralateral lateral lemniscus but also sends fibers to the contralateral lateral superior olivary nucleus, ventral and dorsal nuclei of the lateral lemniscus, and central nucleus of the inferior colliculus. The intermediate acoustic stria projects fibers to the ipsi- and contralateral retro- and periolivary nuclei and contralateral ventral nucleus of the lateral lemniscus and inferior colliculus. The lateral lemniscus consists of tertiary fibers from the superior olivary complexes and crossed secondary fibers from the three auditory stria, but no direct fibers from the ipsilateral cochlear nuclei. The lateral lemniscus, therefore, will predominantly transmit impulses from the contralateral cochlear nucleus, though it will also transmit some impulses from the ipsilateral side via the superior olivary complex.

The bilateral representation of auditory input (above the cochlear nucleus), the extensive interconnections of the brain stem auditory pathways, and the amplification of neurons in the brain stem nuclei, have significant implications for the localization of pathologic conditions of the auditory system. For example, unilateral lesions of the auditory pathways above the level of the cochlear nucleus result in no detectable loss of hearing. Also, destruction of auditory cortices bilaterally results in no change in pure tone hearing thresholds. On the other hand, destruction of inferior colliculi results in a 15-dB loss of threshold and destruction of the auditory system from midbrain to cortex results in a 40-dB loss of threshold. Thus, the auditory cortex is not required to perceive pure tone stimuli, and the auditory sensitivity to pure tones is primarily below the inferior colliculus. Owing to amplification and modulation in the brainstem auditory pathways, nearly normal audiograms can be obtained with a 75% loss of neurons in the cochlear nerve.

### 5.3.12 The Primary Auditory Cortex

The cerebral cortex receives transmissions from the brain stem, but the functional and anatomic details related to sound processing and hearing may be even more enigmatic than the brain stem. As one ascends the auditory pathways, it becomes more and more difficult to predict the responses to complex signals on the basis of nuclear responses to pure tones, and at the level of the cortex selectivity becomes a more critical factor in sound processing. Primary and association auditory cortical neurons respond to incoming amplitude, frequency, and temporal sound characteristics, but how the cortex processes such patterns in unclear. The primary auditory cortex is a landmark, however, that can be identified even though all cortical areas responsible for processing all facets of sound and language have yet to be completely elucidated.

The primary auditory cortex is located within the transverse temporal gyrus (TTG), also known as the gyrus of Heschl (Fig. 5.12). This gyrus of Heschl forms part of the superior surface of the temporal lobe, which is buried within the sylvian (lateral) fissure and difficult to see from the lateral aspect. The superior surface of the temporal lobe is revealed by removal of the lateral-inferior portions of the frontal and parietal lobes, which form the superior margin (operculum) of the sylvian fissure. Three distinct parts can then be visualized (Fig. 5.12). The most anterior component of the superior temporal gyrus (STG) surface is the planum polare, which is a gyrus that is separated from the adjacent insular cortex by the inferior circular sulcus. The gyrus of Heschl is immediately posterior to planum polare. Heschl's gyrus can be either one or two gyri (frequently single on the left but double on the right). When two gyri are present, the anterior and posterior temporal gyri are separated by the intermediate transverse temporal sulcus. The transverse temporal gyri are usually obliquely oriented, with a more posterior medial margin and more anteriorly positioned lateral aspect forming a visible lobule on the lateral surface of the temporal lobe grooved by the sulcus acousticus, which is a short, superiorly oriented branch from the superior temporal sulcus.

The primary auditory cortex (Brodmann's area 41) is located on Heschl's gyrus. Auditory association cortex surrounds the primary auditory areas in adjacent cortical areas of the superior temporal gyrus (including portions of the TTG). When two Heschl's gyri are present, the primary auditory cortex is found on the anterior temporal gyrus while the posterior temporal gyrus is largely an auditory association area (Brodmann's area 42). Functional neuroimaging studies to date have had little success in differentiating primary from association cortex within the TTG, and thus, auditory association areas in the TTG are presumed on the basis of cytoarchitectural studies. Other association areas are located in the middle sector of the STG and just below in the middle temporal gyrus. The most posterior component of the STG superior surface is the planum temporale (Fig. 5.12), which is separated from the TTG by the transverse temporal sulcus and is frequently also visible on the lateral surface of the temporal lobe. The planum temporale is variable in size, but is commonly larger on the left compared to the right, corresponding to a solitary Heschl's gyrus on the left. The planum temporale also probably contains auditory association cortex, but is in close proximity to cortex identified as receptive language areas in the farthest posterior aspect of the STG and the supramarginal gyrus.

## 5.4 Echoplanar Acoustic Scanner Noise

Though many of the reported FMRI paradigms are similar in design to those used in PET imaging, FMRI techniques are unique and contain potential confounding variables that are not associated with other techniques. For echoplanar FMRI investigations of the auditory system, background acoustic scanner

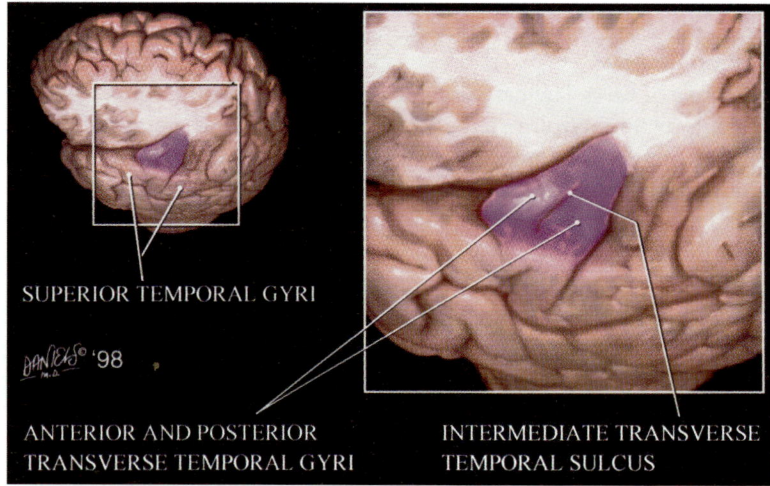


**Fig. 5.12.** Anatomic specimen with frontal and parietal opercular regions removed to expose the TTG (*purple highlight*). On the superior surface of the STG, the TTG is bordered by the planum polari anteriorly and the planum temporali posteriorly. The intermediate transverse temporal sulcus may be absent, partial or complete, dividing the TTG into two distinct gyri. When this last situation is the case, primary cortex is generally located anteriorly, while auditory association cortex is generally located within the posterior aspect of the transverse temporal gyri. (Modified from Strainer et al. 1997)

noise produced by the pulse sequence is among the most worrisome (ULMER et al. 1996b; BANDETTINI et al. 1997; TALAVAGE and EDMISTER 1998) and warrants special consideration in any discussion of auditory FMRI. Although the potential problems related to acoustic scanner noise have largely been ignored in the FMRI literature, results from many auditory FMRI investigations will remain inconclusive until the problem of acoustic scanner noise is solved. Implicit in the interpretations of much of the FMRI data is the assumption that acoustic scanner noise is a constant experimental condition with saturating effects in limited areas of the auditory cortex and that task-induced activation represents cortical neuronal activity above and beyond that produced by the constant background state. While this may be true in the primary auditory cortex, the full effect of acoustic scanner noise on the auditory and language system, and the ultimate effect on FMRI experiments, remain unclear. Unfortunately, earplugs and other sound-dampening developments have had limited success in neutralizing ambient scanner noise to date.

There are at least two perspectives from which to consider the potential confounding effects of echoplanar acoustic scanner noise. First, scanner noise could interfere with FMRI results by activating the auditory and language cortices (ULMER et al. 1996a; BANDETTINI et al. 1997; TALAVAGE and EDMISTER 1998) during the intended "resting" state of the experiment. Secondly, scanner noise could alter the perceptions of auditory stimuli, which then secondarily change the patterns of brain activation in response to the stimulus (ULMER et al. 1998a, b). Early reports suggest that echoplanar noise may substantially reduce task induced signal changes in the auditory cortex by 30% (TALAVAGE and EDMISTER 1998) and might act to saturate some cortical regions, so that activation to superimposed auditory stimuli is underestimated. However, the response to such auditory stimuli is far too complex to predict the effects of scanner noise on cortical activation patterns. Because most central auditory neurons are spontaneously active, cochlear stimulation can be excitatory or inhibitory, or have little effect. Thus the response of a neuron to cochlear input from one type of stimulus may differ significantly when that same stimulus is superimposed on sounds such as background acoustic scanner noise. The next sections of this chapter address some of the potential confounding effects from acoustic echoplanar scanner noise on FMRI studies of auditory (and language) function.

### 5.4.1 Characteristics of Acoustic Echoplanar Scanner Noise

In echoplanar imaging, the fast switching of gradients in the gradient coil causes acoustic noise. Even though most coils are torque balanced, current flow in the wire of the coil induces an electromagnetic force, which tends to cause the wire to change its position. For each wire that is supplied with a current, a symmetrically opposed wire is also given a similar current to cancel this force. This sudden and very rapid change in gradient field produces the complex acoustic scanner noise observed during an FMRI experiment. As the gradient switching rate is increased, the resulting acoustic noise is also increased. For FMRI using echoplanar techniques (and other fast imaging techniques), the data are acquired in a periodic fashion. The effect of this is to produce acoustic noise that is not random, but is of a patterned nature. The intensity of echoplanar acoustic noise has been reported to reach more than 100 dB in the head coil (TALAVAGE and EDMISTER 1998), spanning frequencies in the optimal hearing range (125-8000 Hz) and those present in conversational speech (ULMER et al. 1996a, b). The potential sources of the periodic signals present in the echoplanar sequence are several, including the gradient switching, slice acquisition, and RF excitation rates incorporated in the pulse program. The faster the imaging data is acquired, the louder and higher in pitch the resulting acoustic noise will sound. Also, the pattern and pitch of the noise can be altered by adjusting the TR or TE, or by using interleaved sequences. Thus, altering the imaging pulse sequence parameters can change the character of the acoustic scanner noise considerably (ULMER et al. 1998b).

In addition to encoding FM signals, the auditory system in mammals is capable of encoding the periodic modulations of sound amplitude (AM signals) present in complex stimuli at the cochlear and brain stem levels, ultimately expressed in the primary auditory cortex and other regional cortical fields (LANGNER 1992). That is to say that the temporal patterns of sound are processed beyond simple sensation and spatially represented in specific cortical fields. The complex sounds produced by the fast switching of gradients in echoplanar imaging are distinctly periodic in nature. The temporal properties, or periodicity, of AM signals in acoustic scanner noise might therefore also activate analogous cortical areas in humans. These complex signals could also alter activation patterns by altering perceptions of stimulus periodicity. For example, amplitude modulations with periodic envelopes at frequencies below approximately 20 Hz are associated with the perception of rhythm and correspond to the periodicity of running speech. Periodic amplitude modulations between 10 and 200 Hz result in an unpleasant perception known as roughness. Faster periodic amplitude modulations result in the perception of periodicity pitch and are present in voiced speech sounds. Depending on the sequence parameters, the periodic signals of echoplanar acoustic scanner noise could overlap with each of these AM frequency ranges and should be considered in the design of FMRI experiments (Ulmer et al. 1998a, b). Interestingly, normal volunteers have reported a range of subjective effects from listening to taped scanner noise, including no effect, an irritating sound, or a rhythm-like sound (Ulmer et al. 1998a). Auditory association cortex activation patterns have been shown to be sensitive to the perceived rate of auditory stimulus presentation (Binder et al. 1994b; Dhankar et al. 1997), which could also be altered by these superimposed periodic scanner noises.

## 5.4.2 Perceptual Effects of Acoustic Scanner Noise

Given the physical characteristics of acoustic echoplanar scanner noise, it is not altogether unreasonable to suggest that auditory perceptions and activation patterns in response to superimposed stimuli may be altered under some experimental conditions. In a recent study, an analysis of echoplanar noise revealed a distribution of tonal frequencies throughout the optimal frequency range (125–8000 Hz) of human hearing (Ulmer et al. 1998a), overlapping with those frequencies comprising normal conversational speech (Northern and Downs 1991). In a follow-up study, scanner noise was shown to inhibit the normal perception of pure tones throughout that same range of optimal frequencies (Fig. 5.13a) (Ulmer et al. 1998b). The threshold effect was dependent on the echoplanar pulse sequence parameters, and was most pronounced at the higher rates of scanner noise production. The observed increase in tone thresholds from background acoustic scanner noise was not linear across the frequency spectrum, but dominant in the range of 750–1500 Hz. Also, recent observations suggest that threshold baselines of patients with high-frequency hearing loss differs from those of normal individuals in the presence of echoplanar scanner noise, but in a manner unlike that observed between these groups in a quiet setting (Fig. 5.14) (Ulmer et al. 1998c).

Functional MRI investigators studying the processing of individual words and speech components in normal and hearing-impaired subjects should consider the nonlinear spectral effects of scanner noise on hearing thresholds of these individuals. Language components that are not evenly distributed throughout the frequency spectrum (Fig. 5.13b), such as consonants, vowels, or various pho-

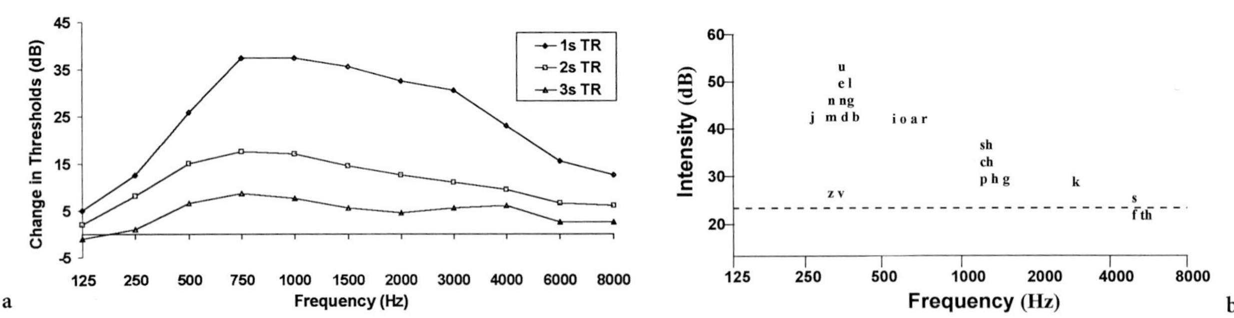


**Fig. 5.13.** **a** Change in pure tone hearing thresholds (dB) of normal individuals ($n$=10) across the optimal hearing frequency spectrum, in the presence of echoplanar acoustic scanner noise produced at three separate noise rates. The rate of noise production was altered by varying only the repetition times (*TR*), while keeping all the parameters including slice number (10 slices) constant. The effect on pure tone hearing thresholds is increased as the rate of scanner noise is increased (i.e. short TR). However, the threshold effect is nonlinear across the frequency spectrum, with peak effects at 750 and 1000 Hz. (Modified from Ulmer et al. 1998b) **b** Frequency distribution of letters and language sounds. Vowels comprise lower frequency sounds, while consonants necessary for distinguishing words comprise primarily higher frequency sounds. *Straight dotted line* represents normal upper limit hearing thresholds. Note the potential effects of a nonhorizontal threshold baseline in the presence of scanner noise (**a**), on the perception of various speech components. (Modified from Ulmer et al. 1998b)

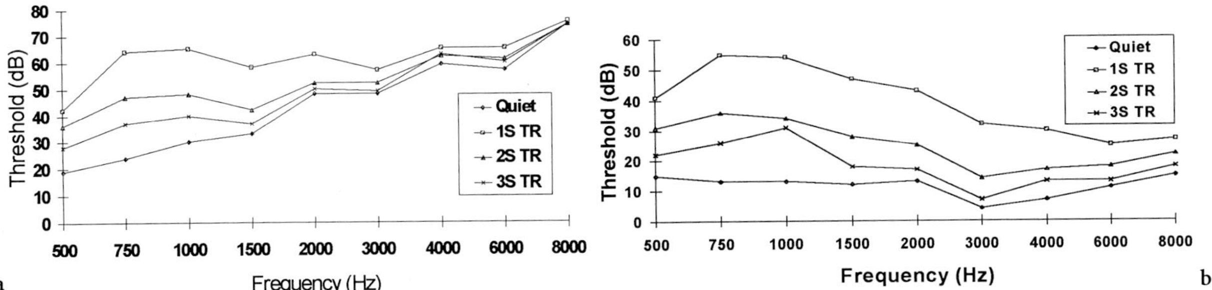


**Fig. 5.14.** Pure tone hearing thresholds **a** in normal hearing individuals ($n$=15) and **b** individuals with high frequency hearing loss ($n$=3) in the presence of echoplanar acoustic scanner noise produced at three separate noise rates. The noise rates are determined by adjusting the repetition times (*TR*) while keeping all other parameters, including slice number (10 slices), constant. Because of the underlying sensorineural hearing loss in the hearing-impaired group, threshold baselines differ between these groups, depending on the rate of background echoplanar acoustic scanner noise

nemes, could be altered in the presence of acoustic scanner noise. Spondees used to test speech thresholds could be perceived with altered syllable emphasis in the presence of acoustic scanner noise as the words span certain frequency spectra. Unequal threshold effects across the frequency spectrum in the presence of high-periodic-rate echoplanar scanner noise could grossly distort the perception of speech spanning the same spectra. Tonotopic mapping and other experiments using a range of frequencies might consider delivering tones at equivalent levels above thresholds determined in the presence of scanner noise, because intensity level impacts on auditory cortical activation patterns (Ulmer et al. 1996a, 1998d; Strainer et al. 1997). Frequency studies using a spectral sweep experimental design should benefit from adjusting intensity levels to the shape of a predetermined threshold curve established for the specific echoplanar sequence to be used in the experiment. Thus, it is clear that standard audiometric tests developed to reference normal-hearing and hearing-impaired individuals in a quiet setting may not be analogous to similar audiometric techniques used for these same individuals in the presence of some types of acoustic scanner noise.

### 5.4.3 Cortical Activation from Acoustic Scanner Noise

A recent FMRI experiment in which taped scanner noise was played to normal-hearing volunteers showed robust activation in primary auditory cortex, as well as auditory association and language cortex in some cases (Fig 5.15) (Ulmer et al. 1998a). The distribution of cortical activity in response to taped acoustic scanner noise was similar to that seen with spoken text, although significantly less. The results of the study suggested that auditory and language cortical activation to taped acoustic scanner noise may have been a response to temporal and spectral properties similar to those present in speech. The cortical activation response was quite variable between subjects (Fig. 5.15) and constant within subjects, suggesting that the perceived character of echoplanar scanner noise may be largely subject dependent. Such sensitivity of the auditory system to acoustic echoplanar noise has important implications for the experimental design and interpretation of FMRI experiments, in which auditory and language tasks are performed. Background acoustic scanner noise could potentially have saturating or synergistic effects in particular cortical areas when combined with various types of auditory task stimuli, by virtue of altered AM and FM perception or other sound interactions. As mentioned previously, cochlear input can have an excitatory or inhibitory effect or no effect on spontaneously active auditory cortical neurons. In effect, ambient acoustic scanner noise could act as a sensitizing stimulus in some experimental conditions and a habituating stimulus in others. Increased complexity of some auditory stimuli has been shown to increase activation within association cortex in FMRI (Ulmer et al. 1996b; Strainer et al. 1997) (Figs. 5.2b, and 5.16) and other functional neuroimaging experiments, but direct effects of scanner noise could also saturate some cortical regions (Talavage and Edmister 1998). These and other questions are subjects for future research.

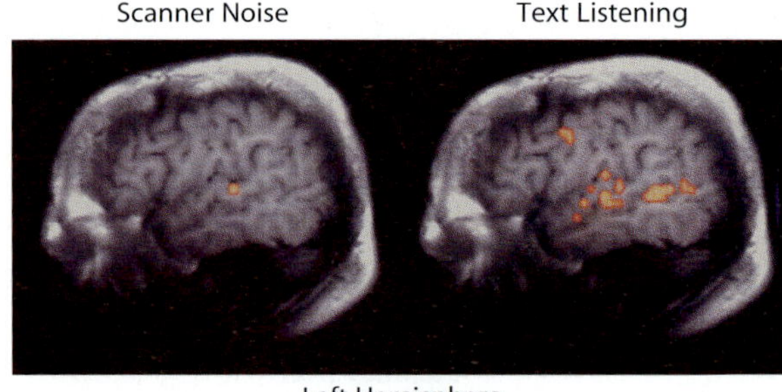


a

Scanner Noise Text Listening

Left Hemisphere

b

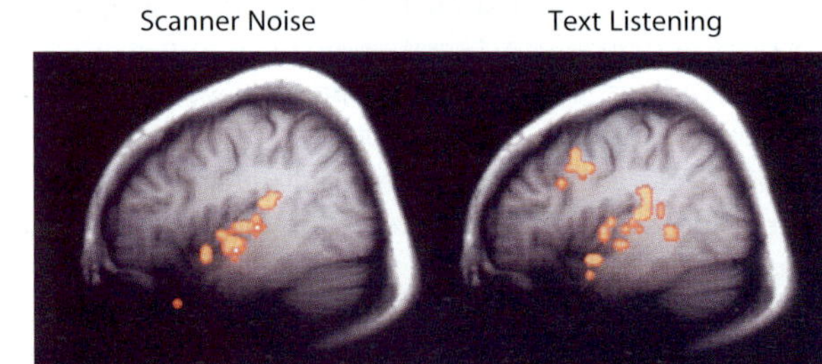


c

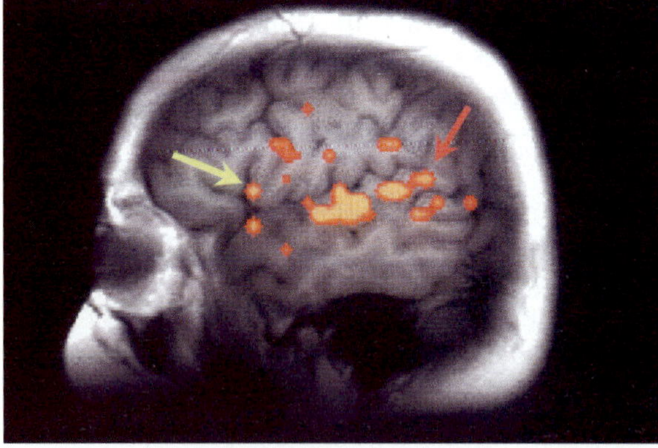

d

**Fig. 5.15a–d.** Cortical activation in response to taped echoplanar acoustic scanner noise and passive text listening in three individuals. In some individuals, scanner noise activated only the transverse TTG (**a**), while in others, primary and auditory association areas were activated by the scanner noise (**b**, **c**). In some individuals (**d**), activation was not only seen in the primary and auditory association cortex but also in posterior (*red arrow*) and anterior (*yellow arrow*) language regions. Activation of language relative cortex in some individuals is presumed to relate to temporal and spectral properties of scanner noise overlapping with those of conversational speech. (Modified from Ulmer et al. 1998a)

## 5.4.4 Reducing Acoustic Scanner Noise

Although echoplanar scanner noise is an experimental condition fraught with uncontrolled variables that potentially may impact on FMRI studies of the auditory system, it is not a problem that should discourage further research in this area. In fact, some influences of acoustic echoplanar scanner noise can be reduced simply by altering the pulse sequence parameters, because some perceptual effects are clearly related to the rate of echoplanar scanner noise production (Ulmer et al. 1998b). The noise-induced increases in hearing thresholds can be minimized by adjusting the pulse parameters to decrease the rate of periodic scanner noise production, thereby increasing the interval between scanner noise bursts (Fig. 5.13a). Lengthening the TR of the echoplanar sequence, which in turn lengthens imaging time, is one way to reduce periodic noise rates. Reducing the slice number for a given TR will also reduce the rate of acoustic noise production. It is important to recognize that a long TR with many slices can produce noise at a high periodic rate, while a short TR with few slices can produce noise at a low periodic rate. Thus, pulse parameters for any FMRI experiment must be tailored to achieve the desired brain coverage, BOLD contrast, and temporal resolution, while at the same time minimizing the confounding variables of acoustic scanner noise. Some effects of acoustic scanner noise may therefore be laboratory specific, affecting the comparison of results between institutions.

The preceeding discussions emphasize the need for further work to improve the techniques used to obtain auditory FMRI data, including delivery systems, earplugs and other sound-dampening measures, and development of coils and fast imaging sequences, which may reduce the level of ambient acoustic scanner noise. Development already under way of sequences that acquire imaging data nonuniformly throughout the TR and leave time for auditory stimuli to be delivered during a quiet period have promise (Talavage and Edmister 1998). These sequences acquire data in the first second or so of the sequence while leaving the remainder of the TR quiet, but such sequences are likely to result in the perception of interrupted speech or other stimuli that extend beyond the TR. Other investigators have recognized the importance of reducing scanner noise and have tackled this problem by altering the gradient coil design (Bowtell and Mansfield 1995; Mansfield et al.

1998). These quieter coils are designed such that the current used to create the gradient magnetic field, which also produces the acoustic noise, is reduced. However, there is a corresponding decrease in gradient strength with a design of this kind. Clearly, continued work is needed to reduce the effects of echoplanar acoustic noise on auditory FMRI experiments of the future.

## 5.5 FMRI of Auditory Cortical Function

Much of the recent FMRI research has centered on activation of the auditory system to a variety of tasks. Activation to pure tone stimuli has been investigated as a means of characterizing the response to changing intensity and the tonotopic organization within the primary auditory cortex (Ulmer et al. 1996b; Talavage et al. 1996, 1997a, b; Strainer et al. 1997). The central processing of speech and language has been investigated by delivering a variety of auditory stimuli including words, non-words, non-speech noise, and spoken text (Binder et al. 1994a, 1996; Berry et al. 1995). Finally, studies have suggested the potential utility of FMRI for preoperative cortical mapping of auditory and language cortex in patients with CNS tumors and epilepsy (Hinke et al. 1993; Desmond et al. 1995; Binder et al. 1995; Yetkin et al. 1996 ). Thus, investigators have used a wide variety of paradigms to study auditory and language function and to develop FMRI techniques for clinical applications. The ultimate aim of many investigators studying hearing is for FMRI to become a useful tool in the characterization and clinical evaluation of subjects with hearing disorders. Investigators have already reported FMRI results indicating the nondominant right STG as the primary site of decoding in prelingually deaf individuals performing lip-reading tasks (Shibata et al. 1998). Auditory association cortical activation to exogenous speech stimuli is reduced in schizophrenia during auditory hallucinations (David et al. 1996). A recent FMRI report also suggested unilaterally altered stimulus-induced activation in the midbrain of patients with tinnitus (Sigalovsky et al. 1998).

### 5.5.1 Auditory Cortical Activation

At this point, it is clear that our understanding of the integration of human primary auditory, auditory association, and language function is still evolving and is undoubtedly a subject for future FMRI research. However, it is important to recognize that these cortical areas are intimately associated spatially and functionally. In fact, FMRI and PET investigations of the auditory cortex have shown activation to simple and complex nonsemantic auditory input extending well into areas identified previously by PET and FMRI to represent posterior (receptive) language cortex (Figs. 5.15d, 5.17) (Roland 1993; Ulmer et al. 1997, 1998a), suggesting dual cortical function in these regions. Auditory processing of a variety of nonword stimuli may also be associated with activation of the inferior frontal gyrus (i.e. anterior language area) (Fig. 5.15d). Of course, anterior and posterior language-relevant cortex will also activate in response to auditory speech stimuli (Fig. 5.18). In general, though, as sounds become more complex activation is propagated from the primary auditory cortical region to immediate surrounding areas of the STG, planum temporale, and middle temporal gyrus containing auditory association cortex (Figs. 5.2b, 5.3, 5.4). Functional imaging studies have shown that the total area of activation within auditory association cortex increases with auditory stimulus complexity (Ulmer et al. 1996b; Roland 1993; Strainer et al. 1997) (Figs. 2b, 16). Because white noise activates essentially only the primary auditory cortex, while other stimuli also activate association cortex, it might be reasonable to conclude that association cortex functions to process patterned sound with nonrandom components (Fig. 5.15d). However, functional imaging investigators have had little success in proving the presence of a field-specific function of the association cortices of humans. Further, a discussion of receptive language function is beyond the scope of this chapter, particularly since Wernicke's area has yet to be precisely localized. The focus of the remainder of this chapter, instead, is on FMRI of the primary auditory cortex. Specifically, the next sections deal with the FMRI appearance of tonotopy and stimulus-intensity-dependent response in the transverse temporal gyrus.

### 5.5.2 FMRI of the Primary Auditory Cortex

The feasibility of FMRI as a technique to image cortical activation in the TTG to simple pure tone stimuli was first substantiated by Millen et al. (1995), showing a consistent activation response in normal-hearing individuals to a 1000-Hz pure tone

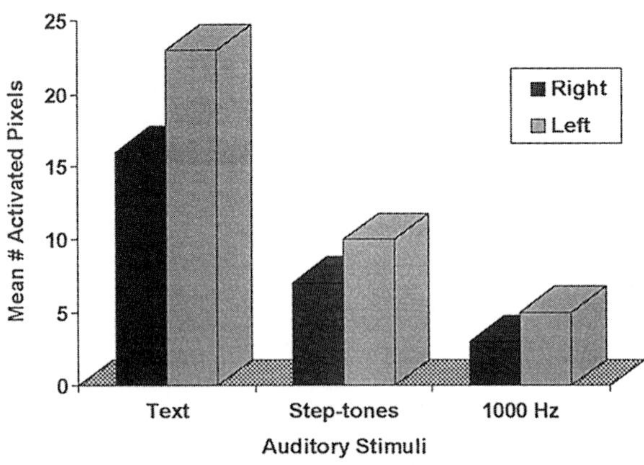


**Fig. 5.16.** Bar graph demonstrating mean number of activated pixels within auditory association cortex in right and left hemispheres of eight normal-hearing individuals. As the complexity of the auditory stimulus is increased from a simple pure tone (1000 Hz) to a series of step-tones and finally to passive text listening, the total area of activation within the auditory association cortex increases. Also note a non-significant trend toward left hemisphere dominance as the complexity of the stimuli is increased. (From Strainer et al. 1997)

stimulus played at 50 dB above threshold (dBSL) when it was determined in the presence of background acoustic scanner noise. Follow-up studies confirmed this technique and revealed a greater cortical response to 1000 Hz than to higher frequency pure tones, characterized by an increased area of TTG activity (Ulmer et al. 1996b, Strainer et al. 1997). In the latter investigation, several explanations that might account for such a phenomenon were suggested, including the possibility of a preferential cortical response to tones in the frequency spectrum dominant in conversational speech (i.e. 500–2000 Hz). Interestingly, other investigators have reported MEG results showing a differential M100 response to 1000 Hz compared with higher and lower frequencies (Roberts and Poeppel 1996). An alternative explanation to account for this effect is that the differences in activation areas were in some way due to sound interactions of the tone stimulus and background acoustic echoplanar scanner noise, which is also dominant in the 1000-Hz frequency range (Fig. 5.13a) (Ulmer et al. 1998b). Also, auditory association cortex contained within the TTG, which might be most sensitive to tones dominant in speech, could add to the increased area of TTG activity. Indeed, 1000-Hz stimuli have also been shown to activate auditory association cortex outside the TTG (Fig. 5.16) (Ulmer et al. 1996b; Strainer et al. 1997). However, neither of these auditory FMRI studies were designed to differentiate processing in the primary cortex from activity reflecting upstream brainstem processing.

Some primate studies have shown proportionally greater cortical activity contralateral to the side of auditory stimulation, but attempts to confirm such an effect with functional neuroimaging techniques in humans have met with variable and contradictory results (Roland 1993). FMRI investigations showing a lack of TTG sidedness in the response to pure tone stimuli, such as those described above, suggest that this relates to the abundance of interconnections and crossing fibers in auditory pathways of the brain stem. FMRI results showing association cortical activity to simple pure tone stimuli also fail to reveal any dominance effect in these areas (Fig. 5.16) (Ulmer et al. 1996b; Strainer et al. 1997). These findings are supported by lesion studies showing no effect on hearing acuity with unilateral insults to the auditory pathways above the level of the cochlear nucleus. Unilateral destruction of even the primary auditory cortex does not produce pure tone hearing loss in either ear.

### 5.5.3 Tonotopic Organization of the Primary Auditory Cortex

The tonotopic organization in the primary cortex is a reflection of tonotopy in the cochlea, which is maintained throughout the complex auditory pathways of the brain stem. Typically, the tonotopic organization of the primary auditory cortex is modeled with low frequencies activating the lateral aspect of the obliquely oriented TTG, while higher frequencies activate the medial aspect of the TTG. This general arrangement has been confirmed with PET and FMRI investigations (Lauter et al. 1985; Roland 1993; Ulmer et al. 1996b; Talavage et al. 1996; Strainer et al. 1997), but the results of these two imaging techniques differ somewhat. One early FMRI investigation of tonotopy indicated that lower frequency tones (i.e. 1000 Hz) were represented primarily in the lateral TTG, but also had significant representation in the medial aspect of the TTG (Ulmer et al. 1996b; Strainer et al. 1997). Also, low frequency tones activated cortex outside of the TTG, in areas traditionally defined as association cortex. Conversely, higher frequency tones (i.e. 4000 Hz) were represented almost exclusively in the medial aspect of the TTG. While the general low-frequency-

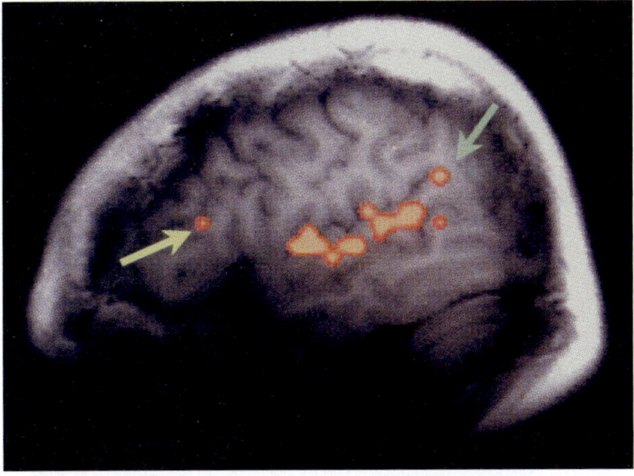

**Fig. 5.17.** Cortical activation map of auditory and language relevant cortex in the left hemisphere of a normal-hearing individual in response to random tones delivered via an audiometer. Note that in addition to primary and association auditory cortical activity in the temporal lobe, activation is present in the posterior language region (**green arrow**) and just anterior to the anterior language region (*yellow arrow*). These areas of activation may be immediately adjacent to language cortex or may represent dual cortical function within language cortex (cf. Fig. 5.18)

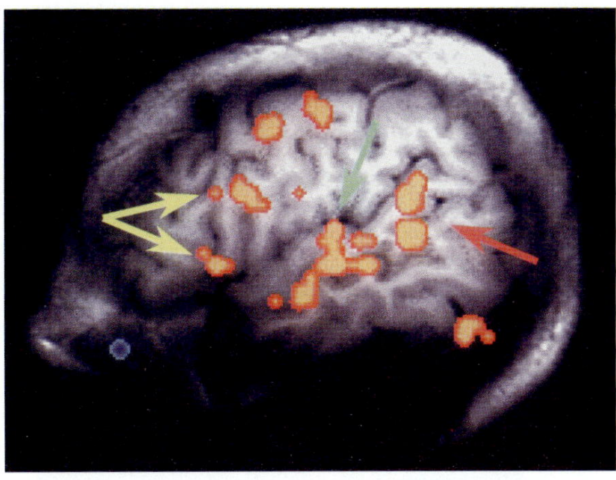

**Fig. 5.18.** Activation of primary (*green arrow*) and surrounding association auditory cortex, as well as posterior (*red arrow*) and anterior (*yellow arrow*) language areas of the left hemisphere in a normal-hearing individual in response to passive text listening

lateral and high-frequency-medial TTG representation held, these FMRI results suggested that the cortical tonotopic arrangement was more complex than is typically believed.

Since the initial FMRI studies of the primary cortex, more detailed high-resolution investigations of tonotopy in the auditory cortex have been carried out by Talavage et al. (1997a, b). These investigators used a frequency sweep stimulus to determine the orientation of shifting cortical activity, and flat mapping techniques to eliminate localization problems from the obliquely oriented regional sulci. Also, a much wider range of stimulus frequencies (125–8000 Hz) was used to map the cortical tonotopy than in the earlier investigations. Consequently, refinement of the FMRI technique in this way allowed these investigators to delineate frequency selectivity within the auditory cortex more precisely. The results of this study suggest that in fact there are multiple frequency-selective, tonotopically organized fields within the auditory cortex (Fig. 5.19). Some low-frequency representations were actually localized outside of the TTG, just anterior and posterior to Heschl's gyrus. In addition, the results showed low-frequency activity to be located primarily on the dome of the TTG and high-frequency activity, primarily in cortex lining the sulci that surrounds the TTG (Fig. 5.20a, b). Though the results are preliminary, they also suggest that the frequency-dependent shift in cortical activity could be divergent or convergent toward some frequency-selective fields at opposite spectral limits. In other words, some high-frequency zones are tonotopically oriented with respect to more than one low-frequency field, and some low-frequency zones are tonotopically oriented toward more than one high-frequency field (Fig. 5.19b). This work is clearly still evolving, but these intriguing and important findings will undoubtedly contribute significantly to our understanding of tonotopy in primary and surrounding auditory cortex.

### 5.5.4 Stimulus Intensity and Cortical Activation

In addition to coding frequency information, the cochlea codes information on sound amplitude, or intensity. Increased intensity of an auditory stimulus results in an increased rate of hair cell stimulation and an increased number of activated hair cells. The cochlear potential then reflects the intensity of the incoming stimulus. Corresponding evoked potentials can be detected in the cochlear nerve and various brain stem pathways and nuclei, with the appearance of individual system components dependent on the intensity of the stimulus. However, the

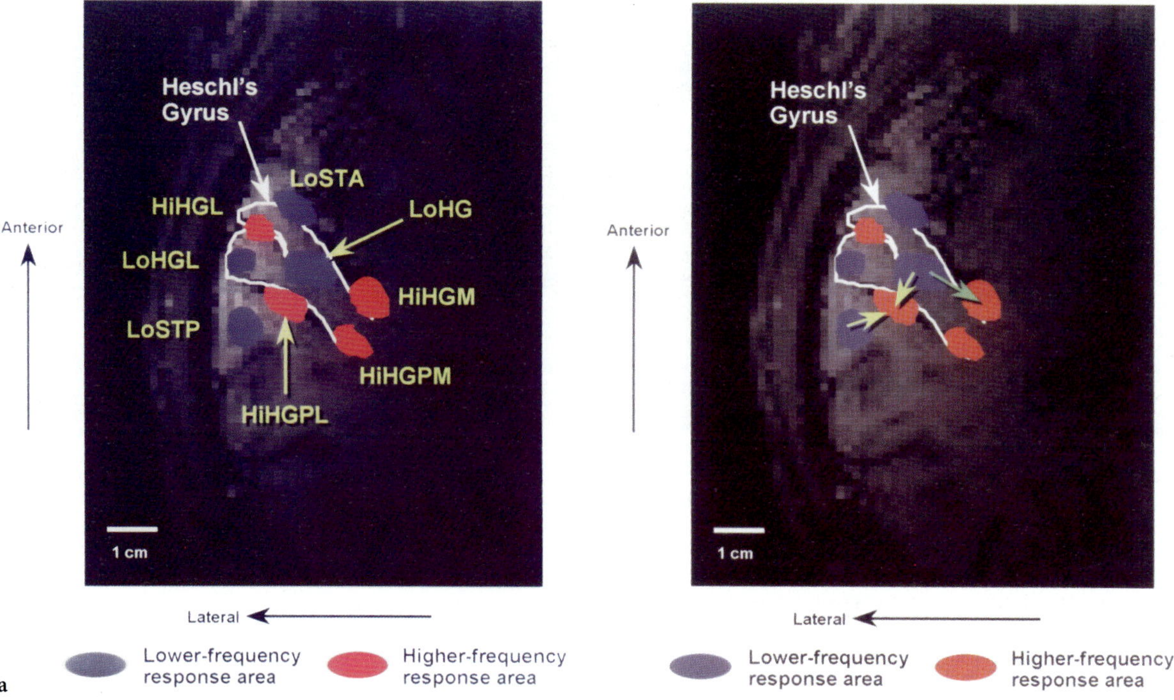


**Fig. 5.19.** **a** Summary of tonotopic cortical activation maps in and about the transverse temporal gyrus (Heschl's gyrus), illustrating multiple frequency-selective regions within the STG. Low frequency selectivity is located in the mid-portion of Heschl's gyrus (*LoHG*), laterally in Heschl's gyrus (*LoHGL*), in the planum polare (LoSTA) and in the planum temporale (*LoSTP*). High frequency selectivity is located within cortex lining the sulci about the TTG. Specific frequency-selective fields are designated in relation to Heschl's gyrus: *Lo* low frequency selectivity, *Hi* high frequency selectivity, *HG* Heschl's gyrus, *ST* superior temporal gyrus, *A* anterior, *P* posterior, *L* lateral, *M* medial. **b** While the exact tonotopic distribution of frequency-selective fields is still under investigation, the tonotopic orientation may be divergent or convergent from some low and high frequency selective areas. (From Talavage et al. with permission)

extent of sound intensity processing, or the lack thereof, in the primary auditory cortex is unclear. What is clear at this point is that cortical activation in the TTG, as measured by FMRI, is influenced by stimulus intensity. Recent FMRI studies have shown differing activation responses in Heschl's gyrus to changing pure tone intensities delivered monaurally (Ulmer et al. 1996b; Strainer et al. 1997; Ulmer et al. 1998d). The total area of activation in the TTG increased significantly as 1000-Hz stimuli determined in the presence of ambient acoustic scanner noise increased from threshold to 50 dB above threshold (Fig. 5.21). The activation response was graded as the intensity of the pure tone stimulus was increased in this range in a group of normal-hearing subjects. However, when the individual subject responses were analyzed separately, a step-wise increase in TTG activation area was generally observed, occurring at around 40– 50 dB above threshold in most cases. Also, the likelihood of bilateral activation increased with increasing tone intensity.

The reason for the increasing TTG activation with increasing tone intensities in FMRI studies is uncertain and awaits the results of ongoing research. Several possible explanations for this phenomenon come to mind. It is possible that the increased activity observed in the TTG is simply a reflection of the cochlear and/or brain stem response to increasing intensity. However, the step-wise cortical response to a graded intensity suggests processing at least above the level of the cochlea and auditory nerve. It is certainly possible that cortical processing is taking place, although the results of FMRI studies designed to answer this particular question are pending. Because acoustic echoplanar scanner noise is dominant in the optimal hearing range for humans, potential interactions with superimposed pure tone stimuli also have to be considered in the interpretation of such findings. For example, the coding of AM periodicity of animals, which is ultimately reflected in the primary cortex, is influenced by sound intensity of optimal ranges. The confounding effects of in-

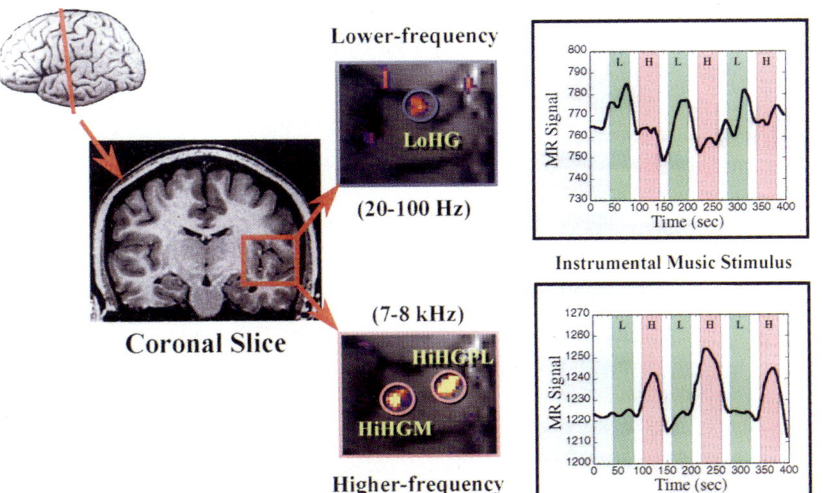


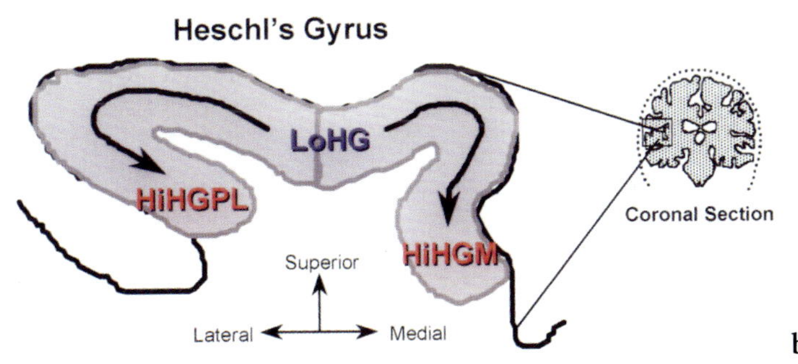


**Fig. 5.20. a** Summary of location and time course of frequency selectivity on Heschl's gyrus (TTG) in response to band-filtered instrumental music. Low frequency selectivity is located on the dome of Heschl's gyrus, while high frequency selectivity is located in the cortex lining the sulci about Heschl's gyrus. **b** Illustration of frequency selectivity on the TTG, with low frequency selectivity on the dome of the gyrus and high frequency selectivity located in cortex lining the sulci about the gyrus, located medially (*HiHGM*) and posterolaterally (*HiHGPL*), relative to the orientation of Heschl's gyrus. (From Talavage et al. with permission)

creasing tone intensity on sound interactions with periodic acoustic scanner noise are not known, but are a potential factor influencing the intensity-dependent cortical responses observed in the TTG. Finally, increasing tone intensity could increase attention to the stimulus, particularly in the presence of distracting background acoustic scanner noise. Second- and third-order brain stem auditory neurons give off collaterals to the reticular formation, providing an indirect sensory input to the cortex. The extent to which a loud tone might increase attention or startle the auditory system in this setting is unknown, but this pathway may certainly influence cortical activity (Grady et al. 1997). Ultimately, more research will be needed to explain the mechanisms underlying the intensity-dependent TTG response in FMRI experiments.

As an observed phenomenon, the intensity-dependent activation of the auditory cortex has significant implications for the design and interpretation of FMRI studies using auditory stimuli. Care must be taken to deliver all auditory stimuli studied and compared with one another with equivalent intensities. This is particularly true where language components are broken down and delivered separately. Because language components are not evenly distributed across the frequency spectrum, this potential confounding effect is made even more complex by the nonlinear properties of acoustic scanner noise spanning the same spectrum (Fig. 5.13). Take, for example, a theoretical scenario where consonants, which are primarily made up of higher frequency sounds are delivered at the same intensity as vowels, which are primarily made up of lower frequency sounds. In this scenario, the auditory cortical response to consonants could be enhanced relative to that induced by the vowels, based purely on differences in sound intensity relative to a nonlinear background state (i.e. acoustic scanner noise). Conclusions concerning differing activation patterns to different words, speech components, or other auditory stimuli, may in fact be invalid when this confounding variable has not been considered.

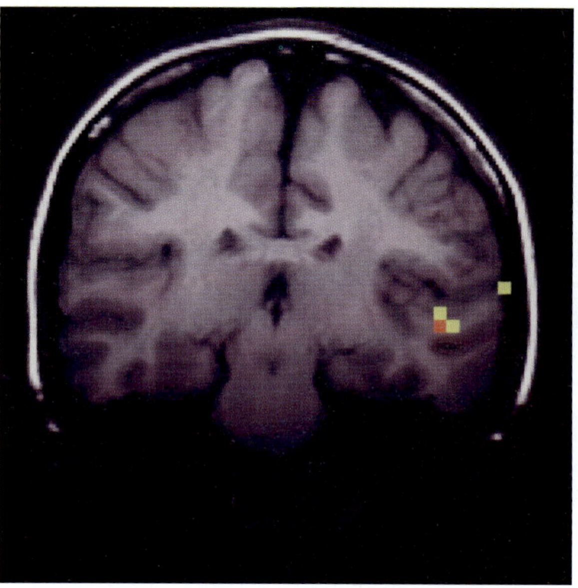


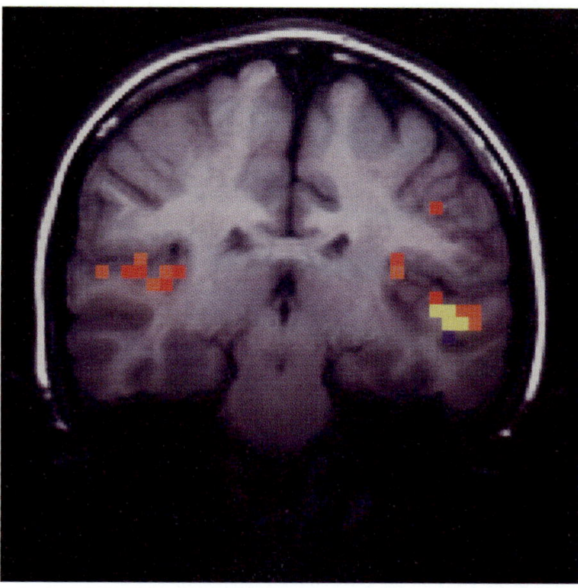


**Fig. 5.21.** Superior temporal gyrus activation in response to 1000 Hz pure tone at **a** 20 dBSL and **b** 50 dBSL. Increasing tone intensity results in increased area of activation within the superior temporal gyrus. Also, bilateral activation is present only at the 50-dBSL pure tone intensity. Activated regions were determined with a cross-correlation analysis and a correlation coefficient threshold of 0.7 (*yellow pixels*), 0.6 (*orange pixels*), and 0.5 (*red pixels*)

## 5.6 Summary

As a noninvasive technique, FMRI has significant potential to enhance our understanding of human audition and will probably provide a mechanism by which hearing dysfunction can be studied in future clinical settings. The availability and potential for widespread utility of this technique will undoubtedly drive further research and the likeliood of clinical applications. However, it is important to recognize that the development of FMRI for the study of human auditory function is only in its infancy, and that significant refinement must be achieved before the full potential of the technique can be realized. Investigators would do well not to ignore the fact that most of the new information concerning auditory function will continue to be derived by non-FMRI techniques, and they should continue to look to animal studies and human investigations (e.g. PET and MEG) for confirmation of their FMRI findings. Because of the unique technical limitations of auditory FMRI, investigators should not be too quick to disregard research from other non-FMRI investigators in favor of their own results.

## References

Bandettini PA, Wong EC, Hinks RS, et al (1992) Time course EPI of human brain function during task activation. Magn Reson Med 25:390–397

Bandettini PA, Jesmanowicz A, Wong EC, et al (1993) Processing strategies for time-course data sets in functional MRI of the human brain. Magn Reson Med 30:161-73

Bandettini PA, Jesmanowicz A, Van Kylen J, et al (1997) Functional MRI of scanner acoustic noise induced brain activation. Neuroimage 5:S193

Bannister LH, Berry MM, Collins P, et al (1995) Gray's Anatomy, 38th edn. Churchill Livingstone, Edinburgh, pp 1024-1027

Baumgartner R, Scarth G, Teichtmeister C, et al (1997) Fuzzy clustering of gradient-echo functional MRI in the human visual cortex. I. Reproducibility. J Magn Reson Imaging 7:1094-1101

Belliveau JW, Kennedy DN, McKinstry RC, et al (1991) Functional mapping of the human visual cortex by magnetic resonance imaging. Science 254:716–719

Berry I, Demonet JF, Warach S, et al (1995) Activation of association auditory cortex demonstrated with functional MRI. Neuroimage 2:215-219

Binder JR, Rao SM, Hammeke TA, et al (1994a) Functional magnetic resonance imaging of human auditory cortex. Ann Neurol 35:662–672

Binder JR, Rao SM, Hammeke TA, et al (1994b) Effects of stimulus rate on signal response during functional magnetic resonance imaging of auditory cortex. Cogn Brain Res 2:31-38

Binder JR, Rao SM, Hammeke TA, et al (1995) Lateralized human brain language systems demonstrated by task subtraction functional magnetic resonance imaging. Arch Neurol 52:593-601

Binder JR, Frost JA, Hammeke TA, et al (1996) Function of the left planum temporale in auditory and linguistic processing. Brain 119:1239–1247

Biswal B, Hyde J S (1997b) Contour-based registration technique to differentiate between task-activated and head motion-induced signal variations in FMRI. Magn Reson Med 38:470-476B

Biswal B,. DeYoe EA, Jesmanowicz A (1994) FMRI analysis for aperiodic task activation using non-paramagnetic statistics. Proceedings of the Society of Magnetic Resonance, San Francisco, p 624

Biswal B, DeYoe AE, Hyde JS (1996) Reduction of physiological fluctuations in fMRI using digital filters. Magn Reson Med 35:107-113

Biswal B, Jesmanowicz A, Hyde JS (1997a) High temporal resolution FMRI. Proceedings of the Fifth ISMRM, Vancouver, p 1629

Bowtell RW, Mansfield P (1995) Quiet transverse gradient coils: Lorentz force balanced designs using geometrical similitude. Magn Reson Med 34:494–497

Boxerman JL, Hamberg LM, Rosen BR, et al (1995) MR contrast due to intravascular magnetic susceptibility perturbations. Magn Reson Med 34:555-566

Brammer MJ, Bullmore ET, Simmons A, et al (1997) Generic brain activation mapping in functional magnetic resonance imaging: a nonparametric approach. Magn Reson Imaging 15:763-770

Brugge JF (1991) Neurophysiology of the central auditory and vestibular systems. In: Paparella MM (ed) Otolaryngology, vol 1. Saunders, Philadelphia, pp 281-301

Buchel C, Wise RJ, Mummery CJ, et al (1996) Nonlinear regression in parametric activation studies. Neuroimage 4:60-66

Celesia GG (1976) Organization of auditory cortical areas in man. Brain 99:403–414

Chen W, Novotny EJ, Zhu XH, et al (1993) Localized $^{1}$H NMR measurement of glucose consumption in the human brain during visual stimulation. Proc Natl Acad Sci USA 90:896-900

David AS, Woodruff PW, Howard R, et al (1996) Auditory hallucinations inhibit exogenous activation of auditory association cortex. Neuroreport 22;7:932–936

Desmond JE, Sum JM, Wagner AD, et al (1995) Functional MRI measurement of language lateralization in Wada-tested patients. Brain 118:1411–1419

Detre JA, Williams DS, Leigh JS, et al (1991) Quantitative measurement of tissue perfusion and diffusion. Magn Reson Med 19:266–269

Dhankhar A, Wexler BE, Fulbright RK, et al (1997) Functional magnetic resonance imaging assessment of the human brain auditory cortex response to increasing word presentation rates. American Physiological Society, Baltimore, pp 476–481

Edelman RR, Siewert B, Darby DG, et al (1994) Qualitative mapping of cerebral blood flow and functional localization with echo-planar MR imaging and signal targeting with alternating radio frequency. Radiology 192:513-520

Forman SD, Cohen JD, Fitzgerald M, et al (1995) Improved assessment of significant activation in functional magnetic resonance imaging (fMRI): use of a cluster-size threshold. Magn Reson Med 33:636-647

Frahm J, Kruger G, Merboldt KD, et al (1996) Dynamic uncoupling and recoupling of perfusion and oxidative metabolism during focal brain activation in man. J Magn Reson Med 35:143-148

Fransson P, Kruger G, Merboldt KD, et al (1997) A comparative FLASH and EPI study of repetitive and sustained visual activation. NMR Biomed 10:204-207

Friston KJ, Williams S, Howard R, et al (1996) Movement-related effects in fMRI time-series. Magn Reson Med 35:346-355

Grady CL Van Meter JW Maisog JM et al (1997) Attention-related modulation of activity in primary and secondary auditory cortex Neuroreport. 8:2511-16

Greenberg S (1988) The ear as a speech analyzer. J Phon 16:139-149

Hinke RM, Hu X, Stillman AE, et al (1993) Functional magnetic resonance imaging of Broca's area during internal speech. Neuroreport 4:675–678

Kim SG (1995) Quantification of relative cerebral blood flow change by flow-sensitive alternating inversion recovery (FAIR) technique: application to functional mapping. Magn Reson Med 34:293-301

Kim SG, Tsekos NV, Ashe J (1997) Multi-slice perfusion-based functional MRI using the FAIR technique: comparison of CBF and BOLD effects. NMR Biomed 10:191-196

Kim T, Ulmer J, Haughton V, et al (1997) The effect of postprocessing algorithm on the pattern and intensity of activation in functional MR imaging. Proceedings of the 35th Annual Meeting of the American Society of Neuroradiology, 18-22May 1997, p145

Knudsen EI, Brainard MS (1995) Creating a unified representation of visual and auditory space in the brain. Annu Rev Neurosci 18:19-43

Kwong KK, Belliveau JW, Chesler DA, et al (1992) Dynamic magnetic resonance imaging of human brain activity during primary sensory stimulation. Proc Natl Acad Sci USA 89:5675–5679

Kwong KK, Chesler DA, Weisskoff RM, et al (1995). MR perfusion studies with T1-weighted echo planar imaging. Magn Reson Med 34:878–887

Langner G (1992) Periodicity coding in the auditory system (review article). Hear Res 60:115-142

Lauter JL, Herscovitch P, Formby C, et al (1985) Tonotopic organization in human auditory cortex revealed by positron emission tomography. Hear Res 20:199-205

Malonek D, Grinvald A (1996) Interactions between electrical activity and cortical microcirculation revealed by imaging spectroscopy: implications for functional brain mapping. Science 272:551-554

Mansfield P, Glover PM, Beaumont J (1998) Sound generation in gradient coil structures for MRI. Magn Reson Med 39:539-550

Mark LP, Ulmer JL, Daniels DL, et al (1998) Anatomic moment. The brainstem auditory system: an overview. AJNR Am J Neuroradiol (in press).

Masterton RB (1992) Role of the central auditory system in hearing: the new direction. Trends Neurosci15:280-285

Millen SJ, Haughton VM, Yetkin FZ (1995) Functional magnetic resonance imaging of the central auditory pathway following speech and pure-tone stimuli. Laryngoscope 104:1305-1310

Moser E, Diemling M, Baumgartner R (1997) Fuzzy clustering of gradient-echo functional MRI in the human visual cortex. II. Quantification. J Magn Reson Imaging 7:1102-1108

Musiek FE, Hoffman DW (1990) An introduction to the functional neurochemistry of the auditory system. Ear Hear 11:395-402

Newby HA, Popelka GR (1992) What and how we hear. In: Audiology, 6th edn. Prentice-Hall, Englewood Cliffs

Nieuwenhuys R (1984) Anatomy of the auditory pathways, with emphasis on the brain stem. Adv Otorhinolaryngol 34:25-38

Nieuwenhuys R, Voogd J, van Huijzen C (1988) The human central nervous system, 3rd edn. Springer, Berlin Heidelberg New York, pp 172-179

Noll DC, Cohen JD, Meyer CH, et al (1995) MR imaging of cortical activation. J Magn Reson Imaging 5:49-56

Northern JL, Downs MP (1991) Hearing in children, 4th edn. Williams & Wilkins, Baltimore

Ogawa S, Tank DW Menon R, et al (1992) Intrinsic signal changes accompanying sensory stimulation: functional brain mapping with magnetic resonance imaging. Proc Natl Acad Sci USA 89:5951–5955

Ogawa S, Menon RS, Tank DW, et al (1993) Functional brain mapping by blood oxygenation level-dependent contrast magnetic resonance imaging. Biophys J 64:803–812

Plomp R (1983) The role of modulation in hearing. In: Klinke R, Hartmann R (eds) Hearing – physiological bases and psychophysics. Springer, Berlin Heidelberg NewYork, pp 270–275

Roberts TPL, Poeppel D (1996) Latency of auditory evoked M100 as a function of tone frequency. Neuroreport 7:1138–1140

Roland PE (1993) Language. In: Roland PE (ed) Brain activation. Wiley-Liss, New York, pp 158–163

Sigalovsky I, Levine RA, Melcher JR, et al (1998) Tinnitus studied using functional magnetic resonance imaging: development of methods. Proceedings of the Twenty-First Midwinter Meeting of the Association for Research in Otolaryngology, p 51

Stehling MK, Turner R, Mansfield P (1991) Echo-planar imaging: magnetic resonance imaging in a fraction of a second. Science 254:43-50

Strainer JC, Ulmer JL, Yetkin FZ, et al (1997) Functional MR of the primary auditory cortex: an analysis of pure tone activation and tone discrimination. AJNR Am J Neuroradiol 18:601–610

Swartz JD, Daniels DL, Harnsberger HR, et al (1996a) Hearing. I. The cochlea. AJNR Am J Neuroradiol 17:1237-1241

Swartz JD, Daniels DL, Harnsberger HR, (1996b) Hearing. II. The retrocochlear auditory pathway. AJNR Am J Neuroradiol 17:1479-1481

Talavage TM, Edmister WB (1998) Measuring and reducing the impact of imaging noise on echo-planar functional magnetic resonance imaging (fMRI) of auditory cortex. Abstracts of the Twenty-first Midwinter Research Meeting of the Association for Research in Otolaryngology, no 138

Talavage TM, Ledden PJ, Sereno MI, et al (1996) fMRI evidence of tonotopic organization in human auditory cortex. Human Brain Mapping

Talavage TM, Ledden PJ, Sereno MI, et al (1997a) Evidence for multiple frequency-selective fields in human auditory cortex obtained by functional magnetic resonance imaging. Abstracts of the Twentieth Midwinter Research Meeting of the Association for Research in Otolaryngology, no 818

Talavage TM, Ledden PJ, Sereno MI, et al (1997b) Multiple phase-encoded tonotopic maps in human auditory cortex. Neuroimage 5:S8

Tan SG, Song AW, Wong EC, et al (1997) High resolution FMRI with interleaved EPI. Proceedings of the Fifth ISMRM, Vancouver, p 796, April 12-18, 1997

Ulmer JL, Estkowski LD, Yetkin FZ, et al (1996a) Functional MR imaging of the auditory cortex: cortical activation response to acoustic scanner noise. Radiology 201[Suppl]:373

Ulmer JL, Strainer JC, Yetkin FZ, et al (1996b) Functional MR imaging of the auditory cortex: pure tone activation and auditory cortical function. Radiology 201(P):451

Ulmer JL, Akansel G, Yetkin FZ, et al (1997) A functional MR imaging investigation of language comprehension: a comparison of passive text listening between intelligible and unintelligible languages. Proceedings of the 35th Annual Meeting of the American Society of Neuroradiology, 18-22 May, p 329

Ulmer JL, Biswal BB, Yetkin FZ, et al (1998a) Cortical activation response to acoustic echoplanar scanner noise. J Comput Assist Tomogr 21:111–119

Ulmer JL, Biswal BB, Mark LP, et al (1998b) Acoustic echoplanar scanner noise and pure tone hearing thresholds: the effects of sequence repetition times and acoustic noise rates. J Comput Assist Tomogr 22:480–486

Ulmer JL, Mark LP, Mathews VP, et al (1998c) Auditory activation and perceptual effects from acoustic echoplanar scanner noise (exhibit). Proceedings of the 36th Annual Meeting of the American Society of Neuroradiology, 17-21 May 1998

Ulmer JL, Millen SJ, Mark LP, et al (1998d) Functional magnetic resonance imaging of the primary auditory cortex: a study of activation patterns with varying pure tone intensity levels. Proceedings of the 36th Annual Meeting of the American Society of Neuroradiology, 17–21May 1998

Villringer A, Dirnagl U (1995) Coupling of brain activity and cerebral blood flow: basis of functional neuroimaging. Cerebrovasc Brain Metab Rev 7:240–276

Williams DS, Detre JA, Leigh JS, et al (1992) Magnetic resonance imaging of perfusion using spin inversion of arterial water. Proc Natl Acad Sci USA 89:4220–4226

Wong EC, Buxton RB, Frank LR (1997) Implementation of quantitative perfusion imaging techniques for functional brain mapping using pulsed arterial spin labeling. NMR Biomed 10:237-249

Woods RP, Cherry SR, Mazziotta JC (1992) Rapid automated algorithm for aligning and reslicing PET images. J Comput Assist Tomogr 16:620-633

Worsley KJ, Poline JB, Vandal AC, et al (1995) Tests for distributed, nonfocal brain activations. Neuroimage 2:183-194

Yetkin FZ, Mueller W, Cox RW, et al (1996) Dependence of postoperative neurologic deficit on distance from lesion to eloquent cortex as measured by functional MR imaging. In: Proceedings of the 34th Annual Meeting of the American Society of Neuroradiology, Seattle, p 61, June 21-27

Yetkin FZ, Mueller W, Morris G, et al (1997) Activation in FMRI correlated with intraoperative cortical mapping. AJNR Am J Neuroradiol 18:1311–1315

# 6 Functional Imaging of Swallowing

K. MOSIER

CONTENTS



## 6.1 Introduction

Swallowing is a phylogenetically old yet highly complex physiological function. Swallowing serves primarily to transport a liquid or solid bolus from the oral cavity to the stomach, while at the same time preventing penetration of the nasopharyngeal or laryngeal airways. Thus, safe and effective swallowing requires the coordinated interaction of twenty-six muscles and five cranial nerves (JONES and DONNER 1991; LOGEMANN 1988).

Traditionally, swallowing is clinically assessed by means of history, physical examination and imaging. Clinical history focuses on complaints of dsyphagia, odynophagia, reports of "food sticking in the throat," frequent coughing or gagging while swallowing, nasal regurgitation, history of aspiration, or pneumonia. Physical examination focuses on evaluation of oral masticatory function, tongue movement, velopharyngeal function, and where indicated, direct visualization of the supraglottis, glottis, and subglottis (SONIES and BAUM 1988).

Imaging in the evaluation of dysphagia is traditionally performed with fluoroscopy or videofluoroscopy (CURTIS and CRUESS 1985). In fact, since the first reported use of fluoroscopy in the evaluation of swallowing (BARCLAY 1930) fluoroscopy has been the mainstay of the imaging evaluation of swallowing. Improvements in recording dynamic movements observed under fluoroscopy, such as cine methods, first reported in 1949 (FRENCKNER 1949), and more recently the advent of video methods in the 1970s (SEAMAN 1976; KILMAN and GOYAL 1976; EKBERG and NYLANDER 1982; CURTIS and CRUESS 1984) have provided the temporal resolution to resolve individual events in swallowing. With the introduction of CT and MRI technologies in the 1970s and 1980s, cross-sectional and multi-planar imaging of the upper aerodigestive tract became possible and has furthered our understanding of pathophysiological processes in swallowing.

Nevertheless, fluoroscopic examination of the swallow remains an important means of evaluating swallowing function. Videofluoroscopy, or standard pharygo- or esophograms, however, only provide information on the function of peripheral structures in swallowing and do not provide information on the function, and integration of function, of the central nervous system elements responsible for the control of swallowing.

## 6.2 Neuroanatomical Overview of Swallowing

The central nervous system control of swallowing function occurs through three levels: cerebral cortex, brain stem and peripheral neuromuscular junction. Briefly, sensory input from receptors in the oral cavity, pharynx and larynx synapses in the nucleus of the tractus solitarius (NTS) located in the dorsal brain stem at the level of the pontine-medullary

K. MOSIER, DMD, PhD, Division of OMF Radiology and Department of Oral Pathology and Diagnostic Sciences, New Jersey Dental School, and Department of Radiology, University Hospital, University of Medicine and Dentistry of New Jersey, Rm C-829, 110 Bergen Street, Newark, NJ 07103-2400, USA

junction. The NTS, via input to the swallowing central pattern generator in the reticular formation, is believed to generate the reflexive, patterned response to this peripheral sensory input and projects to the ventrally located nucleus ambiguus (NA) in the medulla. The NA then activates the cranial motor nuclei innervating the oral cavity, pharynx and larynx (Miller 1986).

At a central level, the cortical representation of swallowing is generally situated at the inferior extent of the lateral precentral gyrus, overlapping and inferior to the areas representing the face, tongue, pharynx and larynx (Pansky et al. 1988). Efferent projections from the cortex converge in the corona radiata and descend with the pyramidal tract corticobulbar fibers through the genu and posterior limb of the internal capsule. The origin of these efferent projections are somewhat diffuse as it is estimated that 30% of the fibers of the corticobulbar tract arise from the premotor cortex (Brodmann's area 6), 30% from the precentral gyrus (primary motor cortex; Brodmann's area 4) and the remaining 40% from the parietal cortex (somatosensory cortex; Brodmann's areas 3, 1, and 2) (Ghez 1985).

In the mesencephalon, the corticobulbar fibers pass through the medial aspect of the middle two-thirds of the cerebral peduncles (Pansky et al. 1988). The majority of fibers in the corticobulbar tract descend from the cerebral peduncles into the medullary pyramids, but some fibers of the corticobulbar tract descend through the mid-brain or pons and reach their respective cranial nerve nuclei through the medial lemniscus or medial longitudinal fasciculus (Ghez 1985). While most of the cortical bulbar fibers remain uncrossed, fibers of the hypoglossal nerve cross, as do fibers innervating the facial nucleus supplying muscles of the lower face. Fibers to the motor nucleus of the trigeminal nerve and the portion of the facial nucleus supplying the upper facial muscles are bilateral (Lewine 1995; Pansky et al. 1988).

## 6.3 Functional Imaging of Swallowing: Clinical Implications

### 6.3.1 Clinical Syndromes Associated with Dysphagia

Dysphagia resulting from cerebrovascular accident (CVA) or other ischemic insults produces a spectrum of signs and symptoms clinically classified into a variety of syndromes. Pseudobulbar palsy, anterior operculum syndrome and the lateral medullary syndrome are three of the most common clinical presentations associated with dysphagia following focal central nervous system injury.

Pseudobulbar palsy, or supranuclear palsy, refers to a cranial nerve palsy originating in the supra-pontine cortical bulbar tracts and nuclei. Usually pseudobulbar palsy results from ischemia, infarction, or degenerative disease involving the subcortical diencephalon, and the corticobulbar fibers running through the internal capsule, corona radiata and cerebral peduncles (Besson et al. 1991). Pseudobulbar palsy can further divided into three subtypes: the Foix-Chavany-Marie syndrome consisting of faciopharyngoglossomasticatory diplegia with disassociation of automatic and voluntary functions, and a striatal variant characterized by faciopharyngoglossomasticatory diplegia with concomitant pyramidal symptoms, emotional liability and intellectual impairment. Lastly, the pontine variant is characterized by faciopharyngoglossomasticatory palsy with pyramidal and occasional cerebellar signs but without the cognitive impairment (Besson et al. 1991; Weller 1993).

The anterior operculum syndrome clinically presents with features of the Foix-Chavany-Marie syndrome and in adults is usually associated with infarction involving the anterior frontal and /or temporal opercular cortex. Less commonly, in children, virally mediated encephalitis or congenital defects have been associated with this syndrome (Gropman et al. 1997).

Lastly, the lateral medullary syndrome results from compromise of a vertebral artery or more distally from involvement of the pontine branches of the basilar artery which supply the medulla oblongata (Osborn 1991; Ramsey 1987; Kim et al. 1994). The lateral medullary syndrome consists of an array of symptoms depending on the area of medulla affected and includes dysphagia, hoarseness, nystagmus, nausea/vomiting, gait ataxia, and facial and hemicoroporal sensory disturbances (Kim et al. 1994).

### 6.3.2 Imaging of Clinical Syndromes Associated with Dysphagia

MRI is the modality of choice for identification of small lacunar infarcts, which are associated with pseudobulbar palsy, a significant cause of neurogenic dysphagia (Besson et al. 1991; Jones and Donner 1991). Lacunar infarcts are readily identified on T2-weighted images typically as ovoid or geometric shaped areas of increased signal intensity in the basal ganglia, thalamus, internal capsule, deep white matter or brain stem, and are often hypointense to brain on T1-weighted images (Jacobs and Brant-Zawadzki 1992; Atlas 1996). Despite the ability to resolve focal sites of infarction that in some cases correlate with clinical presentation, most ischemic origins of neurogenic dysphagia are not well correlated with the peripheral deficit. A number of studies have attempted to correlate infarction involving a particular vascular territory with specific peripheral deficits such as oral phase dysfunction (e.g. lingual propulsion), pharyngeal dysfunction, cricopharyngeal dysfunction or aspiration (Horner et al. 1990; Robbins et al. 1993; Veis and Logemann 1985). However, the results of these investigations have been disappointing in that no consistent correlation between the affected vascular territory and a specific deficit was observed.

Similar results have been reported with imaging in the lateral medullary syndrome. Kim et al. (1994) found correlation of peripheral deficits with a generalized rostral-caudal lesion identification in the medulla, although specific correlation between the medullary site of involvement and the peripheral dysfunction was equivocal.

Aside from differences in study design and individual degrees of ischemia, the difficulty in correlating cortical, subcortical or brain stem morphological abnormalities with peripheral deficits may lie in our lack of understanding of the central nervous system control of swallowing.

The introduction of functional magnetic resonance imaging (fMRI) techniques affords the opportunity to study the functional role of cortical, subcortical and brain stem areas in the control of swallowing. In our laboratory, we have applied fMRI to study the cortical, subcortical and brain stem representation of swallowing and other oro-pharyngeal maneuvers.

## 6.4 Functional Imaging in Swallowing: Image Acquisition and Paradigm Design

### 6.4.1 Image Acquisition

In our institution, all subjects are imaged on a 1.5 T GE SIGNA 5x Horizon echo-speed MRI system using gradient echo echo-planar sequences with the following acquisition parameters: 64 × 64 matrix, 24 cm FOV, repetition time (TR) = 2000 / time to echo (TE) = 60, 5-mm-thick contiguous slices, and a 90° flip angle. For fMRI of swallowing, echo-planar images are acquired in the axial and coronal planes at 14 slice locations with a standard quadrature "birdcage" head coil and standard fMRI blood oxygen level dependent (BOLD) techniques. Spin-echo (TR = 300/TE = 14) high-resolution anatomic images are acquired in the axial and coronal planes in the same slice locations during the same imaging session. Subjects' heads are immobilized to prevent head motion.

While many fMRI studies are predicated on whole-brain image acquisition, the slice number is limited to 14 in order to keep the TR to 2000 ms for data sampling. Thus, for every TR, cortical changes associated with a single swallow are acquired. However, a number of single swallows should be acquired to ensure adequate data sampling (see Section 6.4.2). Increasing the TR to permit whole brain image acquisition (i.e. to 4000 ms for this system) would tend to average at least two swallows for each TR. In order to image cortical activity as a function of peripheral events, individual "snapshots" of those events (i.e. a single swallow) should be acquired instead of a synthesis of events. The rationale for this approach is that it theoretically permits more accurate comparison of concurrent central and peripheral events, since peripheral actions in swallowing are typically captured as single events, i.e. as a series of single frames on videofluoroscopy or on videoendoscopy exmainations.

Axial images are acquired from the level of the diencephalon to the convexity, approximately parallel to the AC–PC line (0 angle). Coronal images are acquired from the anterior commissure to a plane bisecting the temporoparietooccipital junction, parallel with the long axis of the spinal cord (0 angle).

### 6.4.2 Paradigm Design

In order to stimulate cortical activity associated with swallowing, subjects perform paradigms based on a 10- or 15-s "ON" period and a 30-s "OFF' period, with four cycles. The 10-s epoch permits adequate sampling of motor activity during swallowing. A normal swallow typically takes approximately 1.5–2.0 s to complete (Jones and Donner 1991); hence a 10-s epoch samples approximately five swallows. Previous investigations have quantified the variability in motor output over five or more swallows in normal subjects (Gay et al. 1994; Mosier 1997). Although it is technically possible to acquire data over the time-course of a single swallow, this may result in an incomplete representation of cortical activity due to this intrasubject variability. Moreover, recent studies indicate that lower limit of the flow hemodynamic response of the BOLD mechanism (used in these experiments) is at 2 seconds (Hathout et al. 1998). Thus, obtaining data for a single swallow in a single TR of 2000 ms may result in no statistical activation.

Both a 10-s "dry" swallow (in which the subjects swallow their own saliva) and a 10-s "wet" swallow are performed. During the wet swallow the subjects self-administer approximately 3 cc of sterile water through a plastic catheter. Hand movement is restricted during self-administration to avoid motion artifacts and contamination of the signal by a different motor movement. The use of both a dry and a wet swallow permits comparison of cortical activation during nonbolus and bolus swallows. It is well established that there are different patterns of peripheral motor activity for nonbolus and bolus swallows (Kahrilas et al. 1993; Ekberg et al. 1988). Moreover, comparison of non-bolus and bolus swallows has important clinical implications in that the degree and/or presentation of dsyphagia may differ for nonbolus and bolus swallows depending on the site or nature of dysfunction (i.e. neurogenic vs tumor mass).

In addition to the 10-s epoch, the subjects also performed dry swallows with a 15-s "ON" period and a 30-s "OFF" period, with four cycles. The use of a 15-s epoch introduces an increased task load, or a motor challenge to the swallowing motor control system. Performing dry swallows repeatedly over 15 s is difficult and thus presents a motor challenge.

Although it is not possible to directly visualize the subjects swallowing, it is nevertheless important to verify that the subjects swallowed during the ON epochs and did not swallow during the OFF epochs. This is to ensure that the cortical activation detected with these paradigms is associated with swallowing and that baseline measures are not contaminated by movement. To record swallowing with the paradigms, we place MRI-compatible electrodes over the thyroid cartilage and thyrohyoid membrane to measure movement of the hyoid–laryngeal complex, and record the signals on a monitor.

In addition to the swallowing task paradigms, the subjects also perform a self-paced finger-tapping task. The finger-tapping task serves as a positive control for identification of the primary motor cortex since this task is routinely used to identify the primary motor cortex in functional brain mapping (Yousry et al. 1995). Subjects tap the fingers against the opposing thumb on both hands simultaneously, at maximum speed for 30 s with a rest period of 30 s, for two cycles.

## 6.5 Data Analysis

Image reconstruction and analysis is performed using software routines written in IDL (instructive data language; Research Systems, Boulder, CO) with application of an in-plane least-squares motion correction algorithm. A cross-correlation analysis is then applied to the EPI (echo-planar imaging) data sets to create statistical maps of activation associated with each motor task and the resultant images overlaid on the spin-echo anatomic images (Maldjian et al. 1996). A cross-correlation statistical analysis is applied to these data sets in order to statistically determine activation associated with the task paradigms and to eliminate spurious or artifactual activation. Motor or sensory function is typically associated with a 3–5% signal change using BOLD techniques (Ogawa et al. 1993). Thus, signal changes less than, or in excess of this range, due to motion or physiologic (vessel or CSF) pulsation, can be excluded from further data analysis. The statistical maps of activation for the different paradigms are generated using an identical statistical threshold.

## 6.6 Functional Mapping of Swallowing

Swallowing during the 10 (both dry and wet) and 15-s paradigms results in bilateral activation in the mid-lateral to inferior precentral gyrus (primary motor cortex) in all subjects. Activation in this area corresponds to the motor homunculus maps of facial, tongue, and pharyngeal/laryngeal function (Ghez 1985). Moreover, activation in this area corresponds to neuronal activity identified with electrophysiological techniques during swallowing in primates and humans (Martin and Sessle 1993; Martin et al. 1997; Penfield and Rasmussen 1950). Activation is also identified in the supplementary motor cortex, thalamus, internal capsule, superior and middle frontal gyrus, superior temporal gyrus, insula, primary somatosensory cortex, and the hypoglossal nucleus (cranial nerve XII) in the medulla. Figure 6.1 shows the coronal image of a 10-s dry swallowing task for one subject. This subject

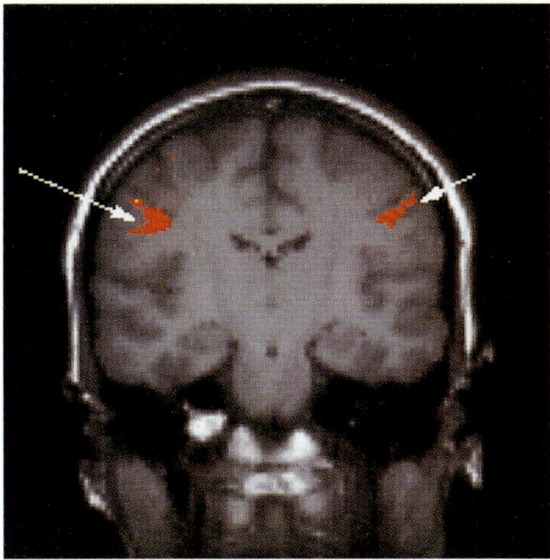

**Fig. 6.1.** Coronal image of a normal subject obtained with a 10-s dry swallow paradigm. Activation is seen in the right (*long arrow*) and left (*small arrow*) mid-inferior lateral primary motor cortex

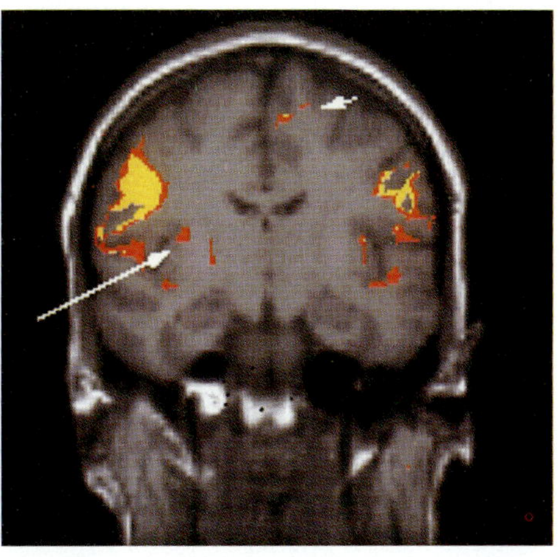

**Fig. 6.2.** Coronal image of a normal subject obtained with a 15-s dry swallow paradigm. Activation is seen in the left supplementary motor area (*short arrow*), and in the right (*long arrow*) and left insular cortices. Large areas of activation are noted bilaterally in the mid and inferior lateral primary motor cortices

demonstrates bilateral activation in the mid-inferior lateral primary motor cortex. In general, the majority of normal subjects show robust activation of the primary motor cortex during the 10-s and 15-s swallowing paradigms.

While the volume of activation varies among subjects, in general, the area of activation in the lateral precentral gyrus overlaps portions of the gyrus spatially represented in the homuncular maps as the tongue, pharynx and larynx. The overlap in activation for these cortical areas is likely attributable to a combination of several factors specific to functional imaging, paradigm design and cortical motor organization. First, the BOLD technique relies on signal change produced by focal changes in blood flow or oxygenation (Ogawa et al. 1993) to neuronally active areas. This area of the cortex is supplied via the terminal branches of the central sulcal and operculofrontal branches of the middle cerebral artery (Jacobs and Brant-Zawadzki 1992; Osborn 1991); thus there is not one to one correspondence between the vascular territory and the specific neuronal populations activated. Secondly, the paradigm stimulates a function with several concurrent oral and pharyngeal events, and given the limit of temporal resolution for this paradigm (approximately 100 ms), discrete temporal sequencing of cortical activity is unlikely to be measured with the cross-correlation analysis. Lastly, other studies using electrode recording in primates have demonstrated functional overlap of specific neuronal popluations in this area of the cortex during swallowing and other oropharyngeal behaviors (Martin et al. 1997).

In our studies, activation of the primary motor cortex during swallowing tasks is consistently located at least 5 mm anterior and inferior to the motor cortex areas identified by finger-tapping. Again, these findings are consistent with the known topographical representations on the motor cortex of different anatomical sites.

Activation of other cortical sites such as the supplementary motor area (or premotor area), represented in the superior and middle frontal gyri and associated with motor planning (Tanji et al. 1996), suggests involvement of multiple cortical sites for the planning and execution of motor output for swallowing (Fig. 6.2).

Intuitively, activity of the supplementary motor areas would be expected during a motor movement, particularly in planning for sequential movements, as occurs with swallowing. However, activity of the supplementary motor areas during swallowing is not a well-characterized feature of the motor control of swallowing in the literature (Martin and Sessle 1993). This may be partially attributable to the classification of swallowing into different "phases." Generally, the oral phase of swallowing is considered to be the only voluntary phase of swallowing, while the pharyngeal and esophageal phases are generally considered to be under automatic or reflexive control (Jones and Donner 1991; Kirshner 1989; Martin

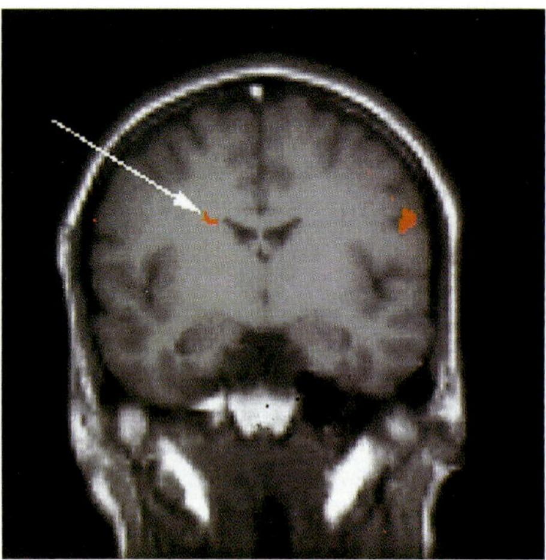

**Fig. 6.3.** Coronal image of a normal subject obtained with a 10-s dry swallow paradigm. Activation is seen in the right internal capsule (*long arrow*) and left primary motor cortex

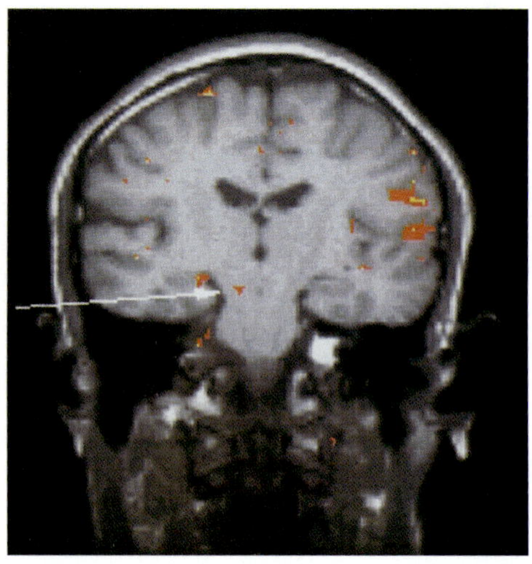

**Fig. 6.4.** Coronal image of a normal subject obtained with a 10-s dry swallow paradigm. Activation is noted in the right cerebral peduncle (*arrow*) and also in the left inferior primary motor cortex and superior temporal gyrus

1986). Thus, the oral phase is thought to be controlled by descending cortical inputs and the pharyngeal and esophageal phases mediated through the brain stem central pattern generator (Jones and Donner 1991; Kirshner 1989; Martin 1986). Differences in swallowing phase control is addressed by having the subjects perform both dry and wet swallows. Stimulation of the anterior tonsillar pillars by a bolus is believed to stimulate the pharyngeal (automatic) phase of swallowing (Jones and Donner 1991). Thus, the cortical activation observed in the wet swallows is likely to be representative of cortical activity during all phases of swallowing. Activation during the wet swallows shows essentially identical patterns of activation to those in the 10-s dry and 15-s tasks.

In subcortical areas, activation of the posterior limb of the internal capsule, the insular cortex and the thalamus is consistently observed in the subjects during swallowing tasks. Activation of the internal capsule (Fig. 6.3) is an important functional feature in swallowing as the internal capsule essentially serves as the "highway" between cortical and brain stem nuclei. Further caudal, activation is also identified in the cerebral peduncle (Fig. 6.4) representing the mesencephalic portion of the corticobulbar fibers.

The insular cortex serves as a sensory and motor integration site between primary cortex and other subcortical (thalamic) nuclei or limbic areas. The anterior portion of the insula has been implicated in gustatory sensation, although neuronal reception to specific taste stimuli was found to be nonspecific. Moreover, the insular cortex has been postulated as having a role in visceral motor activity and motor association (Augustine 1996). Lastly, the insular cortex is thought to be involved with the processing of "routine" or "overlearned" motor associated tasks. Thus activation of the insular cortex (Fig. 6.2) during swallowing tasks may be linked to its visceral motor functions.

The nuclei of the thalamus subserve a variety of roles, with some nuclei serving as relays for cortical areas and others generally serving as association areas (Netter 1995). The ventral anterior nucleus receives input from the basal ganglia and projects to the precentral (primary motor) cortex. This nucleus also receives descending input from the cerebral cortex, and ascending input from the mesencephalic reticular formation (Netter 1995). The posterior group, specifically the ventropostero-lateral and medial nuclei (VPL/VPM) receive from sensory input (touch, pressure, pain, temperature) via the medial lemniscus, trigeminal lemnisci and neospinothalamic tract and projects to the primary somatosensory cortex. The ventral lateral and ventral intermedial nuclei receive input from the cerebellum, substantia nigra and nuclei of the basal ganglia and project to the primary motor cortex (Netter 1995; Lewine 1995). Activation of thalamic nuclei (Fig. 6.5) during swallowing tasks indicates the necessary role of sensory and motor input processing via thalamo-cortical or thalamo-striatial pathways in swallowing. Disruption of these pathways (e.g. is-

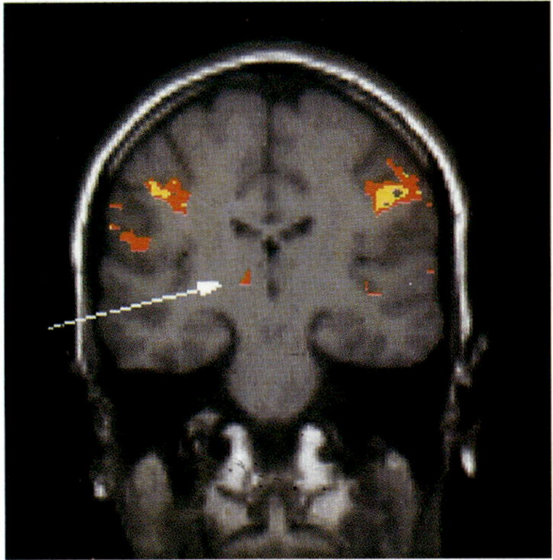

**Fig. 6.5.** Coronal image of a normal subject obtained with a 15-s dry paradigm. Activation is noted in the right thalamus (*arrow*) and in the primary motor cortex bilaterally

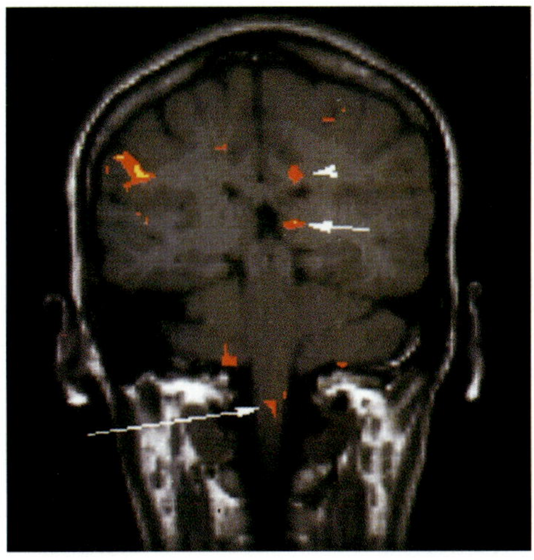

**Fig. 6.6.** Coronal image of a normal subject obtained with a 10-s tongue tapping paradigm. Activation is seen in the putative location of the hypoglossal nucleus (*long arrow*), and also in the pulvinar (*short arrow*), corpus callosum (*arrowhead*), and the right primary somatosensory cortex

chemic disease, degenerative disease) may result in inability to integrate sensory input with the appropriate motor output during swallowing.

Lastly, activation in nuclei of the brainstem was also identified using these methods (Fig. 6.6). To specifically stimulate the hypoglossal nucleus, subjects performed a "tongue-tapping" task in which they tapped the tongue against the palate as fast as possible in a 10 ON/30 OFF, 4-cycle paradigm. Activation is identified in the putative location of the hypoglossal nucleus (Fig. 6.6) at the cervicomedullary junction. Identification of hypoglossal nerve function is important in the evaluation of swallowing, as dysfunction or palsy of the hypoglossal nerve is associated with both oral and pharyngeal phase abnormalities (Logemann 1988).

## 6.7 Summary

Functional magnetic resonance imaging of swallowing provides a means of assessing the functional role of various cortical, subcortical and brain stem areas in the control of swallowing. Activation of primary motor and sensory cortical areas, supplementary motor areas and insular cortex, and activation of subcortical structures such as the thalamus and internal capsule, and activation of specific cranial nerve nuclei (e.g. the hypoglossal nucleus) can be identified with fMRI methods. FMRI provides the ability to image patients presenting with various types of neurogenic dysphagia, and may provide more specific information to correlate the central area of dysfunction with the peripheral deficit. This places the head and neck radiologist in a central role in the evaluation of patients presenting with neurogenic dysphagia. Moreover, fMRI examinations of swallowing function underscore the importance of correlating anatomical, functional and clinical data in the evaluation of swallowing disorders.

*Acknowledgements.* I am indebted to Joseph Maldjian, MD, for his input on study design and image analysis, and to Wen-Ching Liu, PhD, for his assistance in scanning and data processing. In addition, I am very grateful to Andrew Kalnin, MD, for his assistance in interpretation and his helpful comments on this manuscript. Also, I am grateful to Andrea Sawczuk, DDS, PhD, for her constant encouragement and constructive comments. Lastly, this work would not be possible without the vision of Stephen Baker, MD, in developing and supporting the Functional Imaging Laboratory in the Department of Radiology at the University of Medicine and Dentistry of New Jersey.

## References

Atlas SW (1996) Magnetic resonance imaging of the brain and spine, 2nd edn. Lippincott-Raven, Philadelphia, pp 595–600

Augustine JR (1996) Circuitry and functional aspects of the insular lobe in primates including humans. Brain Res Rev 22:229–244

Barclay AE (1930) The normal mechanism of swallowing. Br J Radiol 3:534–546

Besson G, Bogousslavsky J, Regli F, Maeder P (1991) Acute pseudobulbar or suprabulbar palsy. Arch Neurol 48:501–507

Curtis DJ, Cruess DF (1984) Pharyngoesophageal swallowing: a review of 618 videorecorded cases. Milit Med 149:545–549

Curtis DJ, Cruess DF (1985) Videofluoroscopic identification of two types of swallowing. Radiology 152:305–308

Ekberg O, Nylander •• (1982) Cineradiography in the pharyngeal stage of deglutition in 250 patients without dysphagia. Br J Radiol 55:258–262

Ekberg O, Olsson R, Sundgren-Borgstrom P (1988) Relation of bolus size and pharyngeal swallow. Dysphagia 3:69–72

Frenckner P (1949) X-ray cinematografic demonstration of the swallowing procedure in normal and pathologic cases. Acta Otolaryngol [Suppl] 78:83–88

Gay T, Rendell J, Spiro J, Mosier K, Lurie A (1994) Coordination of oral cavity and laryngeal movements during swallowing. J Appl Physiol 77:357–365

Ghez C (1985) Introduction to the motor systems. In: Kandel ER, Schwartz JH (eds) Principles of neural science, 2nd edn. Elsevier Science, New York, pp 437–440

Gropman A, Barkovich AJ, Vezina LG, Conry JA, Dubovsky EC, Packer RJ (1997) •• Neuropediatrics 28:198–203

Hathout GM, Bigoni BJ, Varjavand B, Gopi R, Gambhir S (1998) The hysteresis phenomenon in functional MR imaging: a mathematical model of the BOLD mechanism. Proc Am Soc Neuroradiol 36:159

Horner J, Massey EW, Brazer SR (1990) Aspiration in bilateral stroke patients. Neurology 40:1686–1688

Jacobs BC, Brant-Zawadzki M (1992) Ischemia. In: Stark DD, Bradley WG (eds) Magnetic resonance imaging, 2nd edn. Mosby Year Book, St Louis, pp 636–669

Jones B, Donner M (eds) (1991) Normal and abnormal swallowing: imaging in diagnosis and therapy. Springer, Berlin Heidelberg New York

Kahrilas PJ, Shezhang L, Logemann JA, Ergun GA, Facchini F (1993) Deglutitive tongue action: volume accommodation and bolus propulsion. Gastroenterology 104:152–162

Kilman WJ, Goyal RK (1976) Disorders of the pharyngeal and upper esophageal motor function. Arch Intern Med 136:592–601

Kim JS, Lee JH, Suh DC, Myoung CL (1994) Spectrum of lateral medullary syndrome correlation between clinical findings and magnetic resonance imaging in 33 subjects. Stroke 25:1405–1410

Kirshner HS (1989) Causes of neurogenic dysphagia. Dysphagia 3:184–188

Lewine JD (1995) Introduction to functional neuroimaging: functional neuroanatomy. In: Orrison WW, Lewine JD, Sanders JA, Hartshorne MF (eds) Functional brain imaging. Mosby Year Book, St Louis, pp 45–88

Logemann JA (1988) Swallowing physiology and pathophysiology. Otolaryngol Clin North Am 21:613–623

Maldjian J, Howard R, van Buchem M, et al. (1996) Functional magnetic resonance imaging of regional brain activity in patients with intracerebral arteriovenous malformation before surgical or endovascular therapy. J Neurosurg 84:477–483

Martin RE, Murray GM, Kemppainen P, Masuda Y, Sessle BJ (1997) Functional properties of neurons in the primate tongue primary motor cortex. J Neurophysiol 78:1516–1530

Martin RE, Sessle BJ (1993) The role of the cerebral cortex in swallowing. Dysphagia 8:195–202

Miller AJ (1986) Neurophysiological basis of swallowing. Dysphagia 1:91–100

Mosier KM (1997) The motor control of swallowing. UMI Publications, Ann Arbor, pp 247–249

Netter FH (1995) The Ciba collection of medical illustrations, vol 1: Nervous system. 1. Anatomy and physiology. Ciba Pharmaceuticals, West Caldwell, NJ

Ogawa S, Lee TM, Kay AR (1990) Brain magnetic resonance imaging with contrast dependence on blood oxygenation. Proc Natl Acad Sci 87:9869–9872

Ogawa S, Menon RS, Tank DW (1993) Functional brain mapping by blood oxygenation level dependent contrast magnetic resonance imaging. Biophys J 64:803–812

Osborn AG (1994) Diagnostic neuroradiology. Mosby Year Book, St Louis

Pansky B, Allen D, Budd GC (eds) (1988) Review of neuroscience, 2nd edn. Macmillan, New York, pp 204, 208, 408

Penfield W, Rasmussen T (1950) The cerebral cortex of man. Macmillan, New York

Ramsey RG (1987) Neuroradiology, 2nd edn. Saunders, Philadelphia, pp 164–168

Robbins J, Levine FL, Maser A, Rosebek JC, Kempster G (1993) Swallowing after unilateral stroke of the cerebral cortex. Arch Phys Med Rehabil 74:1295–1300

Seaman WB (1976) Pharyngeal and upper esophageal dysphagia. JAMA 235:2643–2646

Sonies BC, Baum BJ (1988) Evaluation of swallowing pathophysiology. Otolaryngol Clin North Am 21:637–648

Tanji J, Shima K, Mushiake H (1996) Multiple cortical motor areas and temporal sequencing of movements. Cogn Brain Res 5:117–122

Veis SL, Logemann JA (1985) Swallowing disorders in persons with cerebrovascular accident. Arch Phys Med Rehabil 66:372–375

Weller M (1993) Anterior opercular cortex lesions cause dissociated lower cranial nerve palsies and anarthria but no aphasia: Foix-Chavany-Marie syndrome and "automatic voluntary dissociation" revisited. J Neurol 240:199–208

Yousry T, Schmidt U, Jassoy AG (1995) Prospective study with functional MR imaging and direct motor mapping at surgery. Radiology 195:23–29

# 7 PET Scanning of Head and Neck Cancer

P. Lindholm, M. Lapela, S. Leskinen, and H. Minn

CONTENTS



## 7.1 Introduction to Positron Emission Tomography (PET)

Positron emission tomography (PET) is a unique noninvasive method of measuring regional biochemical and physiological processes in vivo. High-contrast spatial and temporal resolution, sensitivity and quantification make PET superior to conventional isotope imaging methods. Advanced morphological imaging modalities reveal changes in macrostructures, while PET may give information about the characteristics of cancer tissue and assist in distinguishing malignant from benign or therapy-induced changes. Modern PET devices have a spatial resolution of 5 mm or less, a 15-cm-wide field of view (FOV) and a three-dimensional (3-D) imaging capability (DeGrado et al. 1994), they and can produce whole-body images. Computed tomography (CT) or magnetic resonance (MR) scans can be digitally fused with PET for co-registration of morphological and metabolic images (Wahl et al. 1993), which will further improve the efficacy of PET in cancer detection.

### 7.1.1 Principles of PET

PET measures the radiation from a compound labelled by a positron-emitting radionuclide externally as a function of time and space. In tissue the radionuclide releases a positively charged electron or positron that travels 2–3 mm before it collides with an electron. An energy-liberating process called annihilation ensues, which gives origin to two 511-keV photons that are emitted at opposite angles. Radiation detectors arranged in a circular array around the patient are coupled to identify coincidence photons with a set of opposing detectors, while other radiation events are rejected. The coincidence data are integrated for each pair of the coincidence detectors, and the distribution of the radioactivity is reconstructed into tomographic images. The measured data need to be corrected for calibration, decay, dead time losses and random coincidence events. Accurate quantification of radioactivity requires correction for tissue attenuation that is obtained by transmission scanning with a positron-emitting source.

The highest resolution of the PET method is approximately 2–3 mm, owing to physical limitations. The line spread function (LSF) is a measure of the spatial accuracy of the PET device, and it is referred


P. Lindholm, MD, Ph.D, M. Lapela, MD, S. Leskinen, MD, H. Minn, MD, Ph.D, Department of Oncology and Radiotherapy, and Turku PET Centre, Turku University Central Hospital, PL 52, FIN-20521 Turku, Finland

to in terms of full width at half maximum: FWHM (HOFFMAN and PHELPS 1986). When the object being observed has at least one dimension smaller than 2 × FWHM, the isotope concentration is underestimated (the partial volume effect). The transaxial resolution is most accurate over the central third of the FOV, while the accuracy is impaired with increasing distance from the central axis. A recovery coefficient (RC), which is the ratio of observed to true isotope concentration in the PET image, can be used to correct count rates in small objects.

In whole-body PET imaging the axial FOV is extended by imaging at multiple bed positions and acquiring data for short periods at each position (DAHLBOM et al. 1992). Two-dimensional planar images that can be displayed as transaxial, sagittal and coronal tomographic images give an overview of the distribution of the tracer. The whole-body PET method is useful primarily as a qualitative indicator of cancer distribution, insofar as the imaging is performed without attenuation correction. New methods of attenuation correction using simultaneous emission and transmission measurements are being evaluated (MEIKLE et al. 1995).

### 7.1.2 Quantification in PET

Before a PET study, a patient should preferably be in the fasting state. After the patient has been positioned for the scanning, transmission images are usually obtained. The tracer is then injected intravenously, and emission scanning is initiated immediately using multiple dynamic time frames; alternatively it can be carried out over a shorter period, for example 40–60 min after the injection.

The sensitivity of the PET technique allows nanomole and picomole levels of the tracer to be used, which minimizes pertubation of the system being observed. The PET image measures the local concentration of a tracer, for example as kilobecquerels per millilitre of tissue. Areas of high and low tracer concentration are visualized as "hot spots" and photopenic areas, respectively.

The PET data can be analysed in several ways. The activity in a target area at a fixed time point can be determined by summing over a region of interest (ROI). Tumour-to-normal tissue or tumour-to-muscle uptake ratios may be used, but the tracer uptake is often reported as standardized uptake values (SUV), also referred to as differential uptake ratios (DUR) or differential absorption ratios (DAR), which adjust the tracer concentration in a ROI to the injected dose and the patient's weight.

$$\mathrm{SUV} = \frac{\text{Radioactivity Concentration in ROI } \left(\mathrm{Bq\ cm^{-3}}\right)}{\text{Injected Dose (Bq)} / \text{Patient's Weight (g)}}$$

To overcome the weight dependence a SUV can be corrected for the body surface area ($SUV_{bsa}$; LESKINEN-KALLIO et al. 1992a, 1994a; MINN et al. 1993a; KIM et al. 1994) or the predicted lean body mass ($SUV_{lean}$; ZASADNY and WAHL 1993). SUVs can be measured from a single scan of 5–10 min at a predetermined time point thought to represent the steady state of tracer uptake. However, the time frame for SUV determination and the ROI technique, like other methodological issues (HAMBERG et al. 1994; KEYES 1995), need to be considered when PET results from different centres are compared.

When the metabolic pathways of the tracer are known kinetic modelling may be performed, but this requires serial blood sampling and dynamic frames after the tracer injection. The time–activity curve is used as the input function for kinetic analyses. When the concentration of the tracer in the tissue measured by PET and the tracer concentration in the blood are known, the kinetics of a physiological phenomenon can be traced. The rate constant or influx constant ($K_i$ value), according to the graphical approach of PATLAK et al. (1983), is the fraction of the tracer transported from plasma to tissue per unit of time (1/time). Tissue heterogeneity and diverse biochemical pathways must be considered in the interpretation of cancer PET studies (HERHOLTZ et al. 1990). Since SUVs and kinetic measurements seem to be closely related (LESKINEN-KALLIO et al. 1992a; MINN et al. 1993a), determination of SUVs appears to be sufficient in clinical cancer PET studies.

### 7.1.3 Tracers for PET Imaging of Head and Neck Cancer

Different aspects of tumour metabolism have been exploited for oncologic PET imaging, but not all of them have been useful for clinical purposes. First, a sufficiently high gradient of tracer uptake between tumour and ambient normal tissues must be achieved. Secondly, uptake of radioactivity should be low in nonmalignant cellular compartments.

Thirdly, a good tracer has predictable pharmacokinetics, since quantitative analysis for differential diagnosis or follow-up of treatment requires at least some understanding of tracer kinetics. In this chapter we have concentrated on radiopharmaceuticals that have already shown promising clinical applicability, paying less attention to those that have not yet emerged into patient imaging.

### 7.1.3.1 Fluorine-18 Fluorodeoxyglucose (FDG)

Of all the tracers available for PET, fluorine-18-labelled 2-fluoro-2-deoxy-D-glucose (FDG) is the most widely used tumour-seeking agent (Conti et al. 1996; Rigo et al. 1996). The use of FDG for cancer imaging is based on studies first described by Warburg (1926), who found that neoplastic cells favoured glycolysis over respiration for their energy metabolism. Later experimental studies have supported this in essence (Weinhouse 1976; Flier et al. 1987). FDG is a glucose analogue, which shares membrane transport sites with its natural counterpart and is subsequently phosphorylated by hexokinase. As cancer cells have up-regulated glucose carrier mechanism and a specific high-affinity hexokinase isoenzyme promoting glycolysis, FDG accumulation is enhanced in tumour cells. Importantly, FDG is retained intracellularly in its phosphorylated form, since it is not a substrate for further metabolism, whereas glucose proceeds down the glycolytic pathway (Gallagher et al. 1978). The association between FDG uptake and malignant potential is discussed in Section 7.3.

In the image interpretation it is critical to know the sites of physiological uptake of FDG in different metabolic states. According to Jabour et al. (1993), FDG uptake is highest in the sublingual gland, followed by the lymphoid tissues in Waldeyer's ring, the parotid and submandibular glands, which contrast with low tracer uptake in the neck muscles of a fasting patient. For example, laryngeal cancer is easily detected in a fasting PET study (Fig. 7.1). However, muscular activity, such as speaking and chewing, during the FDG uptake period may enhance the physiological accumulation (Engel et al. 1996), and speech-related visualization of laryngeal muscles, for example, may interfere with the image interpretation (Kostakoglu et al. 1996). A relatively low uptake in the thyroid does not hamper tumour detection in the nearby tissues. The bones and fat are photopenic.

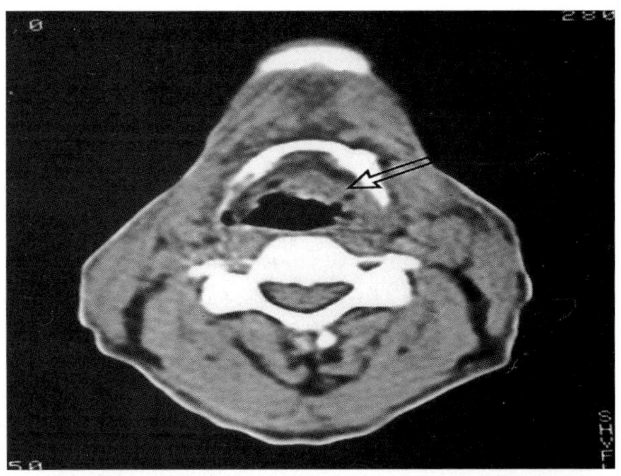
a

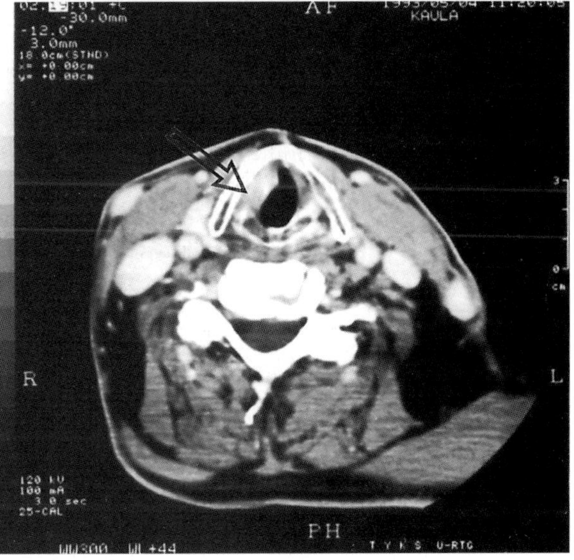

b

**Fig. 7.1.** Squamous cell glottic carcinoma (*arrow*) is clearly visible in the FDG (fluorine-18-fluorodeoxyglucose) image (**a**) when the patient is in the fasting state. Because of the spillover phenomenon the tumour seems to overlap with the airway as the high radioactivity concentration spills over to the neighbouring areas causing overestimation of tracer uptake in the surrounding areas (please see also Figs. 7.7, 7.12). In the corresponding CT image (**b**) the tumour has been marked with an *arrow*

Hyperglycaemia can markedly decrease tumour FDG uptake and impair visualization and delineation of both primary tumour and metastatic lymph nodes because of the increased uptake in the neck muscles (Lindholm et al. 1993a). Most head and neck tumours are squamous cell carcinomas, which do not express insulin-sensitive glucose transport sites and are thus best studied in the fasting state (Minn et al. 1993a; Mellanen et al. 1994). At least 4–6 h of fasting before FDG PET is a general recommendation.

### 7.1.3.2 Carbon-11 Methionine (MET)

Metabolism is altered in cancer cells as compared with normal cells of the same origin. An increased need for glucose, fatty acids, pyrimines and pyrimidines reflects the overall increased demand of nutrients and enhanced metabolism in actively proliferating cells. The transport of amino acids and the rate of protein synthesis are also accelerated, and the transport of amino acids may play a major part in the regulation of protein turnover (SHOTWELL et al. 1983; CHRISTENSEN 1990; BONADONNA et al. 1993).

Several amino acids can be labelled with positron emitters, but the best tumour-to-background ratio has been achieved with carbon-11-labelled methionine, usually labelled at the methyl position (L-methyl-[$^{11}$C]methionine, MET). Amino acid transport systems across the cell membranes are complex, and transportation is partly under hormonal regulation. MET is mainly transported from plasma to tissue by the ubiquitous system A carrier that is a sodium-ion-dependent, strongly energized pump for the transport of most dipolar amino acids. System A is characterized by hormonal regulation in vitro (SHOTWELL et al. 1983; CHRISTENSEN and KILBERG 1987). Insulin stimulates the transport of amino acids specific for system A in human muscle tissue (BONADONNA et al. 1993). MET can also be transported by system L, which is not sodium dependent and cannot transport amino acids against the concentration gradient. System L also seems to work in reverse to get rid of the excess of neutral amino acids in the cell.

MET is further metabolized in humans (ISHIWATA et al. 1991). By 60 min after the injection, 40% of the radioactivity is in the protein-bound fraction, and most of the metabolites result from the methylation of large molecules by the carbon-11-labelled methyl group. The amount of protein products at 60 min after the injection has not been clearly estimated, but for the first 30 min more than 80% of the radioactivity is still bound to MET. Thus, the first 30 min represent the transport of MET (ISHIWATA et al. 1993). Individual measurement of the metabolites is necessary for kinetic analysis.

Although MET is effective in imaging various types of cancer, its transportation is nonspecific in nature and its metabolism complex. Therefore, MET cannot be considered as a tracer of choice for basic physiological studies. An ideal tracer for amino acid transport systems would not be metabolized during the study.

The sites of physiological uptake are critical when the images are interpreted. High MET uptake can be detected in the liver and in exocrine glands such as the pancreas and the salivary and lacrimal glands (Fig. 7.2). MET uptake is also high in the bone marrow and the pituitary, while uniformly low uptake in the normal brain facilitates the detection of brain tumours. The sites of high physiological accumulation may serve as landmarks but can be confusing in

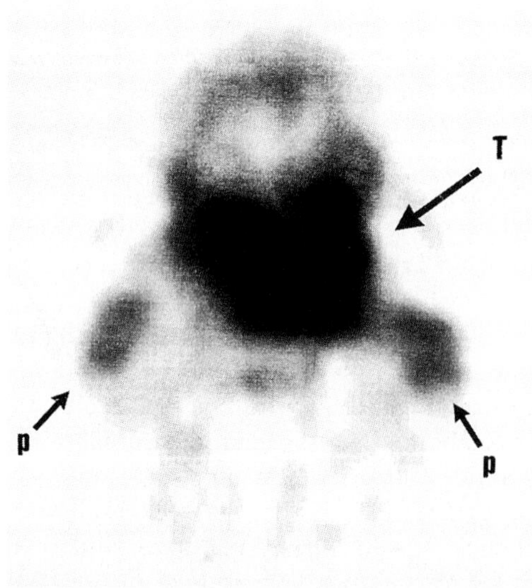


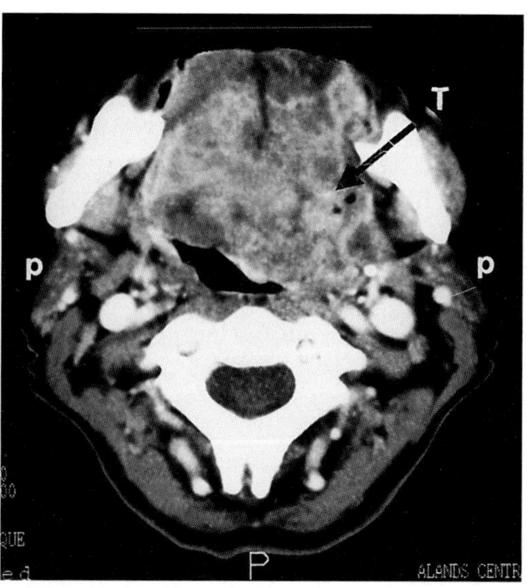


Fig. 7.2. Advanced lingual carcinoma (*large arrow, T*) imaged **A** by MET (carbon-11 methionine) positron emission tomography (PET) and **B** by CT. The parotid glands (*p*) also accumulate MET and can be used as landmarks. The physiological uptake of MET does not disturb the image interpretation

the image interpretation if a tumour is located close to these sites.

In contrast to the situation in FDG studies, the average MET uptake in head and neck cancer did not decrease markedly after food ingestion (LINDHOLM et al. 1994). In spite of the increased postprandial uptake in the salivary glands the PET image quality remained good and all malignant lesions detectable. However, for comparable results it is recommended that the patients are in the fasting state during a MET study.

## 7.2 Detection of Head and Neck Cancer

The role of PET in the diagnosis and staging of head and neck cancer is currently under assiduous investigation. Since head and neck cancers tend to disseminate regionally rather than distantly, the whole area of interest can be covered in one imaging session. Furthermore, the prospect of a noninvasive evaluation of suspicious lymph nodes seen by CT or MRI is attractive. This may have impact on the planning of the therapy.

### 7.2.1 Detection of Primary Tumour by FDG PET

The feasibility of FDG imaging in the pretherapeutic detection of head and neck cancer was first reported by MINN et al. (1988a,b), who found a sensitivity of 100% with a gamma camera adapted for 511-keV photons. In the initial study by HABERKORN et al. (1991), 46 patients with advanced head and neck cancer were investigated with FDG PET. High FDG uptake was found in all malignant lesions (SUVs, 1.8–6.0), while the uptake in normal neck tissues was clearly lower (SUVs 0.8–1.0). Similar sensitivities up to 100% have been obtained in several investigations (Figs. 7.3, 7.4) (HABERKORN et al. 1991, 1993; REISSER et al. 1992, 1993; LINDHOLM et al. 1993b; MINN et al. 1997).

In the summarized results from UCLA, USA (BAILET et al. 1992; CHAIKEN et al. 1993; JABOUR et al. 1993; REGE et al. 1993, 1994), FDG PET was reported to reveal 97% of all known primary tumours, whereas only 77% of them were found on MR images. GREVEN et al. (1994a) from Winston-Salem, USA, investigated 25 patients by FDG PET. All tumours larger than 1 cm in diameter were detected (sensitivity 89%), while three smaller lesions were not visualized. According to the same group, FDG PET was as reliable as CT or MR imaging in identifying laryngeal cancer. The sensitivity was 88%, but three supraglottic lesions were missed (MCGUIRT et al. 1995a). Furthermore, even visual analysis of FDG PET images may reveal a sensitivity of 100% for primary tumours, as stated by WONG et al. (1995, 1997) of London, UK. Several studies have also demonstrated that a previously unknown primary tumour can be identified with FDG PET. This has been successful in 30–50% (REGE et al. 1994; GREVEN et al.

a 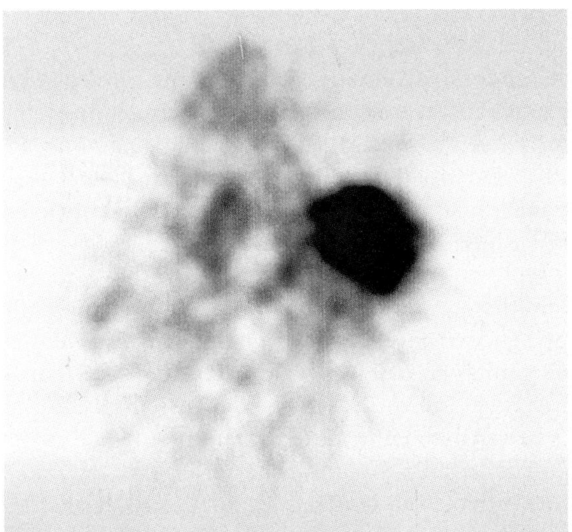

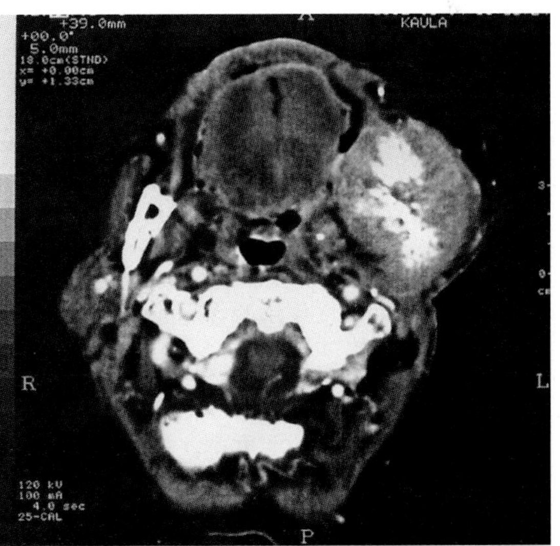 b


**Fig. 7.3.** **a**AFDG PET scan of advanced squamous cell cancer (UICC stage T4) in the left mandibular gum and **B** the corresponding CT scan

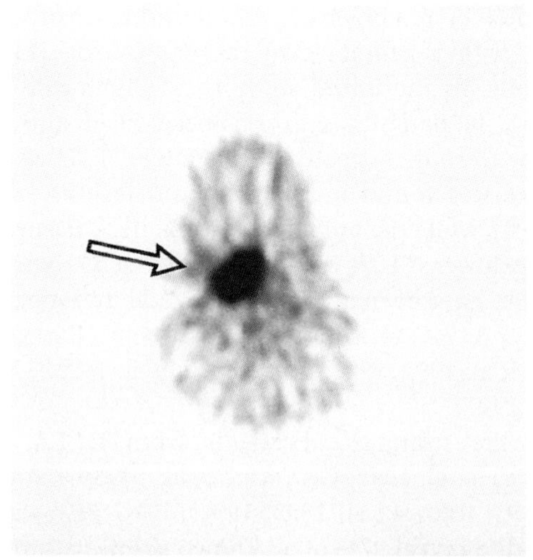

a

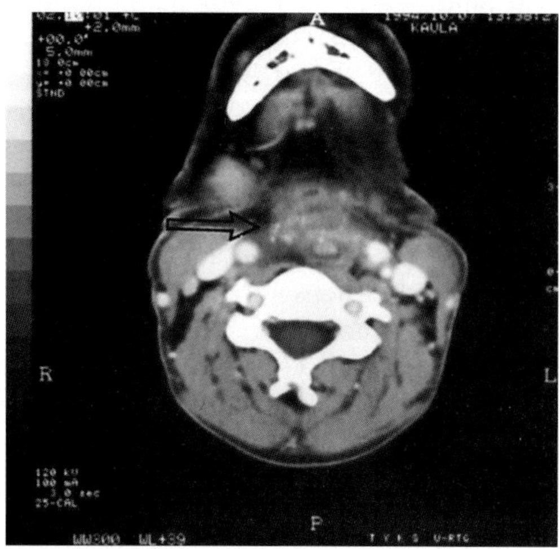

b

**Fig. 7.4.** **A** FDG PET and **B** CT images of a large supraglottic carcinoma (*arrow*)

**Table 7.1.** Identification of neck node status in patients with head and neck cancer

| No. of patients | Accuracy of PET (%) | Accuracy of CT/MRI (%) | Reference |
|---|---|---|---|
| 34 | 94 | 91 MRI | Rege et al. 1994 |
| 17 | 81 | 81 MRI/CT | McGuirt et al. 1995a |
| 49 | 82 | 84 CT | McGuirt et al. 1995b |
| 16 | 75 | 56 MRI/CT | Wong et al. 1997 |
| 17 | 94 | 65 MRI | Laubenbacher et al. 1995 |

1994a; Wong et al. 1995; Schipper et al. 1996; Braams et al. 1997) of patients with cervical metastases.

The results presented above have been based on the overall capability of FDG PET to detect primary head and neck cancer. In the clinical setting more distinct tumour staging is needed. The limited anatomical information obtained by PET puts it in a complementary position, since CT and MRI are essential for detailed planning of therapy. Both FDG PET and MRI may over or underestimate tumour size, compared with endoscopy and histological findings (Laubenbacher et al. 1995). However, potentially better depiction of tumour margins with PET and disclosure of additional tumour deposits may be highly valuable for local management. Coregistration with PET may assist CT/MRI imaging in tumour delineation (Wong et al. 1996).

In conclusion, PET with FDG can effectively detect and delineate primary head and neck cancer. However, clinical examination of a patient in whom head and neck cancer is suspected is usually successful when completed with CT or MRI and confirmed by biopsy. PET may be recommended as a complementary evaluation in patients with unknown primary tumour and metastatic lymph nodes, situation regarded as a "mostly acceptable" indication for PET by an Interdisciplinary Consensus Conference (Reske et al. 1996). In cases where clinical or imaging findings are in disagreement with biopsy findings, PET may be used to direct the site of a new biopsy. The potential of PET in delineation of tumours for planning of radiation therapy (Fig. 7.5) is of interest and needs further study.

## 7.2.2 Detection of Lymph Node Metastases by FDG PET

As node involvement represents the most powerful prognostic factor in head and neck cancer, there have been several studies on nodal staging by FDG PET. Potentially, PET may be able to detect malignant spread in normal-sized lymph nodes but should not show abnormal uptake in enlarged reactive lymph nodes. Several investigators have reported that the accuracy of FDG PET in identification of the presence or absence of lymph node involvement may be similar to or even better than that of CT or MR imaging (Tables 7.1, 7.2), while any of these methods is better than clinical examination only.

The results by published Rege et al. (1994), McGuirt et al. (1995a,b), and Wong et al. (1997) were based on histology of the nodal sites, whereas Jabour et al. (1993), Braams et al. (1995), and Laubenbacher et al. (1995) evaluated the detection

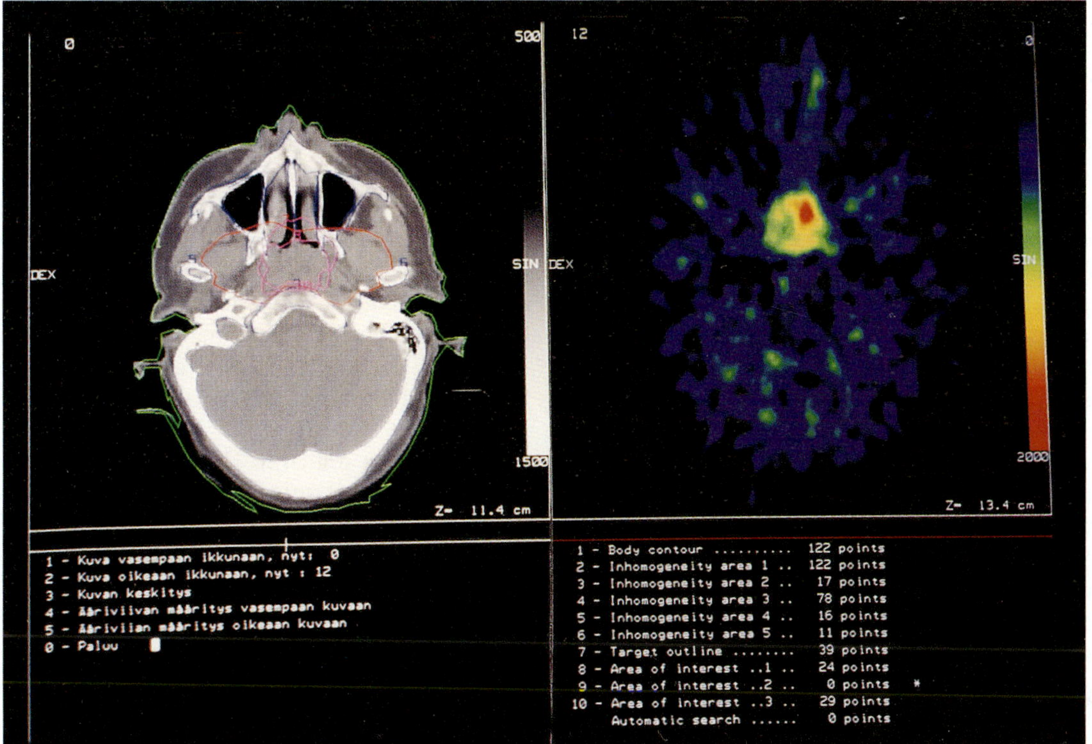


**Fig. 7.5.** In planning of radiotherapy the margins of a large nasopharyngeal adenocystic carcinoma (UICC stage T4) are clearly visualized by MET PET, and the MET image can assist in tumour delineation. The same fixation system (head holder) has to be used when the information yielded by PET and CT studies is to be combined

**Table 7.2.** Sensitivity and specificity of PET and MRI/CT in detection of diseased lymph nodes in patients with head and neck cancer

| No. of nodes (patients) | Malignant/benign nodes | Accuracy | PET | MRI/CT | Reference |
|---|---|---|---|---|---|
| 203 (8) | 17/186 | Sensitivity | 71 | 59 | Bailet et al. 1992 |
| | | Specificity | 98 | 98 | |
| 256 (9) | 34/222 | Sensitivity | 74 | 71 | Jabour et al. 1993 |
| | | Specificity | 99 | 98 | |
| 199 (12) | 22/177 | Sensitivity | 91 | 36 | Braams et al. 1995 |
| | | Specificity | 88 | 94 | |
| 521 (17) | 83/438 | Sensitivity | 90 | 78 | Laubenbacher et al. 1995 |
| | | Specificity | 96 | 71 | |
| 468 (48) | 54/414 | Sensitivity | 72 | 67 | Benchaou et al. 1996 |
| | | Specificity | 99 | 97 | |

of individual nodes. They carefully identified lymph nodes on MR and FDG PET images in patients undergoing neck dissection, and marked the nodes intraoperatively so that the pathologist could report on them individually. In the results by Jabour et al. (1993) all nodes that were falsely positive on MR imaging were negative on PET, and all that were falsely positive on PET were negative on MRI.

In the study by Braams et al. (1995) the preoperative PET images revealed 42 positive lesions; 20 of them proved to be malignant, 16 were reactive, and 6 were normal lymph nodes. Correspondingly, 18 nodes were considered to be malignant on MRI; 8 of them were metastatic, 2 were reactive, and 8 were normal. The FDG uptake was significantly higher in the metastatic lymph nodes than in the normal nodes, but there was no significant difference in uptake between metastatic and reactive nodes. Two metastatic lymph nodes were falsely negative on PET (2 mm and 3.5 mm in diameter), and 14 on MRI. The investigators also evaluated the justification for neck dissections. With the results obtained by preoperative PET, for 19 of the 24 necks a correct decision would have been made. All the necks deemed positive according to histology would have been operated on, but so would 5 necks without cancer. The MRI data would have led to a correct decision about 16 of the 24 necks; 4 necks with malignant lymph nodes would not have been operated on; and 4 unnecessary neck dissections would have taken place. It is of clinical value that 9 of the neck dissections were done electively (staged clinically as N0). In 6 of these, there were a total of nine metastatic nodes. All these nodes were detected by PET, whereas only 3 of the 6 necks were found to be malignant by MRI.

In the study of LAUBENBACHER et al. (1995) the sensitivity and specificity in detecting lymph node metastases was significantly higher for PET than for MRI. The positive predictive values of FDG PET and MRI were 80% and 34%, respectively. Similar results have been obtained by BENCHAOU et al. (1996), who reported a higher diagnostic accuracy for FDG PET than for palpation or CT.

Different lymph nodes of the same patient, and a primary tumour and its metastasis can show different FDG uptake (HABERKORN et al. 1993; LAUBENBACHER et al. 1995). The clinical impact of this phenomenon is currently unsettled. Distant metastases of head and neck cancer have not been investigated with PET, but metastases in other sites than lymph nodes, e.g. in bones, may be depicted within the field of view (HABERKORN et al. 1993).

These reports on staging of head and neck cancer suggest but do not confirm that PET is superior to anatomical imaging. Results based on identification of individual nodes are very interesting but probably lack clinical significance. Sensitivity in depicting the spread of cancer in the neck is clinically more relevant. FDG PET may be used in selected cases to confirm negative nodal disease if radical local therapy without treatment of the neck is planned. However, the whole-body mode should probably not be routinely applied for imaging head and neck cancer, which seldom shows distant metastases at diagnosis. Adequate coverage of the upper respiratory tract with PET may still complement endoscopy in finding occult disease or concurrent second primaries.

### 7.2.3 Differential Diagnosis

Most PET studies on head and neck tumours have been performed to compare PET with other imaging modalities or to relate the metabolic activity of cancer to other biological parameters. Data on the differential diagnostic capacity of PET are more limited. For example, FDG PET does not seem to be able to distinguish squamous cell carcinoma from other histological types of malignancies in the head and neck, such as anaplastic carcinoma and non-Hodgkin's lymphoma (HABERKORN et al. 1993; REISSER et al. 1992).

Since FDG is not a tumour-specific substance, the uptake in benign lesions with increased glucose metabolism can cause false-positive results (Fig. 7.6). FDG may accumulate in inflammatory lesions such as abscesses, osteomyelitis, reactive lymph nodes and postglossectomy sites. There is no reliable way of differentiating between the uptake in malignant and in inflammatory cells in human PET studies (STRAUSS 1996). Larger series are needed to find out whether quantification of FDG uptake can resolve this dilemma. Nevertheless, false-positive findings due to reactive cervical lymph nodes seem to be more frequent with CT and MRI (LAUBENBACHER et al. 1995; WONG et al. 1997).

FDG may preferentially accumulate in excretory tissue. In the study by KEYES et al. (1994) malignant parotid tumours were detectable (SUV, 2.1–24.2), but increased FDG uptake was also found in most of the benign lesions, such as Warthin tumours, adenopathy caused by toxoplasmosis, and benign mixed tumours (SUV, 2.6–13.1). Hence, FDG PET may not be suitable for differential diagnosis of parotid masses.

In conclusion, there are no tumour-specific tracers. Both FDG and MET (LINDHOLM et al. 1995) can accumulate in inflammatory tissue. Morphological imaging is needed for comparison in interpretation of the PET image. Moreover, clinical symptoms and signs have to be considered.

### 7.2.4 Detection of Head and Neck Cancer by MET PET

MET has shown its usefulness in the imaging of head and neck cancer (Fig. 7.7). In the initial study by LESKINEN-KALLIO et al. (1992b) all primaries and metastatic neck nodes were detected in 23 patients. No correlation was found between MET uptake and

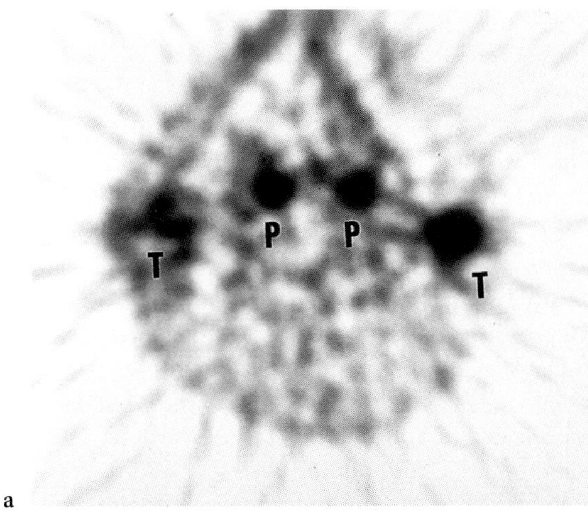


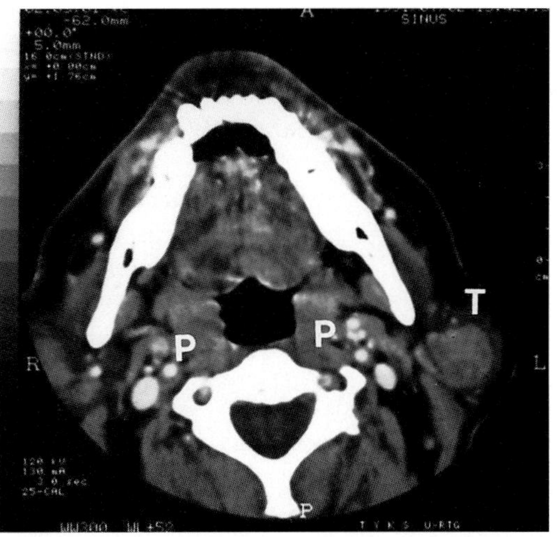


**Fig. 7.6.** A bilateral Warthin tumour (*T*) of the parotid gland is benign, but has increased FDG uptake, as shown in the FDG PET image (**a**). The palatine tonsils (*P*) also accumulate FDG. (**b**) On the corresponding CT scan a cervical tumour (*T*) is detected and the palatine tonsils are marked

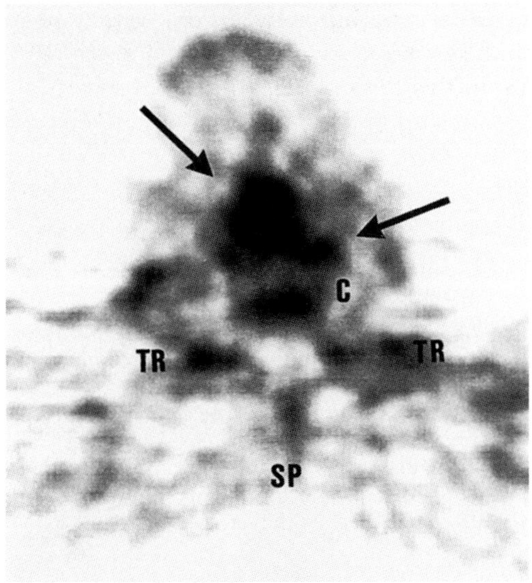


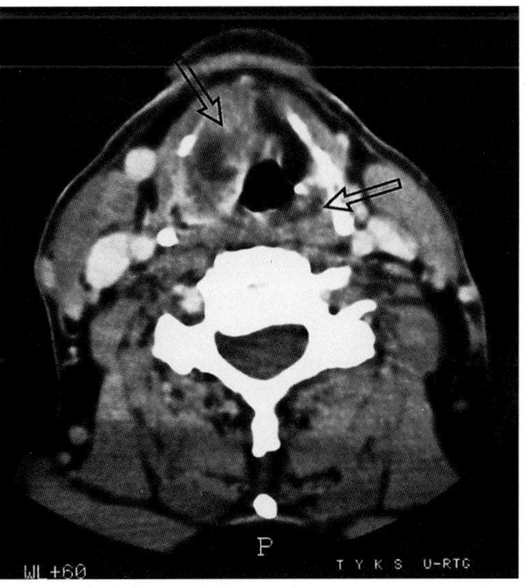


**Fig. 7.7.** (**a**) MET and (**b**) CT images of squamous cell laryngeal cancer extending adjacent to the thyroid cartilage (*arrows*). Because of the spillover the tumour seems to overlap with the airway (please see also Figs. 7.1, 7.12). The corpus (*C*), processus spinosus (*SP*) and transversi (*TR*) of the cervical vertebra are also visualized with MET

the size of the tumour. Later, 46 of 47 malignant tumours with a diameter larger than 1 cm were visualized, but no MET uptake was found in a benign pleomorphic adenoma (LESKINEN-KALLIO et al. 1994b). MET seems to be as effective as FDG in detecting head and neck cancer (LINDHOLM et al. 1993b). Twenty-one malignant lesions in 14 patients were studied with both tracers (Fig. 7.8), and one malignant lymph node was missed by each tracer. The mean SUVs were surprisingly equal (7.7 ± 4.2 for FDG; 7.7 ± 2.5 for MET).

## 7.3 Evaluation of the Biological Nature of Head and Neck Cancer by PET

The tumour stage correlates with prognosis in head and neck cancer (WANG 1997), whereas no such relationship has been demonstrated with histopathological grading (PETERS et al. 1986). Still, head and neck cancers that are similar in stage and histomorphometric appearance may have different clinical behaviour. At present those tumours that are

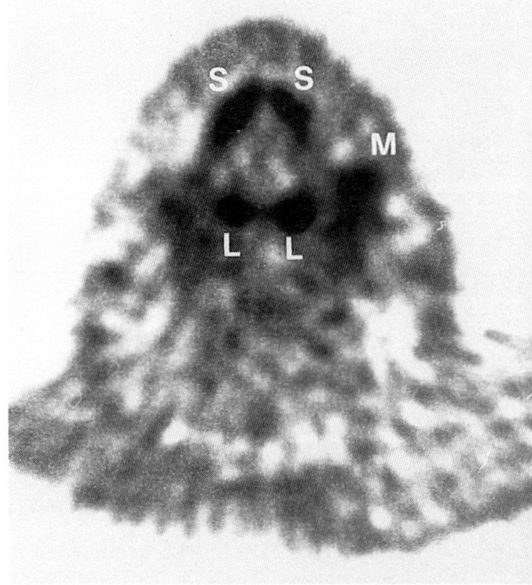


a

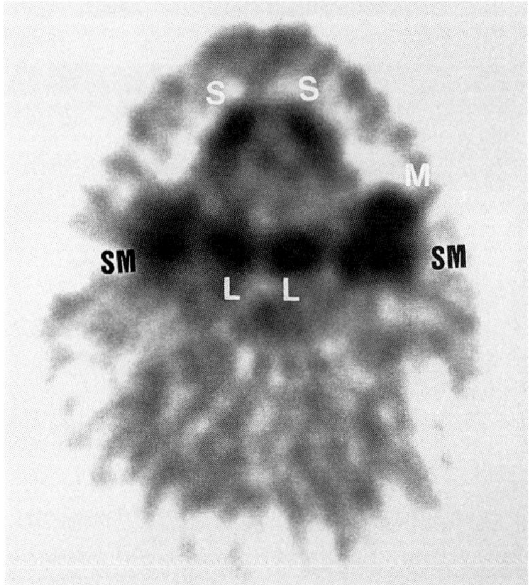


b

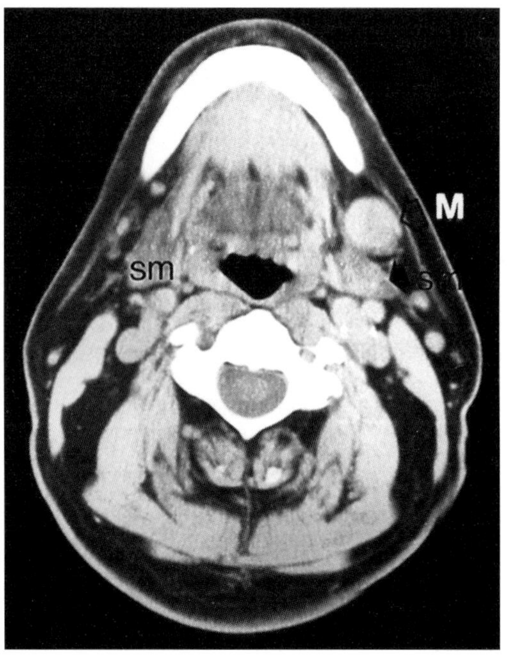


c

**Fig. 7.8 a–c.** Usually FDG and MET have different sites of physiological uptake, but both may accumulate in the sublingual glands and lingual tonsils. PET images of a metastatic lymph node (*M*) on the left side of the neck studied with (**a**) FDG and (**b**) MET, and (**c**) the corresponding CT image. The sublingual glands (*S*) and lingual tonsils (*L*) accumulate both FDG and MET, while the submandibular glands (*SM*) are visualized only in the MET image

biologically the most aggressive cannot be reliably recognized. Thus, clinicians need new methods for planning a more individualized cancer therapy.

### 7.3.1 Assessment of Cell Proliferation

Head and neck tumours are usually treated with surgery and radiotherapy, but advanced head and neck cancers often recur after conventional therapy. Recent randomized trials have proved the efficacy of intense radiotherapy protocols, which yield a larger than standard total dose or give a total dose over a shorter overall treatment time by using smaller fractions given two or three times daily (Ang et al. 1997). Hyperfractionated radiotherapy may further improve local control when individual differences in tumour proliferation, oxygenation and intrinsic radiosensitivity can be characterized (Hall 1994). Tumours with a short potential doubling time ($T_{pot}$) may benefit from hyperfractionated radiotherapy to negate the effect of cell repopulation during the therapy (Begg 1995). Since a biopsy is needed for the determination of $T_{pot}$, and the subsequent flow cytometry (FCM) may be technically challenging, PET has been suggested for assessment of tumour proliferative status. Tumour oxygenation will be discussed in Section 7.6.

A relationship between FDG uptake in untreated head and neck cancer and the proportion of cells synthesizing DNA (S-phase fraction, SPF) was ini-

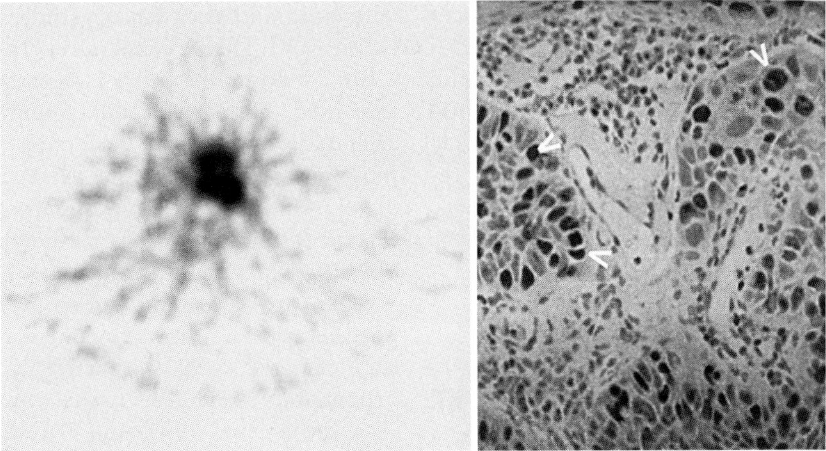

**Fig. 7.9.** Advanced glottic cancer with high FDG uptake ($SUV_{lean}$ 10.4) shows positive labelling of tumour cells with Ki-67 antibody (*white arrowheads*), indicating high proliferative activity

tially found using a specially collimated gamma camera (Minn et al. 1988a). The tumours with a high SPF seemed to have high FDG uptake to conform with enhanced energy metabolism. In the PET study by Haberkorn et al. (1991) such a linear relationship between FDG uptake and SPF was not found, but instead there were two subgroups individually associated with FDG uptake and with tumour proliferation.

A strong association of in vitro FDG uptake with viable cell number has been shown for ovarian carcinoma, melanoma (Higashi et al. 1993) and head and neck squamous cell carcinoma (Minn et al. 1995). Tumour FDG uptake was not linked to SPF or proportion of cells preparing to go into mitosis, while thymidine labelling was closely related to SPF, as measured by FCM (Higashi et al. 1993). On the other hand, proliferating cells seemed to have a preferential uptake of radiolabelled methionine analogous to that of thymidine (Reinhardt et al. 1997). Different uptake patterns for these tracers and their relationship with proliferation have also been studied in rodents (Sato et al. 1992). Imaging with labelled thymidine is discussed in Section 7.7.

Owing to controversial results, the role of FDG PET for the assessment of proliferation has not been confirmed in head and neck cancer. Nonetheless, tumour FDG uptake was strongly correlated with the number of mitoses in 37 untreated patients with squamous cell head and neck cancer (Minn et al. 1997). FDG-avid tumours tended to have a high proliferative index, as assessed by Ki-67 antibody labelling (Fig. 7.9). The relative discrepancies observed in different clinical and experimental studies on tumour metabolism and proliferation may depend partly on the different analytical methods, and they underline the need for careful validation and development of cytometric techniques (Ensley 1996).

### 7.3.2 Grading of Malignancy and Prediction of Prognosis

Glucose utilization is increased in cancer, and it seems to be associated with the malignant potential of the tumour. Protein synthesis and amino acid transport are also enhanced in malignant cells. These findings have encouraged researchers to investigate whether tumour uptake as measured by PET is able to describe biological aggressiveness and predict the final outcome of patients with head and neck cancer.

Reisser et al. (1993) found no correlation between histological grading and tumour FDG uptake in 48 patients with squamous cell head and neck cancer. In contrast, moderately or poorly differentiated squamous cell carcinomas had a larger FDG uptake than well-differentiated ones ($P = 0.046$) in a series of 37 untreated patients (Minn et al. 1997). Moreover, the overall 3-year survival of the patients with a tumour $SUV_{lean}$ smaller than or equal to the median was significantly better than that of the patients with a tumour $SUV_{lean}$ greater than the median (73% vs 22%; $P = 0.002$) after the median follow-up of 43 months. This is in line with another study by Reisser et al. (1992), who found an association between high tumour FDG uptake and poor survival in a series of 50 patients. These results suggest that FDG PET may have a role as a noninvasive predictor of prognosis in squamous cell head and neck cancer.

In contrast, there was no correlation between the grade of malignancy and tumour MET uptake in 30 patients with squamous cell head and neck cancer (Leskinen-Kallio et al. 1994b). Similarly, no correlation was found between tumour MET uptake and the survival time of 39 untreated patients with squamous cell head and neck carcinoma (Lindholm et al., 1998). Apparently, MET uptake in tumour reflects amino acid transport rather than protein synthesis rate. Tumour MET uptake seems to have little prognostic value.

## 7.4 Evaluation of Treatment Response by PET

Head and neck cancers have a high tendency to recur locally and to generate distant metastases at a relatively late phase. Hence, complete loco-regional control is particularly important. The rate of regression varies substantially in tumours with a similar stage and histology, and it may not correlate with the final outcome of the therapy. On the other hand, repeated biopsies should be avoided, since they impair the healing of normal tissues. A reliable method of predicting response to therapy should assist the clinician to identify those patients who require intensified cancer treatment.

### 7.4.1 Response to Radiotherapy

FDG imaging with a specially collimated gamma camera proved to be useful in assessing the treatment response in 19 patients with head and neck cancer (Minn et al. 1988b). A rapid reduction in tumour FDG uptake during radiotherapy indicated a good radiation response. In line with these findings, Chaiken et al. (1993) were reliably able to detect head and neck cancer persisting after radiotherapy by FDG PET. In a PET study performed 2–12 weeks after the completion of radiotherapy, a marked decrease in FDG uptake was found in seven patients with responding tumours, while nonresponding tumours of two patients had increased uptake and histologically confirmed persistent disease.

A rapid and sensitive response to radiotherapy was observed as a decrease in MET uptake in tumour-bearing rodents, and the decrease in the uptake appeared to be dependent on irradiation dose (Kubota et al. 1989, 1992a). In agreement with these findings, a significant decrease in MET uptake was recorded in tumour sites with complete histological response to radiotherapy in a series of 15 patients with head and neck cancer studied with MET PET before and after preoperative radiotherapy (Fig. 7.10). Tumours in which SUV was higher than the threshold value always still contained viable cancer after radiotherapy, whereas most (70%) of the tumour sites with a smaller SUV responded completely. In addition, a good treatment response was related to a low ratio of posttherapy to pretherapy SUV (0.50 or smaller; Lindholm et al. 1995).

There are important issues to be considered when posttherapy PET scans are interpreted. Inflammatory changes such as reactive lymph nodes and oedematous laryngeal tissue can take up MET (Lindholm et al. 1995) and FDG after radiotherapy (Chaiken et al. 1993; Rege et al. 1994). The decrease in tumour FDG uptake at 1 month after radiotherapy may not be an accurate indicator of good response, whereas an FDG study 4 months after radiotherapy seem to predict the response better (Greven et al. 1994b). Similarly, a relatively high MET uptake was found in ring-like laryngeal oedema in a posttherapy scan performed soon after the completion of radiotherapy (Fig. 7.10). Thus, the tracer accumulation in reactive tissue and its temporal relationship to PET studies must be considered when oncological PET images are interpreted.

Rege et al. (1993) recorded no radiation-induced changes of FDG uptake with such normal tissues as the tonsils, nasal turbinates, soft palate and gingiva after radiotherapy of head and neck cancer. In contrast, MET uptake decreased clearly in the salivary glands (30–46%) and in the bone marrow (average 22%). However, a higher uptake was found in the salivary glands imaged within the first week after the completion of radiotherapy, possibly because of an inflammatory reaction (Lindholm et al. 1995).

In summary, a high uptake of FDG or MET after radiotherapy of head and neck cancer suggests the presence of persistent cancer. However, the time interval between the completion of therapy and the PET study appears to be important. It is currently not known whether early changes in the tracer uptake of tumours during radiotherapy can predict the treatment response.

### 7.4.2 Response to Chemotherapy

There are few studies on the evaluation of response to chemotherapy in head and neck cancer. Haberkorn et al. (1993) studied 18 patients with advanced head and neck cancer by FDG PET before

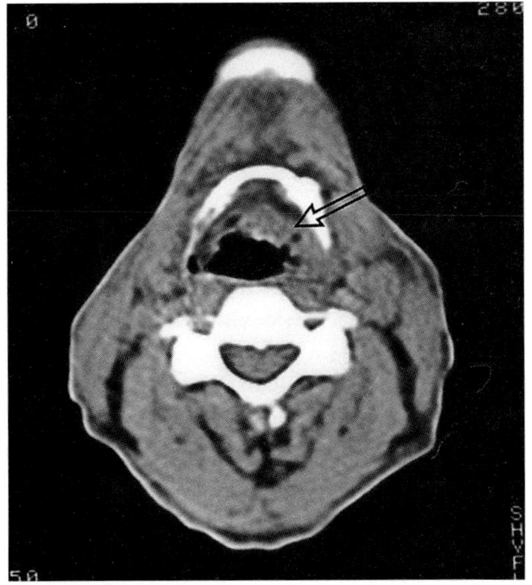

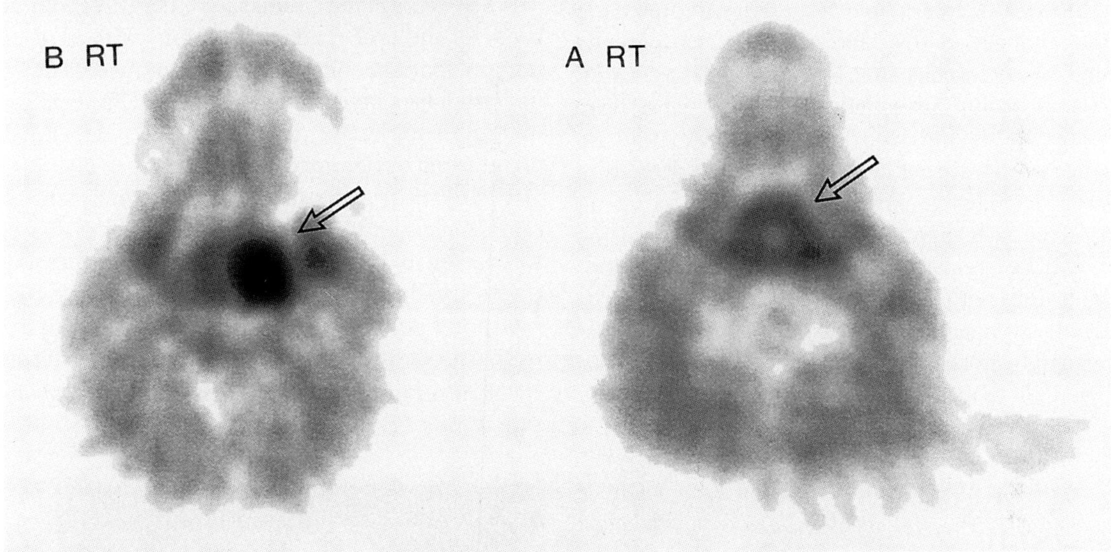


**Fig. 7.10.** A CT and **B** MET images of supraglottic cancer (*arrow*) studied with MET before (*B RT*) and after (*A RT*) radical radiotherapy. The patient was thought on clinical assessment to have persistent cancer, but complete histological response was confirmed. The tumour MET uptake decreased from 10.2 to 2.2. Moderate ring-like laryngeal oedema was found in the posttherapeutic MET image

the first chemotherapeutic cycle with cisplatin and 5-fluorouracil, and a second PET scan was performed 1 week after the first cycle in 11 patients. Volumetric data was collected by CT, and the macroscopic growth rate of the malignant lesions was compared with the PET data. The tumour growth rate and the change in FDG uptake were found to be closely correlated. However, because of the heterogeneity of tumours, different metastatic lymph nodes of the same patient possessed different metabolic activity and, consequently, responded to chemotherapy in different ways. Long-term follow-up data were not reported.

Berlangieri et al. (1994) performed serial FDG PET studies on six patients with advanced squamous cell head and neck cancer treated with hyperfractionated radiotherapy and concurrent chemotherapy. The PET studies were performed prior to and 4 weeks after the beginning of the therapy and 2 years after. The decrease in tumour uptake paralleled the good clinical response to treatment in all except 1 patient, in whom complete response was not achieved. Diffusely increased FDG uptake in peritumour tissue after therapy was noted in several patients and correlated clinically with radiation-induced mucositis.

Apparently, it may be possible to evaluate responses of head and neck cancer to chemotherapy by PET. However, a much greater body of data is needed before any conclusions can be made.

## 7.5 Detection of Recurrent Head and Neck Cancer

Radiotherapy and surgical procedures can cause a variety of changes in the normal anatomy, and radiography, CT, and MRI cannot always help in distinguishing residual or recurrent tumours from benign posttreatment masses consisting of inflammation, fibrosis, oedema, or necrosis. Thus, accurate assessment of cancer viability in posttreatment masses is difficult with morphological modalities, and new methods such as PET seem to be exceptionally attractive.

The efficacy of FDG PET in the identification of viable cancer in the head and neck was demonstrated in a patient with a recurrence in an irradiated mandible (Minn et al. 1993b). Rege et al. (1994) found that FDG PET differentiated recurrent tumours from benign changes better than MRI in 18 patients studied 2.5–192 weeks after radiation therapy. Later, the UCLA group investigated patients who were suspected of having recurrences but who had no evidence of disease on clinical or MRI examination or had inconclusive MRI findings (Bailet et al. 1995). Recurrences were reliably confirmed by using a PET-MRI co-registration technique to direct biopsies of lesions with enhanced FDG uptake. Similarly, recurrent laryngeal cancer was more accurately distinguished from radionecrosis by qualitative analysis of FDG PET (85%) than by CT or MRI (42%). One PET finding was visually equivocal, and one was a false negative, whereas there was no overlap of quantitative FDG uptake values (McGuirt et al. 1995a).

FDG PET has shown significantly better sensitivity (88–100%) and specificity (100%) for recurrent cancer than has CT/MRI (sensitivity, 25–75%; specificity, 75–80%) (Anzai et al. 1996; Wong et al. 1997). In the study of 15 patients in whom recurrent head and neck cancer was suspected (Lapela et al. 1995), the difference in FDG uptake between malignant and benign lesions was statistically significant when measured as SUVs or regional metabolic rates for FDG ($P = 0.008$ and 0.002, respectively). Comparison of CT and FDG PET supported their use as complementary imaging methods (Figs. 7.11, 7.12). The only malignant lesion not found by CT was clearly visible on FDG PET. The three false-positive lesions on CT had an FDG uptake smaller than the threshold value used. Of the four malignant lesions with SUV overlapping that of benign tissues, a tumour was detected in both cases studied by CT. Visual interpretation was more subjective, and its accuracy depended on the grading system chosen.

FDG PET appears to differentiate between recurrent cancer and posttreatment sequelae. There is some controversy about whether quantification of tracer uptake is necessary or not (Braams et al. 1995). For clinical purposes, measurement of SUVs, which are easy to obtain and are more objective than visual analysis, may be most reliable. Quantification

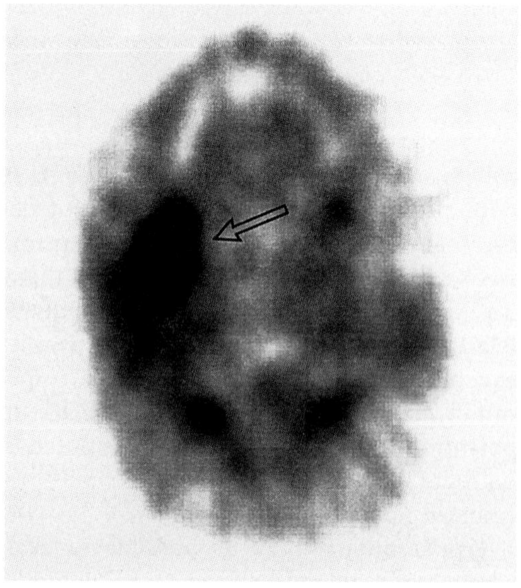

a

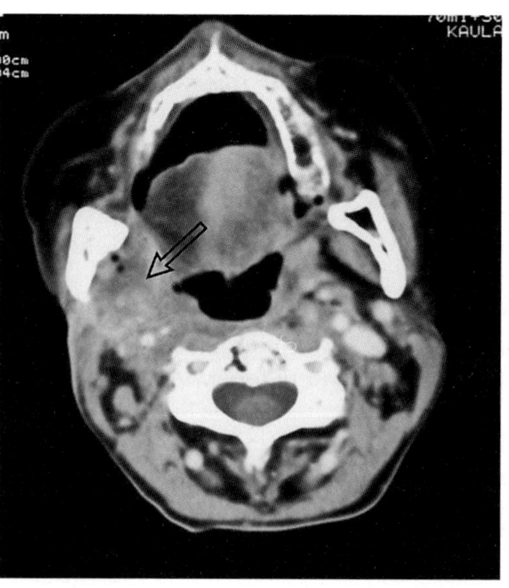

b

**Fig. 7.11.** Recurrent carcinoma (*arrow*) of the right submandibular gland as imaged by **A** FDG and **B** CT. The large tumour originates from the submandibular gland but extends to the right parotid gland

is always advisable if correlations with other patient or tumour characteristics are planned. However, more data are needed to determine the optimal cut-off level of FDG uptake for differentiation between benign and malignant lesions.

In summary, FDG PET is recommended for evaluation of tumour recurrence when physical examination does not reveal the aetiology of a patient's symptom(s) or when a suggestive lesion with a negative biopsy is found (ANZAI et al. 1996). PET may prove valuable in cases where CT/MRI is inconclusive, and PET can be used to direct biopsies to confirm a recurrence. On the other hand, continued clinical follow-up of patients with negative PET is mandatory, since microscopic deposits of cancer may not be found. The sequence of serial PET scans needed is not known. Still, some centres with wide experience of FDG PET in head and neck cancer already use the method as a part of their standard evaluation to detect tumour recurrence after radiotherapy (MCGUIRT 1997).

## 7.6 Imaging of Hypoxia

Hypoxia contributes markedly to the failure of radiotherapy and chemotherapy. Recently, a meta-analysis of data relating to more than 10 000 patients and 40 clinical trials indicated that a modification of hypoxic fraction significantly improved local control and survival in head and neck cancer (OVERGAARD and HORSMAN 1996). Even small cancers with a diameter of 20 mm or less can be significantly hypoxic, according to the polarographic microelectrode apparatus (VAUPEL et al. 1991; RALEIGH et al. 1996). Owing to the limited access of microelectrodes in deep-seated tumours and the invasiveness of the polarographic method, interest has been aroused in studying tissue oxygenation with PET and magnetic resonance spectroscopy.

Fluorine-18-labelled misonidazole (FMISO) is the only hypoxia-avid PET tracer studied in head and neck cancer. FMISO is reduced to a stable compound in hypoxic tissues, but washed out rapidly in well-oxygenated ones. The association of FMISO binding with hypoxia has been validated in animal studies (RASEY et al. 1989). FMISO tumour-to-blood ratios up to 2.5 can be expected after an accumulation period of 2–3 h.

All untreated cancers had positive FMISO PET scans in the first clinical study by KOH et al. (1992), and after radiotherapy FMISO uptake decreased below a preselected tumour-to-blood threshold value of 1.4, suggesting reoxygenation during treatment. Regional FMISO uptake showed wide variations in individual fractional hypoxic tumour volumes (RASEY et al. 1996). Recently, all primary nasopharyngeal tumours and 58% of metastatic neck nodes were found to be FMISO positive when a threshold value of 1.24 was used for tumour-to-muscle retention ratio (YEH et al. 1996). The high number of hypoxic head and neck tumours indicated by FMISO PET is in line with the results of microelectrode studies, which have mostly measured oxygen partial pressure of metastatic neck nodes or oral cavity primaries (RASEY et al. 1996).

FDG metabolic imaging may also contribute to the assessment of tumour oxygenation. In vitro studies showed increased FDG uptake under decreasing oxygen atmospheres in cell lines derived from squamous cell head and neck cancer (CLAVO et al. 1995; CLAVO and WAHL 1996; MINN et al. 1996). Methionine uptake was unchanged, while retention of leucine, depicting the rate of protein synthesis, was decreased in relation to the degree of hypoxia (CLAVO and WAHL 1996; MINN et al. 1996). Thus, FDG PET may have a role in the evaluation of effects

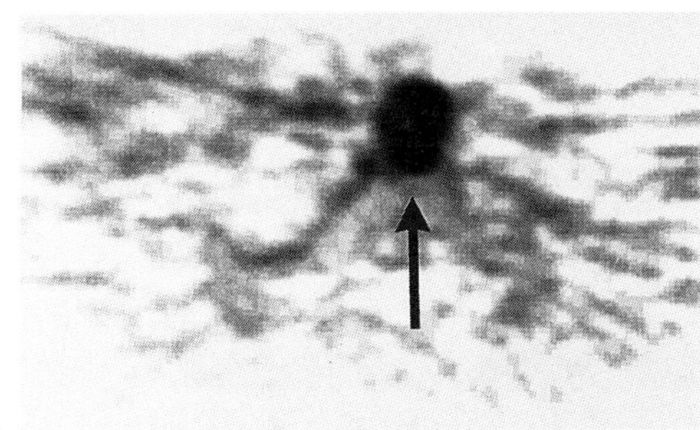
a

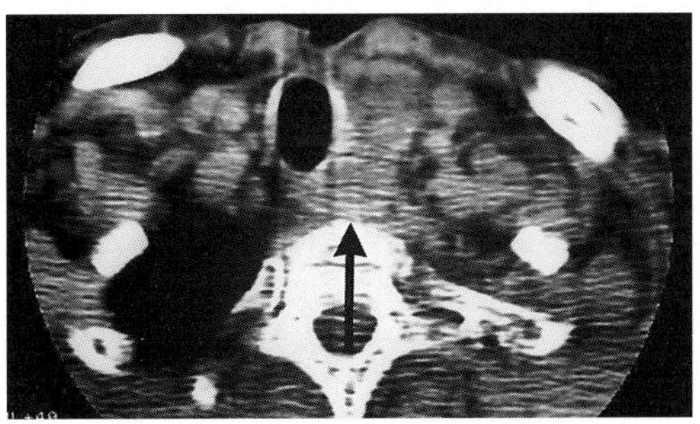
b

**Fig. 7.12.** Recurrent laryngeal carcinoma (*arrow*) imaged with **A** FDG PET and **B** CT at tracheal level. Owing to the spillover the tumour seems to overlap with the airway (please see also Figs. 7.1, 7.7)

targeted towards sensitizing hypoxic tumour cells, since FDG uptake is likely to react to changes in the tumour microenvironment.

## 7.7 Other Tracers for Imaging of Head and Neck Cancer

More than 40 different compounds have been introduced for cancer PET studies. One of the most interesting is carbon-11-labelled thymidine, which has been suggested for measurement of the proliferative activity of tumours. However, the complicated metabolism of the tracer and the short half-life of the positron-emitting isotope have made it difficult to model the incorporation of thymidine into nucleic acids (Shields et al. 1987).

Different drugs have been labelled with short-lived isotopes. However, drugs are metabolized quickly after the injection and metabolic routes are complex; hence, interpretation of the PET data is difficult.

Tyrosine labelled with carbon-11 (L-[1-$^{11}$C]tyrosine, TYR) has been introduced as a marker for protein synthesis. The metabolic routes of TYR have not yet been completely modelled. TYR accumulates avidly in cancer tissue, and a few studies have been performed on head and neck cancer (Fig. 7.13) (Braams et al. 1996). The behaviour of the tracer does not seem to be strikingly different from that of MET in the head and neck region; furthermore, TYR seems to accumulate even more in the salivary glands than MET (Daemen et al. 1991).

## 7.8 Future Aspects

There are at least three essential questions to be addressed when PET is implemented for imaging of head and neck cancer. First: is it likely that PET will alter the management of the patient? If a patient has a suspected recurrence PET may provide information that will lead to a change in management. Pa-

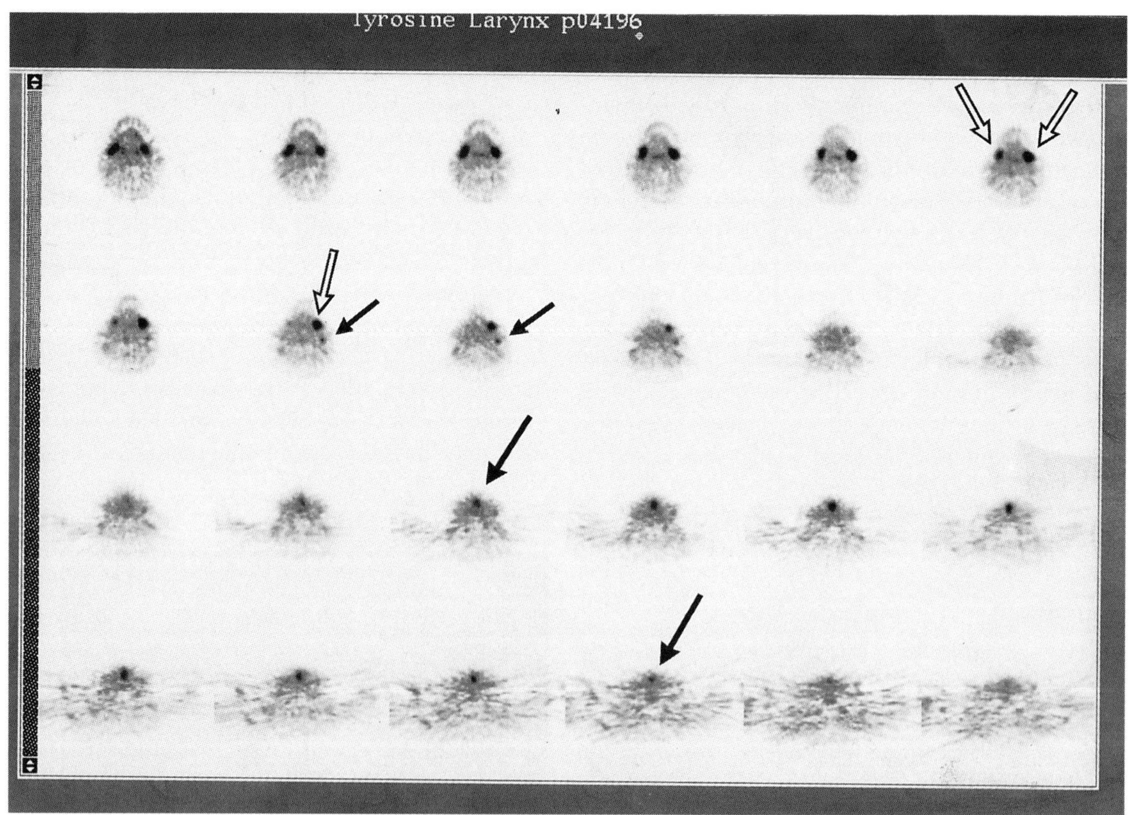

Fig. 7.13. Squamous cell laryngeal cancer (the eight axial planes between the *large arrows*) with a neck node metastasis on the left (*small arrows*), as imaged with $^{11}$C-tyrosine (TYR). The submandibular glands (*open arrows*) also accumulate TYR. Images published courtesy of Dr. Jurjan R. de Boer, University Hospital Groningen, The Netherlands

tients with a probable unknown primary tumour in the head and neck region may also benefit from a PET study. In an era of increasing demands for cost-effectiveness, the second question will be: at what price will PET modify treatment? There are several answers under different health care systems, but with regional radiopharmacy synthesis and delivery centres the prices may become competitive in the very close future, as shown by cost-effectiveness analyses (Valk et al. 1996). Electronic collimators for coincidence imaging with gamma camera may be a solution for regional hospitals that do not invest in a PET scanner. The final question is whether information relevant to tumour biology or prognosis would be at hand with PET. Most patients with head and neck cancer are treated with curative intent, and conventional staging and prognostic methods are not accurate enough to select patients for various treatment regimens. Thus, PET needs to be included in randomized clinical trials, in which pertinent statistical evaluation may reveal the usefulness of PET in the optimization of therapy.

PET is a unique method for functional evaluation both of primary head and neck cancer and lymph node metastases and of normal tissues, and it may provide information relevant to both local and systemic treatment. Different technological innovations, such as high-output image reconstruction algorithms, quantitative analysis based on parametric images, and simultaneous transmission/emission acquisition, should be evaluated in the clinical setting. Despite these new and sophisticated techniques, biological variability caused by the combination of a patient, a tumour and different external variables, such as treatment and the tracer used, remains the major factor affecting interpretation of the PET study.

## References


Ang KK, Thames HD, Peters LJ (1997) Altered fractionation schedules. In: Perez CA, Brady LW (eds) Principles and practicles of radiation oncology, 3rd edn. Lippincott-Raven, Philadelphia, pp 119–142

Anzai Y, Carroll WR, Quint DJ et al (1996) Recurrence of head and neck cancer after surgery or irradiation: prospective comparison of 2-deoxy-2-[F-18]fluoro-D-glucose PET and MR imaging diagnoses. Radiology 200:135–141

Bailet JW, Abemayor E, Jabour BA et al (1992) Positron emission tomography: a new precise imaging modality for detection of primary head and neck tumors and assessment of cervical adenopathy. Laryngoscope 102:281–288

Bailet JW, Sercarz JA, Abemayor E, Anzai Y, Lufkin RB, Hoh CK (1995) The use of positron emission tomography for early detection of recurrent head and neck squamous cell carcinoma in postradiotherapy patients. Laryngoscope 105:135–139

Begg AC (1995) The clinical status of Tpot as a predictor? Or why no tempest in the Tpot! Int J Radiat Oncol Biol Phys 32:1539–1541

Benchaou M, Lehmann W, Slosman DO et al (1996) The role of FDG-PET in the preoperative assessment of N-staging in head and neck cancer. Acta Otolaryngol 116:332–335

Berlangieri S, Brizel D, Scher R et al (1994) Pilot study of positron emission tomography in patients with advanced head and neck cancer receiving radiotherapy and chemotherapy. Head Neck 16:340–346

Bonadonna RC, Saccomani MP, Cobelli C, DeFronzo RA (1993) Effect of insulin on system A amino acid transport in human skeletal muscle. J Clin Invest 91:514–521

Braams JW, Pruim J, Freling JMF et al (1995) Detection of lymph node metastases of squamous-cell cancer of the head and neck with FDG-PET and MRI. J Nucl Med 36: 211–216

Braams JW, Pruim J, Nikkels PGJ, Roodenburg JLN, Vaalburg W, Vermey A (1996) Nodal spread of squamous cell carcinoma of the oral cavity detected with PET-tyrosine, MRI and CT. J Nucl Med 37:897–901

Braams JW, Pruim J, Kole AC, Nikkels PGJ, Vaalburg W, Vermey A, Roodenburg JLN (1997) Detection of unknown primary head and neck tumors by positron emission tomography. Int J Oral Maxillofac Surg 26:112–115

Chaiken L, Rege S, Hoh CK et al (1993) Positron emission tomography with fluorodeoxyglucose to evaluate tumor response and control after radiation chemotherapy. Int J Rad Oncol Biol Phys 27:455–464

Christensen HN (1990) Role of amino acid transport and countertransport in nutrition and metabolism. Phys Rev 70:43–77

Christensen HN, Kilberg MS (1987) Amino acid transport across the plasma membrane: role of regulation in interorgan flows. In: Yudilevich DL, Boyd CAR (eds) Amino acid transport in animal cells. Manchester University Press, Manchester, pp 10–46

Clavo AC, Wahl RL (1996) Effects of hypoxia on the uptake of tritiated thymidine, L-leucine, L-methionine and FDG in cultured cancer cells. J Nucl Med 37:502–506

Clavo AC, Brown RS, Wahl RL (1995) 2-fluoro-2-deoxy-D-glucose uptake into human cancer cell lines is increased by hypoxia. J Nucl Med 36:1625–1632

Conti PS, Lilien DL, Hawley K, Keppler J, Grafton ST, Bading JR (1996) PET and [$^{18}$F]-FDG in oncology: a clinical update. Nucl Med Biol 23:717–735

Daemen BJG, Zwertbroek R, Elsinga PH, Paans AMJ, Doorenbos H, Vaalburg W (1991) PET studies with L-[1-$^{11}$C]tyrosine, L-[methyl-$^{11}$C]methionine and $^{18}$F-fluorodeoxyglucose in prolactinomas in relation to bromocryptine treatment. Eur J Nucl Med 18:453–460

Dahlbom M, Hoffman E, Hoh C et al (1992) Whole-body positron emission tomography. I. Methods and performance characteristics. J Nucl Med 33:1191–1199

DeGrado T, Turkington T, Williams J, Stearns C, Hoffman J, Coleman R (1994) Performance characteristics of a whole-body PET scanner. J Nucl Med 35:1398–1406

Engel H, Steinert H, Buck A, Berthold T, Huch Böni RA, von Schulthess GK (1996) Whole-body PET: physiological and artifactual fluorodeoxyglucose accumulations. J Nucl Med 37:441–446

Ensley JF (1996) The clinical application of DNA content and kinetic parameters in the treatment of patients with squamous cell carcinomas of the head and neck. Cancer Metastasis Rev 15:133–141

Flier JS, Mueckler MM, Usher P, Lodish HF (1987) Elevated levels of glucose transport and transporter messenger RNA are induced by *ras* or *src* oncogenes. Science 235:1492–1494

Gallagher BM, Fowler JS, Gutterson NI, MacGregor RR, Wan CN, Wolf AP (1978) Metabolic trapping as a principle for radiopharmaceutical design: some factors responsible for the biodistribution of (18F)2-deoxyglucose. J Nucl Med 37:502–506

Greven KM, Williams DW III, Keyes JW Jr et al (1994a) Positron emission tomography of patients with head and neck carcinoma before and after high dose irradiation. Cancer 74:1355–1359

Greven K, Williams D, Keyes J et al (1994b) Distinguishing tumor recurrence from irradiation sequelae with positron emission tomography in patients treated for larynx cancer. Int J Radiat Oncol Biol Phys 29:841–845

Haberkorn U, Strauss LG, Reisser C et al (1991) Glucose uptake, perfusion, and cell proliferation in head and neck tumors: relation of positron emission tomography to flow cytometry. J Nucl Med 32:1548–1555

Haberkorn U, Strauss LG, Dimitrakopoulou A et al (1993) Fluorodeoxyglucose imaging of advanced head and neck cancer after chemotherapy. J Nucl Med 34:12–17

Hall EJ (1994) Time, dose and fractionation in radiotherapy. In: Hall EJ (ed) Radiobiology for the radiologist, 4th edn. Lippincott, Philadelphia, pp 211–229

Hamberg L, Hunter G, Alpert N, Choi N, Babich J, Fischman A (1994) The dose uptake ratio as an index of glucose metabolism: useful parameter or oversimplification? J Nucl Med 35:1308–1312

Herholtz K, Wienhard K, Heiss W-D (1990) Validity of PET studies in brain tumours. Cerebrovasc Brain Metab Rev 2:240–265

Higashi K, Clavo A, Wahl RL (1993) Does FDG uptake measure proliferative activity of human cancer? In vitro comparison with DNA flow cytometry and tritiated thymidine uptake. J Nucl Med 34:325–329

Hoffman E, Phelps M (1986) Positron emission tomography: Principles and quantitation. In: Phelps M, Mazziotta J, Schelbert H (eds) Positron emission tomography and autoradiography: principles and applications for the brain and heart. Raven, New York, pp 237–286

Ishiwata K, Kameyama M, Hatazawa J, Kubota K, Ido T (1991) Measurement of L-[methyl-$^{11}$C]methionine in human plasma. Appl Radiat Isot 42:77–79

Ishiwata K, Kubota K, Murakami M et al (1993) Re-evaluation of amino acid PET studies: can the protein synthesis rates in brain and tumor tissues be measured in vivo? J Nucl Med 34:1936–1943

Jabour BA, Choi Y, Hoh CK et al (1993) Extracranial head and neck: PET imaging with 2-[F-18]fluoro-2-deoxy-D-glucose and MR imaging correlation. Radiology 186:27–35

Keyes JW (1995) SUV: standard uptake or silly useless value? J Nucl Med 36:1836–1839

Keyes JW Jr, Harkness BA, Greven KM, Williams DW III, Watson NE Jr, McGuirt WF (1994) Salivary gland tumors: pretherapy evaluation with PET. Radiology 192:99–102

Kim C, Gupta N, Chandramouli B, Alavi A (1994) Standardized uptake values of FDG: body surface area correction is preferable to body weight correction. J Nucl Med 35:164–167

Koh WJ, Rasey JS, Evans ML et al (1992) Imaging of hypoxia in human tumors with [F-18]fluoromisonidazole. Int J Radiat Oncol Biol Phys 22:199–212

Kostakoglu L, Wong JCH, Barrington SF, Cronin BF, Dynes AM, Maisey MN (1996) Speech-related visualization of laryngeal muscles with fluorine-18-FDG. J Nucl Med 37:1771–1773

Kubota K, Matsuzawa T, Takahashi T et al (1989) Rapid and sensitive response of carbon-11-L-methionine tumor uptake to irradiation. J Nucl Med 30:2012–2016

Kubota K, Ishiwata K, Yamada S et al (1992a) Dose-responsive effect of radiotherapy on the tumor uptake of L-[methyl-$^{11}$C]methionine; feasibility for monitoring recurrence of tumor. Nucl Med Biol 19:27–32

Kubota R, Yamada S, Kubota K, Ishiwata K, Tamahashi N, Ido T (1992b) Intratumoral distribution of fluorine-18 fluorodeoxyglucose in vivo: high accumulation in macrophages and granulation tissues studied by microautoradiography. J Nucl Med 33:1972–1980

Lapela M, Grénman R, Kurki T et al (1995) Head and neck cancer: detection of recurrence with PET and 2-[F-18]fluoro-2-deoxy-D-glucose. Radiology 197:205–211

Laubenbacher C, Saumweber D, Wagner-Manslau C et al (1995) Comparison of fluorine-18-fluorodeoxyglucose PET, MRI and endoscopy for staging head and neck squamous-cell carcinomas. J Nucl Med 36:1747–1757

Leskinen-Kallio S, Någren K, Lehikoinen P, Ruotsalainen U, Teräs M, Joensuu H (1992a) Carbon-11-methionine and PET is an effective method to image head and neck cancer. J Nucl Med 33:691–695

Leskinen-Kallio S, Huovinen R, Någren K et al (1992b) [$^{11}$C]Methionine quantitation in cancer PET studies. J Comput Assist Tomogr 16:468–474

Leskinen-Kallio S, Minn H, Zasadny K (1994a) Standardized uptake values of FDG. J Nucl Med 35:1564

Leskinen-Kallio S, Lindholm P, Lapela M, Joensuu H, Nordman E (1994b) Imaging of head and neck tumors with positron emission tomography and [$^{11}$C]methionine. Int J Radiat Oncol Biol Phys 30(5):1195–1199

Lindholm P, Minn H, Leskinen-Kallio S, Bergman J, Ruotsalainen U, Joensuu H (1993a) Influence of the blood glucose concentration on FDG uptake in cancer – a PET study. J Nucl Med 34:1–6

Lindholm P, Leskinen-Kallio S, Minn H et al (1993b) Comparison of fluorine-18-fluorodeoxyglucose and carbon-11-methionine in head and neck cancer. J Nucl Med 34:1711–1716

Lindholm P, Leskinen-Kallio S, Kirvelä O et al (1994) Head and neck cancer: effect of food ingestion on [$^{11}$C]methionine uptake. Radiology 190:863–867

Lindholm P, Leskinen-Kallio S, Grénman R et al (1995) Evaluation of response to radiotherapy in head and neck cancer by positron emission tomography and [$^{11}$C]methionine. Int J Radiat Oncol Biol Phys 32(3):787–794

Lindholm P, Leskinen S, Lapela M (1998) [11C]Methionine uptake in squamous cell head and neck cancer. J Nucl Med 39:1393-1397

McGuirt WF (1997) Laryngeal radionecrosis versus recurrent cancer. Otolaryngol Clin North Am 30:243–250

McGuirt WF, Greven KM, Keyes JW Jr, Williams DW III, Watson NE Jr, Geisinger KR, Cappellari JO (1995a) Positron emission tomography in the evaluation of laryngeal carcinoma. Ann Otol Rhinol Laryngol 104:274–278

McGuirt WF, Williams DW III, Keyes JW Jr, Greven KM, Watson NE Jr, Geisinger KR, Cappellari JO (1995b) A comparative diagnostic study of head and neck nodal metastases. Laryngoscope 105:373–375

Meikle S, Bailey D, Hooper P et al (1995) Simultaneous emission and transmission measurements for attenuation correction in whole-body PET. J Nucl Med 36:1680–1688

Mellanen P, Minn H, Grénman R, Härkönen P (1994) Expression of glucose transporters in head-and neck-tumors. Int J Cancer 56:622–629

Minn H, Joensuu H, Ahonen A, Klemi P (1988a) Fluorodeoxyglucose imaging: a method to assess the proliferative activity of human cancer in vivo. Comparison with DNA flow cytometry in head and neck tumors. Cancer 61:1776–1781

Minn H, Paul R, Ahonen A (1988b) Evaluation of treatment response to radiotherapy in head and neck cancer with fluorine-18 fluorodeoxyglucose. J Nucl Med 29:1521–1525

Minn H, Aitasalo K, Happonen RP (1993) Detection of cancer recurrence in irradiated mandible using positron emission tomography. Eur Arch Otorhinolaryngol 250:312–315

Minn H, Leskinen-Kallio S, Lindholm P et al (1993) [$^{18}$F]Fluorodeoxyglucose uptake in tumors: kinetic vs. steady-state methods with reference to plasma insulin. J Comput Assist Tomogr 17:115–123

Minn H, Clavo AC, Grénman R, Wahl RL (1995) In vitro comparison of cell proliferation kinetics and uptake of tritiated fluorodeoxyglucose and L-methionine in squamous-cell carcinoma of the head and neck. J Nucl Med 36:252–258

Minn H, Clavo AC, Wahl RL (1996) Influence of hypoxia on tracer accumulation in squamous-cell carcinoma: in vitro evaluation for PET imaging. Nucl Med Biol 23:941–946

Minn H, Lapela M, Klemi P et al (1997) Prediction of survival with fluorine-18-fluorodeoxyglucose and PET in head and neck cancer. J Nucl Med 38:1907–1911

Overgaard J, Horsman MR (1996) Modification of hypoxia-induced radioresistance in tumors by the use of oxygen and sensitizers. Semin Radiat Oncol 6:10–21

Patlak C, Blasberg R, Fenstermacher J (1983) Graphical evaluation of blood-to-brain transfer constants from multiple-time uptake data. J Cerebrovasc Blood Flow Metab 3:1–7.

Peters L, Brock W, Johnson T, Meyn R, Tofilon P, Milas L (1986) Potential methods for predicting tumor radiocurability. Int J Radiat Oncol Biol Phys 12:459–467

Raleigh JA, Dewhirst MW, Thrall DE (1996) Measuring tumor hypoxia. Semin Radiat Oncol 6:37–45

Rasey JS, Koh W-J, Greirson JR, Grunbaum Z, Krohn KA (1989) Radiolabeled fluoromisonidazole as an imaging agent for tumor hypoxia. Int J Radiat Oncol Biol Phys 17:985–991

Rasey JS, Koh W-J, Evans ML et al (1996) Quantifying regional hypoxia in human tumors with positron emission tomography of [$^{18}$F]fluoromisonidazole: a pretherapy study of 37 patients. Int J Radiat Oncol Biol Phys 36:417–428

Rege S, Chaiken L, Hoh CK et al (1993) Change induced by radiation therapy in FDG uptake in normal and malignant structures of the head and neck: quantitation with PET. Radiology 189:807–812

Rege S, Maass A, Chaiken L et al (1994) Use of positron emission tomography with fluorodeoxyglucose in patients with extracranial head and neck cancers. Cancer 73:3047–3058

Reinhardt MJ, Kubota K, Yamada S, Iwata R, Yaegashi H (1997) Assessment of cancer recurrence in residual tumors after fractionated radiotherapy: a comparison of fluorodeoxyglucose, L-methionine and thymidine. J Nucl Med 38:280–287

Reisser C, Haberkorn U, Strauss LG (1992) Stoffwechseldiagnostik bei HNO-tumoren – eine PET Studie. HNO 40:225–231

Reisser C, Haberkorn U, Strauss LG (1993) The relevance of positron emission tomography for the diagnosis and treatment of head and neck tumors. J Otolaryngol 22(4):231–238

Reske SN, Bares R, Büll U, Guhlmann A, Moser E, Wannenmacher MF (1996) Klinische Wertigkeit der Positronen-Emissions-Tomographie (PET) bei onkologischen Fragestellungen: Ergebnisse einer interdisziplinären Konsessuskonferenz. Nucl Med 35:42–52

Rigo P, Paulus P, Kaschten BJ et al (1996) Oncological applications of positron emission tomography with fluorine-18-fluorodeoxyglucose. Eur J Nucl Med 23:1641–1674

Sato K, Kameyama M, Ishiwata K, Katakura R, Yoshimoto Y (1992) Metabolic changes of glioma following chemotherapy: an experimental study using four PET tracers. J Neuro-Oncol 14:81–89

Schipper JH, Schrader M, Arweiler D, Müller S, Sciuk J (1996) Die Positronenemissionstomographie zur Primärtumorsuche bei Halslymphknotenmetastasen mit unbekanntem Primärtumor. HNO 44:254–257

Shields AF, Lim K, Grierson J, Link J, Krohn KA (1987) Utilization of labeled thymidine in DNA synthesis: studies for PET. J Nucl Med 28:1435–1440

Shotwell MA, Kilberg MS, Oxender DL (1983) The regulation of neutral amino acid transport in mammalian cells. Biochim Biophys Acta 737:267–284

Strauss LG (1996) Fluorine-18 deoxyglucose and false-positive results: a major problem in the diagnostics of oncological patients. Eur J Nucl Med 23(10):1409–1415

Valk PE, Pounds TR, Tesar RD, Hopkins DM, Haseman MK (1996) Cost-effectiveness of PET imaging in clinical oncology. Clin Nucl Med 23:7373–743

Vaupel P, Cshlenger K, Knoop C, Höckel M (1991) Oxygenation of human tumors: evaluation of tissue oxygen distribution in breast cancers by computerized O2 tension measurement. Cancer Res 51:3316–3322

Wahl R, Quint L, Cieslak R, Aisen A, Koeppe R, and Meyer C (1993) "Anatometabolic" tumor imaging: fusion of FDG PET with CT or MRI to localize foci of increased activity. J Nucl Med 34:1190–1197

Wang CC (1997) Radiation therapy for head and neck neoplasms: indications, techniques, and results, 3rd edn. Wiley, New York, pp 1–13

Warburg O (1926) Über den Stoffwechsel der Tumoren. Springer, Berlin Heidelberg New York

Weinhouse S (1976) The Warburg hypothesis 50 years later. Z Krebsforsch 87:115–126

Wong WL, Chevretton E, McGurk M, Croft D (1995) Pet-FDG imaging in the clinical evaluation of head and neck cancer. J R Soc Med 88:469P–473P

Wong WL, Hussain K, Chevretton E et al (1996) Validation and clinical application of computer-combined computed tomography and positron emission tomography with 2-[18F]fluoro-2-deoxy-D-glucose head and neck images. Am J Surg 172:628–632

Wong WL, Chevretton EB, McGurk M et al (1997) A prospective study of PET-FDG imaging for the assessment of head and neck squamous cell carcinoma. Clin Otolaryngol 22:209–214

Yeh S-H, Liu R-S, Wu L-C et al (1996) Fluorine-18-fluoromisonidazole tumour to muscle retention ratio for the detection of hypoxia in nasopharyngeal carcinoma. Eur J Nucl Med 23:1378–1383

Zasadny K, Wahl R (1993) Standardized uptake values of normal tissues at PET with 2-[fluorine-18]-fluoro-2-deoxy-D-glucose: variation with body weight and a method for correction. Radiology 189:847–850

# 8 Thallium-201 Imaging for Upper Aerodigestive Tract Cancer

M. Gapany and F.M. Grund

CONTENTS



## 8.1 Introduction

Contemporary management of upper aerodigestive tract cancer relies heavily on computed tomography (CT) or magnetic resonance imaging (MRI) for initial staging and long-term follow-up. However, both of these anatomic imaging techniques frequently fall short in their ability to detect unknown primary tumors and occult cervical metastases and to differentiate recurrent tumor from therapy-induced tissue changes. In this respect, functional imaging, which relies primarily on metabolic tissue activity, could be useful in improving the predictive value of CT/MRI for the detection of occult or recurrent head and neck tumors. Several recent reports have suggested that thallium-201 SPECT could be useful for imaging head and neck tumors (El-Gazzar et al. 1988; Togawa et al. 1993). Thallium chloride is utilized primarily for assessment of myocardial perfusion, but it also concentrates avidly in tumors. While the mechanism of accelerated thallium chloride uptake by neoplastic tissue is not completely understood, it is thought to be regulated by the $NA^{+}$-$K^{+}$ adenosine triphosphate-dependent cellular ion exchange pump. Because of this predilection for neoplastic tissue, $^{201}$Tl chloride has been proposed for SPECT imaging of various human cancers (Podoloff et al. 1992). Furthermore, several recent clinical studies have provided evidence that brain tumors and primary tumors of bone treated successfully with radiation or chemotherapy will demonstrate significant reduction or complete resolution on $^{201}$Tl studies (Ramanna et al. 1990; Kaplan et al. 1987; Namba et al. 1995). In lung neoplasms, $^{201}$Tl SPECT is useful in depicting tumors greater than 20 mm in diameter, while the thallium retention index is helpful in differentiating malignant pulmonary lesions from benign ones (Duman et al. 1983; Tonami et al. 1993). There are no comprehensive prospective studies that have assessed the efficacy of $^{201}$Tl SPECT for imaging upper aerodigestive tract cancer. The available data come from relatively small pilot studies or preliminary reports on experience with this imaging modality. The following review will summarize the experience with this imaging modality published in the current literature.

## 8.2 Current Peports on $^{201}$Tl SPECT

In 1988 El-Gazzar et al. published their experience with $^{201}$Tl chloride planar scintigraphy in five cases with advanced squamous cell carcinoma of the head and neck (SCCHN). The authors were successful in imaging cervical lymph node and bone metastases, recurrence of tumor at the skull base, primary tumor in the piriform sinus and persistent cancer of the epiglottis following failure of radiochemotherapy. Togawa et al. (1993) have used $^{201}$Tl SPECT to assess the response of nasopharyngeal carcinoma to radiotherapy. Twelve patients were imaged prior to initiation of treatment. Only three tumors showed $^{201}$Tl uptake. All three hot tumors, however, became negative after successful radiotherapy. Nine patients were available for long-term follow-up, 3 of whom have developed local recurrences. All recurrent tumors were detectable with the help of $^{201}$Tl SPECT. The

M. Gapany, MD, Division of Otolaryngology, Veterans Affairs Medical Center, One Veterans Drive, Minneapolis, MN 55417, USA
F.M.Grund, MD, Department of Nuclear Medicine, Veterans Affairs Medical Center, One Veterans Drive, Minneapolis, Minn., USA

authors felt that $^{201}$Tl SPECT was a useful imaging modality for assessing the response of nasopharyngeal carcinoma to radiotherapy as well as for detection of local recurrence of this tumor. KOSTAKOGLU et al. (1997) monitored the response of nasopharyngeal carcinoma to radiotherapy in 18 patients. $^{201}$Tl SPECT was obtained at 3-month and 6-month follow-up intervals. The accuracy of this imaging modality for detection of residual disease was 72% at 3 months and 71% at 6 months.

MUKHERJI et al. (1994) used $^{201}$Tl SPECT to evaluate five patients with squamous cell carcinoma of tonsil, piriform sinus, nasopharynx and tongue base. They found that tumor detection in the head and neck area was hindered by normal background uptake of $^{201}$Tl by salivary glands and thyroid gland. While four CT-detectable tumors in their series demonstrated enhancement on $^{201}$Tl SPECT, interpretation of the nuclear imaging results was impaired because of the background $^{201}$Tl activity. One CT-negative tongue base tumor showed $^{201}$Tl uptake that was indistinguishable from the uptake in the adjacent salivary glands. None of the four cervical lymph node groups, which were all positive for metastatic involvement according to CT criteria, showed $^{201}$Tl activity distinguishable from adjacent salivary gland uptake.

The most extensive studies on the role of $^{201}$Tl SPECT for imaging head and neck cancer are those performed at the Netherlands Cancer Institute (GREGOR et al. 1996; VALDES OLMOS et al. 1997). A pilot study by GREGOR et al. (1996) suggested that $^{201}$Tl SPECT could be applied in clinical practice for detection of occult primary lesions and of tumor recurrence at the primary site as well as in the cervical lymph nodes. In this study, 25 consecutive patients with tumors of the pharynx, larynx, oral cavity, and unknown primary sites were imaged with $^{201}$Tl SPECT and the results were compared with the results of CT or MRI: $^{201}$Tl SPECT successfully detected 94% of the primary lesions, including 5 T1 tumors. In contrast, only 73% of all primary lesions were detected with the help of CT. In the neck, $^{201}$Tl SPECT correctly predicted metastastatic lymph node status in 12 cervical lymphadenectomy cases, resulting in sensitivity and specificity of 100%, while CT/MRI imaging had a sensitivity of 83% and specificity of only 50%. The authors felt, however, that SPECT gave less information about the number and the anatomy of the lymph nodes than did CT or MRI. Most recently, the same group of authors have published their experience with $^{201}$Tl SPECT in 79 patients studied for primary head and neck cancer and 30 patients investigated for recurrences (VALDES OLMOS et al. 1997). Similar to their result in the preliminary study, in this later series $^{201}$Tl SPECT showed sensitivity of 95% and specificity of 83% for detection of tumors at the primary site and sensitivity of 86% and specificity of 90% for detection of cervical lymph node metastases. In their experience, SPECT proved to be sensitive enough to detect four clinically and radiographically occult primary tumors of the pharynx. Contrary to their earlier data, VALDES OLMOS et al. (1997) reported in their recent publication that $^{201}$Tl SPECT was less sensitive than CT/MRI for detection of cervical lymph node metastases (86% for SPECT vs 97% for CT/MRI) but provided better specificity (90% for SPECT vs 30% for CT/MRI). $^{201}$Tl SPECT appeared particularly useful for detection of recurrent head and neck cancer. In this clinical setting, thallium imaging clearly outperformed anatomical imaging modalities revealing sensitivity of 93%, specificity of 78%, and accuracy of 87% as compared to 76%, 30% and 64% respectively for CT/MRI. The investigators at the Netherlands Cancer Institute reported no difficulties with distinguishing normal uptake in the salivary glands, mouth, nose, and the thyroid gland from enhanced $^{201}$Tl uptake by head and neck neoplasms.

## 8.3 Personal Experience

Our own experience with this imaging modality is based on a prospective pilot study involving 25 patients followed over a period of 2 years. Contrary to the results of the Dutch studies, we found that $^{201}$Tl SPECT was not sensitive enough to detect early (stage T1) primary tumors. Our findings were in accordance with the experience of MUKHERJI et al. (1994) who reported that imaging of small mucosal tumors can be hindered by background uptake of the radionuclide by normal salivary glands and mucous membranes. For similar reasons, difficulty was encountered with interpretation of enhanced $^{201}$Tl uptake in the glottic larynx, because of the intense radionuclide activity in the thyroid gland (Fig. 8.1). In contrast to our findings in early mucosal cancers, imaging with $^{201}$Tl SPECT proved to be successful for tumors staged $T_2$–$T_4$, with a sensitivity of 87%. However, SPECT compared unfavorably with CT imaging, which, in the same group of patients, had a sensitivity of 100%. Although the overall sensitivity of SPECT could possibly be improved through comparison of early and delayed images, our data

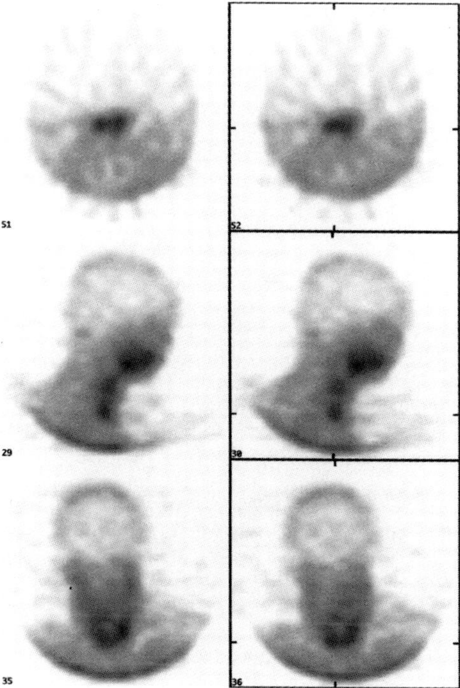

**Fig. 8.1** TL-201 SPECT of T3N0 squamous cell carcinoma of the glottic larynx. Note that the tumor is obscured by intense thyroid uptake. There is also uptake in the salivary glands and pharyngeal mucosa

suggest that SPECT scintigraphy offers no advantage over conventional imaging for the detection of previously untreated primary squamous cell carcinoma of the head and neck (SCCHN). As reported by MUKHERJI et al. (1994) and VALDES OLMOS et al. (1997) SPECT appeared to be less effective for imaging cervical lymph node metastases. In our series, its sensitivity for palpable cervical lymphadenopathy was only 70%, compared with 100% for CT imaging. One could attribute the low thallium affinity for cervical metastases to the poor vascular supply and resulting tumor necrosis often observed in SCCHN metastatic to cervical lymph nodes. In contrast, we found that $^{201}$Tl SPECT may offer advantages in monitoring patients with advanced head and neck tumors after surgery or radiochemotherapy. These findings are in agreement with the reports from the Netherlands Cancer Institute. Especially relevant was the high specificity of SPECT for the detection of recurrent or residual SCCHN (Fig. 8.2), which, in our

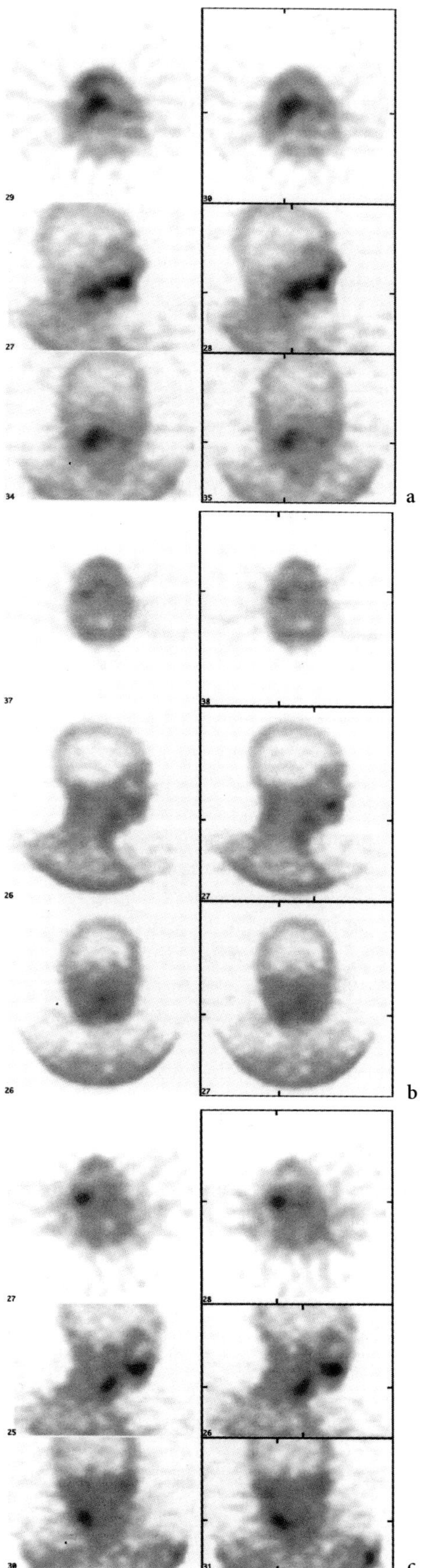

**Fig 8.2 a** T4N2 squamous cell carcinoma of the tongue base prior to therapy. **b** Same patient 9 month after completion of surgery and radiotherapy. The uptake in the tongue base and the right neck has completely disappeared. **c** Same patient 3 month later showing massive tumor recurrence in the right neck

study, was 100% for the primary site and 89% for the neck, compared with 63% and 72%, respectively, for CT scanning. The sensitivity of the study was 83% for the primary site and 100% for the neck, while CT imaging had sensitivity of 100% for both primary and metastatic tumors.

## 8.4 Conclusions

In conclusion, controversy exists as to the value of $^{201}$Tl SPECT for the initial diagnostic assessment of primary head and neck tumors, their staging and the detection of occult primary head and neck cancer. In our opinion, $^{201}$Tl SPECT is not sensitive enough to detect unknown primary tumors and offers no advantage over CT/MRI imaging for evaluation of previously untreated SCCHN. Most authors agree, however, that $^{201}$Tl SPECT is not an accurate imaging modality for detection and staging of cervical lymph node metastases. The main advantage of $^{201}$Tl SPECT may be its accuracy in detecting recurrence of head and neck cancer in previously treated patients. Although the number of patients available for long-term follow-up was small (12 patients in our series and 30 patients reported by Valdes Olmos et al.), the high specificity of $^{201}$Tl SPECT in this clinical setting appears promising. The efficacy of anatomical imaging methods for monitoring the response of head and neck cancer to therapy is hindered by their objective limitations in detecting neoplastic tissue when tissue planes are distorted by previous surgery or radiotherapy. In this respect, complementary utilization of $^{201}$Tl SPECT may substantially improve the predictive value of CT/MRI for the detection of recurrent head and neck cancer. The data in the literature, although preliminary, are sufficiently intriguing to warrant further studies of the value of $^{201}$Tl SPECT for monitoring response and detecting recurrence in advanced SCCHN managed with multimodality therapy.

## References

Duman Y, Burak Z, Erdem S, Tufan M, Unlu M, Haydarogullari A, Ozkok S, Anacak Y, Erdin CE (1993) The value and limitations of $^{201}$Tl scintigraphy in the evaluation of lung lesions and post-therapy follow-up of primary lung carcinoma. Nucl Med Commun 14:446–453

El-Gazzar AH, Sahweil A, Abdel-Dayem HM, Kubasik H, Halker R, Hassan IM, Jamil M, Rageb A, Abdul-Rahim SM, Mahmoud A, Omar YT (1988) Experience with thallium-201 imaging in head and neck cancer. Clin Nucl Med 29:286–289

Gregor RT, Valdes Olmos R, Koops W, Balm AJM, Hilgers FJM, Hoefnagel CA (1996) Preliminary experience with thallous chloride Tl-201-labled single-photon emission computed tomography scanning in head and neck cancer. Arch Otolaryngol Head Neck Surg 122:509–514

Kaplan WD, Takvorian T, Morris JH, Rumbaugh CL, Connoly BT, Atkins HL (1987) Thallium-201 brain tumor imaging: a comparative study with pathologic correlation. J Nucl Med 28:47–52

Kostakoglu L, Uysal U, Ozyar E, Hayran M, Uzal D, Demirkazik FB, Kars A, Atahan L, Bekdik CF (1997) Monitoring response to therapy with thallium-201 and technetium-99m-sestamibi SPECT in nasopharyngeal carcinoma. J Nucl Med 38:1009–1014

Mukherji SK, Drane WE, Tart RP, Landau S, Mancuso AA (1994) Comparison of Thallium-201 and F-18 FDG SPECT uptake in squamous cell carcinoma of the head and neck. AJNR 15:1837–1842

Namba R, Narabayashi I, Matsui R, Sueyoshi K, Nakata Y, TabuchiK, Komori T (1995) Evaluation of Tl-201 SPECT for monitoring the treatment of pulmonary and mediastinal tumors. Ann Nucl Med 9:65–74

Podoloff DA, Kim EE, Haynie TP (1992) SPECT in the evaluation of cancer patients: not quo vadis; rather, ibi fere summus. Radiology 183:305–317

Ramanna L, Waxman A, Binney G, Waxman S, Mirra J, Rosen G (1990) Thallium-201 scintigraphy in bone sarcoma: comparison with gallium-67 and technetium-MDP in the evaluation of chemotherapeutic response. J Nucl Med 31:567–572

Togawa T, Yui N, Kinoshita F, Shimada F, Omura K, Takemiya S (1993) Visualization of nasopharyngeal carcinoma with Tl-201 chloride and a three-head rotating gamma camera SPECT system. Ann Nucl Med 7:105–113

Tonami N, Yokoyama K, Shuke N, Taki J, Kinuya S, Miyauchi T, Michigishi T, Aburano T, Hisada K, Watanabe Y, Takashima T, Nonomura A (1993) Evaluation of suspected malignant pulmonary lesions with $^{201}$Tl single photon emission computed tomography. Nucl Med Communications 14:602–610

Valdes Olmos RA, Balm AJ, Hilgers FJ, Koops W, Loftus BM, Tan IB, Muller SH, Hoefnagel CA, Gregor RT (1997) Thallium-201 SPECT in the diagnosis of head and neck cancer. J Nucl Med 38:873–879

# 9 Evaluation of Predictive Value of CT- and MRI-Dependent Parameters for Recurrence of Laryngeal Cancer After Irradiation Treatment

J.A. Castelijns and R. Hermans

CONTENTS



## 9.1 Introduction

### 9.1.1 Therapeutic Options

Almost all malignancies of the larynx are squamous cell carcinomas. Radiotherapy alone and surgery alone or followed by radiotherapy are the main therapeutic approaches in laryngeal cancer. The choice is influenced by the site and the extent of the lesion. Surgical treatment options for laryngeal cancer are speech-preserving partial laryngectomy in early cancer and total laryngectomy in advanced cancer. The feasibility of voice-sparing partial laryngectomies depends on the position of the tumor relative to potential lines of resection. Correct treatment decisions require an accurate assessment of tumor extent. Both large tumor volume and cartilage invasion are considered to be relative contraindications for radiation therapy.

### 9.1.2 Imaging Modalities

Before the era of CT and MR imaging, laryngeal cancer was evaluated by means of direct visualization, palpation or (plain) radiography or tomography. With the advent of CT, and later MR imaging, clarification of the submucosal extent of disease became possible. As in other areas of the head and neck, the primary role of CT and MR in imaging the larynx is to define the extent of disease. Neither CT nor MR imaging shows mucosal detail, and each is therefore complementary to clinical examination. Soon after the introduction of MR imaging, it was recognized that one of its key advantages over other diagnostic imaging methods was the ability to discriminate between different soft tissue types and between pathologic and normal tissue.

Gradually, the quality of both CT images (particularly since the introduction of high-resolution CT and spiral CT) and MR imaging (particularly since the introduction of faster scanning techniques) has improved substantially.

### 9.1.3 Application of Postprocessing Techniques

In addition, in recent years postprocessing techniques, such as manual tracing and segmentation, have been developed to quantify the volume of

J.A. Castelijns, MD, Academic Hospital Vrije Universiteit, Department of Radiology, Postbus 7057, 1007 MB Amsterdam, The Netherlands
R. Hermans, MD, Catholic University Leuven, Department of Radiology, University Hospitals, UZ Gasthuisberg, Herestraat 49, B-3000 Leuven, Belgium

lesions. Tumor volume can be measured by calculating lesion area on sequential cross-sectional images, outlining the lesions manually, and multiplying the sum of the areas by the slice interval. Consequently tumor volume can be included among the potential prognostic factors used to predict outcome of irradiation treatment.

### 9.1.4 Staging of the Primary Tumor

The two staging systems most frequently used are those proposed by the American Joint Commission on Cancer (AJCC 1992) and by the International Union Against Cancer (UICC 1997) (Tables 9.1, 9.2). Although the two systems differ in several details, they are almost identical with respect to laryngeal tumors. In both staging systems the tumor is classified at T4 (supraglottic, glottic, subglottic) if it invades one of the laryngeal cartilages (thyroid or cricoid cartilage) and/or extends to other tissues beyond the larynx (e.g. oropharynx, soft tissues of the neck).

The issue of staging procedures is important because it is generally recognized that the validity of any classification is dependent on the diagnostic methods employed (Snow and Gerritsen 1993). However, for staging of a given laryngeal tumor

**Table 9.1.** Anatomical sites and subsites according to the International Union Against Cancer (UICC) and the American Joint Commission on Cancer (AJCC)

| Sites | Subsites |
|---|---|
| UICC | |
| 1. Supraglottis | a. Suprahyoid epiglottis (including the tip and lingual and laryngeal surfaces) |
| | b. Ary-epiglottic fold, laryngeal aspect |
| | c. Arytenoid |
| | Supraglottis excluding the epilarynx |
| | d. Infrahyoid epiglottis |
| | e. Ventricular bands (false cords) |
| | f. Ventricular cavities |
| 2. Glottis | a. Vocal cords |
| | b. Anterior commissure |
| | c. Posterior commissure |
| 3. Subglottis | |
| AJCC | |
| Supraglottis | Ventricular bands (false cords) |
| | Arytenoids |
| | Suprahyoid epiglottis (both lingual and laryngeal aspects) |
| | Infrahyoid epiglottis |
| | Arytenoepiglottic folds (laryngeal aspects) |
| Glottis | True vocal cords, including anterior and posterior commissures |
| Subglottis | Subglottis |

**Table 9.2.** Classification of primary tumor in carcinoma of the larynx according to UICC and AJCC

| Site | Classification | Description |
|---|---|---|
| Supraglottis | T1 | Tumor limited to one subsite of supraglottis, with normal vocal cord mobility |
| | T2 | Tumor invades mucosa of more than one adjacent subsite of supraglottis or glottis or region outside the supraglottis (e.g., mucosa of base of tongue, vallecula, medial wall of piriform sinus) without fixation of the larynx |
| | T3 | Tumor limited to the larynx with vocal cord fixation and/or invades any of the following: postcricoid area, pre-epiglottic tissues, deep base of the tongue |
| | T4 | Tumor invades through thyroid cartilage and/or extends into soft tissues of the neck, thyroid, and/or esophagus |
| Glottis | T1 | Tumor limited to vocal cord(s) may involve anterior or posterior commissure(s) with normal mobility |
| | T1a | Tumor limited to one vocal cord |
| | T1b | Tumor involves both vocal cords |
| | T2 | Tumor extends to supraglottis and/or subglottis, and/or with impaired vocal cord mobility |
| | T3 | Tumor limited to the larynx with vocal cord fixation |
| | T4 | Tumor invades through thyroid cartilage and/or extends to other tissues beyond the larynx, e.g. trachea, soft tissues of the neck, thyroid and pharynx |
| Subglottis | T1 | Tumor limited to the subglottis |
| | T2 | Tumor extends to vocal cord(s) with normal or impaired mobility |
| | T3 | Tumor limited to the larynx with vocal cord fixation |
| | T4 | Tumor invades through cricoid or thyroid cartilage and/or extends to other tissues beyond trachea, e.g. trachea, soft tissues of the neck, thyroid, esophagus |

these staging methods are not precise in their recommendations for recently developed imaging methods such as CT and MRI. AJCC, for instance, states that "a variety of imaging procedures are valuable in evaluating the extent of disease, particularly for advanced tumors, and these include laryngeal tomograms, CT scans and MRI scans," but does not indicate when to use any or all of these imaging methods. With no further indications as to the type of imaging, UICC states that imaging should be included in the diagnostic workup.

Eminent oncologists working in the head and neck field have recently expressed their concerns about the weaknesses of staging systems for laryngal cancer (Snow and Gerritsen 1993; Ogura 1975; Hokanson 1991). The difficulty in staging the primary tumor is likely to be one of the main reasons for these shortcomings (Bailey 1991; Hokanson 1991). Consequently, reported cure rates vary widely and prognosis is not sufficiently closely related to TNM values. A more objective staging system is necessary.

Nonetheless, there is a reluctance to change the TNM classification system too hastily. Apart from this, the experts concerned have the feeling that the TNM classification system cannot be changed rapidly to incorporate new facts and new findings. There is a need for a mathematical conceptual framework in the form of a comprehensive equation that can be updated and modified on the basis of either deleted or new information. Increasingly, there are indications that radiologic techniques can provide important prognostic information on tumor volume and cartilage involvement. Tumor volume may have a predictive value for forecasting whether irradiation treatment will be successful, and it may be helpful in monitoring the initial results after irradiation treatment. Invasion of laryngeal structures may also have predictive value in forecasting the success or otherwise of radiation therapy. In particular, invasion of laryngeal cartilages is traditionally considered to be a relative contraindication for radiation therapy. Million (1989) suggested that imaging could help us to detect minor cartilage involvement and that we simply did not know the implications of this finding. The effectiveness of radiation therapy in cases that are positive for cartilage involvement on imaging is not known. Such cartilage abnormality may not be a contraindication to radiation therapy. Comparison of the outcome of radiation therapy and imaging findings would be important. Testing the outcome may be important even without the histological confirmation of radiological findings.

## 9.2 Technique of Laryngeal Imaging

### 9.2.1 Computed Tomography

#### *9.2.1.1 Technical Aspects*

During CT imaging of the larynx, the neck should be slightly hyperextended: the larynx is then drawn a little higher in the neck, and this helps to avoid artifacts from the shoulder region. The patients should be immobilized and instructed not to swallow or cough during image acquisition. The plane of section is chosen parallel to the true vocal cords; if these landmarks are not recognized on the lateral scout view the sections should be made approximately parallel to the midcervical intervertebral disc spaces (Mancuso and Hanafee 1985). Sections made at other angles relative to the true vocal cords can cause interpretation errors, as parts of the false cords may appear at the same level as the true vocal cords.

##### 9.2.1.1.1 Incremental CT Scanning

During conventional CT, different images are generated separately; between each two sections the patients is transported over a certain distance, a prospectively determined table increment.

Section thickness should be no more than 3–4 mm in laryngeal studies. Adjacent sections should be obtained, with the field of view focused on the larynx to maximize spatial resolution. To minimize motion artifacts, the scan time should be 1–2 s. Intravenous contrast medium is always used in studies for laryngeal cancer; most primary tumors will enhance, which will help to delineate any tumor from the surrounding structures, especially muscles (Million et al. 1994).

The patients are asked to breathe quietly during scanning; with the short scanning times possible on modern CT devices, motion artifacts due to breathing rarely occur. Some radiologists prefer breath holding; this may adduct the cords, obliterating the airway and limiting the evaluation of the anterior commissure region.

##### 9.2.1.1.2 Spiral CT Scanning

The essential difference between spiral CT and conventional CT is that during a spiral CT acquisition, with the tube continuously rotating around the patient, the patient is being transported with a constant speed through the gantry. After interpolation of the helical image data, images obtained with a pitch of 1 have nearly the same quality as conventional scans, the only differences being a broadened slice sensitivity profile (SSP) and a different amount of noise. The degree of broadening of the SSP and the amount of noise depend on the algorithm used to interpolate the helical data.

The use of this technique offers a number of advantages, the most obvious being the fast data acquisition. This allows examination of children (for example) without sedation, reduction of motion artifacts in adults, limitation of the dose of injected contrast material in enhanced studies, and optimal use of the short time window of maximal opacification, for example in hypervascular tumors. Another interesting feature of spiral CT is that during transport of the patient through the gantry information is gathered continuously: a volumetric data set is obtained. From this volumetric data set the actual images are calculated. The images can be calculated with an adjacent table position, showing the same amount of information as conventional scans with the same nominal slice thickness. However, spiral CT images can be calculated retrospectively for every possible table position; this means they also can be calculated in an overlapping fashion. The difference in the information in successively calculated images becomes smaller, and a reduction in the partial volume effect is obtained (Hermans et al. 1995). These retrospectively calculated overlapping images allow better multiplanar reconstructions and 3D reconstructions than nonoverlapping incremental scans. These overlapping images are acquired retrospectively, without exposing the patient to any additional irradiation; the only expense is additional computation time. In the larynx, fewer motion and respiratory misregistration artifacts are seen with spiral CT, but somewhat better visualization of laryngeal abnormalities and subtle anatomical structures (such as the paraglottic fat planes) has been reported with dynamic incremental CT (Mukherji et al. 1995a). Other authors have not reported any significant difference between incremental and spiral CT in the visualization of different laryngeal structures (Robert et al. 1996).

Spiral CT examinations of the laryngopharynx always start with a long spiral scan of approximately 30–40 s during quiet respiration. A slice thickness of 2 or 3 mm is generally used, with a table incrementation speed of 3 mm/s. It is important not to start the acquisition too soon after initiation of the contrast injection, because diffusion of the contrast medium into the tumor and the metastatic adenopathies takes some time; good enhancement of the tumor is very important, as it improves the evaluation of its extension. To obtain both good tumoral and good vascular enhancement, a dual injection technique can be used: 50 ml of contrast medium is injected between 120 s and 60 s before the start of the acquisition, leaving enough time for the diffusion to take place into the soft tissues, and then another 30 ml is injected during the 30 s before the start of the acquisition, to give good vascular opacification. The best opacification of both veins and arteries is obtained when this last bolus is further fragmented into two separate injections of 15 s, the last one being administered just before acquisition begins (Dubrulle et al. 1997). Modern injection pumps allow such relatively complex injection schemes to be preprogrammed. Good results can also be obtained with a one-phase injection of contrast medium, e.g. 80 ml of a contrast medium with 300 mg I/ml at 1 ml/s, with the image acquisition started at the end of the contrast medium injection.

Multiplanar and 3D reconstructions give another view of the pathology, possibly with a better demonstration of its extent (Fig. 9.1). Such reconstructions may improve the communication with the clinician (Silverman et al. 1995).

#### 9.2.1.2 *Dynamic Maneuvers*

Dynamic maneuvers during scanning of the larynx and hypopharynx can enhance visualization of particular anatomical structures. During phonation, arytenoidal mobility can be judged and a better visualization of the laryngeal ventricle can be obtained; the slight distension of the piriform sinuses also allows better delineation of the ary-epiglottic folds. A modified Valsalva maneuver (consisting in blowing air against closed lips, puffing out the cheeks) produces a substantial dilatation of the hypopharynx, which may allow better evaluation of the piriform sinuses, including the postcricoid region (Robert et al. 1993). The success rate of these dynamic maneuvers in incremental CT is variable, depending heavily on cooperation from the patient: consistent repetition of the maneuver for each incremental scan is difficult, spatial misregistration being an important

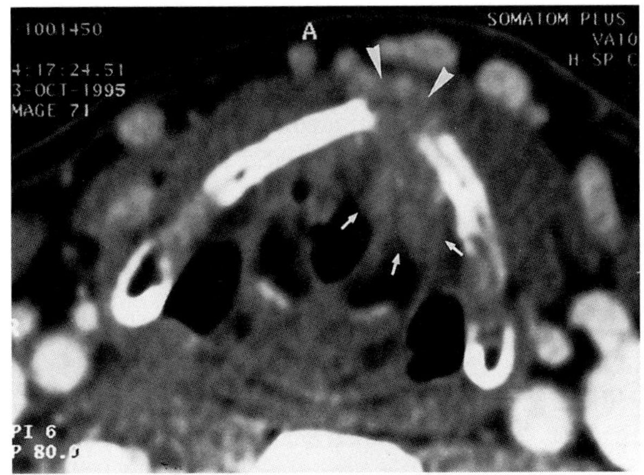


a

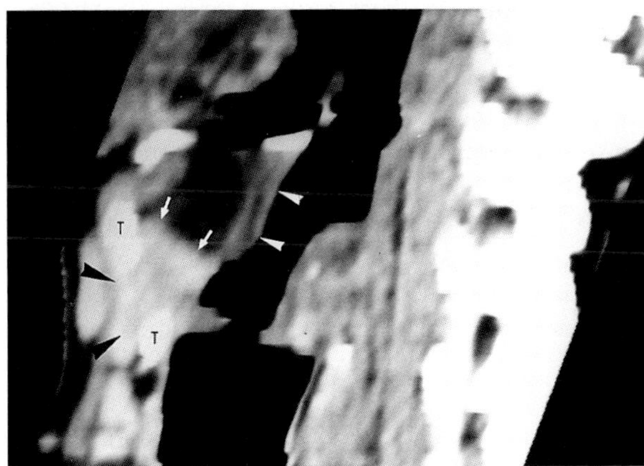


b

**Fig. 9.1 a,b.** Spiral CT images of a patient with a glottic carcinoma involving the anterior commissure, clinically staged as, T1. **a** Axial spiral CT image (2 mm slice thickness, table feed 2 mm/s) at the level of the false vocal cords shows an infiltrative mass in the left paraglottic space and lower pre-epiglottic space (*small arrows*), erosion of the thyroid cartilage angle and early extralaryngeal spread (*large arrowheads*). **b** Sagittal reconstruction through the larynx. This image shows infiltration of the lower pre-epiglottic/paraglottic space (*arrows*) and extralaryngeal extension (*large arrowheads*) through the thyroid cartilage (*T*). The epiglottis is indicated by *small arrowheads*. Based on the CT findings, the tumor was upstaged to T4. The patient was treated by RT, but developed a neck failure 4 months after completing RT

drawback. Furthermore, the incremental acquisition of these additional scans during phonation or Valsalva maneuver is time consuming. These problems can be largely overcome by spiral CT, as the patient has to perform the maneuver only once during a single rapid acquisition. It is difficult for most patients to sustain such a dynamic maneuver for a long time, which means that these dynamic spiral acquisitions are restricted, depending on the patient, to a scan time between 15 s and 24 s. The level scanned is determined from the images acquired during quiet respiration; it is necessary to compensate for the fact that the larynx descends somewhat during the Valsalva maneuver and rises during phonation; the distance over which it moves varies between 0.5 and 1 cm. The patient has to be well informed about what is expected from him or her during the spiral CT study. The dynamic maneuvers need to be practiced with the patient before the examination starts. Often the patients need to be accompanied and encouraged during the actual examination. Investment of this small amount of time yields good results in the majority of cases (Dubrulle et al. 1997).

### 9.2.2 Magnetic Resonance Imaging

#### *9.2.2.1 Technical Aspects*

MR imaging of patients with laryngeal cancer may be difficult owing to dyspnea, coughing and mucous secretion in such patients. A number of requirements need to be fulfilled for diagnostic images to be obtained. The use of a dedicated neck coil is indispensable if optimal results are to be obtained. Ideally, the volume of the neck coil should match the size of the neck as closely as possible. Surface coils are rarely used in the evaluation of patients with laryngeal cancer. As a general rule of thumb, effective penetration by the coil is approximately one half the coil diameter at its narrowest point. To obtain optimal images full account must constantly be to taken of three issues in MR imaging: signal-to-noise ratio, resolution and time. The neck coils make it possible to obtain high resolution and thin section images in spite of relatively short acquisition times. Thinner slices improve the visualization of anatomical detail but require longer scanning times to maintain an equivalent signal-to-noise ratio. Finer matrices, such as 512 × 512, improve the visualization of anatomical detail but involve longer scanning times, in addition to which the signal-to-noise ratio may decrease. Selection of an intermediate matrix size may be appropriate. The field of view should be reduced as much as possible to improve spatial resolution. Signal averaging is the best technique to improve MR image quality. However, benefits of signal averaging must be weighed against the increased scanning time required.

For imaging of laryngeal cancer, spin-echo imaging (SE) is used because of its accurate and reproducible anatomical depiction of laryngeal tissue. However, the intensities of different tissue types in MR images are affected by a number of acquisition parameters, and the contrast can be manipulated by changes in the pulse sequences. The common timing parameters are the sequence repetition time (TR) and the echo time (TE). The flip angle of excitation pulses can also be varied. By altering these parameters it is possible to change the sensitivity of the images to three principal factors: proton density, longitudinal relaxation time (T1) and transverse relaxation time (T2). T1-weighted images appear to be ideal for the study of the larynx. They allow more accurate delineation and characterization of tissue than CT. The higher signal intensity of squamous cell carcinoma on T2-weighted images is a disadvantage in the larynx, because of the high-signal areolar tissue within the larynx, which could obscure the tumor itself. With spin-echo (SE) imaging, the appropriate selection of TR and TE will determine the degree of T1 and T2 weighting. For T1-weighted SE imaging the length of the TR is based on the number of slices required, but must be kept under 800–1000 ms to maintain T1 weighting. A TR within the range of 400–800 ms will allow an adequate number of slices to cover the region of interest. The shortest TE possible (10–20 ms) is selected to attain the best signal-to-noise ratio and to minimize T2 effect. To obtain T2-weighted images we typically use a TR of 2500 ms and TEs of 20–30 ms and 100 ms for the first and second echoes, respectively.

T1-weighted SE images are most appropriate to demonstrate the laryngeal anatomy and to assess the extent of laryngeal pathology. On T2-weighted SE images, tumor is found to have a higher signal intensity than on T1-weighted SE images. The axial imaging technique is most appropriate for study of the location and extent of tumor in intralaryngeal compartments and the laryngeal cartilages, and also in extralaryngeal structures, such as the infrahyoid muscles, piriform sinus, and subcutaneous fat. Fast-SE T2-weighted imaging should be applied rather than conventional SE techniques, by reducing acquisition time and motion artifacts. It is of the utmost importance that both sequences, T1 and fast-T2 SE images, are obtained at exactly corresponding levels. Interpretation of images that have not been obtained at exactly corresponding levels could easily lead to mistakes in interpretation regarding the presence or absence of cartilage invasion.

#### *9.2.2.2 Artifacts*

Motion artifacts are the most common, easily identifiable, phenomena that degrade MR images of the laryngeal area. Motion artifacts caused by respiratory movement and those caused by random patient movement (swallowing, coughing) may be hard to distinguish from each other. Gross movement produces multiple ghosted images, which usually appear as curvilinear crescents of signal. An increase in either TR value or the frequency of motion increases the spacing between parent signal and daughter ghosts. More subtle patient movement results in degraded image quality without obvious ghosting. Motion artifacts are more prominent on images acquired over a longer examination time (i.e., a long repetition time). Motion ghosts are seen along the phase-encoding axis (normally in the vertical direction of the axial image), irrespective of the direction of the motion. A shorter scanning time will reduce motion artifacts caused by coughing and swallowing. The use of turbo SE images is necessary. The use of short examination times necessitates some compromise on image resolution. Most patients can remain sufficiently immobile for approximately 5–8 min. The patient must be encouraged to remain as nearly immobile as possible. Comfortable patient positioning and sedation may both be used to reduce these artifacts. Rigid mounting of the surface coil so it does not rest on the patient eliminates coil motion and improves image quality. The presence of motion artifacts may interfere in approximately 10–15% of examinations with adequate diagnosis (Castelijns et al. 1987a, 1988; Phelps 1992).

Administration of gadolinium to delineate the primary lesion may be an alternative for showing the extent of the lesion. Regions showing moderate intensity on T1-weighted images, high intensity on T2-weighted images, and moderate contrast enhancement probably correspond to tumor tissue on preoperative images. Because of the shorter acquisition times and reduced image degradation from patient movement during scanning, Gd-DTPA-enhanced T1-weighted images are reported to be more useful in the diagnosis of laryngohypopharyngeal cancer than proton-density-weighted and T2-weighted images (Sakai et al. 1993).

#### 9.2.2.3
#### *MRI Protocol*

The patient should be examined in the supine position, with the neck slightly hyperextended, the head immobilized, and the shoulders relaxed and pushed downwards. The patient is positioned so that the laryngeal airway is as near parallel to the table-top as possible. Quiet breathing should be maintained during the examination, with the use of abdominal rather than chest muscles.

We begin with a mid- and parasagittal, T1-weighted SE sequence. This identifies the orientation of the larynx. Axial T1-weighted, proton-density- and relatively T2-weighted images are then obtained at exactly corresponding levels. Section thickness is 4 mm, with no interslice gap. Four measurements are obtained with T1-weighted and two measurements, with T2-weighted images. For detection of lymph node metastasis the neck should also be examined.

## 9.3
## Appearance of Laryngeal Squamous Cell Carcinoma

### 9.3.1
### Appearance on CT

#### 9.3.1.1
#### *Tumor Delineation on CT*

Criteria used for tumor involvement are abnormal contrast enhancement, soft tissue thickening, presence of a bulky mass, infiltration of fatty tissue (even without distortion of surrounding soft tissues), or a combination of these. A soft tissue thickness of more than 1 mm at the anterior commissure is considered pathologic, and any tissue thickening between the airway and the cricoid ring is considered to represent a subglottic tumor. Several studies have compared the CT findings with the results of whole-organ sectioning after total or partial laryngectomy (Mafee et al. 1983; Reid 1984; Hoover et al. 1984; Silverman et al. 1984; Katsantonis et al. 1986; Sulfaro et al. 1989; Becker et al. 1995), showing that CT is an accurate method of visualizing laryngeal pathology. These correlation studies between whole-organ sectioning and CT have also revealed some pitfalls. Small foci of mucosal tumor may be difficult to detect or may be invisible on CT images, and associated inflammatory and edematous changes can cause overestimation of the tumor extent of CT. Distortion of adjacent normal structures may mimic tumoral involvement.

#### 9.3.1.2
#### *Cartilage Invasion on CT*

Gross cartilage invasion can be detected with CT. Owing to the wide variability in the ossification pattern of the laryngeal cartilages, CT often fails to detect early cartilage invasion. Nonossified hyaline cartilage shows the same density values as tumor on CT images. Demonstration of tumor on the extralaryngeal side of the cartilage is a reliable, but late, sign of cartilage invasion. Asymmetrical sclerosis, defined as thickening of the cortical margin and/or greater medullary density, of one arytenoid compared with the other or on one side of the cricoid or thyroid cartilage with the other side, is a sensitive but nonspecific CT finding. In only 45% of thyroid and cricoid cartilages displaying sclerosis are tumor cells found within the bone marrow; the other 55% have only perichondrial invasion or no invasion at all. Only 16% of sclerotic arytenoids display tumor cells within the bone marrow, and 32% have only peripheral invasion of the fibroelastic process of the vocal process or the perichondrium – the remaining 52% showing no neoplastic invasion at all (Becker et al. 1997). Erosion or lysis has been found to be a specific criterion of neoplastic invasion in all cartilages. Other signs, such as cartilaginous blowout or bowing, a serpiginous contour or obliteration of the medullary space, are not very reliable indicators of cartilage invasion. The combination of several diagnostic CT criteria of neoplastic invasion of the laryngeal cartilages seems to constitute a reasonable compromise: when extralaryngeal tumor and erosion or lysis in the thyroid, cricoid and arytenoid cartilages was combined with sclerosis in the cricoid and arytenoid (but not the thyroid) cartilages, an overall sensititivity of 82%, an overall specificity of 79%, and an overall negative predictive value of 91% were obtained (Becker et al. 1997).

#### 9.3.1.3
#### *Volume Estimation on CT: Intra- and Interobserver Reproducibility*

The clinical utility of an imaging study depends not only on the sensitivity, specificity, and accuracy obtained, but also on the consistency of interpretation by the same observer at different times or by different observers. Sometimes observers have different opinions after independent review of the examinations (Becker et al. 1995; Castelijns et al. 1995). The choice of therapy may be influenced by subtle imaging findings, which are prone to interpretation differences. Tumor scores reflecting the anatomical tumor extent are increasingly being investigated as a possible predictor of local outcome after radiation therapy (Lee et al. 1993; Pameijer et al. 1997). Knowledge about the reproducibility of image interpretations is obviously also of interest in patients being considered for surgery, as the decision to operate and the surgical technique selected are influenced by CT findings.

The intra- and interobserver reproducibility of the interpretation of CT studies for laryngeal carcinoma was recently evaluated (Hermans et al. 1997a). Fair to substantial intraobserver reproducibility (kappa = 0.29–0.86), and fair to substantial interobserver reproducibility (average kappa = 0.26–0.74) were found for most laryngeal structures. On average, these kappa values are in the expected range for clinical diagnostic and imaging studies. Even when multiple choices were possible (e.g., degree of invasion of the paralaryngeal space), the reproducibility measured in this study remained within acceptable limits. This indicates that concerns about reproducibility should not discourage a trained radiologist from scoring the involvement of a particular laryngeal structure in subcategories.

Success in controlling a tumor by radiotherapy depends on killing all clonogenic cells. The probability of cure depends, among other factors, on the initial number of clonogenic cells. In clinical situations, the clonogenic cell content can vary widely within a certain tumor stage, and it is not only dependent on tumor volume but also on other factors, such as necrosis or infiltration by normal cells (macrophages, fibrovascular stroma). The number of clonogenic cells also depends on the rate of repopulation during the radiation treatment (Withers 1992). There are indications that the number of clonogens increases linearly with tumor volume (Johnson et al. 1995). Therefore, tumor volume can be an interesting predictor of local outcome.

Tumor volume is difficult to determine clinically, especially in the head and neck, with its complex regional anatomy and the infiltrating behavior of the tumors in this region. Volumetric assessment of soft tissue masses is possible with such cross-sectional imaging techniques as CT.

To determine the volume of a particular structure, its borders are traced on consecutive images, either manually or by some (semi-)automated method. The segmented surface on each image is then calculated. This procedure can be done on the scanner's screen using a mouse-controlled cursor, or indirectly using a digitizer. The surfaces obtained are then multiplied by the slice interval. The total sum of all the volumes obtained represents the total volume of the structure of interest. This technique is called the summation-of-areas technique (Breiman et al. 1982).

A very close relationship was found between CT-determined volume and postoperative weight of enlarged thyroid glands (Hermans et al. 1997b); as the specific gravity of thyroid tissue is close to 1, this means that the thyroid gland's volume can be accurately estimated on the basis of CT imaging. Although thyroid glands are on average (much) larger than most laryngeal tumors, it is likely that with CT the volume of smaller soft tissue lesions can be measured with comparable accuracy.

Before CT-based tumor volume estimations can be incorporated into clinical practice, information about the variability of these volume calculations when done at different times by the same observer or done by different observers is necessary. A statistically significant effect of the observer ($P < 0.0001$) has been demonstrated on the variability of the laryngeal tumor volumes measured (Hermans et al. 1998a). In this study, the most important component of total variabilility was interobserver variability (89.3%), while intraobserver variability contributed 6.4% to the total variability (Fig. 9.2). The variability in the measurements must be reduced as much as possible to obtain sharp classifications of laryngeal tumors based on their volume; only measurements with low variability can usefully be correlated with local outcome after radiation therapy. This can be achieved by always having the same observer performing the measurements; it has been shown that an observer with experience in head and neck radiology can measure laryngeal tumor volumes with significantly less variability than other observers (Hermans et al. 1998a).

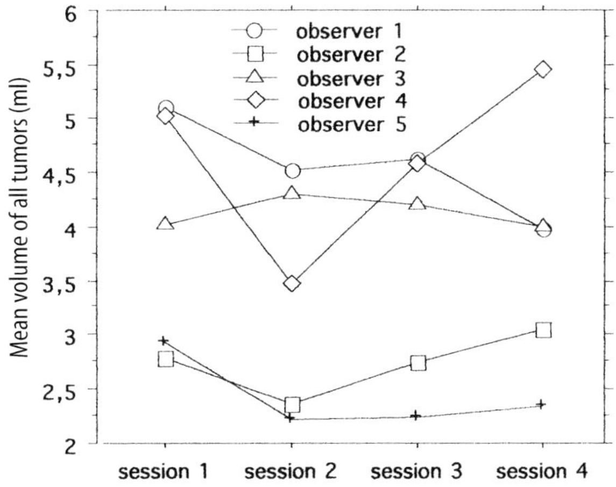


**Fig. 9.2.** Five observers independently measured the volume of 13 randomly chosen laryngeal tumors on CT images. They repeated these measurements four times. The graph shows the interaction of the mean volume (ml) of all tumors and the four measurement sessions. Interobserver variability is seen to be the most important component of total variability. By having the volume calculations done by a single observer, measurement variability can be reduced substantially. Observer 3 (head and neck radiologist) obtained the most stable mean tumor volume over all sessions. Three observers obtained less stable results throughout the different sessions, while one observer (observer 4) obtained fluctuating mean tumor volumes (the other observers were staff radiologists or radiology residents). From Hermans et al. (1998a)

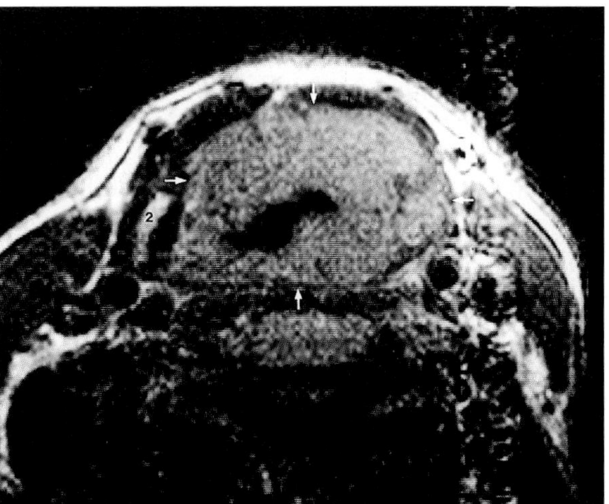


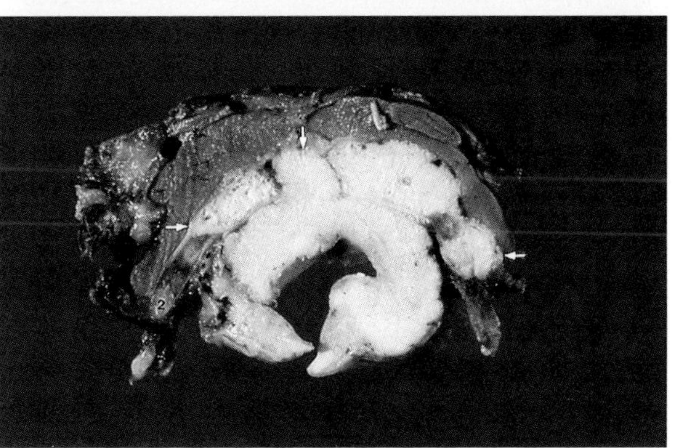


**Fig. 9.3a, b.** MR images of a patient with a previously nontreated laryngeal carcinoma clinically staged as T4. **a** MR T1-weighted image shows a large area (*arrows*) with increased signal intensity surrounding the intralaryngeal lumen almost entirely. This area is found with somewhat higher signal intensity than that of muscular tissue of infrahyoid muscles (*1*), but definitively lower than the high signal intensity of subcutaneous fat and fatty marrow in the nonossified right thyroid lamina (*2*). **b** Sliced surgical specimen. Pathologic tissue (*arrows*) has similar contour and topographic relation to surrounding structures, such as infrahyoid muscles (*1*) and right thyroid lamina (*2*)

## 9.3.2 Appearance on MRI

### *9.3.2.1 Tumor Delineation*

In several previous comparative studies, including comparison with whole-organ sections, it has been suggested that T1-weighted MR images assess the extent of tumor tissue accurately, with high contrast to surrounding fat and much less contrast to surrounding muscular tissue (Castelijns et al. 1987a) (Fig. 9.3). However, inflammation can frequently be seen along the margin of squamous cell carcinoma and may not be differentiated from tumor tissue on T1-weighted images (Becker et al. 1995). Head and neck cancers often display the same signal patterns before and after contrast administration as benign or inflammatory lesions, and it can even happen that they are not differentiated by means of dynamic contrast-enhanced MR imaging (Vogl et al. 1993; Takashima et al. 1993; Yousem 1993). However, on the basis of T1-weighted images it can be maintained that MR images give an accurate depiction of the amount of pathologic tissue.

### *9.3.2.2 Cartilage Invasion on MRI*

Laryngeal cartilages are very difficult to investigate, owing to their irregular pattern of ossification (Isaacs et al. 1988; Yeager and Archer 1982; Curtin 1989). The hyaline cartilages may be variably composed of calcified and noncalcified cartilage, or of bone with a marrow cavity (Isaacs et al. 1988; Hoover et al. 1984). MR imaging shows ossification patterns more accurately than CT does and allows detection of abnormal signal in cartilages

a

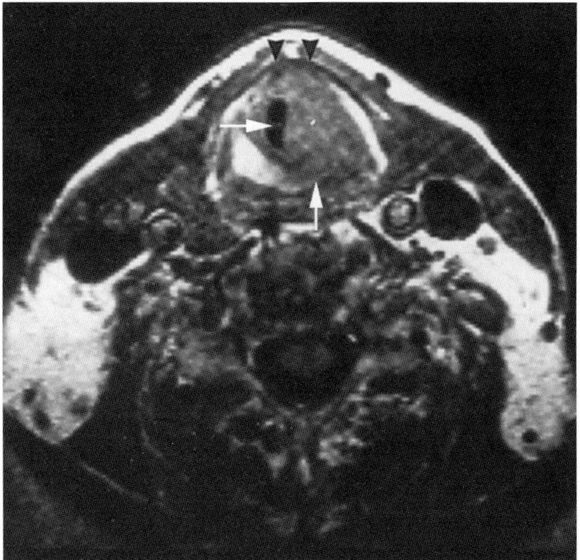

b

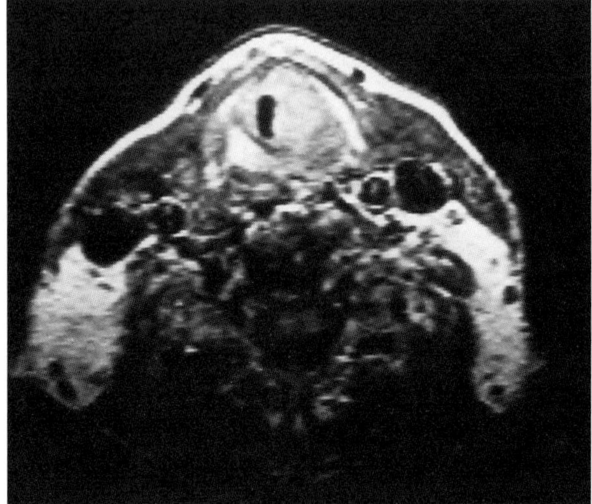

**Fig. 9.4a, b** MR images of a patient with a left-sided, previously untreated glottic tumor, which was initially staged clinically as T4. **a** MR, T1-weighted axial image at the glottic level shows pathologic tissue with intermediate signal intensity (*arrows*). The anterior of the thyroid cartilage (*arrowheads*) and the left part of the cricoid cartilage are also found to have intermediate signal intensity. **b** Pathologic tissue is found with increased signal intensity. Both thyroid and cricoid cartilage appear to be totally ossified and to be invaded by pathologic tissue

(Castelijns et al. 1985; Becker et al. 1995). Cartilage invasion may be best assessed by the combination of unenhanced T1-, proton-density- and T2-weighted images (Fig. 9.4). The use of gadopentate dimeglumine (GdTPA) does not increase the diagnostic accuracy, because contrast enhancement does not make it possible to differentiate between tumor and inflammation. Several articles have explored this issue of detection of cartilage invasion in MRI–histopathological correlation studies. Castelijns et al. (1987b, 1988) have indicated that MR imaging can help to differentiate tumor from nonossified tissue. However, the numbers of sliced specimens in this study are small. Both tumor and nonossified cartilage had low signal intensity with short TR sequences, while tumor had substantially higher signal intensity than nonossified cartilage on more T2-weighted sequences. Castelijns et al. (1988) reported an overall sensitivity of 89% for 0.6-T MR imaging in the detection of neoplastic invasion of cartilage, and a specificity of 88%. The overall results obtained by Becker et al. (1995) at 1.5 T in a much larger MRI–histopathological correlation study were almost identical (sensitivity, 89%; specificity, 84%). However, they found that the ability of MR imaging to help in detecting or excluding neoplastic cartilage invasion varied considerably with the histological degree of invasion, and from one anatomical site to another. They reported that MR imaging was less reliable in the thyroid cartilage than in the cricoid cartilage and arytenoid cartilages, because of a relatively high number of false-positive findings. They claimed that histopathological correlation indicated that these diagnostic errors were caused by nonneoplastic peritumor reactions and changes in the cartilage, namely extensive fibrosis, inflammation, and bone resorption adjacent to the tumor without concomitant neoplastic invasion of the perichondrium. On MR imaging, these changes may result in a high signal intensity on T2-weighted images. As stressed before, it is very important that the T1- and T2-weighted images are at exactly corresponding levels; otherwise interpretation may easily lead to false-positive results relating to the presence of cartilage invasion.

Interpretation of MR examinations in patients with smaller tumors who did not undergo surgical treatment suggested that abnormal MR signal patterns in cartilage may be found in a high percentage of patients with laryngeal carcinoma (Castelijns 1990). In this study a high frequency of abnormal signal in the area of the anterior commissure, suggestive of cartilage invasion, was observed (Fig. 9.5). The study by Becker et al. (1995) allows us to state that MR imaging is very accurate in determining that a cartilage is normal. If the signal intensity in cartilage is abnormal, the cartilage is almost certainly abnormal. However, false-positive findings can be caused by inflammatory disease adjacent to tumor tissue.

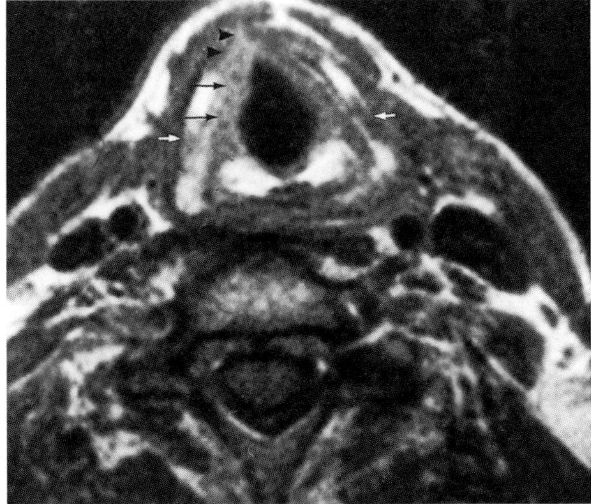
a

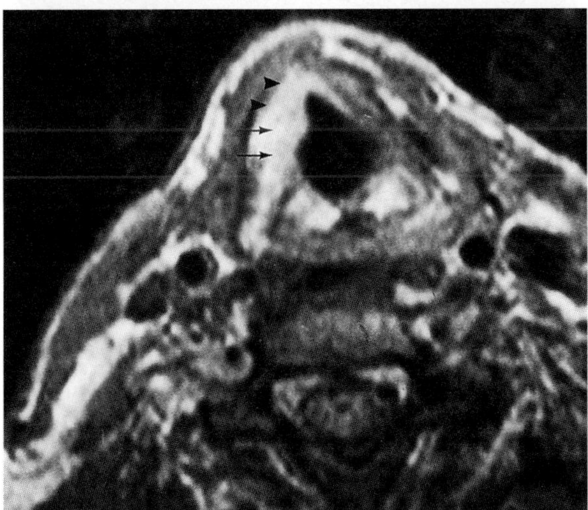
b

**Fig. 9.5 a,b.** MR images of a patient with a previously untreated glottic tumor clinically staged as T1b. **a** MR, T1-weighed axial image at the glottic level shows cricoid and arytenoid cartilage. Muscular tissue of the left vocal cord can easily be differentiated from a small rim of paraglottic high-signal fat. Thyroid lamina are partly ossified and partly nonossified (*white arrows*). A small irregularity can be seen in the anterior part of the right vocal cord, and this area also has intermediate signal intensity (*small arrowheads*), somewhat higher than the signal intensity of muscle. The ventral part of the right thyroid lamina also has abnormal signal intensity (*small arrowheads*) suggestive of invasion by pathologic tissue. **b** MR, T2-weighted axial image shows pathologic tissue with increased signal intensity (*arrows*). Ventral part of the right thyroid lamina is also found to have increased signal intensity (*arrowheads*), confirming abnormal signal intensity in the ventral part of the right thyroid lamina

#### 9.3.2.3 Volume Estimation on MRI: Intra- and Interobserver Reproducibility

To calculate the volume of a tumor, its contour on each slice should be outlined. The volume may be calculated by multiplying together all the above-mentioned areas, summarized over all slices (and interslice gaps) in which the tumor was present. The determination of the size of the tumor on an MRI scan involves subjective elements, and it requires a radiologist with a great deal of experience in the interpretation of laryngeal examinations. In addition, there is likely to be a certain amount of interobserver variability. In our study this variability was low with regard to tumor volume (Castelijns et al. 1995).

Manual outlining of lesions on CT or MR images is moderately accurate when performed by an experienced observer, and has been validated for certain applications. It is relatively straightforward to implement and, in experienced hands, has been shown to give fairly good intra- and interobserver variability (Castelijns et al. 1995, 1996). However, considerable operator–computer interaction time is needed to assess each patient, and the interobserver variability can be considerable. Segmentation, that is automatic delineation and identification of tumor, cannot be performed owing to low contrast with surrounding tissue.

## 9.4 Predictive Value of Pretreatment Imaging Findings for the Frequency of Tumor Recurrence

### 9.4.1 Correlation Between Pretreatment CT Findings and Tumor Recurrence

#### 9.4.1.1 Tumor Volume and Deep Tissue Infiltration on CT

Large primary tumor volume is known to be one reason for a poor local outcome of laryngeal cancer after definitive RT (Fletcher and Hamberger 1974; Fletcher et al. 1975). There was a correlation between clinical estimation of tumor volume in various advanced head and neck cancers treated in a multicenter EORTC trial and survival and loco-regional control after RT (van den Bogaert et al. 1995), but the volume classes defined in this study (<10 cc, 10–30 cc, 30–100 cc, >100 cc) are too rough to be applicable to less advanced head and neck cancers. Overgaard et al. (1986) reported that laryngeal tumor diameter (<2 cm, 2–3.9 cm, >4 cm) was of significant importance to both probability of local control and survival in glottic and supraglottic tumors. Tumor diameters may allow only an inaccurate estimate of tumor volume in a number of head and neck sites, such as the supraglottic region, owing to invisible deep tumor extension (Marks et al. 1979; van den Bogaert et al. 1983). Using a model of cell population kinetics during irradiation, a 10–20% theoretical difference in local control rate was calculated for tumors with a similar largest dimension (5 cm) but different width (3 or 5 cm) (Hjelm-Hansen 1980). This indicates that correct assessment of tumor volume is an important point. Three-dimensional tumor visualization, as offered by modern cross-sectional imaging techniques, allows more accurate estimation of the tumor volume.

Gilbert et al. (1987) were the first to report the prognostic value of CT-determined tumor volume for outcome after definitive radiation therapy. Their study was performed in 37 patients with T2–T4 laryngeal cancer (of both glottic and supraglottic origin). The mean tumor volume was 21.8 ml for patients failing radiotherapy in their study and 8.86 ml for patients primarily controlled; tumor volume was significantly predictive for disease-free interval ($P$ = 0.045) and outcome of radiotherapy ($P$ = 0.02).

Glottic and supraglottic tumors should be considered separately in such studies, as the anatomical situation (and hence the extension pattern) is very different for glottic versus supraglottic tumors; there are also separate staging recommendations for each of the two sites in the AJCC and UICC staging manuals.

Freeman et al. (1990), whose study (31 patients) was updated by Mancuso et al. (1994; 63 patients), were able to identify those patients with T1–T4 supraglottic carcinomas who had a higher likelihood of local control based on pretreatment CT volumetric analysis (tumors of <6 ml had a probability of 83% and 89%, respectively, of local control, while tumors of >6 ml had a control rate of only 46% and 40%, respectively).

Lee et al. (1993), whose study (18 patients) was updated by Pameijer et al. (1997) (42 patients), were able to stratify patients with T3 glottic carcinoma into groups with different likelihood of local control in a similar way (tumors of <3.5 ml had a probability of 92% and 85%, respectively, of local control, while tumors of >3.5 ml had a local control rate of only 33% and 22%, respectively). On the other hand, Mukherji et al. (1995b), in a study on 28 patients with T2 glottic carcinoma, were not able to distinguish groups with significantly different local control rates by CT-determined tumor volume.

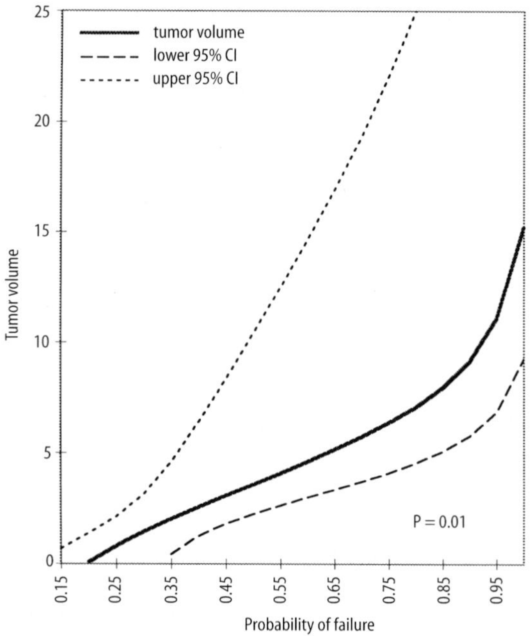


**Fig. 9.6.** Glottic cancer: probability of local failure after definitive RT versus CT-determined primary tumor volume. Local failure rate is significantly higher with larger primary tumor volume. The 95% confidence intervals for tumor volume are indicated. From Hermans (1998)

The results of the study by Hermans (1998) provide good corroboration for these earlier findings. Both for glottic and for supraglottic cancer, tumor volume was found to be a significant prognostic indicator of local control. In glottic cancer, failure probability analysis showed a clear relation between larger tumor volume and increasing risk of local failure (Fig. 9.6); a tumor volume of 3.5 ml correlated with an approximately 50% risk of local failure. From the graph published by Pameijer et al. (1997), an approximately 40% chance of local failure in T3 glottic cancer with a similar tumor volume can be inferred. Hermans (1998) also found a significant relation between tumor volume and risk of local failure for supraglottic cancer (Fig. 9.7). Compared with glottic cancer, larger supraglottic tumor volumes were found for similar local control rates; similar results can be inferred from the publications by the investigators in Gainesville, Fla. (Mancuso et al.

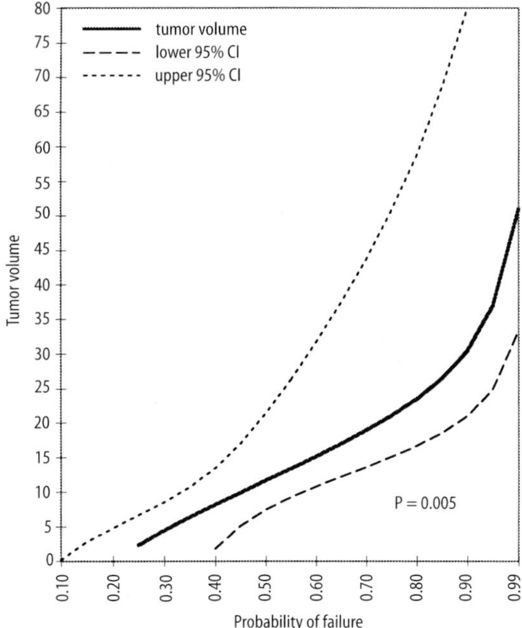


**Fig. 9.7.** Supraglottic cancer: probability of local failure after definitive RT versus CT-determined primary tumor volume. As for glottic cancer, local failure rate is significantly higher with larger primary tumor volume. The 95% confidence intervals for tumor volume are indicated. From HERMANS (1998)

1994; PAMEIJER et al. 1998b). The reason for this difference in critical tumor volume between glottic and supraglottic cancer is not clear; it might be related to a different local environment in the glottic and supraglottic regions, but also (and maybe predominantly) to the more exophytic growth pattern exhibited by supraglottic tumors. In the study by HERMANS (1998), tumor volume was not found to be a independent predictor of local outcome when a multivariate analysis was applied. In glottic carcinoma, involvement of the paraglottic space at the level of the true vocal cord and involvement of the pre-epiglottic space were found to be independent predictors of local outcome; in supraglottic carcinoma, involvement of the pre-epiglottic space and subglottic extension were the strongest independent predictors of local control.

Tumor volume and degree of involvement of the laryngeal deep tissues are correlated to some extent. However, these descriptive CT parameters may also reflect a more aggressive tumor behavior (ISAACS et al. 1988), which could explain their closer association with local recurrence. FLETCHER and HAMBERGER (1974) stated that the pre-epiglottic space was poorly vascularized; they suggested that the anoxic compartment of tumors invading this space must be significant and the tumors thus relatively radioresistant.

PAMEIJER et al. (1997), evaluating pretherapeutic CT studies in patients with T3 glottic carcinomas, found a trend to decreased local control when the paraglottic space at the true vocal cord level was infiltrated ($P = 0.14$), while infiltration of this space at the false cord level was significantly associated with a lower local control rate after definitive RT ($P = 0.01$); however, they did not find that these or other investigated CT parameters provided additional information on the probability of local control when considered simultaneously with tumor volume.

FREEMAN et al. (1990) reported a "trend" towards decreased postirradiation local control rate with increasing percentage of pre-epiglottic space involvement in T3 supraglottic cancer ($P = 0.384$).

### *9.4.1.2*
### *Laryngeal Cartilage Involvement on CT*

Laryngeal cartilage invasion is often considered to be predictive of a low probability of control of the primary tumor site by RT alone and to indicate an increased risk of late complications, such as severe edema or necrosis (LLOYD et al. 1981; SILVERMAN et al. 1985; CASTELIJNS et al. 1990).

Before the era of computer-assisted cross-sectional imaging only gross cartilage destruction, usually occurring in large-volume laryngeal tumors, could be detected clinically or by conventional radiography. More limited laryngeal cartilage invasion can be detected with modern cross-sectional imaging methods (BECKER et al. 1995). Earlier studies revealed an association between CT-depicted cartilage involvement in laryngeal carcinoma and poor outcome after RT (SILVERMAN et al. 1985; ISAACS et al. 1988). However, according to others, involvement of laryngeal cartilage is not necessarily associated with a reduced success rate for RT (MILLION 1989). More recent studies correlating CT-detected laryngeal cartilage abnormalities with local outcome after RT seem to corroborate this last point of view.

The cartilage that most often shows abnormalities is the arytenoid cartilage; usually it appears sclerotic. An abnormal appearance of this cartilage was not found to be associated with poorer local control (TART et al. 1994; HERMANS 1998). As pointed out by TART et al. (1994), tumor invasion of the arytenoid cartilage may be unimportant in terms of prognosis. The majority of sclerotic arytenoid cartilages do not contain tumor within ossified bone marrow, which can help to explain why RT is efficient in a high percentage of patients with isolated arytenoid sclerosis on CT (Becker et al. 1997).

Pameijer et al. (1997) found a lower probability of local control in patients with T3 glottic carcinoma when both arytenoid and cricoid showed sclerosis. These authors assume that if both the arytenoid and the cricoid cartilage are sclerotic, the probability of microscopic cartilage invasion will increase. Hermans (1998) did also find that when there were cricoid cartilage abnormalities in glottic carcinoma a statistically significant lower control rate was obtained; 10 of the 13 patients with sclerosis of the cricoid in this study also had sclerosis of the arytenoid cartilage, corresponding to the "double sclerosis" situation described by Pameijer et al. (1997). The multivariate analysis performed in the study by Hermans (1998) showed that an abnormal appearance of the cricoid cartilage is not an independent predictor of poor local control in glottic carcinoma: it lost significance when paraglottic and pre-epiglottic space involvement were introduced into the statistical model. Even relatively subtle cartilage abnormalities, as detected in this study population (sclerosis of the cartilage being the most frequent alteration seen), seem to be correlated with deep tumor extension. More destructive cartilage changes are associated with bulky tumors, which are not normally selected for RT. There are few data available on the correlation between thyroid cartilage abnormalities as seen on CT and local outcome of glottic cancer after definitive RT. In some studies patients showing evidence of thyroid cartilage involvement were explicitly excluded (Mukherji et al. 1995b; Pameijer et al. 1997). In the study by Hermans (1998), in which tumor visible on both sides of the cartilage and lysis of ossified cartilage were used as signs of thyroid cartilage invasion, only a limited number of patients with glottic carcinoma had an abnormal appearance of this cartilage. No evidence was found that thyroid cartilage involvement in itself, as seen on CT, is associated with a poorer local outcome after definitive RT, but as already seen, the number of patients with signs of neoplastic involvement of this cartilage was low in this study.

No conclusions can be drawn about cricoid or thyroid cartilage abnormalities on CT in supraglottic carcinoma, owing to the limited number of patients selected for RT who have had abnormalities of these cartilages.

#### 9.4.1.3 Involvement of the Anterior and Posterior Commissure on CT; Extralaryngeal Extension

Involvement of the posterior commissure as shown by CT was found to be associated with borderline statistical significance ($P = 0.07$) with a poorer local outcome after RT (Hermans 1998). Involvement of the posterior commissure occurs most often in relatively large glottic cancers.

Involvement of the anterior commissure as shown by CT in glottic cancer was not found to be an independent predictor of local recurrence ($P = 0.4$) (Hermans 1998). In the study on T3 glottic cancer by Pameijer et al. (1997), CT evidence of anterior commissure involvement was also not related to poorer local outcome after RT ($P = 0.5$).

Extralaryngeal spread was found to be associated with a higher recurrence rate of glottic cancer after radiation therapy, but this did not reach significance as only 10/119 patients were found to have such spread on CT (Hermans 1998). In the same study, nearly half the patients with supraglottic cancer had some evidence of an extralaryngeal abnormality on CT, but this was not associated with poorer local control. This is probably related to the subtle character of the extralaryngeal abnormalities (usually in the valleculae or piriform sinuses) detected with CT in most of these patients. According to the UICC classification, extralaryngeal spread should be staged as T4; in supraglottic cancer this probably would be overstaging if based on subtle CT findings.

### 9.4.2 Correlation Between Pretreatment MRI Findings and Tumor Recurrence

In a retrospective analysis a variety of MRI- and non-MRI-dependent prognostic factors in the success of RT in laryngeal carcinoma were evaluated (Castelijns et al. 1995). Age, sex, histopathology, and invasion of the vocal muscle or pre-epiglottic space did not influence the risk of tumor recurrence significantly. In contrast, cord mobility ascertained clinically, and invasion of laryngeal cartilages and tumor volume shown by MRI appeared to influence the risk of tumor recurrence. That tumor volume is important is not surprising, as it has been demonstrated for many tumor sites and is consistent with established radiobiological priciples. Comparison between statistically significant parameters by a logistic regression model revealed three relevant prognostic parameters: cord mobility, tumor volume and, most importantly, cartilage invasion. Our data indicate that information obtained from pretreatment MRI examination can help to predict the rate of local control with irradiation alone.

The ability of RT to cure laryngeal cancer invading bone or cartilage has been questioned by MILLION (1989). The effectiveness of RT in cases that are positive for cartilage involvement at MR imaging, especially in cases with abnormal signal in patients with smaller tumors, has not been extensively explored. Such cartilage involvement may well be not a contraindication for RT. A study comparing the outcome of RT and MR imaging findings is therefore important. In other words, the outcome and the radiological findings would be compared without radiological confirmation that the findings are correct. The false-positive rate is, of course, a concern. The effect of inflammation on the prognosis is another factor that must be considered unknown. Although this inflammatory response is considered to be protective, perhaps this tissue must be treated as tumor and a safe margin must be regarded as being beyond the edema. The spreading inflammation could carry cells and, with them, the potential for a higher recurrence rate. In this case, the effective false-positive rate would be much lower than that indicated by BECKER et al. (1995) Perhaps, on the other hand, the inflammation is less ominous than actual tumor and we have to aim at finding a method to help us in differentiating between tumor tissue and inflammation.

A correlation has been found between an abnormal MR signal pattern in cartilage and the risk of tumor recurrence. However, CASTELIJNS et al. agree with MILLION (1989) that it is incorrect to postulate that RT cannot cure a substantial number of lesions with cartilage involvement. Minimal cartilage involvement in patients with low-stage tumors also does not mean a poor prognosis (CASTELIJNS et al. 1995, 1996). Nor is minimal cartilage involvement in patients with small tumors (under 5 ml) a very ominous finding. On the other hand, an abnormal MR signal pattern in cartilage combined with large tumor volume (above 5 ml) worsens the prognosis significantly. Consequently, an abnormal MR signal pattern in cartilage should not automatically imply laryngectomy, especially in lesions with smaller volumes.

Neoplastic involvement of the yellow fibrocartilage of the epiglottis is amenable to RT (LEDERMAN 1970). Involvement of this type of cartilage was not investigated in this study. Involvement of the thyroid cartilage in the area of the anterior commissure correlated statistically with tumor recurrence. Therefore, an abnormal MR signal pattern in the anterior commissure is of predictive value for tumor recurrence.

In the literature it is stated that patients with glottic tumors primarily staged as T1b have a higher risk of tumor recurrence than those with tumors staged as T1a (MANTRAVADI et al. 1983; KIRCHNER 1970). In our study population, abnormal signal in the thyroid cartilage in the area of the anterior commissure might not explain the increased risk of tumor recurrence in patients with T1b glottic lesions. Tumor recurred in 2 out of 5 patients in whom MRI showed an abnormal signal intensity in cartilage in the area of the anterior commissure, whereas tumor recurred in both patients in whom no abnormal signal was seen (CASTELIJNS et al. 1996).

Owing to selection bias, involvement of the thyroid lamina was found infrequently in this study population. Patients with T3 or T4 lesions in whom CT and/or MRI showed major cartilage involvement of the thyroid cartilage were treated by surgery and consequently were not included in this study. According to our study results, involvement of the thyroid laminae also increases the risk of tumor recurrence. In a relatively high number of patients involvement was diagnosed in the crico-arytenoid joint. Motion artifacts caused by movement of the arytenoid might sometimes interfere with an adequate diagnosis. It is reported that when the arytenoid cartilage is involved the adjacent area of the cricoid cartilage is usually also involved (YEAGER and ARCHER 1982). In agreement with other reports (TART et al. 1994), involvement of cartilages around the crico-arytenoid joint had no clear predictive value for tumor recurrence. An abnormal signal pattern of the thyroid cartilage (both in the area of the anterior commissure and elsewhere in this cartilage) had an even higher predictive value for tumor recurrence than involvement of laryngeal cartilages generally. There was also a correlation between the number of cartilages involved and the risk of tumor recurrence. The risk of tumor recurrence increased if cartilages were destroyed. In agreement with others, we found serious complications, such as radionecrosis, to be rare (KEENE et al. 1982).

In further studies dealing with the prognostic value of MR parameters, glottic and supraglottic tumors should be considered separately.

## 9.5 Correlation Between Imaging After RT and Tumor Recurrence

After RT, clinical examination of the larynx and pharynx is difficult because of radiation effects, which alter the mucosa and produce varying degrees of deeper edema and fibrosis. Residual or recurrent tumor, therefore, can be difficult to detect by physical examination. MR imaging may have an advantage over CT for differentiating persistent or recurrent tumor from posttreatment fibrosis, demonstrating fibrosis with low signal intensity on T2-weighted images (DILLON and HARNSBERGER 1991). However, definite distinctions cannot be made between cancer, edema, and irradiation fibrosis on either CT or MR imaging (CASTELIJNS et al. 1987; MANCUSO 1991). Therefore, diagnostic methods allowing early assessment of residual or recurrent tumor during or after RT for squamous cell carcinoma are urgently needed.

### 9.5.1 Correlation Between Posttreatment CT Findings and Tumor Recurrence

Accurate interpretation of CT studies in patients irradiated for laryngeal cancer requires that the radiographic changes expected to result from treatment not be misinterpreted as residual or recurrent tumor. After RT, complete resolution of the tumor at the primary site is expected, but symmetrical soft tissue thickening and increased attenuation of the pre-epiglottic and paraglottic fat may be visible on follow-up CT (MUKHERJI et al. 1994a).

As described above, a risk profile for local tumor recurrence can be determined on a pretreatment CT. In a recent study (PAMEIJER et al. 1998a) it was shown that patients irradiated for a supraglottic carcinoma, piriform sinus carcinoma or T3 glottic carcinoma can also be stratified in different risk groups for primary site failure based on posttreatment CT studies.

A CT examination obtained between 1 and 6 months after completion of RT and classified as post-RT CT score 1 (expected tissue changes after RT, such as symmetrical thickening of the laryngeal and pharyngeal soft tissue structures and increased attenuation of the paralaryngeal fat; MUKHERJI et al. 1994a), was shown to be a very strong predictor of local control. Patients with such findings on post-RT CT will probably not benefit from further follow-up imaging studies, regardless of their pretreatment risk classification.

Patients with a first follow-up examination classified as post-RT CT score 3 (i.e. focal mass with a maximal diameter of >1 cm, or <50% estimated tumor volume reduction) did very poorly in this study; almost all these patients (18 of 20) developed a local failure. Although most patients in this group belonged, as might be expected, to the pretreatment high-risk CT group, some poor responders identified by follow-up CT initially had a low-risk pretreatment CT profile; the poor response in these patients could be due to an aggressive tumor biology or to a suboptimal tumor–host interaction. Despite the two false-positive cases in this study, these findings strongly suggest that further exploration in such post-RT CT score 3 patients is warranted, even though deep biopsies could aggravate or initiate necrosis (WARD et al. 1975). FDG or thallium imaging may prove to be a useful intermediate step when biopsy is considered too risky. Ongoing studies suggest that radionuclide imaging can detect local recurrences with a higher accuracy than purely anatomically based methods, such as CT and MR imaging (LAPELA et al. 1995; MCGUIRT et al. 1995; GAPANY et al. 1996; GREGOR et al. 1996; KIM et al. 1996).

The local outcome of patients with an initial post-RT CT score of 2 (i.e. focal mass with a maximal diameter of <1 cm and/or asymmetrical obliteration of laryngeal tissue planes) was found to be indeterminate (Fig. 9.8). About 60% of the patients in this group belonged to the pre-RT high-risk group, and half of them had local failure. About 40% of the patients in the post-RT CT score 2 group were at low risk for local failure according to a pre-RT CT study; most of them (78%) had achieved control at the primary site in this study, but this difference in local control between low- and high-risk patients was statistically not significant.

The experience obtained in this study suggests that a first baseline follow-up study should preferably be obtained about 4 months after completion of RT. This takes account of FDG positron emission tomography (PET) studies showing that baseline examinations less than 4 months after RT may not accurately reflect the outcome and that such studies, when done at 4 months and later, result in a more accurate prediction of the ultimate outcome (GREVEN et al. 1994).

The study by PAMEIJER et al. (1998a) also showed that in about 40% of local failures, follow-up CT revealed this event earlier than clinical examination; in these patients the CT diagnosis of local failure was

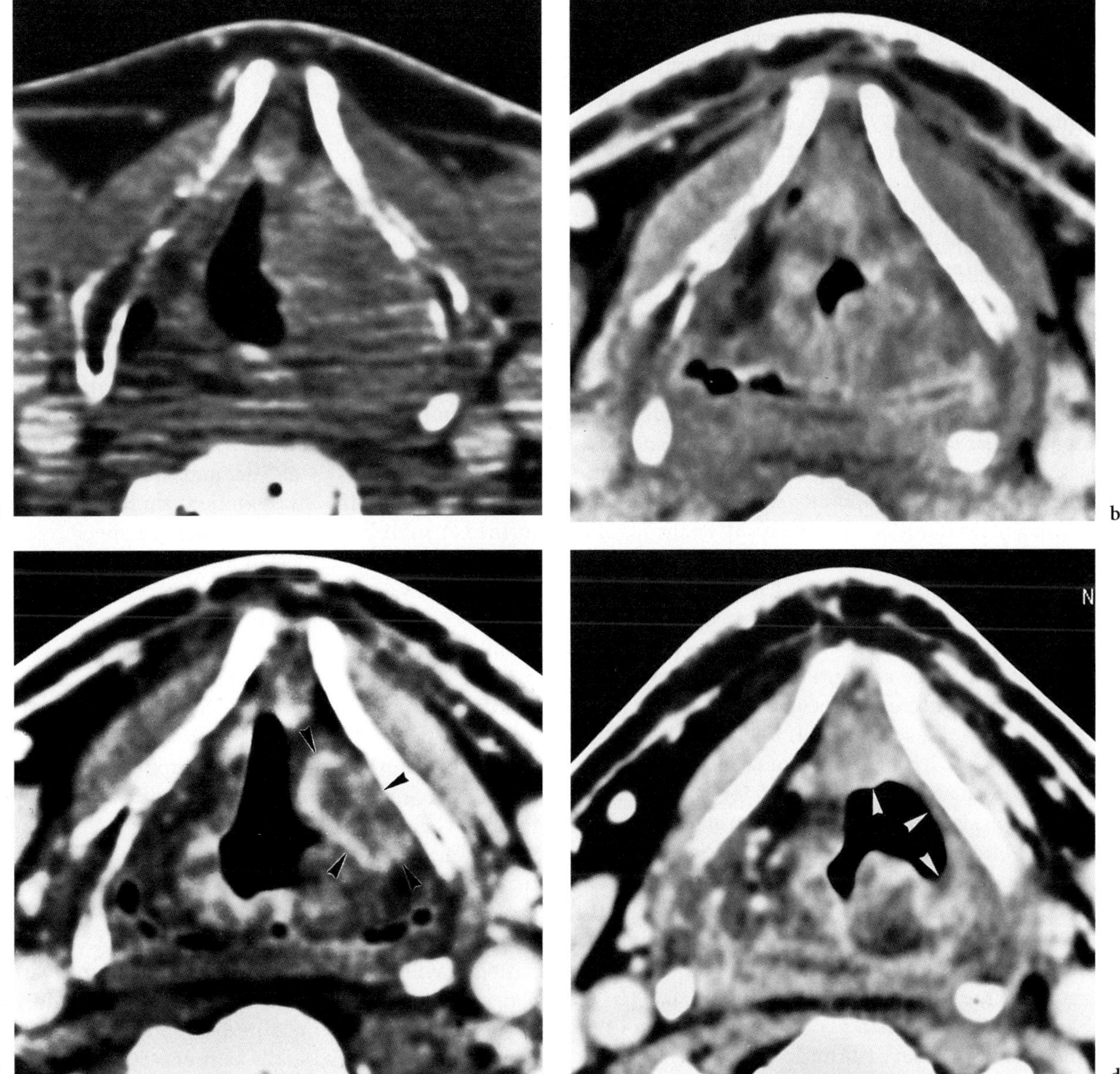


**Fig. 9.8 a–d.** CT images of a patient with a T3 supraglottic carcinoma and a low pretreatment risk profile. **a** Pretreatment CT image: tumor is seen in region of left false cord and paraglottic space. **b** CT image obtained at 2.5 months after RT. The tumor has regressed, but there is persistent obliteration of the deep fatty tissue at the left, without an obvious focal mass. This can be given a post-RT CT score of 2. **c** Five months after RT. A focal mass with a maximal diameter something over 1 cm (*arrowheads*) is seen in the original tumor bed: post-RT CT score 3. **d** Ten months after RT. Further progression and ulceration of the mass (*arrowheads*). Post-RT CT score 3. Laryngectomy performed at the same time confirmed the presence of local recurrence. Patient has no evidence of disease 2 years 8 months after RT. From Pameijer et al. (1998a)

eventually confirmed with a mean delay of 5.5 months. Use of this imaging-based information could lead to more prompt salvage surgery and potentially improve the survival of these patients. Proof of such a survival benefit requires further study. In a prospective study an improved survival following surgery for local recurrence was shown for those cases with less extensive local failure after RT alone or combined with chemotherapy (Keane et al. 1993); these patients underwent examination under anesthesia and biopsy of the original primary tumor site 8–12 weeks after completion of RT. The predictive value of a negative biopsy for local control was reported to be 70%. These authors support routine biopsy reassessment 8–12 weeks after completion of RT in an effort to detect recurrence as early as possible (Keane et al. 1993). Use of a baseline follow-up CT could substantially reduce the number of patients needing a biopsy; furthermore, CT could be used to target the biopsy into the radiologically most suggestive area.

New or progressive laryngeal cartilage alterations after RT are often associated with local failure and are attributed either to local tumor recurrence or to chondroradionecrosis (Mukherji et al. 1994b). These cartilage alterations can occur without a focal mass with a diameter of more than 1 cm: such cartilage changes may be due to limited chondronecrosis, without structural collapse of the laryngeal framework, and are predominantly seen in the arytenoid cartilage (Hermans et al. 1998b). It seems justified to adopt a wait-and-see policy in patients with progressive, arytenoid cartilage changes and minimal soft tissue asymmetry. Close follow-up, both clinically and radiologically, is necessary to detect progressive soft tissue changes, since such progression is associated with tumor recurrence or severe laryngeal necrosis (Hermans et al. 1998b).

Follow-up CT is probably not cost effective in patients who have been irradiated for a small carcinoma of the larynx, as the local control rates for such tumors after RT are very high. However, there are strong indications that patients with a higher likelihood of local failure, such as those with supraglottic, T3 or T4 glottic, and hypopharyngeal carcinomas, may benefit from a baseline follow-up CT study about 4 months after completion of RT. If the baseline CT study shows complete resolution of the tumor at the primary site and a symmetrical appearance of laryngeal and hypopharyngeal tissues (i.e., expected RT-related changes), it is very likely that local control has been achieved and further follow-up CT studies are not necessary. If less than 50% estimated volume reduction or a focal mass with a diameter larger than 1 cm is found, immediate further investigation is warranted, as the likelihood of local failure is high. If the laryngeal tissues appear asymmetrical, or a focal mass with a diameter smaller than 1 cm is found, unless clinical examination has already suggested the suspicion of local failure, further follow-up CT studies are needed; intervals of 3–4 months are recommended, to be continued for up to 2 years after completion of RT. In a substantial number of cases it seems possible to detect local failure earlier by CT than by clinical examination alone. These patients can then be salvaged at an earlier stage of local recurrence (Pameijer et al. 1998a).

### 9.5.2 Correlation Between Posttreatment MRI Findings and Tumor Recurrence

The prognostic value of posttreatment MR imaging for the risk of tumor recurrence has not yet been explored in a large study. However, it might be expected that results will be comparable with those of previously mentioned CT results. To obtain prognostic information regarding outcome of irradiation treatment of patients with larger tumors, such as supraglottic, T3 or T4 glottic, and hypopharyngeal carcinomas an MRI examination should be performed 4 months after completion of the RT. To date, reports on the use of MR spectroscopy for monitoring RT planning are also scarce.

## 9.6 Discussion

Whether CT or MR imaging is the preferred modality for imaging of laryngeal cancer has to be determined. Generally, MR imaging seems to be the optimal method of examination in cooperative patients. CT is recommended in patients who may have rapid breathing or coughing as a result of chronic lung disease or if MR imaging is not a option (e.g., in patients with a pacemaker, surgical clips, or severe claustrophobia). Both modalities can delineate deep tissue anatomy. MR imaging has better soft tissue contrast than CT, especially between fat tissue and pathologic tissue, and may be somewhat better in differentiating between pathologic tissue and surrounding normal tissue. On the other hand, high-resolution CT produces images with thinner slices and higher spatial resolution than MR imaging. Neither modality allows differentiation between tumor tissue and surrounding inflammatory tissue, which may be present in greater or lesser amounts. Both T1-weighted MR images and high-resolution CT are appropriate to assess tumor extent in various laryngeal compartments, such as the pre-epiglottic space, paraglottic space, and the anterior and posterior commissures. They can also be used as a basis for assessment of tumor volume. Tumor volume can be measured by calculating lesion area on a computerized image, outlining the lesions manually. Automatic or even semi-automatic postprocessing is not possible, owing to low contrast between tumor tissue and surrounding normal tissue, especially muscular tissue. With both techniques volume can be assessed by trained observers with acceptable intraobserver reproducibility. Consequently tumor volume, as shown by MR imaging or CT, may be included as a potential prognostic factor in predicting the outcome of RT. As the availability of techniques of postprocessing (access to workstation, ease of operation) increases, assessment of tumor volume can be expected to become a more essential part of routine diagnostic work-up.

In contrast to tumor volume, CT and MRI differ clearly in the possibilities they offer for detection of cartilage invasion. CT criteria for presence of cartilage invasion are based mainly on bony abnormalities, which may be detected as sclerotic changes or destruction. Sclerotic changes are thought to be caused by adjacent inflammatory or tumorous tissue.

On the other hand, MR imaging shows alterations in the cartilage directly. Consequently, changes in bony marrow are seen as abnormal signal, especially on T1-weighted images. CT appears to be more specific than MRI in the detection of neoplastic cartilage invasion, but seems to have a somewhat lower sensitivity, especially for thyroid cartilage involvement (Becker et al. 1995; Zbären et al. 1996). Most probably CT findings cause an underestimation, whereas MRI findings produce an overestimation, of the actual presence of cartilage invasion. The choice between CT and MRI may be settled in some cases by the clinical needs: if it is important to exclude cartilage invasion, as it can be when partial laryngectomy is considered, MR imaging may be indicated, while when cartilage invasion needs to be shown with more confidence CT may be more appropriate.

It is self-evidently apparent that the prognostic value of each of the modalities and its defined criteria is also valuable in the choice of treatment. Consequently, studies evaluating the prognostic value of imaging findings are becoming more numerous. At present, this theme has been elaborated more extensively and in more detail for CT than for MRI. In CT studies tumors have been classified for tumor location (glottic, supraglottic) and tumor stage. In further studies dealing with the prognostic value of MR parameters, glottic and supraglottic tumors and various T stages should be considered separately. There appears to be no question but that tumor volume, as determined by CT or MRI, is a predictor for risk of tumor recurrence. CT and MR findings concerning tumor volume should be included in a revised TNM classification. In contrast, results on the presence of cartilage invasion appear to be somewhat contradictory. Generally, in studies evaluating CT, cartilage invasion, as shown by this modality, appears to have a somewhat lower prognostic value, whereas MRI findings for cartilage involvement are reported to be more reliably indicative of an increased risk of tumor recurrence. Anyway, we agree with Million (1989) that the "myth about the radiocurability and bone and/or cartilage" should be replaced by an understanding of relative rates of control by RT. The prognostic value of laryngeal cartilage abnormalities in both CT and MRI studies needs to be examined more extensively, and if possible in multicenter trials.

Radiological information can be used to elaborate a more informed decision-making process when treatment has to be selected for laryngeal cancer; it could be useful to select patients for concomitant treatment during RT (such as chemotherapy or radiosensitizing treatment), and it can help to identify patients who may benefit from post-RT imaging surveillance.

## References


American Joint Committee on Cancer (AJCC) (1992) In: Manual for staging of cancer, 4th edn. Lippincott, Philadelphia

Bailey BJ (1991) Beyond the "new" TNM Classification. Arch Otolaryngol Head Neck Surg 117:369–370

Becker M, Zbären P, Laeng H, Stoupis C, Porcellini B, Vock P (1995) Neoplastic invasion of the laryngeal cartilage: comparison of MR imaging and CT with histopathologic correlation. Radiology 194:661–669

Becker M, Zbären P, Delavelle J, Kurt A-M, Egger C, Rüfenacht DA, Terrier F (1997) Neoplastic invasion of the laryngeal cartilage: reassessment of criteria for diagnosis at CT. Radiology 203:521–532

Breiman RS, Beck JW, Korobkin M, Glenny R, Akwari OE, Heaston DK, Moore AV, Ram PC (1982) Volume determinations using computed tomography. AJR Am J Radiol 138:329–333

Castelijns JA, Doornbos J, Berbeeten B Jr, Vielvoye GJ, Bloem JL (1985) Magnetic resonance imaging of the normal larynx 9(5):919–925

Castelijns JA, Kaiser MC, Valk J, Gerritsen GJ, van Hattum AH, Snow GB (1987a) MRI of laryngeal cancer. J Comput Assist Tomogr 11:134–140

Castelijns JA, Gerritsen GJ, Kaiser MC, Valk J, Jansen W, Meyer CJLM, Snow GB (1987b) MRI of normal and cancerous laryngeal cartilages: histopathological correlation. Laryngoscope 97:1085–1093

Castelijns JA, Gerritsen GJ, Kaiser MC et al (1988) Invasion of laryngeal cartilage by cancer: comparison of CT and MR imaging. Radiology 167:199–206

Castelijns JA, Golding RP, van Schaik C, Valk J, Snow GB (1990) MR findings of laryngeal cartilage invasion by laryngeal cancer: value in predicting outcome of radiation therapy. Radiology 174:669–673

Castelijns JA, van den Brekel MWM, Smit EMT, Tobi H, van Wagtendonk FW, Golding RP, Venema HW, van Schaik C, Snow GB (1995) Predictive value of MR imaging-dependent and non-MR imaging dependent parameters for recurrence of laryngeal cancer after radiation therapy. Radiology 196:735–739

Castelijns JA, van den Brekel MWM, Tobi H, Smit EM, Golding RP, van Schaik C, Snow GB (1996) Laryngeal carcinoma after radiation therapy: correlation of abnormal MR imaging signal patterns in laryngeal cartilage with the risk of tumor recurrence. Radiology 198:151–155

Curtin HD (1989) Imaging of the larynx: current concepts. Radiology 173:1–8

Dillon WP, Harnsberger HR (1991) The impact of radiologic imaging on staging of cancer of the head and neck. Semin Oncol 18:64–79

Dubrulle F, Robert Y, Delerue C, Chevalier D, Gaillandre L, Rocourt N, Lemaitre L (1997) Intérêt du scanner spiralé dans la pathologie du larynx et de l'hypo-pharynx. Feuill Radiol 37:118–131

Fletcher GH, Hamberger AD (1974) Causes of failure in irradiation of squamous-cell carcinoma of the supraglottic larynx. Radiology 111:697–700

Fletcher GH, Lindberg RD, Hamberger A, Horiot JC (1975) Reasons for irradiation failure in squamous cell carcinoma of the larynx. Laryngoscope 85:987–1003

Freeman DE, Mancuso AA, Parsons JT, Mendenhall WM, Million RR (1990) Irradiation alone for supraglottic larynx carcinoma: can CT findings predict treatment results? Int J Radiat Oncology Biol Phys 19:485–490

Gapany M, Grund F, Faust R, Fehling S, Hildebrandt W (1996) Thallium-201 SPECT imaging of head and neck tumors. Presented at the 4th international conference on head and neck cancer, Toronto, Canada, 28 July–1 Aug

Gilbert RW, Birt D, Shulman H, Freeman J, Jenkin D, Mackenzie R, Smith C (1987) Correlation of tumor volume with local control in laryngeal carcinoma treated by radiothereapy. Ann Otol Rhinol Laryngol 96:514–518

Gregor TR, Valdés Olmos R, Koops W, Balm AJM, Hilgers FJM, Hoefnagel CA (1996) Preliminary experience with Thallous Chloride T1 201-labeled single-photon emission computed tomography scanning in head and neck cancer. Arch Otolaryngol Head Neck Surg 122:509–514

Greven KM, Williams DW III, Keyes JW, McGuirt WF, Watson NE, Randall ME, Raben M, Geisinger KR, Cappelari JO (1994) Positron Emission Tomography of patients with head and neck carcinoma before and after high dose irradiation. Cancer 74:1355–1359

Hermans R, Marchal G, Feenstra L, Baert AL (1995) Spiral CT of the temporal bone: value of image reconstruction at submillimetric table increments. Neuroradiology 37:150–154

Hermans R, Van der Goten A, Baert AL (1997a) Image interpretation in CT of laryngeal carcinoma: a study on intra-and interobserver reproducibility. Eur Radiol 7:1086-1090

Hermans R (1998) Value of computed tomography as treatment outcome predictor of head and neck cancer treated with irradiation. Doctoral dissertation, Catholic University of Leuven

Hermans R (1998) Value of computed tomography as treatment outcome predictor of head and neck cancer treated with irradiation. Doctoral dissertation, Catholic University of Leuven

Hermans R (1998) Value of computed tomography as treatment outcome predictor of head and neck cancer treated with irradiation. Doctoral dissertation, Catholic University of Leuven

Hermans R, Bouillon R, Laga K, Delaere PR, De Foer B, Marchal G, Baert AL (1997b) Estimation of thyroid gland volume by spiral computed tomography. Eur Radiol 7:214–216

Hermans R (1998) Value of computed tomography as treatment outcome predictor of head and neck cancer treated with irradiation. Doctoral dissertation, Catholic University of Leuven

Hermans R, Feron M, Bellon E, Dupont P, Van den Bogaert W, Baert AL (1998a) Laryngeal tumor volume measurements determined with CT: a study on intra- and interobserver variability. Int J Radiat Oncol Biol Phys 40:553–557

Hermans R, Pameijer FA, Mancuso AA, Parsons JT, Mendenhall WM (1998b) Computed tomography findings in chondroradionecrosis of the larynx. AJNR Am J Neuroradiol 19:711-718

Hjelm-Hansen M (1980) Laryngeal carcinoma. IV. Analysis of treatment results using the Cohen model. Acta Radiol Oncol 19:3–12

Hokanson J (1991) Discussion/Perspective of "Beyond the 'New' TNM Classication". Arch Otolaryngol Head Neck Surg 117:371

Hoover LA, Calcaterra TC, Walter GA, Larsson SG (1984) Preoperative CT scan evaluation for laryngeal carcinoma: correlation with pathological findings. Laryngoscope 94:310–315

International Union Against Cancer (UICC) (1997) TNM classification of malignant tumors, 5th edn. Hermanek P, Sobin LH (eds). Wiley, New York

Isaacs JH, Mancuso AA, Mendenhall WM, Parsons JT (1988) Deep spread patterns in CT staging of T2–4 squamous cell laryngeal carcinoma. Otolaryngol Head Neck Surg 99:455–464

Johansen LV, Overgaard J, Hjelm-Hansen M, Gadeberg CG (1990) Primary radiotherapy of T1 squamous cell carcinoma of the larynx: analysis of 478 patients treated from 1963 to 1985. Int J Radiat Oncol Biol Phys 18:1307–1313

Johnson CR, Thames HD, Huang DT, Schmidt-Ullrich RK (1995) The tumor volume and clonogen number relationship: tumor control predictions based upon tumor volume estimates derived from computed tomography. Int J Radiat Oncol Biol Phys 33:281–287

Katsantonis GP, Archer CR, Rosenblum BN, Yeager VL, Friedman WH (1986) The degree to which accuracy of preoperative staging of laryngeal carcinoma has been enhanced by computed tomography. Otolaryngol Head Neck Surg 95:52–62

Keane TJ, Cummings BJ, O' Sullivan B, Payne D, Rawlinson E, MacKenzie R, Danjoux C, Hodson I (1993) A randomized trial of radiation therapy compared to split course radiation therapy combined with Mitomycin C and 5 Fluorouracil as initial treatment for advanced laryngeal and hypopharyngeal squamous carcinoma. Int J Radiat Oncol Biol Phys 25:613–618

Keene M, Harwood AR, Bryce DP, van Nostrand AWP (1982) Histopathological study of radionecrosis in laryngeal carcinoma. Laryngoscope 92:173–180

Kim KH, Sung M-W, Jang JY, Yun JB, Chung J-K (1996) F-18 FDG whole body PET in the evaluation of recurrence of head and neck cancer patients. Presented at the 4th international conference on head and neck cancer, Toronto, Canada, 28 July–1 Aug

Kirchner JA (1970) Cancer at the anterior commissure of the larynx. Results with radiotherapy. Arch Otolaryngol 91:524

Lapela M, Grénman R, Kurki T, Joensuu H, Leskinen S, Lindholm P, Haaparanta M, Ruotsalainen U, Minn H (1995) Head and neck cancer: Detection of recurrence with PET and 2-[F-18] Fluoro-2-deoxy-D-glucose. Radiology 197:205–211

Lederman M (1970) Radiotherapy of cancer of the larynx. J Laryngol Otol 84:867–896

Lee WR, Mancuso AA, Saleh EM, Mendenhall WM, Parsons JT, Million RR (1993) Can pretreatment computed tomography findings predict local control in T3 squamous cell carcinoma of the glottic larynx treated with radiotherapy alone? Int J Radiat Oncol Biol Phys 25:683–687

Lloyd GAS, Michaels L, Phelps PD (1981) The demonstration of cartilaginous involvement in laryngeal carcinoma by computerized tomography. Clin Otolaryngol 6:171–177

Mafee MF, Schild JA, Valvassori GE, Capek V (1983) Computed tomography of the larynx: correlation with anatomic and pathologic studies in cases of laryngeal carcinoma. Radiology 147:123–128

Mancuso AA (1991) Evaluation and staging of laryngeal and hypopharyngeal cancer by computed tomography and magnetic resonance imaging. In: Silver CE (ed) Laryngeal cancer. Thieme Medical, New York, pp 46–95

Mancuso AA, Hanafee WN (1985) Larynx and hypopharynx. In: Computed tomography and magnetic resonance imaging of the head and neck, 2nd edn. Williams and Wilkins, Baltimore, p 247

Mancuso AA, Mukherji SK, Mendenhall WM, Kotzur I, Freeman D (1994) Value of pretreatment CT as a predictor of outcome in supraglottic cancer treated with radiotherapy alone. Radiology 193(P):262

Mantravadi RVP, Liebner EJ, Haas RE, Skolnik EM, Applebaum EL (1983) Cancer of the glottis: prognostic factors in radiation therapy. Radiology 149:311–314

Marks JE, Freeman RB, Lee F, Ogura JH (1979) Carcinoma of the supraglottic larynx. AJR 132:255–260

McGuirt WF, Greven KM, Keyes JW, Williams DW III, Watson NE, Geisinger KR, Cappellari JO (1995) Positron emission tomography in the evaluation of laryngeal carcinoma. Ann Otol Rhinol Laryngol 104:274–278

Million RR (1989) The myth regarding bone or cartilage involvement by cancer and the likelihood of cure by radiotherapy. Head Neck 11:30–40

Million RR, Cassisi NJ, Mancuso AA (1994) Larynx. In: Million RR, Cassisi NJ (eds) Management of head and neck cancer: a multidisciplinary approach. Lippincott, Philadelphia, p 447

Mukherji SK, Mancuso AA, Kotzur IM, Mendenhall WM, Kubilis PS, Tart RP, Lee WR, Freeman D (1994a) Radiologic appearance of the irradiated larynx, part I. Expected changes. Radiology 193:141–148

Mukherji SK, Mancuso AA, Kotzur IM, Mendenhall WM, Kubilis PS, Tart RP, Freeman D, Lee WR (1994b) Radiologic appearance of the irradiated larynx, part II. Primary site response. Radiology 193:149–154

Mukherji SK, Castillo M, Huda W, Suojanen J, Kubilis P, Tart RP, Dhillon G (1995a) Comparison of dynamic and spiral CT for imaging the glottic larynx. J Comp Assist Radiol 19:899–904

Mukherji SK, Mancuso AA, Mendenhall W, Kotzur IL, Kubilis P (1995b) Can pretreatment CT predict local control of T2 glottic carcinomas treated with radiation therapy alone? AJNR Am J Neuroradiol 16:655–662

Ogura JH, Sessions DG, Spector GJ (1975) Conservation surgery for epidermoid carcinoma of the supraglottic larynx. Laryngoscope 85:1808–1813

Overgaard J, Hansen HS, Jørgensen K, Hjelm-Hansen M (1986) Primary radiotherapy of larynx and pharynx carcinoma – an analysis of some factors influencing local control and survival. Int J Radiat Oncol Biol Phys 12:515–521

Pameijer FA, Mancuso AA, Mendenhall WM, Parsons JT, Kubilis MS (1997) Can pretreatment computed tomography predict local control in T3 squamous cell carcinoma of the glottic larynx treated with definitive radiotherapy? Int J Radiat Oncol Biol Phys 37:1011–1021

Pameijer FA, Hermans R, Mancuso A, Mendenhall W, Parsons J, Stringer S, Kubilis P (1998a) Post radiotherapy computed tomography surveillance in laryngeal and hypopharyngeal cancer. Int J Radiat Oncol Biol Phys (submitted)

Pameijer FA, Mancuso AA, Mendenhall WM, Parsons JT, Mukherji SK, Hermans R, Kubilis PS (1998b) Evaluation of pretreatment computed tomography as predictor of local control in T1/T2 pyriform sinus carcinoma treated with definitive radiotherapy. Head Neck 20:159–168

Phelps PD (1992) Review: carcinoma of the larynx- the role of imaging in staging and pre-treatment assessments. Clin Radiol 46:77–83

Reid MH (1984) Laryngeal carcinoma: high-resolution computed tomography and thick anatomic sections. Radiology 151:689–696

Robert YH, Chevalier D, Rocourt NL, Lemaitre LG (1993) Dynamic manoeuver acquired with spiral CT in laryngeal disease. Radiology 189(P):298–299

Robert Y, Rocourt N, Chevalier D, Duhamel A, Carcasset S, Lemaitre L (1996) Helical CT of the larynx: a comparative study with conventional CT scan. Clin Radiol 51:882–885

Sakai F, Sone S, Kiyono K, Maruyama A, Kawai T, Oguchi M, Shikama N, Izuno I, Aoki J, Ueda H, Ishii K, Taguch K (1993) MR evaluation of laryngohypopharyngeal cancer: value of gadopentate dimeglumine enhancement. AJNR Am J Neuroradiol 14:1059–1069

Silverman PM, Bossen EH, Fisher SR, Cole TB, Korobkin M, Halvorsen RA (1984) Carcinoma of the larynx and hypopharynx: computed tomographic-histopathologic correlations. Radiology 151:697–702

Silverman PM, Zeiberg AS, Sessions RB, Troost TR, Zeman RK (1995) Three-dimensional imaging of the hypopharynx and larynx by means of helical (spiral) computed tomography. Comparison of radiological and otolaryngological evaluation. Ann Otol Rhinol Laryngol 104:425–431

Snow GB, Gerritsen (1993) TNM classification according to the UICC and AJCC. In: Ferlito A (ed) Neoplasms of the larynx. Churchill Livingstone, Edinburgh, pp 425–434

Sufaro S, Barzan L, Querin F, Lutman M, Caruso G, Comoretto R, Volpe R, Carbone A (1989) T staging of the laryngohypopharyngeal carcinoma. Arch Otolaryngol Head Neck Surg 115:613–620

Takashima S, Noguchi Y, Okumura T, Aruga H, Kobayashi T (1993) Dynamic MR imaging in the head and neck. Radiology 189:339–346

Tart RP, Mukherji SK, Lee WR, Mancuso AA (1994) Value of laryngeal cartilage sclerosis as a predictor of outcome in patients with stage T3 glottic cancer treated with radiation therapy. Radiology 192:567–570

Van den Bogaert W, Ostyn F, van der Schueren E (1983) The different clinical presentation, behaviour and prognosis of carcinomas originating in the epilarynx and the lower supraglottis. Radiother Oncol 1:117–131

Van den Bogaert W, van der Schueren E, Horiot JC, De Vilhena M, Schraub S, Svoboda V, Arcangeli G, de Pauw M, van Glabbeke M (1995) The EORTC randomized trial on three fractions per day and misonidazole in advanced head and neck cancer: prognostic factors. Radiother Oncol 35:100–106

Vogl TJ, Mack MG, Juergens M et al (1993) Skull base tumors: gadodiamide injection-enhanced MR imaging- drop-out effect in the early enhancement pattern of paragangliomas versus different tumors. Radiology 188:339–346

Ward PH, Calcaterra TC, Kagan AR (1975) The enigma of post-radiation edema and recurrent or residual carcinoma of the larynx. Laryngoscope 85:522–529

Whiters HR (1992) Biologic basis of radiation therapy. In: Perez CA, Brady LW (eds) Principles and practice of radiation oncology, 2nd edn. Lippincott, Philadelphia, pp 64–96

Yeager VL, Archer CR (1982) Anatomical routes of cancer invasion of laryngeal cartilages. Laryngoscope 92:449

Yousem DM (1993) Dynamic MR imaging in the head and neck: an idea whose time has come . . . and gone? Radiology 189:659–660

Zbären P, Becker M, Laeng H (1996) Pretherapeutic staging of laryngeal cancer: clinical findings, computed tomography and magnetic resonance imaging versus histopathology. Cancer 77:1263–1273

# 10 New Developments in Imaging of Neck Node Metastases

M.W.M. Van Den Brekel and J.A. Castelijns

CONTENTS



## 10.1 Introduction

In patients with squamous cell carcinomas of the mucosal linings in the head and neck, lymphatic metastasis is the most important mechanism in the spread of their tumors. In general, lymph nodes are rather poor barriers to tumor cells (Fisher and Fisher 1967), and clinical practice has shown that lymph nodes quite often appear to be a fertile soil for tumor growth. The rate of metastasis probably reflects the aggressiveness of the primary tumor. In carcinomas of the head and neck the presence of lymph node metastases is an important prognosticator (Jones et al. 1994; Snow et al. 1982). Not only the presence, but also the number of nodal metastases, the level in the neck, the size of the nodes and the presence of extranodal spread are important prognostic features. In many institutions throughout the world, the neck is staged mainly by palpation. Although palpation has the advantage of being both easy and inexpensive to perform and repeat, it is generally accepted that it is inaccurate. Both sensitivity and specificity are in the range of 60–70%, depending on the tumor studied (Sako et al. 1964; Ali et al. 1985). Neck staging is performed according to UICC (International Union Against Cancer) and AJCC (American Joint Committee on Cancer) guidelines (Table 10.1). As a consequence of the known low sensitivity of palpation, a neck side without palpable metastases is at risk of harboring occult metastasis. This risk is not only dependent on the clinician, but to a large extent on the size and site and other characteristics of the primary tumor (Martinez Gimeno et al. 1995; Ghouri et al. 1994; Kowalski et al. 1995; Jones et al. 1992). For example, in small glottic carcinomas and in sinonasal carcinomas the risk of occult metastases is far below 10%. On the other hand, with nasopharyngeal carcinomas and, to a lesser extent, hypopharyngeal carcinomas the risk is 50% or higher. For most T1–3 oral, oropharyngeal and supraglottic tumors this risk of occult metastases is in the range of 20–50%, with significant differences between different sites and studies (Levendag et al. 1989; Ho et al. 1992; Spiro et al. 1988; Shingaki et al. 1995; McGuirt et al. 1995; Kligerman et al. 1994; Ramadan and Allen 1993). In many head and neck primaries not only the ipsilateral site of the neck is at risk, but the contralateral site also has a significant risk of harboring metastases, especially when the primary has grown close to or extends over the midline. Because of the high false-negative rate of palpation, it is widely accepted for the neck to be treated electively if the risk of occult metastases is high. The optimal balance of risk between performing and refraining from elective treatment is very hard to define and is to a large extent related to the prognostic impact of this policy versus a wait-and-see policy. As most clinicians do not treat the neck electively in the case of small T1 oral carcinomas, which carry around a 15% risk of occult metastases, these risk figures are often quoted in the literature. However, in a recent meta-analysis using a decision analysis on the basis of prognostic


M. W. M. Van Den Brekel, MD, Department of Otolaryngology, Free University Hospital Amsterdam P.O. Box 7057, 1007 MB Amsterdam, The Netherlands

J. A. Castelijns, MD, Department of Radiology, Free University Hospital Amsterdam, P.O. Box 7057, 1007 MB Amsterdam, The Netherlands

**Table 10.1.** International Union Against Cancer (UICC) and American Joint Committee on Cancer (AJCC) staging of lymph node metastases in neck

| | |
|---|---|
| Nx | The neck cannot be assessed |
| N0 | No regional lymph node metastases |
| N1 | One ipsilateral metastasis, 3 cm or smaller |
| N2a | One ipsilateral metastasis larger than 3 cm, smaller than 6 cm |
| N2b | Multiple ipsilateral metastases smaller than 6 cm |
| N2c | Contra- or bilateral metastases smaller than 6 cm |
| N3 | Regional metastasis larger than 6 cm |

literature data, a risk of occult metastases higher than 20% was calculated to be optimal for elective treatment (Weiss et al. 1994).

## 10.2 Neck Anatomy and Patterns of Metastases

The neck nodes are divided into six levels, five of which are routinely dissected in a comprehensive neck dissection (Fig. 10.1). An advantage of uniform numbering of the different levels is that the operation report and the pathological and radiological reports can easily be compared. Most tumors originating from the mucosal lining of the upper aerodigestive tract have a well-defined and predictable pattern of metastasis to the neck (Shah 1990; Candela et al. 1990a,b). Although skip metastases do occur, these are quite rare (Candela et al. 1990a,b; Davidson et al. 1993; Byers er al. 1997). Many studies have been published on this subject, some deriving their data from—unreliable—clinical findings (Bataini et al. 1985) and others from the pathological reports obtained from therapeutic (Lindberg 1972; Kinsey et al. 1958) or elective (Byers et al. 1988; Shah 1990) neck dissections. These studies allow the inference that all primary carcinomas can eventually spread to all levels of the neck. The pathological studies performed on specimens from elective neck dissections give clues about the first- (and second)-echelon lymph nodes that are at highest risk of harboring occult metastases from the various sites of primary tumors within the mucous membranes of the head and neck. It is important for radiologists to know these patterns of metastasis, as this makes the search for metastases on axial scans easier. Furthermore, it is essential if

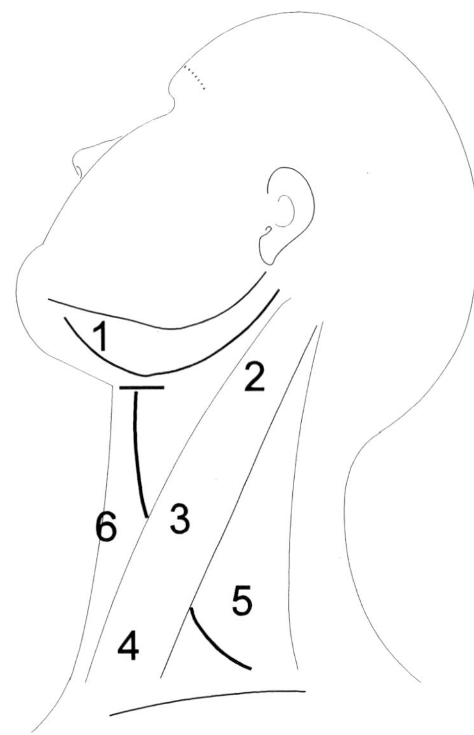


**Fig. 10.1.** Six lymph node levels in the neck according to the Memorial Sloan-Kettering Cancer Center

ultrasound-guided fine needle aspiration cytology (US-FNAC) is used.

Level 1 corresponds to the submental and subdigastric area and is the drainage region for anterior oral carcinomas, lip and sinonasal carcinomas. Level 2 corresponds to the subdigastric or high jugular region and is the most frequently involved level of the neck. Most tumors originating from the oropharynx, posterior oral cavity and supraglottic larynx metastasize primarily to this level. However, even anterior oral cavity carcinomas and glottic and hypopharyngeal carcinomas, frequently metastasize to this level. Level 3 corresponds to the midjugular region and is the first drainage level for glottic, subglottic and hypopharyngeal carcinomas. Leve 4 corresponds to the low jugular region and is very rarely the only level involved in head and neck primaries. In the case of lymph node metastases at this level, the primary tumor can have a subglottic localization or be sited in the thyroid gland or the cervical esophagus. Occasionally, mid- or low-esophageal carcinomas, breast, lung or gastric carcinomas present with level 4 metastases. Level 5 corresponds to the posterior triangle, behind the sternocleidomastoid muscle. This level is only rarely involved in head and neck cancer patients whose disease is not advanced (DAVIDSON et al. 1993). Only in nasopharyngeal carcinomas and skin carcinomas of the neck or occipital skull is this level frequently involved. Level 6 corresponds to the juxtavisceral area, containing the parapharyngeal and paratracheal lymph nodes. The para- and retropharyngeal nodes can be involved in pharyngeal and less frequently in sinonasal carcinomas (MCLAUGHLIN et al. 1995; HASEGAWA and MATSUURA 1994; WATARAI et al. 1993). Paratracheal metastases are frequently seen in thyroid, subglottic, hypopharyngeal and esophageal cancers (WEBER et al. 1993; NOGUCHI et al. 1993; CHANDAWARKAR et al. 1996).

## 10.3 Clinical Impact of Nodal Imaging

### 10.3.1 Clinically Negative (N0) Neck

Accurate pretreatment knowledge about the status of both neck sides is of the utmost importance for the surgeon or radiotherapist (VAN DEN BREKEL et al. 1994a, 1996a). Imaging can be indicated if no metastases are palpable, to detect occult metastases or to ascertain that the neck is pathologically N0 and thus can be observed. If metastases are palpable, imaging can be indicated to assess ingrowth into vital structures or to assess the contralateral, clinically N0, side. Assessment of the number and levels of involved lymph nodes or the presence of extranodal spread is less important, as most clinicians will treat all levels of the neck if a metastasis is obvious. Imaging of the clinically N0 neck, however, is indicated only if the imaging results are to be used in treatment planning. In this respect, depiction of suggestive nonpalpable lymph nodes can allow selective neck treatment or a wait-and-see policy to be rejected in favor of a more secure comprehensive treatment of all levels of the neck. Negative imaging results, on the other hand, can be used as an argument for refraining from elective treatment of the neck if the risk of radiologically occult metastases is considered to be low enough and the primary tumor is not excised through the neck (WEISS et al. 1994; VAN DEN BREKEL et al. 1993; BAATENBURG DE JONG et al. 1991).

Because imaging of the N0 neck can diminish the risk of occult metastases but never reduce this risk to zero, and because radiologically occult metastases will inevitably develop into manifest disease if left alone, decision making requires that two important issues be addressed: first, the prognostic impact of a wait-and-see policy versus elective treatment, and secondly the risk of occult metastases. The impact of a wait-and-see policy versus elective treatment on prognosis has not been determined unequivocally. Although a negative influence can indeed be anticipated, it is likely to be dependent on the duration of the time-lapse before the treatment of any neck node metastases that develop during follow-up. In this respect, both the intervals between follow-up examinations and the technique used for assessment of the neck are crucial. Many retrospective studies have been performed, which have (SPIRO and STRONG 1973; MCGUIRT et al. 1995; MARTIS et al. 1979), or have not (HUGHES et al. 1993; LYDIATT et al. 1993; HO et al. 1992) shown a difference in survival. Retrospective studies, however, are hampered by patient selection and other biases. Thus far a prognostic influence has not been proven unequivocally in three small prospective studies (VANDENBROUCK et al. 1980; FAKIH et al. 1989; KLIGERMAN et al. 1994), one of which (VANDENBROUCK et al. 1980) even showed a nonsignificant advantage of a wait-and-see policy. Currently a nationwide Canadian prospective randomized study is ongoing that might give more definitive answers, although even this sample might not be large enough to give definitive answers. For the prognosis after a neck relapse, the salvage rate is crucial. As the salvage rate depends on the metastatic burden (ALVI and JOHNSON 1996), the time-lapse to diagnosis of the neck failure seems crucial. In this respect, short intervals between postoperative controls and an accurate assessment method for the neck might increase the salvage rate. The second issue concerns the risk of occult metastases. This risk is dependent both on characteristics of the primary tumor and on the sensitivity of the assessment method. As a 20% risk of occult metastases is considered an acceptable basis for observation of the neck rather than elective treatment, and because most T2 oral carcinomas carry about a 30–40% risk of palpably occult metastases (WEISS et al. 1994; HO et al. 1992; SPIRO et al. 1988; SHINGAKI et al. 1995), the sensitivity of any imaging technique should be at least around 50% to detect half of the occult metastases and diminish the postimaging risk of occult metastases accordingly.

One should realize that it will never be possible to detect all occult metastases. As the incidence of micrometastases exclusively in clinically N0 necks with occult metastases is 25%, we should realize that no imaging technique can ever reach a sensitivity over 75% without losing a high specificity (Van Den Brekel et al. 1996b).

So far, our experience with this wait-and-see policy, in which we follow up the patient by palpation and US-FNAC, have been encouraging. Of the 77 patients who underwent a transoral excision without neck treatment, 14 failed with metastasis in the neck (18%), 10 of whom were salvaged (71% salvage rate) and are alive without tumor (Van Den Brekel et al. 1998a).

### 10.3.2 Tumor-Positive Neck

Although radiological assessment of the clinically N0 neck is the most important issue in neck node imaging, several other indications can be of importance. Identification of false-positive findings at physical examination can have significant therapeutic consequences for the patient, although almost all clinicians will treat the neck if nodes are clearly palpable irrespective of imaging findings. The relevance of depiction of extranodal spread or the exact number and levels of metastases is of less importance if the patient is treated surgically, because the final histopathology report will guide further therapy, and most surgeons treat all levels of the neck once a positive lymph node is detected. However, accurate depiction of these features becomes more important when selective neck dissections are considered for limited disease (Spiro et al. 1996) or when radiotherapy is the primary treatment and no histopathology will become available. CT, US and MRI are not very accurate in assessment of the exact number of metastases in the neck or the number of levels involved (Van Den Brekel et al. 1991a), as relatively large detectable metastases are very often accompanied by small undetectable micrometastases (Van Den Brekel et al. 1996b). For US-FNAC it seems highly impractical and less tolerable for the patient to aspirate from more than two or three lymph nodes per side, and thus it is often impossible to make an exact estimate of the number of lymph nodes involved.

#### *10.3.2.1 Extranodal Spread*

Extranodal spread is radiologically characterized by ablation of fat planes and irregular nodal borders. For this feature, Yousem et al. (1992) reported an accuracy of 90% for CT, whereas MRI had an accuracy of 78% in their study. Som (1992) even reported an estimated sensitivity of 100% for CT. On the other hand, Close et al. (1989) reported that CT could only identify extranodal spread in large nodes. Carvalho et al. (1991) studied the value of CT in detecting extranodal spread and found a sensitivity of 63% and a specificity of 60%. In our opinion, only major macroscopic extranodal spread (infiltration) can be detected by preoperative imaging. As even pathologists do not always agree on the presence of microscopic extranodal spread, and because it is very often a discrete histopathological sign, radiological assessment should be considered unreliable.

#### *10.3.2.2 Carotid Artery Invasion*

Assessment of the invasion of vital structures can have implications for both prognosis and treatment, as the resectability becomes uncertain and prognosis very poor once vital structures are invaded. In this respect, invasion of the common or internal carotid artery is probably the most important (Brennan and Jafek 1994), although invasion of both internal jugular veins, the skull base or the thoracic inlet poses similar therapeutic challenges. The reported accuracy of CT, MRI and US in detecting tumor invasion into the carotid artery varies widely (Langman et al. 1989; Pradeep et al. 1991; Mann et al. 1994; Gritzmann et al. 1990; Yousem et al. 1995). Some authors have successfully tried the use of US palpation to detect carotid wall invasion (Mann et al. 1994; Gritzmann et al. 1990). In general, a tumor encircling over 270° of the vessel's perimeter on CT or MRI (Yousem et al. 1995), or a tumor that cannot be moved away from the vessel using sono-palpation indicates involvement of the vessel wall and often unresectability. However, this involvement does not necessarily mean the tumor cannot be peeled off from the vessel.

#### 10.3.2.3
#### *Retropharyngeal and Paratracheal Metastases*

Pretreatment depiction of retropharyngeal metastases or paratracheal metastases can alter the extent of the neck dissection or radiotherapy fields (McLaughlin et al. 1995; Watarai et al. 1993). Although these nodes are a poor prognosticator, their presence can certainly indicate more extensive dissections or wider fields of radiotherapy (McLaughlin et al. 1995; Hasegawa and Matsuura 1994). Involvement of paratracheal lymph nodes in laryngeal and hypopharyngeal cancer is a sign of poor prognosis that warrants a paratracheal resection (Weber et al. 1993; Batsakis et al. 1975). Very few studies have addressed the radiological aspects of this issue as yet. Chandawarkar et al. (1996) have found that paratracheal lymph nodes are better depicted with either endosonography or CT than with MRI. Olmi et al. (1995) found MRI superior to CT in depicting retropharyngeal nodes. However, our experience in detecting paratracheal metastases preoperatively has so far been disappointing. As a consequence, a paratracheal lymph node dissection should routinely be carried out in piriform sinus carcinomas and laryngeal cancers with subglottic extension.

#### 10.3.2.4
#### *Recurrent Disease in the Neck*

Radiation therapy and surgery can lead to changes that mask recurrent disease on physical examination. Very often, recurrent disease in the neck after surgery and radiotherapy can no longer be treated with curative intent. Only very early detection, especially if only one of the two treatment modalities was employed, will enable salvage treatment in selective patients.

CT and MRI have been disappointing in the early detection of recurrent or residual disease in the neck. As a consequence, their role in evaluating the post-treatment neck is controversial. Attempts at early detection of recurrences have been frustrating (Dillon and Harnsberger 1991; Gussack and Hudgins 1991). Tumor tissue generally displays higher signal intensity on T2-weighted images than normal fat or muscle. Unfortunately, the specificity of this finding is poor, as radiation or postsurgical edema are depicted with similar signal intensities. Contrast enhancement with Gd-DTPA can be of help for the evaluation of recurrent head and neck tumors. Malignant disease is known to enhance with Gd-DTPA. However, scar tissue and inflammatory disease may also enhance in the first few months after treatment (Gong et al. 1991; Gussack and Hudgins 1991). In patients who have a primary tumor with a high likelihood of loco-regional recurrence, a baseline MRI or CT can be obtained 3–4 months after the initial treatment. Using the baseline scan, certain abnormalities that develop later can then be interpreted more reliably (Dillon and Harnsberger 1991). The use of US or duplex Doppler for follow-up of the treated neck has been reported by several authors (Westhofen 1987; Ahuja et al. 1996; Szmeja et al. 1998; Steinkamp et al. 1993, 1994a; Hessling et al. 1991). Westhofen showed that US-FNAC was superior to CT in detecting neck recurrences after previous treatment. Recently, Anzai et al. (1996) showed that PET is more sensitive than CT and MRI in detecting early recurrences.

### 10.4
### Radiological Criteria for Metastases

The accuracy of imaging techniques for the neck is largely restricted by the criteria used for lymph node metastases (Van Den Brekel et al. 1994b; Som 1992; Don et al. 1995). In general, none of the currently available imaging techniques is able to depict small tumor deposits inside lymph nodes, nor are any of them able to distinguish reactively enlarged lymph nodes from metastatic lymph nodes. The characteristics of metastatic lymph nodes that can be depicted are size (Fig. 10.2) and presence of non-contrast-enhancing parts inside metastatic lymph

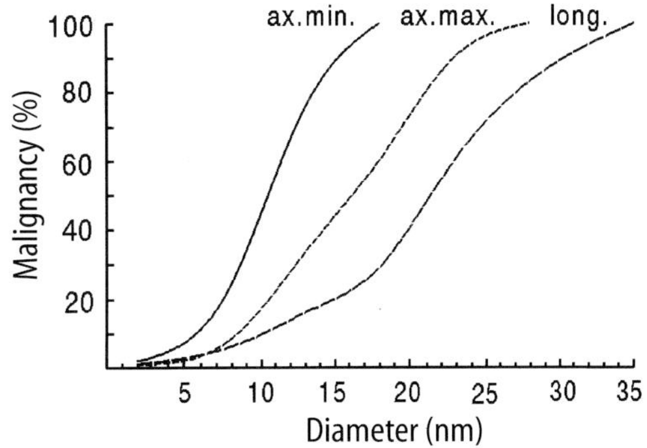


**Fig. 10.2.** Percentage of lymph nodes metastatic versus their respective diameters (*Ax.min.* minimal axial diameter, *ax.max.* maximal axial diameter, *long.* longitudinal diameter)

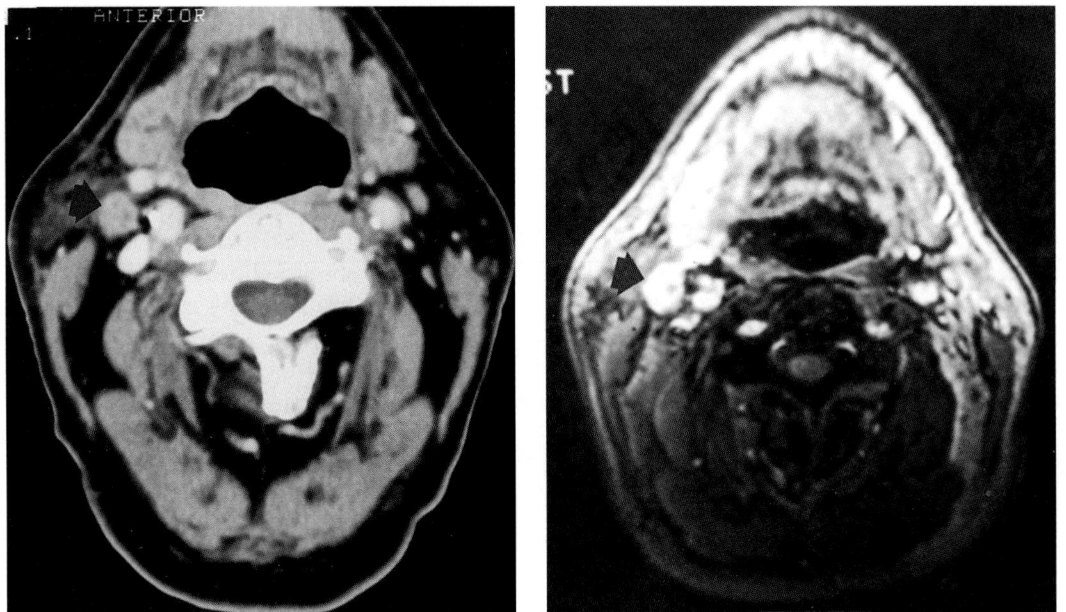


**Fig. 10.3.** **a** Axial CT scan of a patient with a T2N1 oral carcinoma on the right. The subdigastric lymph node metastasis is clearly depicted (*arrow*). Inside the lymph node a small hypodense area corresponds to tumor necrosis. This area, about 3 mm large, is still clearly recognizable and can be used with certainty as a criterion for metastasis. It should be realized that smaller areas cannot be reliably distinguished from artifacts or nonspecific variation in contrast uptake, thus limiting the sensitivity of this criterion. **b** Gd-DTPA-enhanced T1-weighted gradient echo image at the same level clearly demonstrating that "necrosis" is about equally well visualized on well-performed MR images (*arrow*)

nodes (Fig. 10.3) caused by tumor necrosis, tumor keratinization and cystic areas inside the tumor. Only rarely does tumor tissue enhance more than reactive lymph node tissue, and in these rare cases the tumor tissue can be visualized inside a reactive lymph node (Fig. 10.4, 10.5). With the use of modern MRI contrast agents that are selectively accumulated in the reticuloendothelial cells in reactively enlarged lymph nodes the depiction of tumor in contrast to this lymphatic tissue should become possible (Anzai and Prince 1997). However, the current spatial resolution and contrast do not seem to enable the depiction of small metastases inside lymph nodes. Grouping of lymph nodes is also used as a criterion by several authors. Some authors claim that the presence of extranodal spread (unsharp borders and obliteration of fat planes) can be used as a criterion for metastases. However, this criterion is seldom met in small lymph nodes and, as explained above, does not seem to correlate well with histopathological extranodal spread. Very often extranodal spread in small metastatic nodes is a subtle microscopic phenomenon that cannot be detected with any available imaging technique. Nodal shape is also used by several authors (Steinkamp et al. 1995). In general, a round shape is considered more grounds for suspicion than an oval or flat shape (Fig. 10.6). The shape can be defined either in the vertical plane (longitudinal/maximal or minimal axial diameter; L/T) or in the axial plane (minimal axial diameter/maximal axial diameter). As a criterion, shape is generally used in combination with the maximal diameter, to prevent very small nodes (smaller than 5 mm) from being interpreted as positive. In reactive nodes, the L/T ratio is 2 or higher in 86% of cases (Bruneton et al. 1994). As in round nodes the maximal diameter is the same as the minimal diameter, and because we previously found this diameter to be superior (Van Den Brekel et al. 1990a), instead of using the maximal axial diameter in combination with shape we prefer to use the minimal nodal diameter (Fig. 10.2). Morphological criteria such as focal cortical widening (Vassallo et al. 1992) will become more important as the contrast and spatial resolution of imaging techniques increases.

Although very-high-resolution CT and MRI with fewer artifacts, immuno-imaging with SPECT and PET, and more specific contrast agents are becoming available (Yousem and Hurst 1994; Anzai and Prince 1997; Meijs et al. 1997; Quak et al. 1993; Bruneton et al. 1994), either these techniques are too expensive and impractical for routine use, or

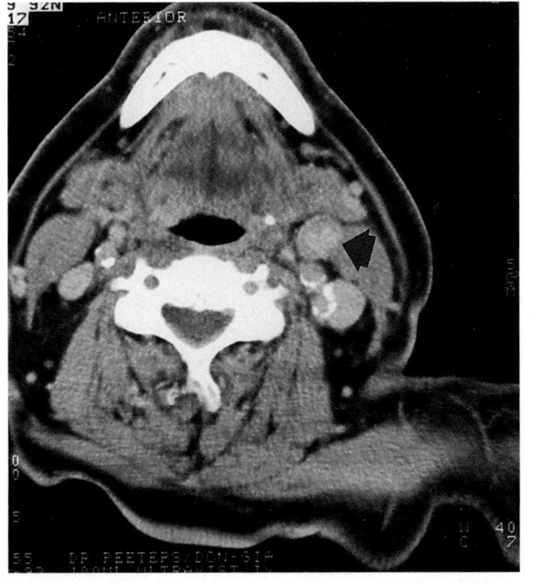


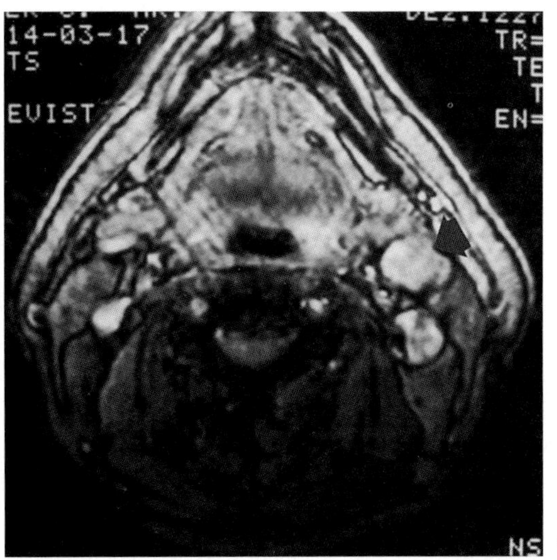


**Fig. 10.4.** A Contrast-enhanced axial CT scan, using 5-mm section thickness depicting a lymph node metatasis (*arrows*) of an oral carcinoma in the subdigastric area (level 2). The hyperdense area inside the lymph node is clearly depicted, corresponding to a very highly vascular metastasis. This finding of tumor tissue depicted with higher density than reactive lymph node tissue is quite rare, however. **B** T1-weighted gradient echo image after Gd-DTPA at the same level. The lymph node with metastasis and the configuration of the metastasis are still recognizable on this MRI (*arrow*). However, the metastasis is depicted with less, but clearly different, signal intensity than the surrounding reactive lymph node tissue. Unfortunately, this finding is also still quite rare.

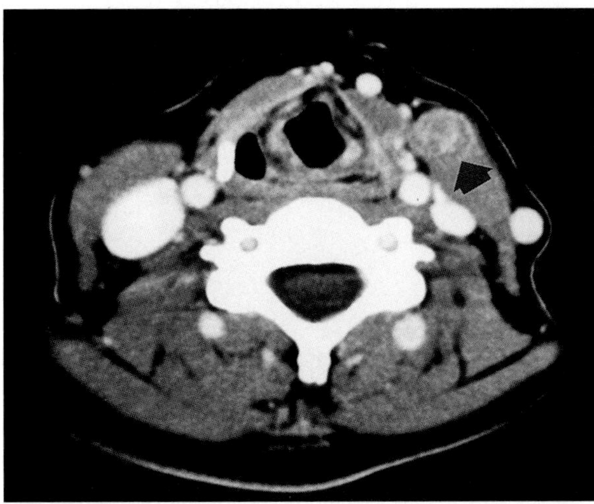

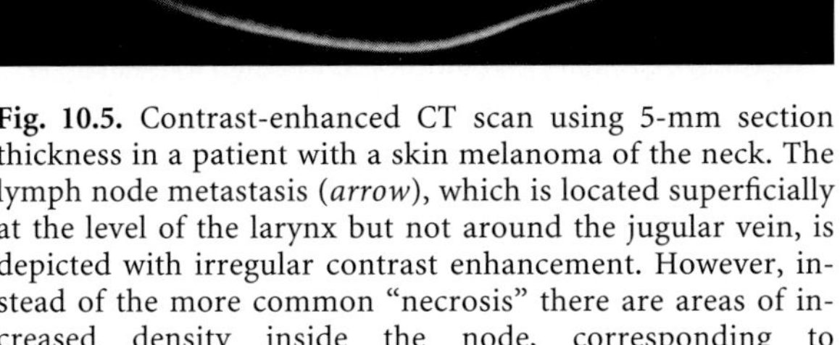

**Fig. 10.5.** Contrast-enhanced CT scan using 5-mm section thickness in a patient with a skin melanoma of the neck. The lymph node metastasis (*arrow*), which is located superficially at the level of the larynx but not around the jugular vein, is depicted with irregular contrast enhancement. However, instead of the more common "necrosis" there are areas of increased density inside the node, corresponding to hypervascular tumor tissue, which is more common in melanoma metastases

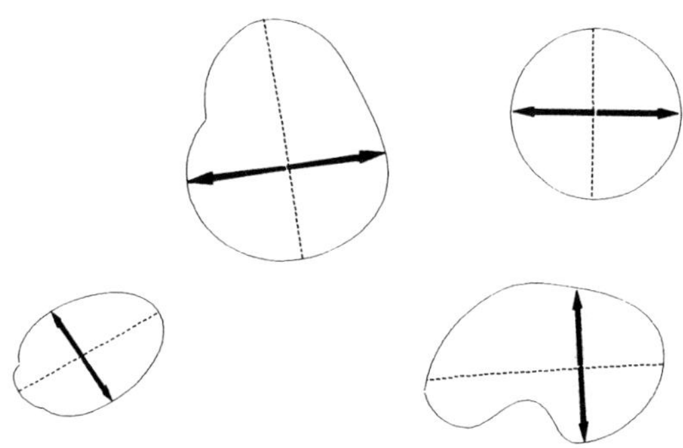

**Fig. 10.6.** The minimal and maximal axial diameter. Note that the minimal axial diameter (*thick arrows*) is the widest diameter at a right angle to the maximal axial diameter

they still rely on known radiological criteria for metastases, such as nodal size and depiction of necrosis. Necrosis, to a radiologist, is defined as irregular contrast enhancement and can be caused by tumor necrosis, extensive tumor keratinization or cyst formation (Fig. 10.3, 10.7). This radiological finding is much more common in head and neck cancer than in other lymph node metastases in the body. Only metastases from undifferentiated nasopharyngeal carcinomas are less frequently necrotic. Whereas necrosis is a very reliable criterion

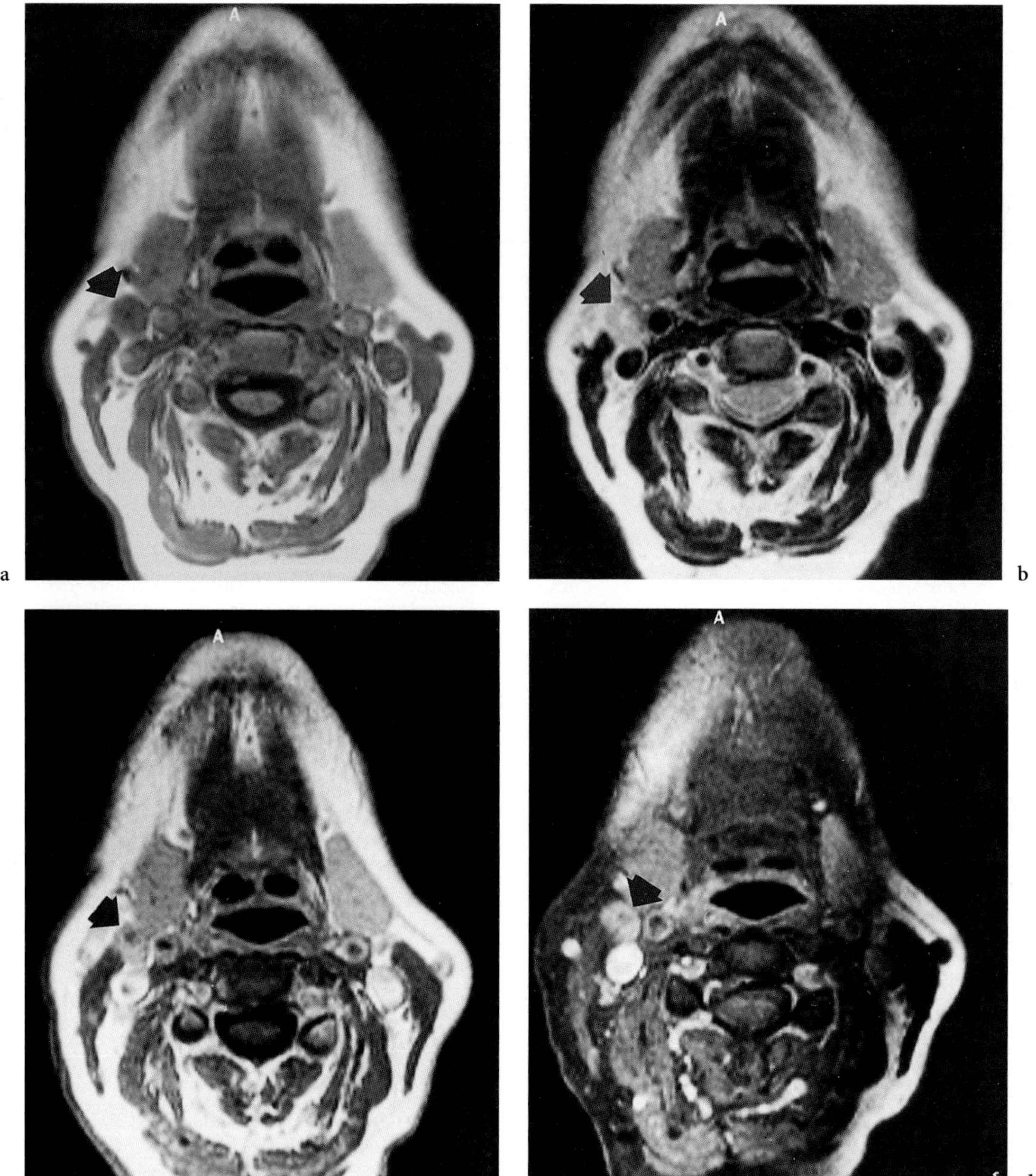

**Fig. 10.7. a** Axial T1-weighted spin echo image of a patient with an oropharyngeal carcinoma. Note the 1 cm subdigastric lymph node, depicted with low-intermediate signal intensity (*arrow*). Inside the lymph node a small central low signal intensity area can just be visualized. **b** T2-weighted spin echo-image of the same lymph node metastasis (*arrow*), clearly showing a high-signal-intensity area inside the lymph node corresponding to the low-signal-intensity area on the T1-weighted image. This is almost proof of liquid-filled cystic tumor degeneration. **c** T1-weighted Gd-DTPA-enhanced image depicting the node (*arrow*) less clearly as the contrast with the submandibular gland deminishes. Inside the node the very-low-signal-intensty area corresponds to the cystic degeneration. **d** Fat suppression T1-weighted spin echo image after Gd-DTPA administration clearly increases the contrast between the lymph node and its surroundings and still depicts the central low signal intensity, improving the contrast of the image without fat suppression

for lymph node metastases, it is unfortunately rare in small lymph node metastases (Don et al. 1995; Friedman et al. 1993). Although very small irregularities in contrast enhancement are present in many lymph nodes, it is very difficult to distinguish these small irregularities from artifacts or anatomic variations in blood supply inside reactive lymph nodes (Fig. 10.8). There are some reports that different pat-

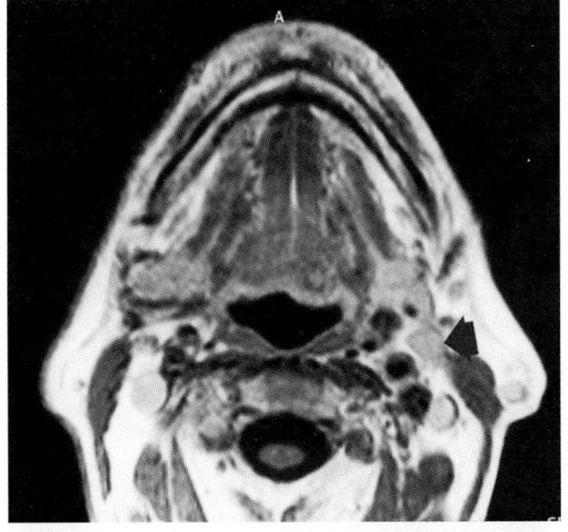


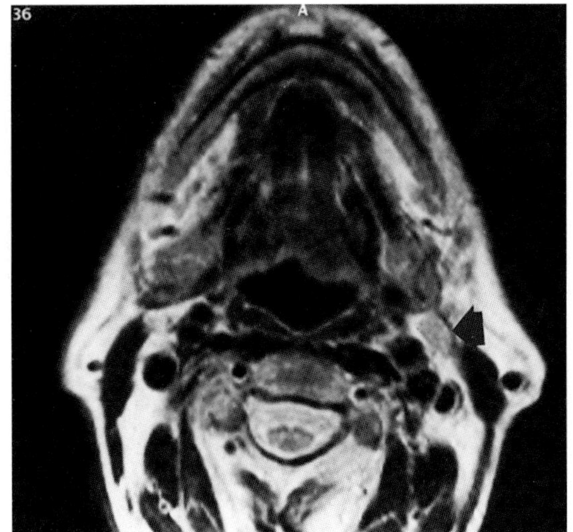


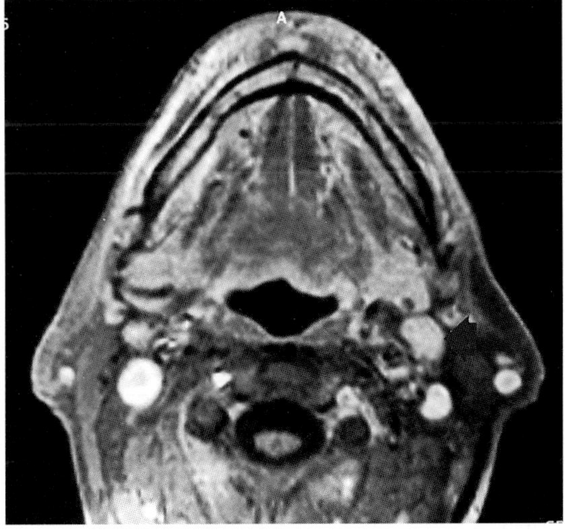


**Fig. 10.8.** **a** Patient with an oral carcinoma and a small palpable lymph node at the left subdigastric level. This T1-weighted nonenhanced spin echo image shows a 7-mm lymph node with no irregularities (*arrow*). **b** T2-weighted spin echo image at the same level shows the same lymph node with slightly more signal intensity but no irregularities, suggesting a reactive lymph node. **c** Gd-DTPA-enhanced, fat-suppressed STIR image depicting the same lymph node (*arrow*). Note the small irregularities in contrast enhancement. However, at histopathology this was found to be a reactive lymph node, demonstrating that very tiny irregularities cannot be interpreted as tumor tissue or necrosis

terns of internal echoes on ultrasound correlate better with histopathology than size criteria (Lee et al. 1992; Steinkamp et al. 1993; Vassallo et al. 1992, 1993; Ahuja et al. 1997). However, these inhomogeneities are very seldom encountered (less than 5%) in lymph nodes smaller than 1 cm and can thus not be frequently used as a criterion in the N0 neck. These irregularities might be caused by either a difference in nodal reflection patterns between tumor and lymph nodes tissue or necrosis and lymph node tissue (Fig. 10.9). Apart from being used as a radiological criterion, necrosis inside a lymph node metastasis is also a prognostic feature in patients treated with chemotherapy or radiotherapy. In the case of extensive necrosis, poor tumor oxygenation is probably the cause of resistance to chemo- and radiotherapy (Gatenby et al. 1988; Janot et al. 1993).

Because irregular contrast enhancement is seldom present in palpably N0 sides of the neck, the size (and shape) of lymph nodes plays an important part in assessment of their nature (Steinkamp et al. 1995). As the size of lymph nodes varies according to the level in the neck and because small metastatic deposits inside lymph do not always cause enlargement of a lymph node, it is very difficult to define the optimal size. As a consequence, the size cutoff points used vary between 5 and 30 mm (Table 10.2) (Stern et al. 1990; Som 1992; Mancuso et al. 1983; Hillsamer et al. 1990; Friedman et al. 1990; Close et al. 1989; Bruneton et al. 1994; Steinkamp et al. 1994b; Vassallo et al. 1992; Van Den Brekel et al. 1990a; Tachimori et al. 1994). Some authors take the lymph node level into account. Because lymph nodes in level II tend to be larger in the general population as well as in head and neck cancer pa-

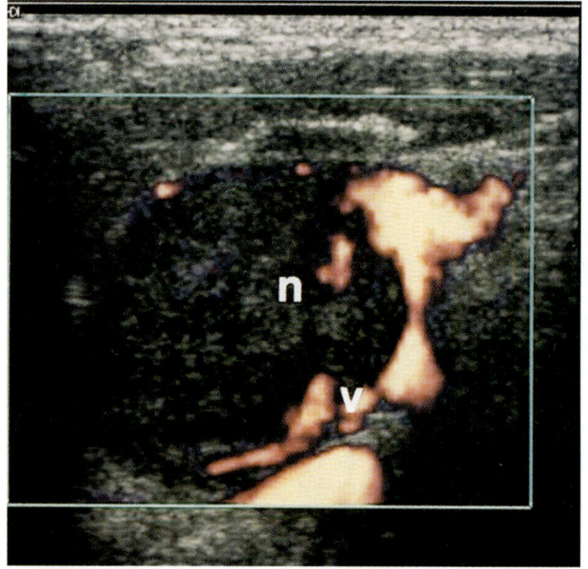


a

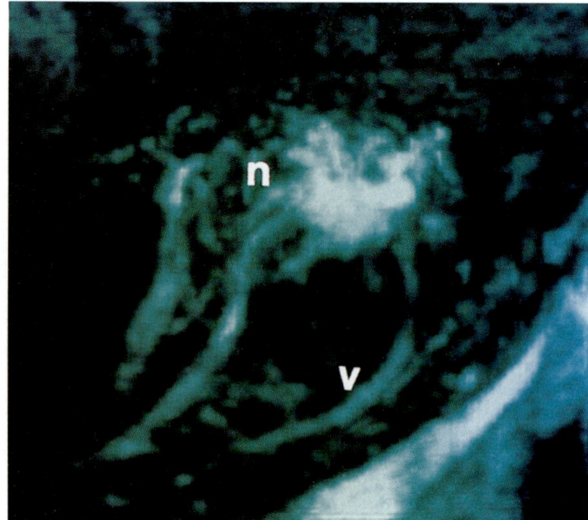


b

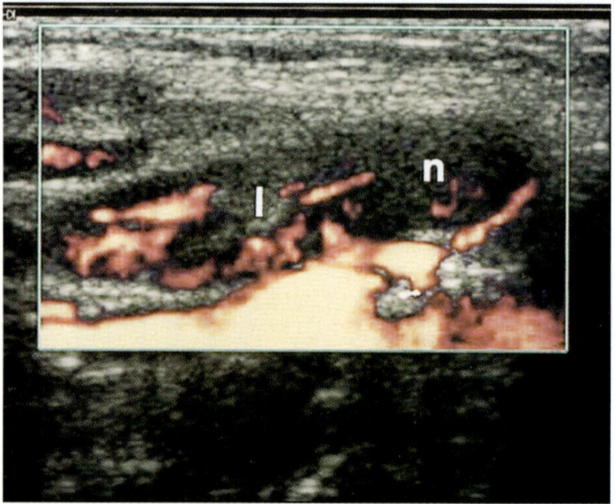


c

**Fig. 10.9.** **a** Power duplex doppler of a metastatic lymph node measuring over 2 cm (*n*). The avascular area, also characterized by a higher echogeneity, is visualized and corresponds to necrotic tumor. **b** Three-dimensional power duplex doppler showing the same node with 3 feeding vessels. Vessel (*v*) corresponds to "v" in Fig. 10.8a. **c** A similar image also depicting an irregular echogeneity (*i*) and vascularization inside a metastatic lymph node (*n*). These areas, however, are very seldom depicted in small lymph nodes with small metastases and are thus less useful as criteria in the N0 neck

tients, many authors agree that the size criterion for lymph nodes in level II is larger. In places where reactively enlarged nodes are seldom encountered, such as the retropharyngeal nodes, it was previously recommended that 8-mm nodes (maximal axial diameter) should be categorized as metastatic (Mancuso et al. 1983). Any size cutoff point is a compromise, as a small size criterion has a high sensitivity and low specificity whereas a large size criterion gives high specificity and low sensitivity (Fig. 10.3, Tables 10.3, 10.4). As a consequence, it is crucial to define the optimal compromise between sensitivity and specificity. If a clinician is inclined to be influenced by imaging results in the palpably N0 neck, and thus to treat the upstaged neck and observe or perform less radical therapy if the neck remains N0 after imaging, he or she is best served by a very sensitive imaging technique. As before the era of imaging most clinician performed elective neck treatment for the great majority of clinically N0 neck sides, overtreatment and the morbidity are well accepted. On the other hand, undertreatment, and the consequent development of neck node metastases that are not treated until after some delay, should be kept to a minimum. As a consequence, high sensitivity is more important than high specificity.

So far, only in four studies has the calculation of criteria been attempted by evaluating nodal size and the histopathological outcome in neck dissection specimens (Don et al. 1995; Friedman et al. 1993; Van Den Brekel et al. 1990a, 1998b). Although the most important question for the clinician concerns the clinically negative neck, radiologists currently

**Table 10.2.** Criteria concerning size and shape according to different authors (*ax-max* maximum axial diameter, *ax-min* minimum axial diameter, *long* longitudinal diameter)

| | |
|---|---|
| Stern et al. 1990 | 15 mm all levels |
| Som 1992 | 15 mm levels I & II or 10 mm elsewhere |
| Mancuso et al. 1983 and Hillsamer et al. 1990 | 8 mm retropharyngeal or 15 mm all other levels or grouping of 3 or more of 8–15 mm |
| Friedman et al. 1990 | 10 mm all levels |
| Close et al. 1989 | 30 mm ovoid shape or 10 mm round shape or grouping of 2 or more of 10–30 mm |
| Bruneton et al. 1994 | 8 mm ax-max and long/ax-max <1.5 |
| Steinkamp et al. 1994b | 8 mm ax-min or 8 mm ax-max and long/ax-min <2 |
| Vassallo et al. 1992 | no size criterion, long/ax-min <2 or absence of a hilus or focal cortical widening |
| Van Den Brekel 1990a | ax-min 11 mm level II or 10 mm elsewhere or grouping of 3 or more 8–10 mm |
| Tachimori et al. 1994 | 5 mm minimal diameter and long/ax-min <2 |

**Table 10.3.** Sensitivity and specificity of different size criteria for 131 elective neck dissections (51 positive, 80 negative)

| Minimal axial diameter (level 2: 1 mm larger) | Sensitivity (%) | Specificity (%) |
|---|---|---|
| 4 mm | 90 | 33 |
| 5 mm | 86 | 44 |
| 6 mm | 80 | 59 |
| 7 mm | 61 | 76 |
| 8 mm | 41 | 84 |
| 9 mm | 27 | 95 |
| 10 mm | 16 | 98 |

**Table 10.4.** Sensitivity (%) for different size cutoff point for different levels in the neck. Figures without brackets are percentages for the whole patient population (248 sides); those in brackets the percentages for the 131 electively operated sides

| Minimal axial diameter | Level 1 | Level 2 | Level 3–5 |
|---|---|---|---|
| 4 mm | 82 (79) | 92 (87) | 81 (68) |
| 5 mm | 77 (71) | 91 (87) | 80 (63) |
| 6 mm | 67 (57) | 89 (81) | 76 (53) |
| 7 mm | 56 (43) | 87 (77) | 72 (43) |
| 8 mm | 46 (21) | 81 (58) | 61 (32) |
| 9 mm | 44 (14) | 73 (39) | 49 (11) |

base their criteria on findings in random head and neck cancer populations. Friedman et al. studied the maximal axial diameter and found a cutoff point of 1 cm. Don et al. studied the longitudinal diameter and concluded that this diameter is highly inaccurate as a size criterion. By comparing three lymph node diameters we previously found that the minimal axial diameter was a better criterion than the more widely used maximal axial diameter or the longitudinal diameter (Van Den Brekel et al. 1990a) (Fig. 10.2). This minimal diameter is also accepted as a better criterion in mediastinal lymph nodes (Glazer et al. 1985). We also established that size criteria for level II lymph nodes are optimally 1 mm larger than for nodes elsewhere in the neck. Don et al. found that 68 out of 102 (67%) metastatic nodes had a longitudinal diameter smaller than 1 cm, whereas in our study the corresponding proportion was 48/144 (33%). For the minimal axial diameter we even found that 102/144 (71%) were smaller than 1 cm. We recently performed a US study comparing the sensitivity and specificity of different size criteria for different levels in the neck and in patients with positive or negative clinical findings (Van Den Brekel et al. 1998b). This study shows that most of the currently used size criteria have a low sensitivity and are not optimal for the palpably N0 neck. It also shows that the use of different criteria for different levels of the neck is justified (Tables 10.3, 10.4). For US of the palpably N0 neck, for level II a criterion of 7 mm renders an optimal compromise between sensitivity and specificity, whereas for the rest of the neck, lymph nodes with a minimal diameter of 6 mm should be considered suggestive. These small size criteria are in agreement with the reports of Steinkamp et al. (1994b), who studied CT and Bruneton et al. (1994), who studied US. In spite of these refinements it is clear that size, shape and grouping are not accurate criteria for the clinically N0 neck. As a consequence, it is our opinion that lymph nodes should be aspirated to obtain accurate cytological criteria. This will be discussed further below.

## 10.5 Imaging Techniques

### 10.5.1 Ultrasound

Ultrasound is gaining popularity because of its high sensitivity and its price. US of the neck was first used in the 1970s and gained popularity in the 1980s (Wiley et al. 1975; Scheible 1981; Bruneton et al.

1984). In general US is reported to be superior to palpation in detecting lymph nodes and its metastases (Bruneton et al. 1984; Baatenburg De Jong et al. 1989; Prayer et al. 1990; Chang et al. 1992; Ishii et al. 1991). Whereas some authors report that it is superior to contrast-enhanced CT and MRI (Furukawa et al. 1991; Quetz et al. 1991), others have found similar accuracy levels (Ishii et al. 1991; Van Den Brekel et al. 1993) or regard endoscopic US as superior for partracheal node detection (Chandawarkar et al. 1996). Advantages of US over the other imaging techniques are its price, low patient burden and the possibility of on-screen nodal measurements. Furthermore, US is the only imaging technique available that can be used for frequent routine follow-up (Steinkamp et al. 1993). For US, many authors use different criteria than for CT and MRI. In general the size criteria are smaller (7–8 mm) and sonomorphological criteria are used. Focal cortical widening, a very low echogenic pattern or irregularities, and a round shape and an absent hilus are suggestive of metastasis (Steinkamp et al. 1995; Vassallo et al. 1992, 1993; Grimm et al. 1992; Lee et al. 1992; Ahuja et al. 1997). Using duplex doppler or power duplex some authors claim that irregular patterns of vascularization are indicative of metastasis (Leuwer et al. 1997; Tschammler et al. 1996; Giovagnorio et al. 1997; Gosepath et al. 1994). However, these irregularities, probably caused by necrosis, are seldom visible in lymph nodes smaller than 1 cm (Fig. 10.9, 10.10). One preliminary report was very positive about using a contrast enhancer, D-galactose microbubbles, which increases contrast in duplex doppler US (Maurer et al. 1997).

A transducer of 7 MHz or more should be used. In general, more nodes can be detected with higher frequency transducers and more details can be visualized inside the lymph nodes. Lymph nodes as small as 3–4 mm can often be detected, depending on their location. The optimal technique involves axial imaging of the lymph nodes around the jugular vein and coronal and/or sagittal imaging of the submandibular lymph nodes. On US, lymph nodes are in general depicted as low echogenic oval or round structures. Small lymph nodes are visualized in almost all patients. A hilus, containing vessels and fat, is visualized in 90% of all reactively enlarged lymph nodes and is seen as a central area of higher echogeneity. Further inhomogeneities are not present in reactively enlarged lymph nodes. As lymph node metastases are more often missed in level 1, this level is assumed to be more difficult to examine with US (Takes et al. 1996; Righi et al. 1997). This might be caused by the presence of the submandibular gland, which is not always easy to distinguish from the surrounding lymph nodes. Lymph node metastases in this level are most often located in front of the submandibular gland and around the facial artery adjacent to the mandible. The subdigastric lymph nodes (level 2) are generally the largest and have to be distinguished from the many vascular branches and suprahyoid muscles in this level. Especially when

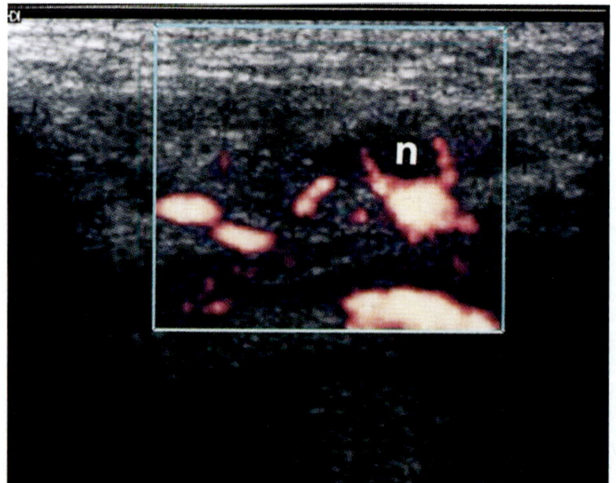

a

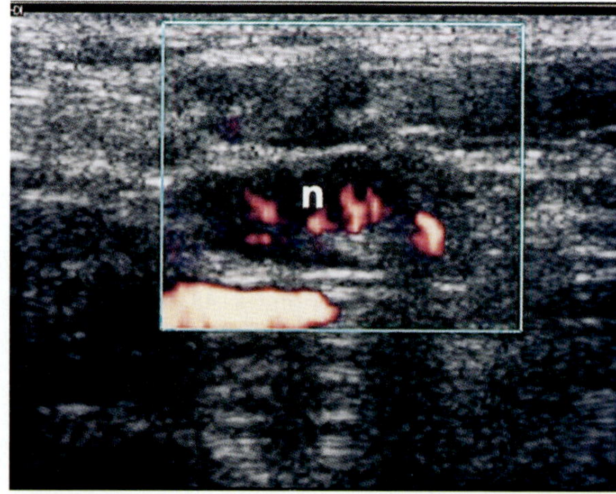

b

**Fig. 10.10.** **a** Power duplex doppler of a reactively enlarged lymph node (*n*). Note the high resolution and sensitivity for flow of this technique. Two separate vessels are supplying the lymph node. Although some authors describe multiple vessels to be a criterion for metastasis, it is our opinion that this is not a reliable criterion. More accurate criteria may become available using these sophisticated techniques. **b** Another tumor negative lymph node of the same patient showing multiple vessels again

nodes in this area are high against the skull base or deep and almost parapharyngeal they are difficult to visualize. However, as both level 1 and 2 are very important metastatic sites, it is of the utmost importance to invest a lot of effort in visualizing nodes in these levels. US imaging of levels 3, 4 and 5 is much easier, and lymph nodes with a minimal diameter of 3 mm are easily visualized in these levels. Imaging of paratracheal lymph nodes, often situated in the fat surrounding the thyroid gland, is possible with US as well as with CT or MRI. However, there are few comparative literature data (Chandawarkar et al. 1996; Tachimori et al. 1994), and in our patients with paratracheal metastases these were seldom seen on US, MRI or CT. Although small nodes were often visible on CT or MRI, these were seldom diagnosed as metastatic. Retropharyngeal nodes are not visualized on US, and in cases of pharyngeal or palatal carcinomas a CT or MRI is indicated to assess these nodes.

For follow-up, repeated US measurements of lymph nodes can be helpful. However, in our experience repeated identical measurements of lymph nodes do not guarantee their benign nature and these lymph nodes can suddenly start growing after many months. As the US criteria for metastases are not accurate enough for the assessment of the neck, in our opinion US-FNAC is mandatory in borderline lymph nodes or lymph nodes that increase in size.

### 10.5.2 Computed Tomography and Magnetic Resonance Imaging

The introduction of CT and MRI has resulted in numerous applications of these modalities in head and neck oncology. MRI is still a rapidly evolving field and has replaced CT in the majority of primary lesions of the extracranial head and neck. Still, CT is often the preferred method, because of its availability and ease of interpretation. Many authors prefer CT to stage laryngeal carcinomas and carcinomas in proximity to the mandible and skull base (Katsounakis et al. 1995). In patients who are dyspneic or cannot lie still, CT is less hampered by motion artifacts. Furthermore, CT is indicated in patients with claustrophobia or with contraindications for MRI. Although CT is in general regarded as easier to interpret than MRI, low interobserver agreement is reported for it in mediastinal lymph node metastases (Bollen et al. 1994). Similar studies have never been done for the neck. For the assessment of neck node metastases there are proponents for CT as well as for MRI. In general, the technique used to image the primary tumor should be used to stage the neck as well.

Most authors agree that CT has a higher accuracy than palpation (Sham et al. 1993; Ishii et al. 1991; Merrit et al. 1997). However, the difference in accuracy is sometimes reported to be very small, and some authors see no benefit of CT over palpation at all (Bergman et al. 1994). In spite of this higher accuracy, there are hardly any clinicians who rely on CT or MRI for their decision-making about the N0 neck, and very often the images are used mainly for the staging of the primary tumor.

Although the number of authors who have reported on the accuracy of CT and MRI for the assessment of the neck is quite large (Reed and Bergeron 1982; Mancuso et al. 1983; Dooms et al. 1984; Stevens et al. 1985; Heppt et al. 1989; Hillsamer et al. 1990; Jabour et al. 1990; Moreau et al. 1990; Feinmesser et al. 1990; Carvalho et al. 1991; Friedman et al. 1993; Lenz et al. 1993; Wilson et al. 1994; Shingaki et al. 1995; van den Brekel et al. 1991a, 1998c), fewer authors have reported their results on the important issue of accuracy of CT or MRI for the assessment of the N0 neck (Stern et al. 1990; Hillsamer et al. 1990; Feinmesser et al. 1990; Friedman et al. 1990; Ishii et al. 1991; van den Brekel et al. 1993; Yucel et al. 1997; Atula et al. 1997; Righi et al. 1997). In these studies on the N0 neck the specificity and sensitivity of CT, MRI, US and US FNAC varies considerably (Table 10.5). As a rule, 40–60% of all occult metastases are found using either CT or MRI, at the cost of some false positives. Studies comparing the accuracy of CT and of MRI for the assessment of the neck generally found comparable figures or some superiority of CT and no statistically significant differences (Lydiatt et al. 1989; Heppt et al. 1989; Hillsamer et al. 1990; van den Brekel et al. 1993; Friedman et al. 1993; Lenz et al. 1993).

Yousem et al. (1992), Friedman et al. (1993), and Chong et al. (1996) found that CT was more sensitive and accurate than MRI in depicting nodal necrosis (Fig. 10.3). However, Chong et al. only studied contrast-enhanced and non-contrast-enhanced spin echo techniques, whereas Friedman et al. did not use gadolinium-DTPA at all. Contrast-enhanced MRI is certainly more sensitive in detecting necrosis than unenhanced MRI (van den Brekel et al. 1990b; Som 1992; Hudgins 1994; Chong et al. 1996) (Figs. 10.3, 10.7). Unenhanced T2-weighted MRI enables only the detection of cystic tumor necrosis, and

**Table 10.5.** Sensitivity and specificity of different imaging modalities found by several auhors for the palpatory N0 neck (electively operated on)

| Author | Modality | Sensitivity | Specificity | No. of patients |
|---|---|---|---|---|
| Stern et al. 1990 | CT | 40 | 92 | 53 |
| Watkinson et al. 1991 | CT | 14 | 89 | 16 |
| | T-99 | 43 | 67 | 16 |
| Stevens et al. 1985 | CT | 83 | 90 | 16 |
| Friedman et al. 1990 | CT | 68 | 90 | 68 |
| | MRI | 80 | 82 | 16 |
| Feinmesser et al. 1990 | MRI | 29 | – | 12 |
| Van Den Brekel et al. 1993 | CT | 49 | 78 | 86 |
| | US | 58 | 75 | 88 |
| | MRI | 55 | 88 | 83 |
| | US-FNAC | 73 | 100 | 43 |
| Hillsamer et al. 1990 | CT | 60 | 83 | 11 |
| | MRI | 66 | 83 | 9 |
| Lydiatt et al. 1989 | CT/MRI | 100 | 100 | 8 |
| John et al. 1993 | US | 50 | 82 | 28 |
| Takes et al. 1996 | US-FNAC | 42 | 100 | 118 |
| Righi et al. 1997 | CT | 60 | 100 | 25 |
| | US-FNAC | 50 | 100 | 25 |
| Moreau et al. 1990 | CT | 50 | 86 | 32 |
| Yucel et al. 1997 | MRI | 57 | 92 | 20 |

is not sensitive for the detection of other causes of necrosis and keratinization (Fig. 10.7). Contrast-enhanced T1-weighted spin echo techniques are less sensitive than T1-weighted gradient echo images in the depiction of small areas of tumor necrosis (van den Brekel et al. 1990b). Neither CT nor MRI allows the distinction of reactively enlarged lymph nodes from moderately enlarged metastatic lymph nodes without necrosis (Fig. 10.8). Furthermore, no currently available imaging technique can depict small metastatic deposits inside reactively enlarged lymph nodes. Very occasionally, tumor is visualized with higher contrast uptake than surrounding lymph node tissues on contrast-enhanced CT scans (Fig. 10.4, 10.5). Because necrosis thus remains the most reliable criterion, it is of the utmost importance that a MRI and CT technique that is optimal for the depiction of necrosis be used. Although necrotic foci of 3 mm or more are present in almost three-quarters of all tumor-positive sides of the neck (van den Brekel et al. 1990a), this figure is much lower in electively operated sides of the neck with small metastatic lymph nodes.

False-positive CT and MRI findings are most often caused by reactive enlargement of lymph nodes. Irregular nodal contrast enhancement, which is visible to a certain extent in many lymph nodes at high-resolution imaging, is rarely mimicked by cysts or abscesses and is thus a very reliable criterion. On CT, central fat inside a lymph node is mostly easily recognized, but can sporadically mimic a metastasis (Elson et al. 1994; van den Brekel et al. 1990b). False-negative findings are usually caused by small metastases without necrosis or metastases outside the imaged volume.

Ideally, reactive lymphatic tissue should be depicted in high contrast to tumor tissue. Unfortunately, this contrast is seldom obtained with the techniques currently available. New MRI techniques focus on better contrast, higher resolution, fat suppression and faster sequences to minimize motion artifacts (van den Brekel et al. 1990b; Panush et al. 1993; Castelijns and van den Brekel 1993; Held and Breit 1994; Barakos 1994; Bruning et al. 1994; Lewin et al. 1994; Fulbright et al. 1994; Yousem and Hurst 1994; Guckel et al. 1996). However, although artifacts can be diminished and resolution and the detection rate of lymph nodes are improving, no better means of tissue diagnosis has been found. Yousem et al. (1994), Held and Breit (1994), and Fulbright et al. (1994) have shown that T2-weighted fast spin-echo techniques diminish artifacts and imaging time and increase lymph node detectability. Panush et al. (1993) showed that inversion recovery fast spin-echo techniques increased contrast even more and thus improved conspicuity of small lymph nodes. However, none of these authors reported better tissue differentiation. Frequency-selective fat suppression and fat saturation techniques have been used by several authors

(Lewin et al. 1994; Muller-Lisse et al. 1996; Tien and Robbins 1992; Vogl et al. 1994). Most of them report better tumor delineation and contrast and superior lymph node detection. However, again, none of these authors has reported improved tissue characterization using these techniques. Furthermore, artifacts, such as chemical shift artifacts and water saturation and fat suppression heterogeneity, limit the routine use of these techniques. Recently developed superparamagnetic lymphographic MRI contrast agents have been offered to improve the ability of MRI to differentiate metastatic from benign cervical lymph nodes (Harika et al. 1996; Lee et al. 1991; Vassallo et al. 1995; Anzai and Prince 1997; Bengele et al. 1994). Dextran-coated, ultrasmall superparamagnetic iron oxide is selectively accumulated in the reticuloendothelial cells in liver and lymph nodes. In this way, reactive lymph node tissue is depicted with low signal intensity on T2-weighted images, whereas tumor tissue is depicted with high signal intensity. The initial results have been encouraging, but the costs associated with multiple MRI studies and the logistical problems associated with the need for delayed imaging may prevent this technique from gaining wide acceptance. Furthermore, owing to the paramagnetic effect of the contrast medium, overshadowing of neighboring structures occurs. As a consequence, small metastases inside reactive lymph nodes are potentially masked on these highly T2-weighted gradient images. Other techniques, such as magnetization transfer imaging and spin lock imaging have been shown to give some clues in differentiating different parotid tumors (Gillams et al. 1996; Markkola et al. 1996; Yousem et al. 1994). However, thus far no tissue characterization has been reported inside small lymph nodes. A more detailed description of these techniques is given by Yousem in Chapter 3. Guckel used dynamic snapshot gradient-echo techniques after gadolinium-DTPA injection and showed that the optimal imaging times are between 6 s and 18 s and between 1 min and 3 min after injection (Guckel et al. 1996). However, no tumor-specific enhancement pattern was found.

#### *10.5.2.1 Technique*

Our protocol for MRI of the neck uses a neck coil. Dramatic improvement in the quality of neck images has been shown in all imaging systems when surface coils are used. Circumferential coils are most useful for deeper structures in the neck that are not easily reached with planar coils.

First, a sagittal T1-weighted localizer scan is obtained. Fast sagittal T1-weighted spin echo techniques are used for this purpose. The cranial and caudal ends of the region of interest are identified to ensure thorough slice coverage of the study volume. At least one precontrast examination of T1-weighted images is obtained in the axial plane from skull base to clavicle. T1-weighted images offer the best anatomic resolution because of the high signal-to-noise ratio per unit of time and their relative freedom from motion artifacts. Additionally, for most primary tumors axial T2-weighted images and sometimes sagittal or coronal T2-weighted examinations are performed. T2-weighted images allow better discrimination of tumor tissue from surroundings or inflammatory changes. Depending on the primary tumor, other techniques might be necessary. Gadolinium-DTPA is necessary to depict tumor necrosis inside lymph nodes and is often helpful in delineating the primary tumor as well. After intravenous injection, T1-weighted spin echo or gradient echo images are obtained. Alternatively, short TI inversion recovery sequences or fat suppression techniques can be used, and these images can be directed to the lymph nodes of interest. Resolution of the detailed head and neck region requires thin sections. The slice thickness should be 3–5 mm, with an interslice gap of 1–2 mm, on a 256 × 256 matrix or 192 × 256 matrix. The field of view should be as small as possible.

For CT scanning of the neck, the same rules apply to the field of interest and the volume to be imaged. Intravenous contrast as an initial bolus followed by a drip infusion is necessary to obtain enough contrast. Slice thickness should preferably be 3–4 mm without an interslice gap to obtain high resolution and depict small nodes with central necrosis. The patient is asked to stop breathing and swallowing while the scans are obtained. Spiral CT, apart from being faster, does not seem to have an advantage over conventional CT. Dynamic studies have also so far not proven their usefulness (Som et al. 1985; Gay et al. 1991).

#### *10.5.2.2 Artifacts*

Artifacts caused by dental amalgam, surgical clips, or other hardware can severely limit the diagnostic possibilities of CT. Surgical clips usually produce no artifacts and are not detected by MRI. Dental amalgam and dense bone of the mandible will not degrade MRI. Unlike CT, very few metals cause artifacts on MRI; essentially ferromagnetic materials (stainless steel root canal prostheses or metal bridgework), which alter the magnetic field homogeneity, are the only ones. Ferromagnetic materials result in image distortion that is limited to the immediate area of the material. Motion artifacts due to respiration and swallowing reduce the image quality of the neck MRI. To minimize motion artifacts, patients are instructed to breathe normally and refrain from moving the tongue and swallowing. When the phase-encoding gradient direction is changed to the antero-posterior direction, pulsation artifacts arising from the bloodstream in the carotid sheath appear in the antero-posterior direction and thus do not blur diagnostic structures.

### 10.5.3 Ultrasound-Guided Aspiration Cytology

Because many authors have found that borderline lymph nodes cannot be reliably scored using CT, MRI or US, and because radiological criteria are not as reliable as cytological, US-FNAC is gaining in popularity (Fig. 10.11). It has been shown that US-FNAC has a very high specificity, approaching 100%, as false-positive aspirates are rare. Causes of false positives are radiation changes, inadvertent aspirations from inflamed salivary glands, branchiogenic cysts or extraparotid warthin tumors (van den Brekel et al. 1991c). In a previous study, we found US-FNAC to have a sensitivity of 73% with a specificity of 100% in N0 necks (van den Brekel et al. 1991b, 1993), which made it significantly better than CT or MRI in this respect. Atula et al. (1997) also compared US-FNAC with CT and MRI and found it to be superior. Recently, however, following a multicenter study using US-FNAC, a sensitivity of only 42% was reported for the N0 neck (Takes et al. 1996; van den Brekel 1996). However, in this series, relatively few elective neck dissections were included per center, and some patients were radiated before surgery. Righi et al. (1997) found a sensitivity of 50%, which was worse than the 60% for CT in their relatively small study. However, in Righi's study, most false negatives were found at the beginning of the study and some of these were in radiated patients or non-squamous-cell carcinoma patients. Atula et al. (1997), in an even smaller study, detected all but one of the palpably occult metastases. The usefulness of this US-FNAC has further been proven by multiple other studies (Baatenburg de Jong et al. 1991; McIvor et al. 1994; van Overhagen et al. 1991; Lenz et al. 1993; Schoengen et al. 1993; Chang et al. 1992). All these studies have revealed that the accuracy depends to a large extent on the ultrasonographer. The skill of the cytopathologist also influences the overall accuracy.

#### *10.5.3.1 Technique and Risks*

In US-FNAC the lymph nodes at risk of harboring metastases are aspirated. After visualization of the node on real-time US, a 0.7-mm needle is introduced into the lymph node. This needle is attached to a 10-

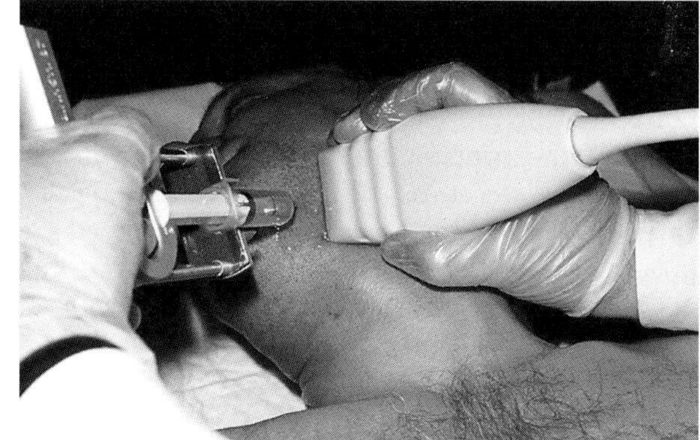

a

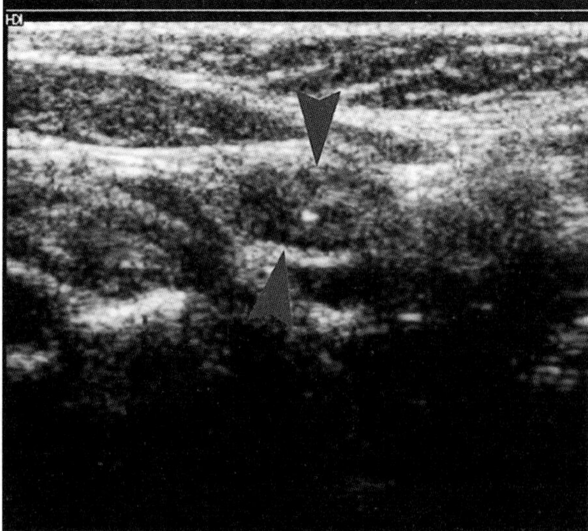

b

Fig. 10.11

to 20-ml syringe in a syringe holder. As soon as the needle is visualized inside the lymph node aspiration is started, while the needle is moved up and down through several areas of the lymph node. After discontinuation of the aspiration, the needle is pulled back and the aspirate is spread over several slides and/or washed into a fixative. The smears can be either air-dried or fixed with ethanol. Although the technique is not difficult, considerable training is required to aspirate from lymph nodes as small as 3–5 mm and still obtain sufficient cells (van den Brekel et al. 1991b; McIvor et al. 1994). The quality of the aspirate can initially be judged either by experience and macroscopic judgment of the smear or by direct microscopic examination. The crucial aspect is the selection of the most suggestive lymph nodes for aspiration. For this it is absolutely necessary to have clinical information on the primary tumor and knowledge about the patterns of metastases from this tumor. In general, the most suggestive node is the largest and/or the most nearly round node in the first echelon.

Because specificity is not a problem, the ultrasonographer's only concern is to obtain a high sensitivity, and thus even small lymph nodes at risk of harboring metastases should be aspirated. Using 5 or 6 mm as a cutoff size in level 2 of the N0 neck, a sensitivity of 87% can be obtained (Tables 10.3, 10.4). For level 1, with a cutoff size of 4 mm sensitivity is 79%, whereas the same threshold size in levels 3–5 has a sensitivity of 68%. When used solely as size criteria these small cutoff points carry a very low specificity. However, as aspiration guarantees a high specificity, aspiration should be obtained from these small nodes to obtain a high enough sensitivity. As a recommendation, lymph nodes of 4 mm or larger should be aspirated in levels 1, 3, 4 and 5 (as well as 6). In level 2, in which the nodes lie deeper, nodes of 5 mm or larger should be aspirated. Although aspirating smaller nodes will probably increase the sensitivity, it becomes difficult to obtain a diagnostic aspirate. In a previous study we found that the percentage of inadequate aspirates grew with decreasing node size. During follow-up, not only the size is important, but also the evolution over time. As the aspirations can be painful, the number of punctures should be limited.

The risks of aspiration are limited. As the carotid artery is clearly visualized, inadvertent damage can easily be avoided. Punctures can be quite painful, especially in the submandibular area, close to the mandible and after radiotherapy. Because of this, some patients refuse regular follow-up with use of US-FNAC. Seeding of tumor cells in the needle tract is very rare if thin needles are used. Seeding is more common with the Tru-Cut needles used for core biopsies. To minimize this risk, it our policy never to aspirate a suspect palpable lymph node, as the impact of the results on treatment is minimal.

### 10.5.3.2 Future Developments

Currently, in melanoma metastases, the possibility of replacing microscopic assessment of the aspirate with molecular biological techniques using reverse transcriptase polymerase chain reaction (RT-PCR) techniques for tyrosinase mRNA is being tested, and the new methods seem more sensitive than cytology (Voit et al. 1998; ven der Velde-Zimmermann et al. 1996; Hofmann et al. 1996). Similar techniques that can be used for squamous cell carcinomas, such as P53 mutational assays (Brennan et al. 1995), might enhance the sensitivity of US-guided aspiration. Another technique to increase the accuracy of US-guided aspiration is better selection of the sentinel node to aspirate from. The use of the sentinel node approach is based on the hypothesis that nodal metastases progress in an orderly manner, with the first site of metastases being in the sentinel node (Fig. 10.12). Similar techniques to the sentinel node procedures used in melanoma and breast cancer can be used (van der Veen et al. 1994; Albertini et al. 1996). The technique involves injecting around the

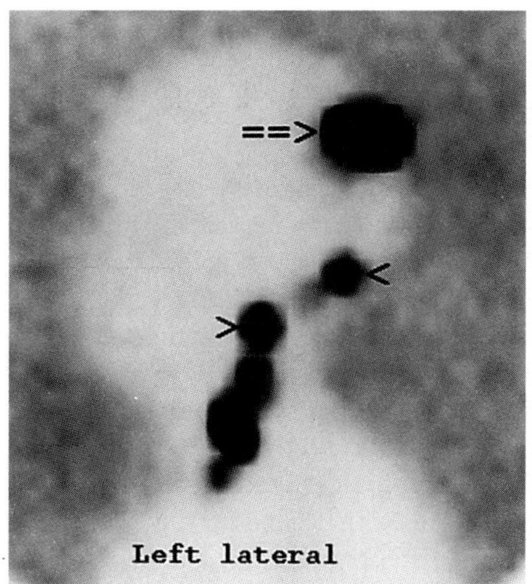


Fig. 10.12

primary tumor site with Tc-99m-labeled sulfur colloid. Localization of the sentinel node is then performed by planar scintigraphy or SPECT and the use of a hand-held gamma camera. Combined use of the hand-held gamma probe and a US transducer could well optimize the identification of the nodes at most risk of harboring metastasis and so allow selective aspiration from these nodes.

### 10.5.4 Positron Emission Tomography and Single Photon Emission Computed Tomography

Small studies have demonstrated that PET may make it possible to detect nodal metastases in lymph nodes that are negative according to size criteria (Braams et al. 1995, 1996; Bailet et al. 1992; Jabour et al. 1993). SPECT imaging with the use of FDG or thallium is reported also to be able to detect nodal disease (Gregor et al. 1996; Mukherji et al. 1994; Nagamachi et al. 1996). However, no studies on the accuracy in the N0 neck are available. The use of PET in combination with immuno-imaging using monoclonal antibodies might further enhance the accuracy (Quak et al. 1993; Meijs et al. 1997). This important application should be further investigated. Although the expense of PET prohibits widespread usage, it is conceivable that PET may be used to evaluate the N0 neck when the results will so good they directly affect treatment. However, it is more likely that these techniques will be used to detect occult recurrences, occult primaries or distant metastases. These topics are further elucidated in Chapters 7, 8 and 11.

## 10.6 Conclusions

As described in the previous paragraphs, many new imaging developments have already influenced decision-making on the N0 neck as well as on the neck with large metastases in which resectability is questionable. As more accurate imaging techniques become available their clinical impact will increase further. Now that healthcare budgets are being cut down, and because elective treatment costs a lot of operating time, imaging might gain importance for the decision-making needed for the N0 neck. If, however, the N0 neck is being observed, the cervical lymph nodes should be closely monitored. In our opinion not all head and neck cancer patients should be evaluated radiologically. First of all, no imaging is needed if no consequences are attached to it. Patients with clear evidence on physical examination of a unilateral mobile metastasis on the side of the primary tumor that is well confined to one side, or with bilateral palpably mobile metastases do not need additional radiological neck node staging. If elective treatment of the neck is carried out irrespective of the imaging findings, this also means that no imaging is indicated. On the other hand, many patients need additional radiological staging of their primary tumors by CT or MRI, and these patients are scanned through the neck at the same time. As in our clinic US-FNAC is the most accurate staging technique for the N0 neck, this technique is primarily used to stage the neck. It is indicated if CT or MRI do not depict clear metastases or if no CT or MRI is carried out and there is a risk of occult metastasis. It is our opinion that US-FNAC is currently the optimal technique to stage the neck and to follow up patients who are not undergoing elective treatment. However, as for any medical technique, because it cannot be read afterwards like CT and MRI, its accuracy is fully dependent on the motivation and skills of the physicians involved. Furthermore, organizing short-interval follow-up visits with US-FNAC takes a lot of effort and cooperation between patients, clinicians and radiologists. Currently in our clinic we use this technique for several indications, irrespective of CT or MRI findings. First of all, if patients can be treated by transoral tumor excisions for T1 and T2 oral, oropharyngeal, and supraglottic ($CO_2$ laser) carcinomas, the neck is not treated electively if US-FNAC is negative. These patients are closely followed up with the use of palpation and US-FNAC every 6–12 weeks after primary tumor excision. Most of these patients are not imaged with CT or MRI. In selected patients treated with laryngectomy for primary or recurrent laryngeal carcinomas (T1–3 supraglottic, T1–4 glottic) the same policy applies. Although most of these patients are staged with CT or MRI, we rely mainly on the results of US-FNAC. The same policy applies for the contralateral neck in most patients undergoing ipsilateral neck dissections. However, as most of these patients will be radiated electively on the contralateral side of the neck, we do not routinely follow these patients with US-FNAC.

## References

Ahuja A, Ying M, Leung SF, Metreweli C (1996) The sonographic appearance and significance of cervical metastatic nodes following radiotherapy for nasopharyngaeal carcinoma. Clin Radiol 51:698–701

Ahuja A, Ying M, King W, Metreweli C (1997) A practical approach to ultrasound of cervical lymph nodes. J Laryngol Otol 111:245–256

Albertini JJ, Cruse CW, Rapaport D, Wells K, Ross M, DeConti R, Berman CG, Jared K, Messina J, Lyman G, Glass F, Fenske N, Reintgen DS (1996) Intraoperative radio-lympho-scintigraphy improves sentinel lymph node identification for patients with melanoma. Ann Surg 223:217–224

Ali S, Tiwari RM, Snow GB (1985) False positive and false negative neck nodes. Head Neck Surg 8:78–82

Alvi A, Johnson JT (1996) Extracapsular spread in the clinically negative neck (n0): implications and outcome. Otolaryngol Head Neck Surg 114:65–70

Anzai Y, Prince MR (1997) Iron oxide-enhanced MR lymphography: the evaluation of cervical lymph node metastases in head and neck cancer. J Magnet Reson Imag 7:75–81

Anzai Y, Carroll WR, Quint DJ, Bradford CR, Minoshima S, Wolf GT, Wahl RL (1996) Recurrence of head and neck cancer after surgery or irradiation: prospective comparison of 2-deoxy-2-[f-18]fluoro-d-glucose PET and MR imaging diagnoses. Radiology 200:135–141

Atula TS, Varpula MJ, Kurki TJI, Klemi PJ, Grenman R (1997) Assessment of cervical lymph node status in head and neck cancer patients – palpation, computed tomography and low field magnetic resonance imaging compared with ultrasound-guided fine-needle aspiration cytology. Eur J Radiol 25:152–161

Baatenburg de Jong RJ, Rongen RJ, Laméris JS, Harthoorn M, Verwoerd CDA, Knegt P (1989) Metastatic neck disease; Palpation vs Ultrasound examination. Arch Otolaryngol Head Neck Surg 115:689–690

Baatenburg de Jong RJ, Rongen RJ, Verwoerd CDA, Overhagen van H, Laméris JS, Knegt P (1991) Ultrasound-guided fine needle aspiration biopsy of neck nodes. Arch Otolaryngol Head Neck Surg 117:402–404

Bailet JW, Abemayor E, Jabour BA, Hawkins RA, Ho C, Ward PH (1992) Positron emission tomography: a new, precise imaging modality for detection of primary head and neck tumors and assessment of cervical adenopathy. Laryngoscope 102:281–288

Barakos JA (1994) Advances in magnetic resonance imaging of the head and neck. Top Magn Reson Imaging 3:155–165

Bataini JP, Bernier J, Brugere J, Jaulerry C, Picco C, Brunin F (1985) Natural history of neck disease in patients with squamous cell carcinoma of oropharynx and pharyngolarynx. Radiother Oncol 3:245–255

Batsakis JG, Hybels R, Rice DH (1975) Laryngeal carcinoma: stomal recurrences and distant metastases. Can J Otolaryngol 4:906–916

Bengele HH, Palmacci S, Rogers J, Jung CW, Crenshaw J, Josephson L (1994) Biodistribution of an ultrasmall superparamagnetic iron oxide colloid, bms 180549, by different routes of administration. Magnet Reson Imaging 3:433–442

Bergman SA, Ord RA, Rothman M (1994) Accuracy of clinical examination versus computed tomography in detecting occult lymph node involvement in patients with oral epidermoid carcinoma. J Oral Maxillofac Surg 12:1236–1239

Bollen EC, Goei R, van't Hof-Grootenboer BE, Versteege CW, Engelshove HA, Lamers RJ (1994) Interobserver variability and accuracy of computed tomographic assessment of nodal status in lung cancer. Ann Thorac Surg 1:158–162

Braams JW, Pruim J, Freling NJ, Nikkels PG, Roodenburg JL, Boering G, Vaalburg W, Vermey A (1995) Detection of lymph node metastases of squamous-cell cancer of the head and neck with FDG-PET and MRI. J Nucl Med 36:211–216

Braams JW, Pruim J, Nikkels PG, Roodenburg JL, Vaalburg W, Vermey A (1996) Nodal spread of squamous cell carcinoma of the oral cavity detected with PET-tyrosine, MRI and CT. J Nucl Med 37:897–901

Brennan JA, Jafek BW (1994) Elective carotid artery resection for advanced squamous cell carcinoma of the neck. Laryngoscope 104:259–263

Brennan JA, Mao L, Hruban RH, Boyle JO, Eby YJ, Koch WM, Goodman SN, Sidransky D (1995) Molecular assessment of histopathological staging in squamous-cell carcinoma of the head and neck. N Engl J Med 332:429–435

Bruneton JN, Roux P, Caramella E, Demard F, Vallicioni J, Chauvel P (1984) Ear nose and throat cancer: Ultrasound diagnosis of metastasis to cervical lymph nodes. Radiology 152:771–773

Bruneton JN, Balu-Maestro C, Marcy PY, Melia P, Mourou MY (1994) Very high frequency (13 MHz) ultrasonographic examination of the normal neck: detection of normal lymph nodes and thyroid nodules. J Ultrasound Med 13:87–90

Bruning R, Heuck A, Naegele M, Seelos K, Vahlensieck M, Reiser M (1994) Fat-suppressing STIR sequences with and without contrast media in the MRT of ENT tumors. Rofo Fortschr Geb Rontgenstr Neuen Bildgeb Verfahr 5:412–416

Byers RM, Wolf PF, Ballantyne AJ (1988) Rationale for elective modified neck dissection. Head Neck Surg 3:160–167

Byers RM, Weber RS, Andrews T, McGill D, Kare R, Wolf P (1997) Frequency and therapeutic implications of "skip metastases" in the neck from squamous carcinoma of the oral tongue. Head Neck 19:14–19

Candela FC, Kothari K, Shah JP (1990a) Patterns of cervical node metastases from squamous carcinoma of the oropharynx and hypopharynx. Head Neck 12:197–203

Candela FC, Shah J, Jaques DP, Shah JP (1990b) Patterns of cervical node metastases from squamous carcinoma of the larynx. Arch Otolaryngol Head Neck Surg 4:432–435

Carvalho P, Baldwin D, Carter R, Parsons C (1991) Accuracy of CT in detecting squamous carcinoma metastases in cervical lymph nodes. Clin Radiol 44:79–81

Castelijns JA, van den Brekel MW (1993) Magnetic resonance imaging evaluation of extracranial head and neck tumors. Magn Reson Q 9:113–128

Chandawarkar RY, Kakegawa T, Fujita H, Yamana H, Hayabuthi N (1996) Comparative analysis of imaging modalities in the preoperative assessment of nodal metastasis in esophageal cancer. J Surg Oncol 61:214–217

Chang DB, Yang PC, Yu CJ, Kuo SH, Lee YC, Luh KT (1992) Ultrasonography and ultrasonographically guided fine-needle aspiration biopsy of impalpable cervical lymph nodes in patients with non-small cell lung cancer. Cancer 5:1111–1114

Chong VF, Fan YF, Khoo JB (1996) MRI features of cervical nodal necrosis in metastatic disease. Clin Radiol 51:103–109

Close LG, Merkel M, Vuitch MF, Reisch J, Schaefer SD (1989) Computed tomographic evaluation of regional lymph node involvement in cancer of the oral cavity and oropharynx. Head Neck 11:309–317

Davidson BJ, Kulkarny V, Delacure MD, Shah JP (1993) Posterior triangle metastases of squamous cell carcinoma of the upper aerodigestive tract. Am J Surg 4:395–398

Dillon WP, Harnsberger HR (1991) The impact of radiologic imaging on staging of cancer of the head and neck. Semin Oncol 18:64–79

Don DM, Anzai Y, Lufkin RB, Fu Y, Calcaterra TC (1995) Evaluation of cervical lymph node metastases in squamous cell carcinoma of the head and neck. Laryngoscope 105:669–674

Dooms GC, Hricak H, Crooks LE, Higgins CB (1984) Magnetic resonance imaging of the lymph nodes: comparison with CT. Radiology 153:719–728

Elson M, Rothman M, Ord RA (1994) False-positive computed tomography scan mimicking metastasis due to fatty hilum in a cervical lymph node. J Oral Maxillofac Surg 12:1334–1336

Fakih AR, Rao RS, Borges AM, Patel AR (1989) Elective versus therapeutic neck dissection in early carcinoma of the oral tongue. Am J Surg 4:309–313

Feinmesser R, Freeman JL, Noyek AM, Birt D, Gullane P, Mullen JB (1990) MRI and neck metastasis: a clinical/radiological/patholo-gical correlative study. J Otolaryngol 91:136–140

Fisher B, Fisher ER (1967) Barrier function of lymph node to tumor cells and erythrocytes; I Normal nodes; II Effect of X-Ray/inflammation/sensitization and tumor growth. Cancer 20:1907–1919

Friedman M, Mafee MF, Pacella BL Jr, Strorigl TL, Dew LL, Toriumi DM (1990) Rationale for elective neck dissection in 1990. Laryngoscope 100:54–59

Friedman M, Roberts N, Kirshenbaum GL, Colombo J (1993) Nodal size of metastatic squamous cell carcinoma of the neck. Laryngoscope 103:854–856

Fulbright R, Panush D, Sze G, Smith RC, Constable RT (1994) MR of the head and neck: comparison of fast spin-echo and conventional spin-echo sequences. AJNR 15:767–773

Furukawa M, Kaneko M, Mochimatsu I, Sawaki S, Igari H, Tsukuda M (1991) Comparative studies of diagnosis with US or CT of the cervical lymph node metastases in head and neck cancer (in Japanese). Nippon Jibiinkoka Gakkai Kaiho 4:577–586

Gatenby RA, Kessler HB, Rosenblum JS, Coia LR, Moldofsky PJ, Hartz WH, Broder GJ (1988) Oxygen distribution in squamous cell carcinoma metastases and its relationship to outcome of radiation therapy. Int J Radiat Oncol Biol Phys 14:831–838

Gay SB, Pevarski DR, Phillips CD, Levine PA (1991) Dynamic CT of the neck. Radiology 178:284–285

Ghouri AF, Zamora RL, Sessions DG, Spitznagel EL Jr, Harvey JE (1994) Prediction of occult neck disease in laryngeal cancer by means of a logistic regression statistical model. Laryngoscope 104:1280–1284

Gillams AR, Fuleihan N, Grillone G, Carter AP (1996) Magnetization transfer contrast mr in lesions of the head and neck. AJNR 17:355–360

Giovagnorio F, Rusticali A, Araneo AL (1997) Color and pulsed doppler evaluation of benign and malignant adenopathy. Clin Imag 21:163–169

Glazer GM, Gross BH, Quint LE, Francis IR, Bookstein FL, Orringer MB (1985) Normal mediastinal lymph nodes: number and size according to american thoracic society mapping. AJR 144:261–265

Gong QY, Zheng GL, Zhu HY (1991) MRI differentiation of recurrent nasopharyngeal carcinoma from postradiation fibrosis. Comput Med Imaging Graph 15:423–429

Gosepath K, Hinni M, Mann W (1994) The state of the art of ultrasonography in the head and neck. Ann Otolaryngol Chir Cervicofac 111:1–5

Gregor RT, Valdes-Olmos R, Koops W, Balm AJ, Hilgers FJ, Hoefnagel CA (1996) Preliminary experience with thallous chloride tl 201-labeled single-photon emission computed tomography scanning in head and neck cancer. Arch Otolaryngol Head Neck Surg 122:509–514

Grimm H, Hamper K, Binmoeller KF, Soehendra N (1992) Enlarged lymph nodes: malignant or not? Endoscopy 24[Suppl 1]:320–323

Gritzmann N, Grasl MC, Helmer M, Steiner E (1990) Invasion of the carotid artery and jugular vein by lymph node metastases: detection with sonography. AJR 154:411–414

Guckel C, Schnabel K, Deimling M, Steinbrich W (1996) Dynamic snapshot gradient-echo imaging of head and neck malignancies: time dependency and quality of contrast-to-noise ratio. Magma 4:61–69

Gussack GS, Hudgins PA (1991) Imaging modalities in recurrent head and neck tumors. Laryngoscope 101:119–124

Harika L, Weissleder R, Poss K, Papisov MI (1996) Macromolecular intravenous contrast agent for MR lymphography: characterization and efficacy studies. Radiology 198:365–370

Hasegawa Y, Matsuura H (1994) Retropharyngeal node dissection in cancer of the oropharynx and hypopharynx. Head Neck 16:173–180

Held P, Breit A (1994) MRI and CT of tumors of the pharynx: comparison of the two imaging procedures including fast and ultrafast MR sequences. Eur J Radiol 18:81–91

Heppt W, Haels J, Lenartz T, Mende U, Gademann G (1989) Nachweis und Beurteilung von Halslymphknotenmetastasen bei Kopf-Hals-Tumoren; ein methodenvergleich. Laryngol Rhinol Otol 68:327–332

Hessling KH, Schmelzeisen R, Reimer P, Milbradt H, Unverfehrt D (1991) Use of sonography in the follow-up of preoperatively irradiated efferent lymphatics of the neck in oropharyngeal tumours. J Cran Max Fac Surg 19:128–130

Hillsamer PJ, Schuller DE, McGhee RB, Chakeres D, Young DC (1990) Improving diagnostic accuracy of cervical metastases with computed tomography and magnetic resonance imaging. Arch Otolaryngol Head Neck Surg 116:1297–1301

Ho CM, Lam KH, Wei WI, Lau WF (1992) Treatment of neck nodes in oral cancer. Surg Oncol 1:73–78

Hofmann S, Remy W, Borelli S Jr, von Reis A, Weidinger S (1996) Detection of tyrosinase mRNA using reverse transcription/polymerase chain reaction with fine needle punctures of melanoma metastases. Hautarzt 47:197–199

Hudgins PA (1994) Contrast enhancement in head and neck imaging. Neuroimaging Clin North Am 1:101–115

Hughes CJ, Gallo O, Spiro RH, Shah JP (1993) Management of occult neck metastases in oral cavity squamous carcinoma. Am J Surg 166:380–383

Ishii J, Amagasa T, Tachibana T, Shinozuka K, Shioda S (1991) US and CT evaluation of cervical lymph node metastasis from oral cancer. J Craniomaxillofac Surg 3:123–127

Jabour BA, Lufkin RB, Layfield LJ, Hanafee WN (1990) Magnetic resonance imaging of metastatic cervical adenopathy. Top Magn Reson Imaging 2:69–75

Jabour BA, Choi Y, Hoh CK, Rege SD, Soong JC, Lufkin RB, Hanafee WN, Maddahi J, Chaiken L, Bailet J (1993) Extracranial head and neck: PET imaging with 2-[f-18]fluoro-2-deoxy-d-glucose and MR imaging correlation. Radiology 186:27–35

Janot F, Cvitkovic E, Piekarski JD, Sigal R, Armand JP, Bensmaine A, Luboinski B (1993) Correlation between nodal density in contrasted scans and response to cisplatin-based chemotherapy in head and neck squamous cell cancer: a prospective validation. Head Neck 15:222–229

John DG, Anaes FC, Williams SR, Ahuja A, Evans R, To KF, King WW, van Hasselt CA (1993) Palpation compared with ultrasound in the assessment of malignant cervical lymph nodes. J Laryngol Otol 107:821–823

Jones AS, Roland NJ, Field JK, Phillips DE (1994) The level of cervical lymph node metastases: their prognostic relevance and relationship with head and neck squamous carcinoma primary sites. Clin Otolaryngol 19:63–69

Jones KR, Lodge-Rigal RD, Reddick RL, Tudor GE, Shockley WW (1992) Prognostic factors in the recurrence of stage I and II squamous cell cancer of the oral cavity. Arch Otolaryngol Head Neck Surg 118:483–485

Katsounakis J, Remy H, Vuong T, Gelinas M, Tabah R (1995) Impact of magnetic resonance imaging and computed tomography on the staging of laryngeal cancer. Eur Arch Otorhinolaryngol 252:206–208

Kinsey DL, James AG, Bonta JA (1958) A study of metastatic carcinoma of the neck. Ann Surg 147:366–374

Kligerman J, Lima RA, Soares JR, Prado L, Dias FL, Freitas EQ, Olivatto LO (1994) Supraomohyoid neck dissection in the treatment of T1/T2 squamous cell carcinoma of oral cavity. Am J Surg 168:391–394

Kowalski LP, Franco EL, de Andrade Sobrinho J (1995) Factors influencing regional lymph node metastasis from laryngeal carcinoma. Ann Otol Rhinol Laryngol 104:442–447

Langman AW, Kaplan MJ, Dillon WP, Gooding GAW (1989) Radiologic assessment of tumor and the carotid artery: Correlation of magnetic resonance imaging/ultrasound and computed tomography with surgical findings. Head Neck 11:443–449

Lee AS, Weissleder R, Brady TJ, Wittenberg J (1991) Lymph nodes: microstructural anatomy at MR imaging. Radiology 178:519–522

Lee N, Inoue K, Yamamoto R, Kinoshita H (1992) Patterns of internal echoes in lymph nodes in the diagnosis of lung cancer metastasis. World J Surg 16:986–993

Lenz M, Kersting-Sommerhoff B, Gross M (1993) Diagnosis and treatment of the N0 neck in carcinomas of the upper aerodigestive tract: current status of diagnostic procedures. Eur Arch Otorhinolaryngol 250:432–438

Leuwer RM, Westhofen M, Schade G (1997) Color duplex echography in head and neck cancer. Am J Otolaryngol 18:254–257

Levendag P, Sessions R, Vikram B (1989) The problem of neck relapse in early stage supraglottic larynx cancer. Cancer 63:345–348

Lewin JS, Curtin HD, Ross JS, Weissman JL, Obuchowski NA, Tkach JA (1994) Fast spin-echo imaging of the neck: comparison with conventional spin-echo, utility of fat suppression, and evaluation of tissue contrast characteristics. Am J Neurorad 15:1351–1357

Lindberg RD (1972) Distribution of cervical lymph node metastases from squamous cell carcinoma of the upper respiratory and digestive tracts. Cancer 29:1446–1449

Lydiatt DD, Markin RS, Williams SM, Davis LF, Yonkers AJ (1989) Computed tomography and magnetic resonance imaging of cervical metastasis. Otolaryngol Head Neck Surg 101:422–425

Lydiatt DD, Robbins KT, Byers RM, Wolf PF (1993) Treatment of stage I and II oral tongue cancer. Head Neck 15:308–312

Mancuso AA, Harnsberger HR, Muraki AS, Stevens MH (1983) Computed tomography of cervical and retropharyngeal lymph nodes: normal anatomy, variants of normal, and applications in staging head and neck cancer. Part II: pathology. Radiology 148:715–723

Mann WJ, Beck A, Schreiber J, Maurer J, Amedee RG, Gluckmann JL (1994) Ultrasonography for evaluation of the carotid artery in head and neck cancer. Laryngoscope 104:885–888

Markkola AT, Aronen HJ, Paavonen T, Hopsu E, Sipila LM, Tanttu JI, Sepponen RE (1996) Spin lock and magnetization transfer imaging of head and neck tumors. Radiology 200:369–375

Martinez Gimeno C, Rodriguez EM, Vila CN, Varela CL (1995) Squamous cell carcinoma of the oral cavity: a clinicopathologic scoring system for evaluating risk of cervical lymph node metastasis. Laryngoscope 105:728–733

Martis C, Karabouta I, Lazaridis N (1979) Incidence of lymph node metastasis in elective neck dissection for oral carcinoma. J Maxillofac Surg 7:182–191

Maurer J, Willam C, Schroeder R, Hidajad N, Hell B, Bier J, Weber S, Felix R (1997) Evaluation of metastases and reactive lymph nodes in doppler sonography using an ultrasound contrast enhancer. Invest Radiol 32:441–446

McGuirt WF Jr, Johnson JT, Myers EN, Rothfield R, Wagner R (1995) Floor of mouth carcinoma. The management of the clinically negative neck. Arch Otolaryngol Head Neck Surg 121:278–282

McIvor NP, Freeman JL, Salem S, Elden L, Noyek AM, Bedard YC (1994) Ultrasonography and ultrasound-guided fine-needle aspiration biopsy of head and neck lesions: a surgical perspective. Laryngoscope 104:669–674

McLaughlin MP, Mendenhall WM, Mancuso AA, Parsons JT, McCarty PJ, Cassisi NJ, Stringer SP, Tart RP, Mukherji SK, Million RR (1995) Retropharyngeal adenopathy as a predictor of outcome in squamous cell carcinoma of the head and neck. Head Neck 17:190–198

Meijs WE, Haisma HJ, Klok RP, Vangog FB, Kievit E, Pinedo HM, Herscheid JDM (1997) Zirconium-labeled monoclonal antibodies and their distribution in tumor-bearing nude mice. J Nucl Med 38:112–118

Merrit RM, Williams MF, James TH, Porubsky ES (1997) Detection of cervical metastasis. A meta-analysis comparing computed tomography with physical examination. Arch Otolaryngol Head Neck Surg 123:149–152

Moreau P, Goffart Y, Collignon J (1990) Computed tomography of metastatic cervical lymph nodes. Arch Otolaryngol Head Neck Surg 116:1190–1193

Mukherji SK, Drane WE, Tart RP, Landau S, Mancuso AA (1994) Comparison of thallium-201 and F-18 FDG SPECT uptake in squamous cell carcinoma of the head and neck. AJNR 15:1837–1842

Muller-Lisse GU, Kretschmar UL, Jager L, Dreher A, Grevers G, Riser M (1996) Value of fat signal suppression mri pulse sequences for diagnosis of malignant tumors in the area of the head-neck. Radiologe 36:199–206

Nagamachi S, Hoshi H, Jinnouchi S, Ohnishi T, Flores LG, 2nd, Futami S, Nakahara H, Watanabe K (1996) 201TL SPECT for evaluating head and neck cancer. Ann Nucl Med 10:105–111

Noguchi M, Kinami S, Kinoshita K, Kitagawa H, Thomas M, Miyazaki I, Michigishi T, Mizukami Y (1993) Risk of bilateral cervical lymph node metastases in papillary thyroid cancer. J Surg Oncol 52:155–159

Olmi P, Fallai C, Colagrande S, Giannardi G (1995) Staging and follow-up of nasopharyngeal carcinoma: magnetic resonance imaging versus computerized tomography. Int J Radiat Oncol Biol Phys 32:795–800

Panush D, Fulbright R, Sze G, Smith RC, Constable RT (1993) Inversion-recovery fast spin-echo MR imaging: efficacy in the evaluation of head and neck lesions. Radiology 187:421–426

Pradeep VM, Padmanabhan V, Sen P, Ramachandran K, Sasidharan K, Krishnamoorthy S, Nair MK (1991) Sonographic evaluation of operability of malignant cervical lymph nodes. Am J Clin Oncol 14:438–441

Prayer L, Winkelbauer H, Gritzmann N, Winkelbauer F, Helmer M, Pehamberger H (1990) Sonography versus palpation in the detection of regional lymph-node metastases in patients with malignant melanoma. Eur J Cancer 26:827–830

Quak J, Gerretsen M, De Bree R, Brakenhof R, van Dongen G, Snow G (1993) Perspectives of monoclonal antibodies for detection and treatment of head and neck tumours. Anticancer Res 13:2533–2539

Quetz JU, Rohr S, Hoffmann P, Wustrow J, Mertens J (1991) B-image sonography in lymph node staging of the head and neck area. a comparison with palpation, computerized and magnetic resonance tomography. HNO 39:61–63

Ramadan HH, Allen GC (1993) The influence of elective neck dissection on neck relapse in N0 supraglottic carcinoma. Am J Otolaryngol 14:278–281

Reed DL, Bergeron RT (1982) CT of cervical lymph nodes. J Otolaryngol 11:411–418

Righi PD, Kopecky KK, Caldemeyer KS, Ball VA, Weisberger EC, Radpour S (1997) Comparison of ultrasound fine needle aspiration and computed tomography in patients undergoing elective neck dissection. Head Neck 19:604–610

Sako K, Pradier RN, Marchetta FC, Pickren JW (1964) Fallibility of palpation in the diagnosis of metastases to cervical nodes. Surg Gynaecol Obstet 118:989–990

Scheible W (1981) Recent advances in ultrasound: high-resolution imaging of superficial structures. Head Neck Surg 4:58–63

Schoengen A, Binder T, Faiss S, Weber L, Zeelen U (1993) Fine needle aspiration cytology of metastatic malignant melanoma. improvement of results with ultrasound control. Hautarzt 11:703–707

Shah JP (1990) Patterns of cervical lymph node metastasis from squamous carcinomas of the upper aerodigestive tract. Am J Surg 160:405–409

Sham JS, Cheung YK, Choy D, Chan FL, Leong L (1993) Computed tomography evaluation of neck node metastases from nasopharyngeal carcinoma. Int J Radiat Oncol Biol Phys 26:787–792

Shingaki S, Kobayashi T, Suzuki I, Kohno M, Nakajima T (1995) Surgical treatment of stage I and II oral squamous cell carcinomas: analysis of causes of failure. Br J Oral Maxillofac Surg 33:304–308

Shingaki S, Suzuki I, Nakajima T, Hayashi T, Nakayama H, Nakamura M (1995) Computed tomographic evaluation of lymph node metastasis in head and neck carcinomas. J Cran Max Fac Surg 23:233–237

Snow GB, Annyas AA, van Slooten EA, Bartelink H, Hart AAM (1982) Prognostic factors of neck node metastasis. Clin Otolaryngol 7:185–192

Som PM (1992) Detection of metastasis in cervical lymph nodes: CT and MR criteria and differential diagnosis. AJR 158:961–969

Som PM, Lanzieri CF, Sacher M, Lawson W, Biller HF (1985) Extracranial tumor vascularity: Determination by dynamic CT scanning. Radiology 154:401–412

Spiro JD, Spiro RH, Shah JP, Sessions RB, Strong EW (1988) Critical assessment of supraomohyoid neck dissection. Am J Surg 156:286–289

Spiro RH, Strong EW (1973) Epidermoid carcinoma of the oral cavity and oropharynx. Eective vs therapeutic radical neck dissection as treatment. Arch Surg 107:382–384

Spiro RH, Morgan GJ, Strong EW, Shah JP (1996) Supraomohyoid neck dissection. Am J Surg 172:650–653

Steinkamp HJ, Knobber D, Schedel H, Maurer J, Felix R (1993) Palpation and sonography in after-care of head-neck tumor patients: comparison of ultrasound tumor entity parameters. Laryngorhinootologie 72:431–438

Steinkamp HJ, Maurer J, Cornehl M, Knobber D, Hettwer H, Felix R (1994a) Recurrent cervical lymphadenopathy: differential diagnosis with color-duplex sonography. Eur Arch Otorhinolaryngol 251:404–409

Steinkamp HJ, Hosten N, Richter C, Schedel H, Felix R (1994b) Enlarged cervical lymph nodes at helical CT. Radiology 191:795–798

Steinkamp HJ, Cornehl M, Hosten N, Pegios W, Vogl T, Felix R (1995) Cervical lymphadenopathy: ratio of long- to short-axis diameter as a predictor of malignancy. Br J Radiol 68:266–270

Stern WBR, Silver CE, Zeifer BA, Persky MS, Heller KS (1990) Computed tomography of the clinically negative neck. Head Neck 12:109–113

Stevens MH, Harnsberger R, Mancuso AA, Davis RK, Johnson LP, Parkin JL (1985) Computed tomography of cervical lymph nodes; staging and management of head and neck cancer. Arch Otolaryngol 111:735–739

Szmeja Z, Wierzbicka M, Kaczmarek J, Kordylewska M (1998) The value of ultrasound examination in early detection of nodal disease in the neck in follow-up patients operated for head and neck cancer. Br J Cancer 77 [Suppl 1]:15

Tachimori Y, Kato H, Watanabe H, Yamaguchi H (1994) Neck ultrasonography for thoracic esophageal carcinoma. Ann Thorac Surg 57:1180–1183

Takes RP, Knegt P, Manni JJ, Meeuwis CA, Marres HAM, Spoelstra HAA, de Boer MF, Bruaset I, van Oostayen JA, Lameris JS, Kruyt RH et al (1996) Regional metastases in head and neck squamous cell carcinoma: revised value of US with US-guided FNAB. Radiology 198:819–823

Tien RD, Robbins KT (1992) Correlation of clinical, surgical, pathologic, and mr fat suppression results for head and neck cancer. Head Neck 14:278–284

Tschammler A, Wirkner H, Ott G, Hahn D (1996) Vascular patterns in reactive and malignant lymphadenopathy. Eur Radiol 6:473–480

van den Brekel MW (1996) US-guided fine-needle aspiration cytology of neck nodes in patients with N0 disease. Radiology 201:580–581

van den Brekel MW, Stel HV, Castelijns JA, Nauta JJ, van der Waal I, Valk J, Meyer CJ, Snow GB (1990a) Cervical lymph node metastasis: assessment of radiologic criteria. Radiology 177:379–384

van den Brekel MW, Castelijns JA, Stel HV, Valk J, Croll GA, Golding RP, Luth WJ, Meyer CJ, Snow GB (1990b) Detection and characterization of metastatic cervical adenopathy by MR imaging: comparison of different MR techniques. J Comput Assist Tomogr 14:581–589

van den Brekel MW, Castelijns JA, Croll GA, Stel HV, Valk J, van der Waal I, Golding RP, Meyer CJ, Snow GB (1991a) Magnetic resonance imaging vs palpation of cervical lymph node metastasis. Arch Otolaryngol Head Neck Surg 117:663–673

van den Brekel MW, Castelijns JA, Stel HV, Luth WJ, Valk J, van der Waal I, Snow GB (1991b) Occult metastatic neck disease: detection with US and US-guided fine-needle aspiration cytology. Radiology 180:457–461

van den Brekel MW, Risse EK, Tiwari RM, Stel HV (1991c) False-positive fine needle aspiration cytologic diagnosis of a warthin's tumor with squamous metaplasia as a squamous-cell carcinoma. Acta Cytol 35:477–478

van den Brekel MW, Castelijns JA, Stel HV, Golding RP, Meyer CJ, Snow GB (1993) Modern imaging techniques and ultrasound-guided aspiration cytology for the assessment of neck node metastases: a prospectie comparative study. Eur Arch Otorhinolaryngol 250:11–17

van den Brekel MW, Bartelink H, Snow GB (1994a) The value of staging of neck nodes in patients treated with radiotherapy. Radiother Oncol 32:193–196

van den Brekel MW, Castelijns JA, Snow GB (1994b) Detection of lymph node metastases in the neck: radiologic criteria. Radiology 192:617–618

van den Brekel MW, Leemans CR, Snow GB (1996a) Assessment and management of lymph node metastases in the neck in head and neck cancer patients. Crit Rev Oncol Hematol 22:175–182

van den Brekel MW, van der Waal I, Meyer CJ, Freeman JL, Castelijns JA, Snow GB (1996b) The incidence of micrometastases in neck dissection specimens obtained from elective neck dissections. Laryngoscope 106:987–991

van den Brekel MW, Reitsma LC, Snow GB, Castelijns JA (1988a) The outcome of a wait and see policy for the neck after negative ultrasound guided cytology results and follow-up with ultrasound guided cytology. Br J Cancer 77 [Suppl 1]:20

van den Brekel MWM, Castelijns JA, Snow GB (1998b) The size of lymph nodes in the neck on sonograms as a radiologic criterion for metastasis: How reliable is it. AJNR Am J Neuroradiol 19:695-700

van den Brekel MW, Pameijer FA, Koops W, Hilgers FJ, Kroon BB, Balm AJ (1998c) Computed tomography for the detection of neck node metastases in melanoma patients. Eur J Surg Oncol 24:51–54

VandenBrouck C, Sancho-Garnier H, Chassagne D, Saravane D, Cachin Y, Micheau C (1980) Elective versus theapeutic radical neck dissection in epidermoid carcinoma of the oral cavity: results of a randomized clinical trial. Cancer 46:386–390

van der Veen H, Hoekstra OS, Paul MA, Cuesta MA, Meijer S (1994) Gamma probe-guided sentinel node biopsy to select patients with melanoma for lymphadenectomy. Br J Surg 81:1769–1770

van der Velde-Zimmermann D, Roijers JF, Bouwens-Rombouts A, de Weger RA, De Graaf PW, Tilanus MG, van den Tweel JG (1996) Molecular test for the detection of tumor cells in blood and sentinel nodes of melanoma patients. Am J Pathol 149:759–764

van Overhagen H, Laméris JS, Zonderland HM, Tilanus HW, van Pel R, Schütte HE (1991) Ultrasound and ultrasound-guided fine needle aspiration biopsy of supraclavicular lymph nodes in patients with esophageal carcinoma. Cancer 67:585–587

Vassallo P, Wernecke K, Roos N, Peters PE (1992) Differentiation of benign from malignant superficial lymphadenopathy: the role of high-resolution US. Radiology 183:215–220

Vassallo P, Edel G, Roos N, Naguib A, Peters PE (1993) In-vitro high-resolution ultrasonography of benign and malignant lymph nodes. A sonographic-pathologic correlation. Invest Radiol 28:698–705

Vassallo P, Matei C, Heston WD, McLachlan SJ, Koutcher JA, Castellino RA (1995) Characterization of reactive versus tumor-bearing lymph nodes with interstitial magnetic resonance lymphography in an animal model. Invest Radiol 30:706–711

Vogl TJ, Mack MG, Juergens M, Stark M, Deimling M, Knobber W, Grevers G, Felix R (194) Fat suppression in contrast-enhanced mrt of the base of the skull and of the head-neck area: its clinical value. Rofo Fortschr Geb Rontgenstr Neuen Bildgeb Verfahr 160:417–424

Voit C, Schoengen A, Peter RU (1998) Increased sensitivity in early detection of submicroscopic lymph node metastases in melanoma patients. Br J Cancer 77 [Suppl 1]:29

Watarai J, Seino Y, Kobayashi M, Shindo M, Kato T (1993) CT of retropharyngeal lymph node metastasis from maxillary carcinoma. Acta Radiol 34:492–495

Watkinson JC, Todd CE, Paskin L, Rankin S, Palmer T, Shaheen OH, Clarke SEM (1991) Metastatic carcinima in the neck: a clinical/radiological/scintigraphic and pathological study. Clin Otolaryngol 16:187–192

Weber RS, Marvel J, Smith P, Hankins P, Wolf P, Goepfert H (1993) Paratracheal lymph node dissection for carcinoma of the larynx, hypopharynx, and cervical esophagus. Otolaryngol Head Neck Surg 108:11–17

Weiss MH, Harrison LB, Isaacs RS (1994) Use of decision analysis in planning a management strategy for the stage N0 neck. Arch Otolaryngol Head Neck Surg 120:699–702

Westhofen M (1987) Ultrasound b-scans in the follow-up of head and neck tumors. Head Neck Surg 9:272–278

Wiley AL, Zagzebski JA, Tolbert DD, Banjavic RA (1975) Ultrasound B-scans for clinical evaluation of neoplastic neck nodes. Arch Otolaryngol 101:509–511

Wilson GR, McLean NR, Chippindale A, Campbell RS, Soames JV, Reed MF (1994) The role of MRI scanning in the diagnosis of cervical lymphadenopathy. Br J Plast Surg 47:175–179

Yousem DM, Hurst RW (1994) MR of cervical lymph nodes: comparison of fast spin-echo and conventional spin-echo T2W scans. Clin Radiol 49:670–675

Yousem DM, Som PM, Hackney DB, Schwaibold F, Hendrix RA (1992) Central nodal necrosis and extracapsular neoplastic spread in cervical lymph nodes: MR imaging versus CT. Radiology 182:753–759

Yousem DM, Montone KT, Sheppard LM, Rao VM, Weinstein GS, Hayden RE (1994) Head and neck neoplasms: magnetization transfer analysis. Radiology 192:703–707

Yousem DM, Hatabu H, Hurst RW, Seigerman HM, Montone KT, Weinstein GS, Hayden RE, Goldberg AN, Bigelow DC, Kotapka MJ (1995) Carotid artery invasion by head and neck masses: Prediction with MR imaging. Radiology 195:715–720

Yucel T, Saatci I, Sennaroglu L, Cekirge S, Aydingoz U, Kaya S (1997) MR imaging in squamous cell carcinoma of the head and neck with no palpable lymph nodes. Acta Radiol 38:810–814

# 11 The Value of Radioimmunoscintigraphy for Detection of Lymph Node Metastases in Head and Neck Cancer Patients

G.A.M.S. VAN DONGEN, R. DE BREE, J.C. ROOS, J.J. QUAK, and G.B. SNOW

CONTENTS



## 11.1 Introduction

Monoclonal antibodies (MAbs) directed against tumor-specific or tumor-associated antigens can be used for selective tumor targeting. If such an MAb is labeled with a radionuclide that emits gamma rays, the localization of a targeted tumor can be visualized with a gamma camera. This imaging technique is called radioimmunoscintigraphy (RIS). Because RIS identifies biological antigenic targets on the tumor cell it differs fundamentally from anatomic imaging modalities, such as computed tomography (CT), magnetic resonance imaging (MRI), and ultrasound (US). The potential of RIS depends on the tumor antigen, the monoclonal antibody, the radionuclide, the tumor and the imaging procedures used. This paper deals with the progress made in the technical development of RIS during recent decades. Furthermore, the diagnostic potential of RIS for tumor detection in general, and for the detection of lymph node metastases in patients with squamous cell carcinoma of the head and neck (HNSCC) in particular, will be outlined. Advantages and disadvantages of RIS relative to other diagnostic modalities will be discussed. Finally, possibilities for further improvement of antibody imaging, for example the use of positron emission tomography (PET), will be indicated.

G.A.M.S. VAN DONGEN, Ph.D, R. DE BREE, MD, J.J. QUAK, M.D., G.B. SNOW, MD, Department of Otolaryngology/Head and Neck Surgery, Free University Hospital, De Boelelaan 1117, 1081 HV Amsterdam, The Netherlands
J.C. ROOS, MD, Department of Nuclear Medicine, Free University Hospital, De Boelelaan 1117, 1081HV Amsterdam, The Netherlands

## 11.2 Factors Influencing Tumor Detection by RIS

Several factors are known to affect the potential of RIS for tumor detection (Table 11.1). These factors are related to the antigenic target, the MAb, the radionuclide, the tumor and the imaging procedures. Before clinical results with RIS are summarized the influence of each of these factors on the efficacy of RIS will be discussed.

### 11.2.1 The Target Antigen

The hybridoma technology introduced in 1975 by KÖHLER and MILSTEIN (1975) made it possible to develop MAbs specifically directed against each particular cellular antigen. In this procedure mice are mostly immunized with tumor cells or a purified tumor antigen. Spleen cells from the immunized mice are fused with myeloma cells, which can be propagated indefinitely and have the machinery for MAb production. As such, the resulting hybridoma cells receive the genetic information for the production of specific MAbs from the splenic B-lymphocytes and the growth potential and MAb production and secretion machinery from the myeloma cells. After the cell

**Table 11.1.** Variables influencing tumor detection by radioimmunoscintigraphy (RIS)

| |
|---|
| Antigen |
| Specificity |
| Distribution in normal tissue |
| Heterogeneity of expression |
| Content/density |
| Shedding |
| Internalization |
| Monoclonal antibody |
| Size |
| Affinity |
| Protein dose |
| Immunogenicity |
| Tumor |
| Site |
| Vascularization |
| Permeability |
| Perfusion |
| Size |
| Interstitial pressure |
| Radionuclide |
| Physical characteristics |
| Imaging procedures |

fusion procedure, a hybridoma cell clone can be selected that produces a MAb with the desired antigen specificity.

An ideal antigenic target for RIS is highly expressed by all tumors in the patient population at the outer cell surface of all tumor cells, and not by normal tissues. Unfortunately, tumor-specific antigens have only been found in experimentally induced tumors and not in so-called spontaneous tumors. Most identified antigens in human tumors represent tumor-associated antigens, which are present on tumor tissue but are also detectable on normal tissues. Expression of the target antigen in normal tissues can be acceptable for RIS when this normal tissue is poorly accessible for MAbs or when it is localized at a site outside the anatomic region of interest. Shedding of an antigen by the tumor into the blood is considered to be a disadvantage, since circulating antigen can trap the injected radiolabeled MAb before the MAb reaches the tumor and this makes RIS less effective. After binding of a MAb to a surface antigen, the antigen–MAb interaction can result in internalization of the antibody. The effect of internalization of a MAb on the efficacy of RIS depends on the conjugated radionuclide. For example, degradation of iodine-123 ($^{123}$I)-, iodine-131 ($^{131}$I)-, and technetium-99m ($^{99m}$Tc)-labeled MAbs will result in a rapid clearance of these radionuclides from the tumor. In contrast, when internalized indium-111 ($^{111}$In)-labeled MAbs become degraded, $^{111}$In will be trapped intracellularly (Mattes et al. 1994). Therefore, the phenomenon of internalization can make RIS in some cases less, and in other cases more sensitive.

### 11.2.2 The Monoclonal Antibody

MAbs can now be produced in large quantities, with a quality that fulfills the US Food and Drug Administration requirements, and at a cost which are acceptable for marketing.

The uptake of a MAb in a tumor depends on the antigen recognized by the MAb, as well as on the molecular size of the MAb. An intact MAb is a large immunoglobulin molecule with a weight of 150 kDa. Such large molecules have a limited capability for penetrating a tumor. Moreover, the residence time of an intact MAb in blood is long, resulting in low tumor-to-nontumor ratios. For RIS the use of smaller MAb fragments such as F(ab′)$_2$ (mol. Wt. ≈ 100 kDa), Fab (mol. Wt. ≈ 50 kDa) and Fv (mol. Wt. ≈ 25 kDa) fragments can be an advantage, because smaller fragments penetrate better than whole immunoglobulin and therefore have the potential for more rapid tumor targeting, with higher tumor-to-nontumor ratios at earlier time points after administration. F(ab′)$_2$ and Fab fragments can be obtained by proteolytic cleavage of the intact MAb. Recombinant DNA technology can be used to produce the smaller derivatives, such as Fv fragments (Hawkins et al. 1992). Whether a MAb should have a low or high affinity, and whether the MAb should be administered at a low or high dose depends heavily on the specific MAb under investigation.

Administration of a murine MAb to a patient usually results in a human anti-mouse antibody (HAMA) response. Owing to the presence of HAMAs, a subsequent administration of the MAb can lead to rapid clearance of the injected MAb from the blood, thus preventing efficient tumor targeting. Moreover, an anaphylactic reaction can occur. To avoid HAMA responses the MAb molecule can be reshaped to human–mouse chimeric (cMAbs) or even humanized (hMAbs) versions by using recombinant DNA techniques (Hazra et al. 1995).

### 11.2.3 The Tumor

After administration to the patient, the large MAb molecules have to pass several physiological barriers before binding to the antigen. When the tumor is reached, the MAb distributes throughout the vascular compartment of the tumor. The vascularization pattern depends heavily on the site of the tumor. Within a tumor the vascularization pattern can be heterogeneous, with extensive vascularization in the vital regions and limited vascularization in the necrotic areas. The average perfusion is lower in tumor tissue than in normal tissue (Jain 1988). To reach the tumor cells, MAbs have to pass blood vessel walls. In normal tissues the barrier offered by endothelial cells varies greatly (Cobb 1989). In liver, spleen and bone there is virtually no barrier, because the endothelium is fenestrated and a basement membrane is lacking. In contrast, endothelium of lung and skin is particularly poorly permeable for macromolecules like immunoglobulins. In tumors, the endothelium is usually fenestrated, even in tumors arising from tissues that normally have no fenestrated capillaries. In addition, the basement membrane of the tumor endothelium is frequently defective and this is likely to give rise to increased permeability (Jain 1990). Once the MAb molecules have crossed the blood vessel wall, they have to move through the extracellular space of the tumor stroma by diffusion and convection (bulky fluid movement) before they reach the tumor cells (Jain 1987). Depending on the composition of such structural proteins as collagen, elastin and proteoglycans, resistance to immunoglobulin diffusion will occur. Another factor influencing antibody movement throughout the tumor is the intratumor pressure (Boucher and Jain 1992). This pressure increases upon tumor growth, and may lead to reduced blood flow and reduced extravasation of the MAb. As a consequence, small tumors show relatively higher MAb uptake levels than large tumors (Behr et al. 1997). When the MAb finally has arrived in the peripheral cell layer of a tumor nest it has to pass intercellular junctions (especially desmosomes in case HNSCC) before reaching inner cell layers.

### 11.2.4 The Radionuclide

The radionuclides most commonly used in RIS are $^{131}$I (half-life: 8 days), $^{123}$I (half-life: 13 h), $^{111}$In (half-life: 68 h) and $^{99m}$Tc (half-life: 6 h). Several comments can be made on the applicability of these radionuclides for RIS of HNSCC. $^{131}$I and $^{123}$I labels are not favorable, because the detachment of iodine from MAbs (dehalogenation) will result in activity uptake in the thyroid, which may disturb HNSCC imaging in this region. Similar considerations can be made for detached $^{111}$In, which can accumulate in lymphocytes present in the lymph nodes. Furthermore, sequestration of $^{111}$In in the liver can hamper the detection of HNSCC metastases in this organ. High costs ($^{111}$In, $^{123}$I), extensive exposure of the patient to radiation ($^{111}$In), limited availability ($^{123}$I), long half-life ($^{131}$I) and poor imaging qualities ($^{131}$I) are considered to be other drawbacks. $^{99m}$Tc has many advantages over the previously mentioned radionuclides: the minimal radiation delivered to the patient (short half-life time and low gamma energy), its ideal properties for gamma cameras (high photon abundance), low costs, and good availability. Simple and suitable labeling methods for $^{99m}$Tc have recently become available (Verbruggen 1990).

### 11.2.5 The Imaging Procedure

In general the first images are acquired within a few minutes after injection of the radioimmunoconjugate. These early images serve as a baseline reference in the interpretation of later images. For head and neck cancer patients whole-body images and planar images of the head and neck region can be acquired. Several aspects should be taken into account when the optimal time point for later images is sought. (a) It takes some time before high MAb levels in the tumor and optimal tumor-to-nontumor ratios are achieved. For smaller MAb fragments this time period is shorter than for intact MAb. (b) The imaging system should receive a sufficiently high count rate from the tumor, as otherwise the resolution and sensitivity of imaging will not be optimal. Radionuclides with a short half-life have an advantage, because these can be administered at a high activity dose. (c) For the patient it is convenient when the total imaging procedure does not take up too much time. For most intact MAbs or fragments labeled with $^{99m}$Tc or $^{123}$I, the time point for optimal imaging is between 4 h and 24 h after injection.

Later images mostly comprise whole-body images and images of the head and neck region. Single photon emission computerized tomography (SPECT) images are often acquired in addition. Axial, coronal and sagittal sections can be used to separate activity in the tumor from uptake in normal tissues including the blood vessels.

## 11.3 Current Status of RIS in General

Radiolabeled antibodies have been safely admistered to several thousands of patients in RIS studies (Delaloye and Delaloye 1995; Zuckier and DeNardo 1997). The potential applications for RIS are diverse and depend on the tumor type. RIS is most commonly used for the presurgical detection of occult tumors or for confirmation of inconclusive diagnostic findings obtained with anatomic imaging modalities such as CT and MRI. Besides that, RIS is used for detection of residual disease after primary therapy. This latter approach is of especial value in the visualization of recurrences in patients with increasing tumor marker titers in the blood. Finally, RIS is used to identify patients who can be considered candidates for radioimmunotherapy. In this case accumulation of the MAb in the tumor is confirmed by RIS, while images are used for making dosimetric predictions.

As indicated in a excellent recent review by Zuckier and DeNardo (1997), three MAbs have been approved by the US Food and Drug Administration for imaging of cancer. In addition, several antibodies are in phase II and III evaluation in FDA-monitored trials. One of the approved MAbs is MAb 72.3 (commercial name: OncoScint, Cytogen, Princeton, N.J.), which is used in colon cancer patients for detection of occult disease in the case of rising serum tumor markers, to detect residual disease after primary therapy, and to confirm findings observed by other diagnostic modalities. Diagnostic results with $^{111}$In-labeled B72.3 intact IgG in phase III studies appeared to be superior to those obtained with anatomic imaging modalities for the detection of pelvic (sensitivity 74% vs 57%; $P$ = 0.035) and extrahepatic intraabdominal lesions (sensitivity 66% vs 34%; $P$ = 0.001), but inferior for the detection of hepatic lesions (sensitivity 84% vs 41%; $P$ < 0.001) (Collier et al. 1992). The poor results for detection of liver metastases can be explained by the nonspecific uptake of $^{111}$In in this organ, as indicated in Section 11.2.4. While these data seem to be very promising, the real impact of B72.3 RIS on patient management was qualified differently in the various studies, ranging from poor to moderate (Doerr et al. 1991; Dominguez et al. 1996). The same MAb also received approval as an RIS agent for the detection of ovarian carcinoma after showing a higher overall sensitivity than CT imaging (68% vs 44%) in the detection of surgically confirmed tumors (Surwit et al. 1993). A second MAb approved as an RIS agent, for the detection of colon cancer, is MAb IMMU-4 (commercial name: CEA scan; Immunomedics, Morris Plains, N.J.). This MAb is used as a $^{99m}$Tc-labeled Fab′ fragment. The sensitivity of RIS with this Mab also appeared to be better than that of conventional imaging techniques in the case of pelvic (69% vs 48%; $P$ = 0.005) and extrahepatic intraabdominal lesions (55% vs 32%; $P$ = 0.007; Moffat et al. 1996). In the detection of liver metastases, RIS with IMMU-4 appeared to do as well as other modalities (sensitivity 63% vs 64%). Finally, NR-LU-10 (commercial name Verluma, NeoRx, Seattle, Wash.), used as a $^{99m}$Tc-labeled Fab for the detection of small cell lung cancer, has been approved by the FDA. Data from phase III studies showed that RIS with NR-LU-10 is as accurate as all other standard diagnostic tests together (Breitz et al. 1993). Verluma also awaits approval for use in the detection of non-small-cell lung cancer.

## 11.4 Monoclonal Antibodies for RIS of Head and Neck Cancer

Squamous cell carcinoma account for the vast majority of malignant tumors of the head and neck (Zarbo and Crissman 1988). While in the last decade MAbs have been administered to thousands of patients with various types of tumors for diagnostic purposes, the application of MAbs for detection of HNSCC has not kept pace. One of the main reasons for this slow progress has been the lack of MAbs with a high specificity for HNSCC and a restricted reaction pattern on normal tissues. So far, at least 30 MAbs directed against HNSCC have been described in the literature (a selection of MAbs is shown in Table 11.2). These MAbs can be divided in two main categories. The first group of MAbs is reactive with squamous cell carcinoma and not with other tumor types. A general shortcoming of this group of MAbs is their reactivity with normal squamous epithelia. When such MAbs are used in RIS, uptake of radioactivity in the normal oral mucosa can occur, and as a result tumor detection in this area might be hampered. A second group of MAbs also recognizes other tumor types besides HNSCC, the so-called pancarcinoma MAbs. A general shortcoming of these MAbs is their heterogeneous reaction pattern with HNSCC and their reactivity with several normal tissues. Many of the MAbs described in literature are

**Table 11.2.** Monoclonal antibodies (*MAb*) directed against squamous cell carcinoma

| MAb | Antigen | Limitations | Reference |
|---|---|---|---|
| *Squamous cell specific* | | | |
| 174H.64 | 48 + 57 kDa | Reactive with basal cells of normal squamous epithelia, cytoplasmic antigen | Samuel et al. (1989) |
| E48 | 16-20 kDa | Reactive with basal and suprabasal cells of normal squamous epithelia | Quak et al. (1990a) |
| INS-2 | 40 kDa | Reactive with normal squamous epithelia, cytoplasmic antigen, IgM | Inoue et al. (1990) |
| U36 | CD44v6/epican | Reactive with basal and suprabasal cells of normal squamous epithelia | Schrijvers et al. (1993) |
| BM2 | 52 kDa | Reactive with basal cells of normal squamous epithelia, IgM | Yoshiura et al. (1993) |
| VFF18 | CD44v6/epican | Reactive with basal and suprabasal cells of normal squamous epithelia | Heider et al. (1996) |
| *Pan-carcinoma* | | | |
| SQM1 | 48 kDa | Reactive with blood vessels, IgM | Boeheim et al. (1985) |
| A9 | $\alpha_6\beta_4$-Integrin | Reactive with blood vessels and basal cells of normal squamous epithelia | Kimmel and Carey (1986) |
| B10 | Various keratins | Reactive with various normal tissues, cytoplasmic antigen, IgM | Myoken et al. (1987) |
| 1H5 | Various keratins | Reactive with various normal tissues, cytoplasmic antigen, IgM | Myoken et al. (1987) |
| 425 | EGF-receptor | Reactive with various normal tissues | Murthy et al. (1987) |
| K931 | Ep-CAM | Reactive with various normal tissues | Quak et al. (1990b) |
| 225 | EGF-receptor | Reactive with various normal tissues | Divgi et al. (1991) |
| K984 | 125 kDa | Reactive with basal cells of normal squamous epithelia and various other normal tissues | Quak et al. (1992) |
| K928 | 50–55 kDa | Reactive with suprabasal cells of normal squamous epithelia and various other normal tissues | Quak et al. (1992) |
| 175F4 | 45–50 kDa | Reactivity with normal squamous epithelia | Balm et al. (1992) |
| 175F11 | 45–50 kDa | Reactivity with normal squamous epithelia | Balm et al. (1992) |
| CAK1 | 40 kDa | Reactivity with mesothelium and basal epithelium of trachea | Chang et al. (1992) |
| HMFG1 | >400 kDa, PEM | Reactive with various normal tissues | Maraveyas et al. (1995) |

poorly characterized with respect to their reactivity profile on normal and malignant tissues. For these MAbs it is difficult to speculate about their suitability for RIS.

Only a few of the MAbs listed in Table 11.2 have been administered to HNSCC patients (Table 11.3). This can be explained by the serious drawbacks of many of the MAbs. Besides that, also the high production costs for a batch of clinical grade MAb restrict their preliminary clinical evaluation in RIS. MAb production is a complex procedure. Mostly a batch of several grams of MAb is produced in one run, and this is enough for RIS studies with hundreds of patients. The following steps have to be followed: hybridoma cells secreting the specific MAb have to be expanded to a so-called production master cell bank. By performing in vitro and in vivo tests it has to be demonstrated that this cell bank is free from microbial contaminants (e.g., bacteria, fungi and mycoplasma) and from any infectious or adventitious viruses. Subsequently, a part of the cell bank is put in a continuous perfusion fermentor for cell expansion and MAb production in the appropriate culture medium. A standardized downstream process is applied for the purification of the MAb from the culture medium under good manufacturing practice conditions. The remaining concentrated bulk harvest has to be tested again for the presence of contaminants, after which final sterile filling of the purified MAb into glass vials can occur. The filled product must then be re-analyzed in detail. After the validation of procedures for radiolabeling of the particular MAb and the performance of safety/toxicity studies in animals, clinical RIS studies can be started.

Despite all these efforts, it may appear at an early stage of clinical studies that the MAb is not suitable for RIS. This can be illustrated by our own experience with an MAb called SF-25. MAb SF-25 had been immunohistochemically characterized and appeared to be reactive with HNSCC, adenocarcinoma of the colon and, among normal tissues, with cells in the distal tubule of the kidney (Takahashi et al. 1988).

**Table 11.3.** Monoclonal antibodies used for imaging of squamous cell carcinoma in patients[a]

| Antibody | No. of patients | No. of patients with neck involvement | Reference |
|---|---|---|---|
| Anti-CEA | 5 | 3 | Tranter et al. (1984) |
| | 13 | 6 | Kairemo et al. (1990a) |
| | 29 | 1 | Kairemo et al. (1990b) |
| | 7 | 3 | Timon et al. (1991) |
| | 20 | 18 | De Rossi et al. (1997) |
| Anti-EGFR | 11 | 3 | Soo et al. (1987) |
| MAb 225/anti-EGFR | 19 | 18 | Divgi et al. (1991) |
| MAb 174H.64 | 21 | 18 | Baum et al. (1993) |
| | 10 | 1 | Heissler et al. (1994) |
| | 40 | 6 | Adamietz et al. (1996) |
| MAb SF-25 | 1 | 1 | De Bree et al. (1994a) |
| MAb 323/A3/anti-Ep-CAM | 3 | 0 | De Bree et al. (1994a) |
| MAb K928 | 6 | 6 | De Bree et al. (1994a) |
| MAb E48 | 32 | 25 | De Bree et al. (1994b) |
| MAb U36/anti-CD44v6 | 10 | 9 | De Bree et al. (1995) |

[a] All studies were performed with head and neck cancer patients, except the study with MAb 225, in which patients with lung cancer were imaged.

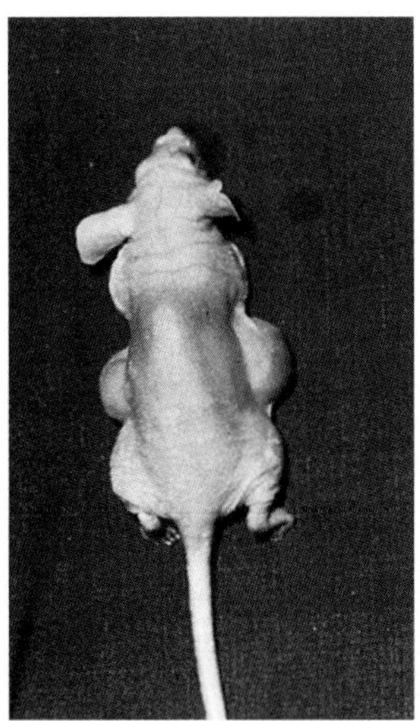
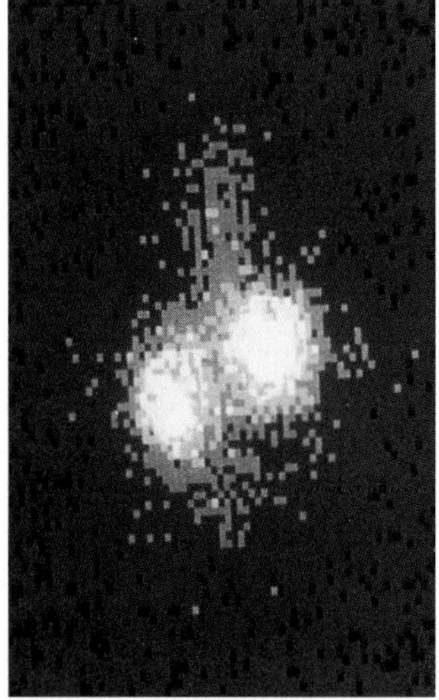

**Fig. 11.1.** Whole-body scintigraphic image of an athymic mouse bearing two subcutaneous HNSCC (squamous cell carcinoma of head and neck) xenografts. This image was taken 3 days after injection of 10 µCi $^{131}$I-labeled anti-HNSCC monoclonal antibodies (MAb)

Moreover, $^{131}$I-labeled MAb SF-25 was shown to be capable of selective tumor targeting in human HNSCC-bearing nude mice. A representative antibody image in this tumor model is shown in Fig. 11.1. On the basis of the above information it was decided to start clinical RIS studies with $^{99m}$Tc-labeled SF-25 for the detection of primary tumors and lymph node metastases in patients with histologically proven HNSCC (De Bree et al. 1994a). Unfortunately, MAb SF-25 was not able to detect HNSCC owing to rapid and extensive accumulation at nontumor sites (Fig. 11.2). Within 15 min after injection 80% of the activity had disappeared from the blood, while preferential uptake was seen in liver, spleen and brain, but not in the tumor. As a result of these images an immunohistochemical re-evaluation of MAb SF-25 was performed. MAb SF-25 appeared to be reactive with Kupffer cells in the liver, the red pulpa and the follicle centre in the spleen, and with endothelium of blood vessels in the brain. Since this experience, the industry-sponsored MAb SF-25 has never been administered to patients again.

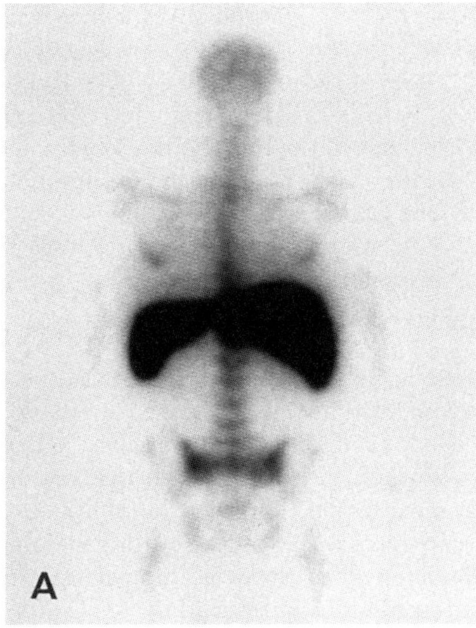


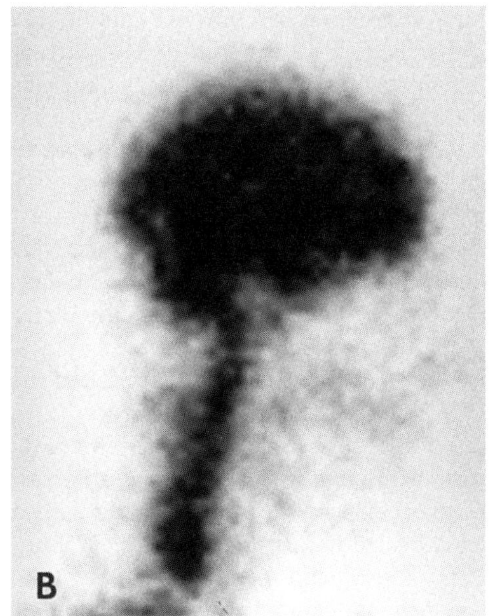


**Fig. 11.2 A,B.** Images of a patient with pharyngeal HNSCC, TNM stage pT2N2c, 15 min after injection of $^{99m}$Tc-labeled MAb SF-25. **A** Planar posterior image of the whole body. Note the extensive uptake in liver, spleen and skeleton. No blood pool activity is seen. **B** Planar right lateral image of the head and neck of the same patient 21 h after injection, showing activity in the whole brain area. The primary tumor in the right tonsillar fossa is not visualized. Since this negative result, MAb SF-25 has not been used for RIS again

## 11.5 Detection of Lymph Node Metastases with RIS in Head and Neck Cancer Patients

### 11.5.1 The Clinical Needs

During 1996 approximately 41 090 Americans developed head and neck cancer, and 12 510 died from it (Parker et al. 1996). Worldwide more than 500 000 new cases are projected annually, and the incidence is rising. HNSCC grow in a locally invasive manner and also have a proclivity to metastasize to regional lymph nodes in the neck rather than to spread by the hematogenous route. The status of the lymph nodes is the single most important tumor-related prognostic factor, and for optimal treatment planning it is essential to know the exact involvement of the nodes. In many institutions, this is still mainly based on palpation. However, palpation is far from reliable for the detection of lymph node metastases (Watkinson et al. 1990). Histopathological evaluations have demonstrated that both the false-positive rate and the false-negative rate are unsatisfactorily high. The overall error of palpation is about 20–30% (Ali et al. 1985). Modern imaging techniques, such as CT, MRI, US, and especially US-guided fine-needle aspiration cytology (FNAC), are more reliable than palpation, but also still leave much room for improvement (van den Brekel et al. 1993). In our department, radiological criteria have been defined for the optimal assessment of cervical lymph node metastases with CT and MRI (van den Brekel et al. 1990). Using these criteria the overall error of CT and MRI in the preoperative detection of lymph node metastases in neck sides is about 20%. For US-guided FNAC this figure is much better, about 10%. Despite this, US-guided FNAC also has some unfavorable aspects: (1) it is an invasive method, (2) it only gives diagnostic information on the neck and not on the primary tumor or distant metastases, and (3) its accuracy is dependent on the skill of the ultrasonographer and the cytopathologist and clinical documentation of the procedure is difficult (van den Brekel et al. 1993). These aspects are discussed more thoroughly in Chapter 10.

One of the novel options for refinement of the staging of head and neck cancer is the use of positron emission tomography (PET). In PET, radioactive tracers are used, which give an elevated accumulation in tissues with high metabolic activity, such as cancer tissue. For imaging of head and neck cancer,

$^{18}$fluorine-fluorodeoxyglucose, $^{11}$carbon-methionine and $^{11}$carbon-tyrosine have been used. The current status of PET in staging of head and neck cancer is reviewed in Chapter 7.

The capability of all of the above techniques to detect small tumor deposits is limited. Moreover, these imaging techniques very often cannot discriminate between normal lymph nodes, reactively enlarged nodes, and tumor-infiltrated lymph nodes. Because of these problems, it may be difficult to decide whether the neck should be treated or not, and this can lead to over- and undertreatment of the neck.

As indicated in Section 11.3, RIS has been recognized as a promising novel option for the improvement of cancer staging. However, up to now only a few MAbs have been administered to a limited number of HNSCC patients, and it is therefore much too early to make firm statements about the diagnostic potential of RIS in head and neck cancer. RIS has mostly been applied in presurgical staging of the extent of disease, to obtain a first impression of the diagnostic potential of the particular radioimmunoconjugate. Comparison of the results obtained in these studies is difficult, because of the variability in (1) the number of patients, which in some studies was too low to make accurate calculation of sensitivity and specificity possible, (2) the control of tumor deposits for antigen expression, (3) the scintigraphic methods used, (4) the methods used for topographical evaluation of the diagnostic findings, and (5) the methods used for confirmation of the diagnostic findings. Furthermore, optimal CT and/or MRI imaging procedures were not used for comparison in all studies, and in cases when they were applied it is not clear whether the examiner for RIS was blinded to the results of the other diagnostic examinations. In Section 11.5.2, we summarize our own data on the detection of lymph node metastases with RIS and give some short comments on the other studies performed in this field.

### 11.5.2 Design of Clinical RIS Studies

Forty-nine patients who were at risk for having neck lymph node metastasis from a histologically proven HNSCC and were scheduled to undergo neck dissection(s) participated in our studies. Prior to enrollment a biopsy of the primary tumor, if available, had to show positive immunoperoxidase staining with the MAbs used for injection, the squamous cell-specific MAbs E48 or U36 (see Table 11.2).

Patients received 1–50 mg E48 $F(ab')_2$ fragment (15 patients), E48 intact IgG (24 patients) or U36 intact IgG (10 patients) labeled with approx. 740 MBq $^{99m}$Tc by intravenous injection in 5 min. Before administration to the patient, the quality of the radioimmunoconjugate was checked by assessment of the radiochemical purity and the immunoreactivity.

All patients were examined by palpation, CT, MRI, and RIS of the neck prior to surgery. Preoperative palpation was performed by the same experienced head and neck surgeon. CT scans were performed with a third-generation Philips Tomoscan 350 (Philips Medical Systems, Best, The Netherlands) or with a fourth-generation Siemens Somaton Plus (Siemens, Erlangen, Germany) after intravenous administration of contrast medium (Ultravist 300 mg iodine/ml, Schering, Germany). Contiguous axial 5- to 6-mm scanning planes were used. MRI examinations were performed on a 0.6 T or 1.0 T imaging system (Teslacon, Technicare – General Electric, Milwaukee, Wis.) using a partial volume coil. Axial T1-weighted spin echo and gadolinium-diethylenetriaminepentaacetic acid (Magnevist, Schering, Germany) enhanced T1-weighted gradient-recalled echo images were made in all patients without claustrophobia. Slice thickness varied from 3 mm to 5 mm, with an interslice gap of 50%. Criteria for the optimal assessment of cervical lymph node metastases by CT or MRI, as defined by Van den Brekel et al. (1990), were used. On CT or MRI, neck levels were considered malignant if nodes with necrosis were depicted, or if the minimal diameter in the axial plane of the node was 11 mm or more for nodes located in level II (subdigastic) and 10 mm or more for all other nodes, or if groups of three or more borderline lymph nodes (1–2 mm smaller) were seen.

The radioimmunoscintigrams were obtained with a large field of view gamma camera (Gemini, General Electric, Milwaukee, Wis., or later with a Dual Head Genesys Imaging System, ADAC laboratories, Milpitas) equipped with a low-energy hole collimator, connected to a computer (Bartec, Farnborough, U.K. or later Pegasys, ADAC laboratories, Milpitas). Whole-body images (anterior and posterior views) and planar images of the head and neck (anterior views) were obtained immediately after and 16 h and 21 h after injection. SPECT images of the head and neck were acquired 16 h after injection, while lateral scans were obtained 21 h after injection. Interpretation of increased uptake of activity was based on asymmetry and retention, specially on late images.

CT, MRI and RIS examinations were each scored by one experienced examiner. All examiners were blinded to the results of other examinations and the pathological outcome. They were informed only of the site of the primary tumor. All patients had uni- or bilateral neck dissections performed 2 days after administration of the radioimmunoconjugate. After fixation, all palpable and visible lymph nodes were dissected from the surgical specimen and cut into 2- to 4-mm-thick slices for microscopic examination by the pathologist. This histopathological examination was used as the "gold standard."

For topographical evaluation the findings were recorded per side as well as per lymph node level (Fig. 11.3) according to the Memorial Sloan-Kettering Cancer Center Classification (Shah et al. 1981). Level I includes the contents of the submental and submandibular triangles. Levels II, III and IV include the contents of the lymph nodes adjacent to the internal vein and the lymph nodes contained within the fibroadipose tissue located medial to the sternocleidomastoid muscle. This area is arbitrarily divided into three equal parts, level II being the highest level and IV the lowest level. Level V includes the contents of the posterior cervical triangle. Lymph nodes outside these levels were considered separately. These lymph nodes are included in the evaluation per side, but are not included in the evaluation per level.

Diagnostic findings were not recorded per deposit. In our experience, evaluation of RIS data per deposit is inaccurate because precise localization of the deposit is impossible owing to the lack of anatomical stuctures on the immunoscintigrams. For this reason, in this paper we will not pair immunoscintigrams with CT or MRI images.

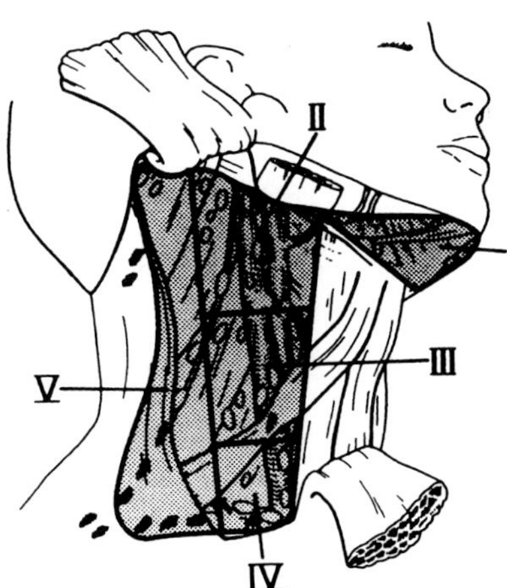


**Fig. 11.3.** Lymph node levels in the neck according to the Memorial Sloan-Kettering Cancer Cancer Classification (*I* submandibular, *II* subdigastric, *III* midjugular, *IV* low jugular, *V* posterior cervical triangle)

### 11.5.3 Results of RIS Studies

All 44 primary tumors in 49 patients were visualized by RIS. Thirty-two patients, underwent unilateral neck dissection and 17 patients, bilateral neck dissection. A total number of 318 levels were histopathologically examined. Fifty-one of the 66 operated sides contained metastases of HNSCC in a total of 77 levels. Five patients refused MRI examination because of claustrophobia, and were not included in the evaluation of MRI results.

The findings on palpation, CT, MRI and RIS are summarized in Table 11.4 and 11.5. Findings were evaluated per lymph node level (Table 11.4) and per side (Table 11.5) and correlated with the histopathological results. RIS detected lymph node metastases in 42 of 77 (sensitivity 55%) levels and in 35 of 51 sides (sensitivity 69%). In addition to the planar images, SPECT images provided extra information for most of the patients. Figure 11.4 provides typical images obtained with $^{99m}$Tc-labeled U36 IgG, of a patient with a carcinoma of the right inferior alveolar processus and a submandibular lymph node metastasis. Figure 11.5 provides typical images obtained with $^{99m}$Tc-labeled E48 IgG, showing a carcinoma of the tongue and a subdigastic and a midjugular lymph node metastasis. In contrast to MAb SF-25, MAbs U36 and E48 appeared to be capable of selective tumor targeting. MAb uptake was also seen in the nasal and oral region, which can be explained by the expression of the antigen in normal squamous mucosa. Besides that, liver, lungs, heart, spleen and kidneys were also visualized, which is not a result of MAb binding to these organs, but of circulating MAb still present in the blood.

Five tumor-free levels in two tumor-free neck sides were scored false positive without any explanation. Thirty-five levels and 16 sides were scored false negative. Interpretation of RIS was correct in 276 of 316 levels (accuracy 87%) and in 47 of 65 sides (accuracy 72%). Accuracy of palpation, CT, and MRI was, per level, 87%, 86%, and 88%, respectively, and per side, 82%, 82%, 77%, respectively. The capability of RIS for the detection of tumor-involved neck levels missed (false negative) or detected (true

**Table 11.4.** Correlation of preoperative diagnostic findings with histopathological findings per level (*TP* true-positive, *FN* false-negative, *FP* false-positive, *TN* true-negative, *PPV* positive-predictive value, *NPV* negative-predictive value.)

| | TP | FN | FP | TN | Sensitivity | Specificity | Accuracy | PPV | NPV |
|---|---|---|---|---|---|---|---|---|---|
| E48 ($n$ = 39) | | | | | | | | | |
| Palpation | 39 | 24 | 10 | 193 | 62 | 95 | 87 | 80 | 89 |
| CT | 39 | 24 | 10 | 193 | 62 | 95 | 87 | 80 | 89 |
| MRI[a] | 35 | 23 | 5 | 166 | 60 | 97 | 88 | 88 | 88 |
| RIS | 35 | 28 | 5 | 198 | 56 | 98 | 88 | 88 | 88 |
| U36 ($n$ = 10) | | | | | | | | | |
| Palpation | 7 | 7 | 0 | 36 | 50 | 100 | 86 | 100 | 84 |
| CT | 7 | 7 | 2 | 36 | 50 | 95 | 83 | 78 | 84 |
| MRI[b] | 7 | 6 | 0 | 32 | 54 | 100 | 87 | 100 | 84 |
| RIS | 7 | 7 | 0 | 36 | 50 | 100 | 86 | 100 | 84 |
| All ($n$ = 49) | | | | | | | | | |
| Palpation | 46 | 31 | 10 | 229 | 60 | 96 | 87 | 82 | 88 |
| CT | 46 | 31 | 12 | 229 | 60 | 95 | 86 | 79 | 88 |
| MRI[c] | 42 | 29 | 5 | 198 | 59 | 98 | 88 | 89 | 87 |
| RIS | 42 | 35 | 5 | 234 | 55 | 98 | 87 | 89 | 87 |

[a] MRI in 34 patients.
[b] MRI in 9 patients.
[c] MRI in 43 patients.

**Table 11.5.** Correlation of preoperative diagnostic findings with histopathological findings per side

| | TP | FN | FP | TN | Sensitivity | Specificity | Accuracy | PPV | NPV |
|---|---|---|---|---|---|---|---|---|---|
| E48 ($n$ = 39) | | | | | | | | | |
| Palpation | 37 | 4 | 4 | 11 | 90 | 73 | 86 | 90 | 73 |
| CT | 35 | 6 | 4 | 11 | 85 | 73 | 82 | 90 | 65 |
| MRI[a] | 30 | 6 | 4 | 8 | 83 | 67 | 79 | 88 | 57 |
| RIS | 29 | 12 | 2 | 12 | 71 | 86 | 75 | 94 | 50 |
| U36 ($n$ = 10) | | | | | | | | | |
| Palpation | 6 | 4 | 0 | 0 | 60 | – | 60 | 100 | – |
| CT | 8 | 2 | 0 | 0 | 80 | – | 80 | 100 | – |
| MRI[b] | 6 | 3 | 0 | 0 | 67 | – | 67 | 100 | – |
| RIS | 6 | 4 | 0 | 0 | 60 | – | 60 | 100 | – |
| All ($n$ = 49) | | | | | | | | | |
| Palpation | 43 | 8 | 4 | 11 | 84 | 73 | 82 | 91 | 58 |
| CT | 43 | 8 | 4 | 11 | 84 | 73 | 82 | 91 | 58 |
| MRI[c] | 36 | 9 | 4 | 8 | 80 | 67 | 77 | 90 | 47 |
| RIS | 35 | 16 | 2 | 12 | 69 | 86 | 72 | 95 | 43 |

[a] MRI in 34 patients.
[b] MRI in 9 patients.
[c] MRI in 43 patients.

positive) by palpation, CT and/or MRI, is shown in Table 11.6. In 3 levels RIS visualized lymph node metastases not detected by any other diagnostic technique.

Of the 77 tumor-containing levels, 35 were missed by RIS. The paraffin slides of the missed metastatic lymph nodes were re-examined histopathologically. The missed lymph nodes all appeared to be small lymph nodes (less than 2 cm in diameter) or to contain small tumor deposits (micrometastases), or metastases containing a large proportion of necrosis, keratin, or fibrin deposits. In two patients a level was scored false negative, probably because of lack of anatomical structures on RIS. In 2 patients lymph nodes were missed because of a close spatial relation to the primary tumor. One submandibular lymph node was missed, probably because of the high MAb uptake in the normal oral mucosa. Histopathological examination revealed that the smallest tumor-involved lymph node detected by RIS had diameters

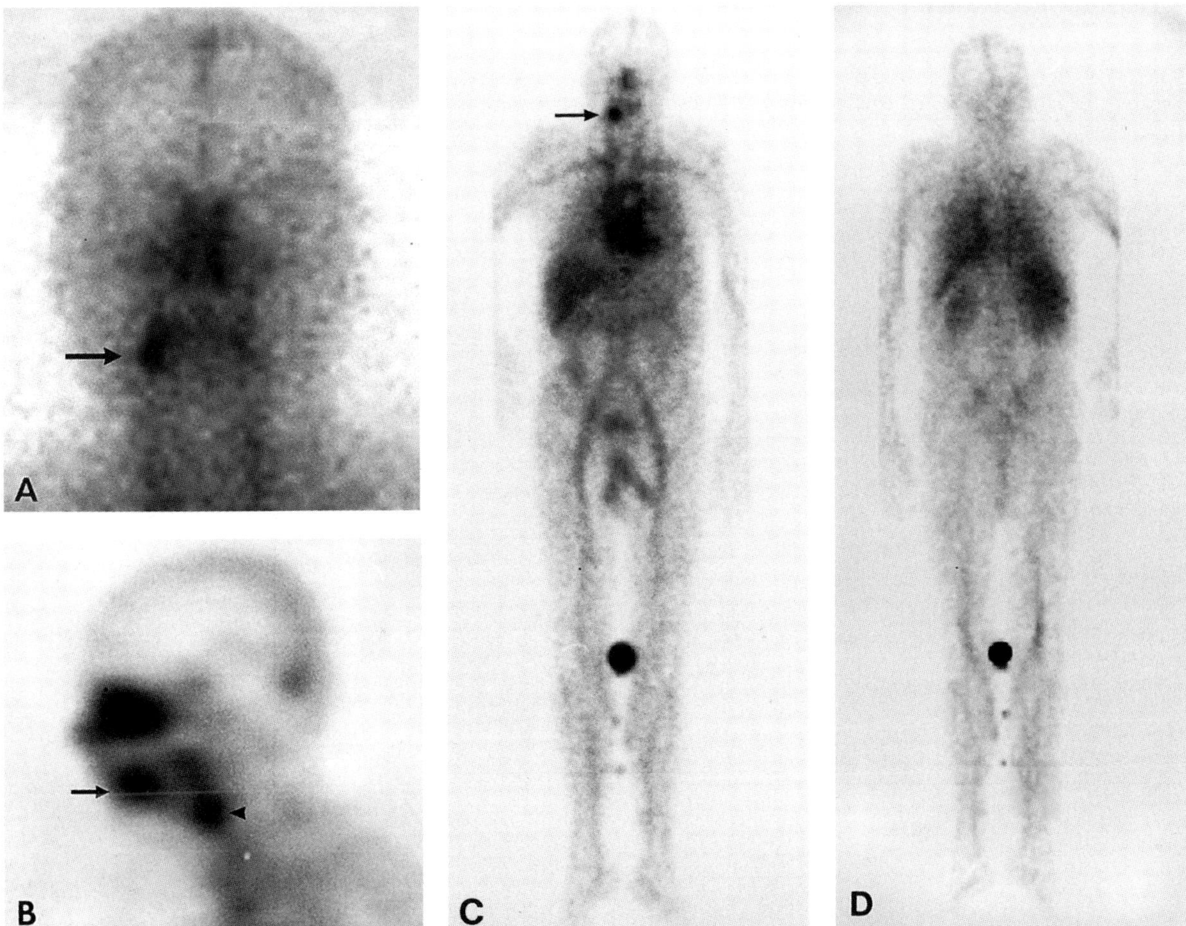


**Fig. 11.4 A–D.** Images of a head and neck cancer patient with a carcinoma of the right inferior alveolar processus, 16h after injection of $^{99m}$Tc-labeled U36 IgG. **A** Planar anterior image. Increased uptake is seen on the right side of the mouth. Only one spot can be distinguished (*arrow*). **B** A sagittal SPECT slice of the same patient shows the two separate spots, representing the primary tumor in the lower jaw (*arrow*) and the subdigastric lymph node metastasis (*arrowhead*). **C** Anterior and **D** posterior whole-body images 16h after injection. Note the clear visualization of the primary tumor (*arrow*)

**Table 11.6.** Results of RIS per level in false-negative and true-positive findings by palpation, CT and MRI

| | False-negative findings by palpation, CT, MRI | | True-positive findings by palpation, CT, MRI | |
|---|---|---|---|---|
| | Seen with RIS | Not seen with RIS | Seen with RIS | Not seen with RIS |
| E48 ($n$ = 39) | | | | |
| Palpation | 6/24 (25%) | 18/24 (75%) | 29/39 (74%) | 10/39 (26%) |
| CT | 5/24 (21%) | 19/24 (79%) | 31/39 (79%) | 8/39 (21%) |
| MRI | 6/23 (26%) | 17/23 (74%) | 26/35 (74%) | 9/35 (26%) |
| Palpation, CT, and MRI | 3/16 (19%) | 13/16 (81%) | 30/43 (70%) | 13/43 (30%) |
| U36 ($n$ = 10) | | | | |
| Palpation | 2/7 (29%) | 5/7 (71%) | 5/7 (71%) | 2/7 (29%) |
| CT | 2/7 (29%) | 5/7 (71%) | 6/7 (86%) | 1/7 (14%) |
| MRI | 0/6 (0%) | 6/6 (100%) | 6/7 (86%) | 1/7 (14%) |
| Palpation, CT, and MRI | 0/5 (0%) | 5/5 (100%) | 7/9 (78%) | 2/9 (22%) |
| All ($n$ = 49) | | | | |
| Palpation | 8/31 (26%) | 23/31 (74%) | 34/46 (74%) | 12/46 (26%) |
| CT | 7/31 (23%) | 24/31 (77%) | 37/46 (80%) | 9/46 (20%) |
| MRI | 6/29 (21%) | 23/29 (79%) | 32/42 (76%) | 10/42 (24%) |
| RIS | 3/21 (14%) | 18/21 (86%) | 37/52 (71%) | 15/52 (29%) |

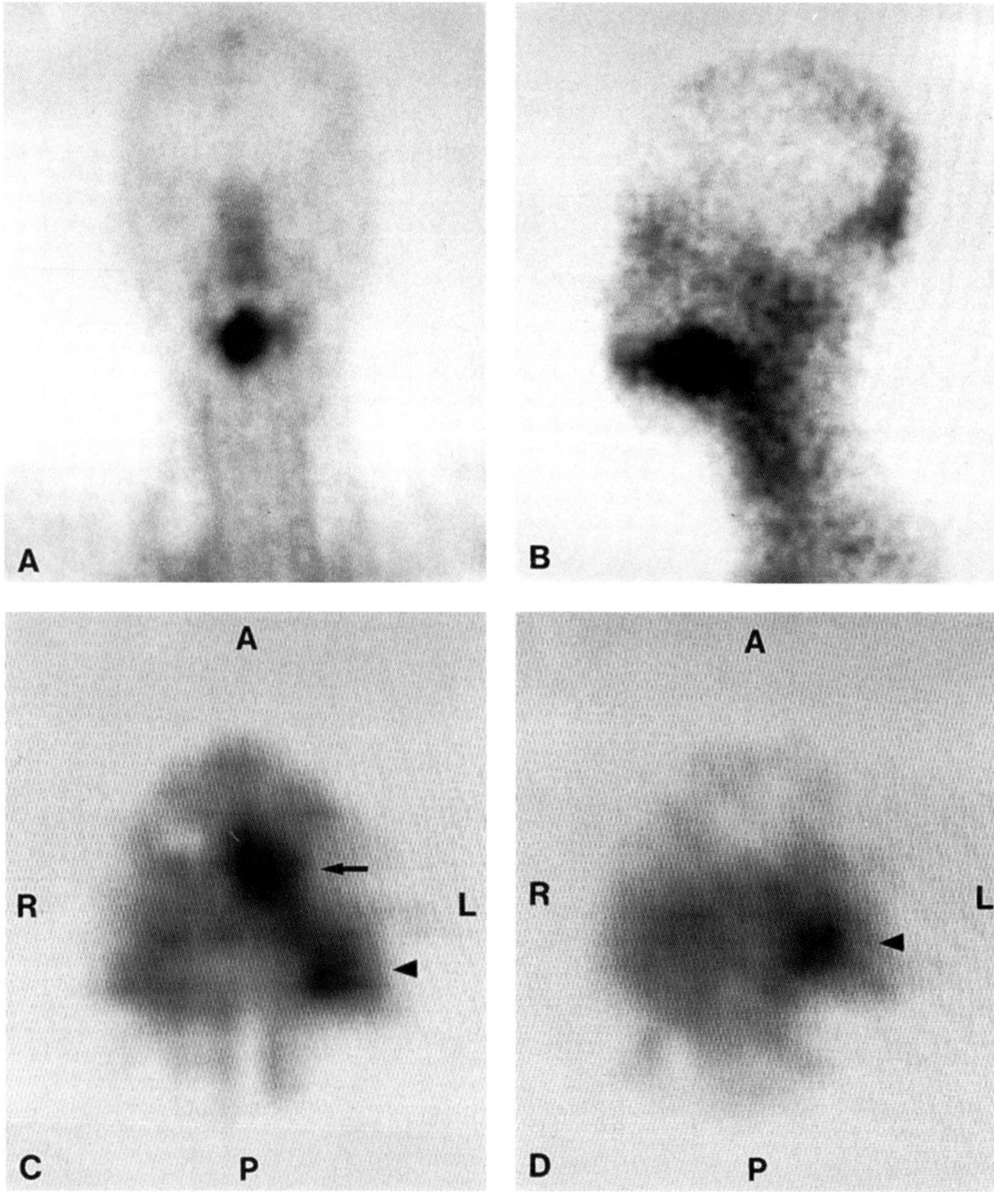


**Fig. 11.5 A–D.** Images of a head and neck cancer patient with a carcinoma of the tongue, 16h after injection of $^{99m}$Tc-labeled E48 IgG. **A** Planar anterior image. Note the high activity in the primary tumor. On this image the lymph node metastases in the left subdigastic and midjugular levels of the neck are not visualized. **B** The left lateral image shows the primary tumor in the tongue. **C** Axial SPECT images show both the primary tumor (*arrow*) and the subdigastric lymph node metastasis (*arrowhead*) in one axial plane and separately, although not clearly; **D** the midjugular lymph node metastasis (*arrowhead*) in a lower axial plane (*A* anterior, *P* posterior, *R* right, *L* left)

of 5mm and 9mm in the axial plane, with a tumor burden of 50%.

Baum et al. (1993), also using $^{99m}$Tc-labeled MAb 174H.64, found in 21 patients that the diagnostic value of RIS was comparable to that of other imaging techniques. In their group of patients 15 of 18 lymph node metastases were visualized by RIS. In 1 patient lymph node metastases were detected by RIS only. Besides that, distant metastases were present in 3 patients, 2 of whom were identified by RIS. Imaging results with MAb 174H.64 were confirmed by others (Heissler et al. 1994; Adamietz et al. 1996). De Rossi et al. (1997) used an $^{111}$In-labeled anti-CEA MAb in 20 patients and detected lymph node metastases in 18 of them. In other studies, the number of HNSCC patients with lymph node involvement was very limited (see Table 11.3).

## 11.6 Discussion

For the detection of lymph node metastases the diagnostic value of RIS with $^{99m}$Tc-labeled E48 IgG, E48 $F(ab')_2$ or U36 IgG is comparable to that of palpation, CT and MRI, as shown by the sensitivity, specificity and accuracy data in Tables 11.4 and 11.5. No clear advantage of any one of the three radioimmunoconjugates for RIS was found (no separate E48 IgG and E48 $F(ab')_2$ data are shown).

The most important question to ask about this approach is whether RIS with MAb E48 or U36 can contribute to the preoperative staging of the neck in HNSCC patients, for example by complementing other methods used to assess nodal involvement? All patients who have nodal involvement will need treatment of the regional lymphatics, while the neck needs no treatment if no metastasis is present. Recently the concept of selective neck dissection has been introduced. Selective neck dissections are used in patients with only minimal nodal disease, with the intention of reducing morbidity. A policy of selective neck dissections requires accurate presurgical assessment of the extent of nodal involvement. Another tendency is a "wait-and-see" policy for the clinically negative neck. This is only acceptable if the assessment of the status of the lymph nodes in the neck is reliably accurate. From our studies we conclude that RIS in its present form is not a diagnostic modality that could justify the above policies, because of the high percentage of false-negative scores. A total of 35 out of 316 levels and 16 out of 51 neck sides were falsely scored negative. All missed tumor-involved lymph nodes were smaller than 2 cm in diameter. Micrometastases, small involved nodes, and tumor-involved nodes containing a large proportion of keratin, necrosis, or fibrosis and only a small proportion of viable tumor cells were not diagnosed. Does this mean that the currently available MAbs are not the "magic bullets" required for detection of HNSCC? We think that there are still perspectives for RIS. This optimism of ours results from immunohistochemical analyses performed during the RIS studies described in this chapter, which revealed that MAbs E48 and U36 had targeted all tumor-involved lymph nodes, and also the deposits that were not visualized by RIS. What is more, the relative tumor uptake of the MAbs, expressed as the percentage of the injected dose per kilogram (%ID/kg), appeared to be higher in the small than in the large tumors. These data indicate that in the case of false-negative observations the MAbs were not failing per se.

## 11.7 Future Perspectives

Are there ways of improving the impact of antibody imaging for the detection of lymph node metastases? It is possible that in the coming years new MAbs will be developed that are better suited to RIS than the currently available MAbs, such as E48, U36 and 174H.64. Besides that, new approaches can be explored to improve the sensitivity, specificity and resolution of RIS. A disadvantage of RIS compared with CT and MRI, which limits its routine application, is the lack of anatomical structures for orientation. Fused images, matching images obtained by different imaging modalities, can be used to improve the interpretation of RIS. When fused with CT or MRI, RIS may benefit from the anatomical precision of these structural images. Another factor limiting the sensitivity and specificity of RIS is the long residence time of radioimmunoconjugates in the bloodstream. With respect to this, the use of smaller MAb fragments, such as Fab or Fv fragments, may lead to improvements (see Section 11.2.2). Another solution to this problem may be the use of so-called pretargeting strategies (Stoldt et al. 1997). The concept of pretargeting is based on the separation in time of antibody localization and radionuclide targeting. Several ligand–receptor systems have been evaluated, the biotin–(strept)avidin system being the most promising of these. The attractiveness of this system lies in the very high affinity of avidin and streptavidin for biotin ($Kd = 10^{-15}$ M). With this system, in a first step, a streptavidin–MAb conjugate is targeted to the tumor, and in a second step, radiolabeled biotin is administered after clearance of the MAb-conjugate from the blood. Since radiolabeled biotin is a small molecule, the radiolabel will rapidly accumulate in the tumor and will rapidly be cleared from the blood, thus resulting in high tumor-to-nontumor ratios.

One of the most challenging approaches to be explored by our group is the use of MAbs in PET technology. For this purpose MAbs must be labeled with positron-emitting radionuclides. Candidate positron emitting radionuclides for labeling are $^{18}$fluorine (half-life time 1.83 h), $^{55}$cobalt ($t_{1/2}$ = 17.5 h), $^{64}$copper ($t_{1/2}$ = 12.8 h), $^{66}$gallium ($t_{1/2}$ = 9.45 h), $^{68}$gallium ($t_{1/2}$ = 1.13 h), $^{76}$bromine ($t_{1/2}$ = 15.9 h), $^{89}$zirconium ($t_{1/2}$ = 78.4 h) and $^{124}$iodine ($t_{1/2}$ = 100.3 h). Most of these radionuclides have a short half-life and can be used in combination with MAb fragments or in pretargeting approaches. In contrast, $^{89}$Zr and $^{124}$I are particularly suitable when used in combination with intact MAbs, since their half-lives fit in well with the half-lives of intact MAbs in serum after injection. $^{124}$I-labeled MAbs have been successfully used for imaging of tumors in animals and humans (Wilson et al. 1991; Larson et al. 1992; Kairemo 1993). Disadvantages of $^{124}$I are its limited availability and the hard $\beta^+$-energy and the hard $\gamma$-photons emitted in coincidence with the positrons, which can interfere with the 511-keV signals. Therefore, at our institute effort is concentrated on the development of $^{89}$Zr-MAb conjugates for the detection of tumors with PET and for quantification of targeted MAbs and their kinetics. To this end, facile procedures for the production of highly pure no-carrier-added $^{89}$Zr and for the coupling of $^{89}$Zr to MAbs have been developed (Meijs et al. 1994, 1997). Studies in tumor-bearing nude mice have shown that $^{89}$Zr-labeled MAbs can easily be visualized with a PET camera, allowing detection of tumors as small as 50 mg. On the basis of these preliminary results we are hopeful that antibody PET may emerge as superior to conventional antibody-SPECT in sensitivity, resolution and quantification. In our department, preparations are in progress for a comparative evaluation of palpation, CT, MRI, $^{18}$FDG-PET and $^{89}$Zr-MAb-PET in the detection of primary and metastatic head and neck tumors.

## References


Adamietz IA, Baum RP, Schemman F, Niesen A, Knecht R, Saran F, Tieku S, Boniface GR, Hör G, Böttcher HD (1996) Improvement of radiation treatment planning in squamous-cell head and neck cancer by immuno-SPECT. J Nucl Med 37:1942–1946

Ali S, Tiwari RM, Snow GB (1985) False positive and false negative neck nodes Head Neck Surg 8:78–82

Balm AJM, Hageman PC, Mulder CJ, Hilkens J (1992) Carcinoma-associated monoclonal antibodies in head and neck carcinoma: immunohistochemistry and biodistribution of monoclonal antibodies 175F4 and 175F11. Eur Arch Otorhinolaryngol 249:237–242

Baum RP, Adams S, Kiefer J, Niesen A, Knecht R, Howaldt H-P, Hertel A, Adamietz IA, Sykes T, Boniface GR, Noujaim AA, Hör G (1993) A novel Technetium-99m labeled monoclonal antibody (174H.64) for staging head and neck cancer by immuno-SPECT. Acta Oncol 32:747–751

Behr TM, Sharkey RM, Juweid ME, Dunn RM, Ying Z, Zhang CH, Siegel JA, Goldenberg DM (1997) Variables influencing tumor dosimetry in radioimmunotherapy of CEA-expressing cancers with anti-CEA and antimucin monoclonal antibodies. J Nucl Med 38:409–418

Boeheim K, Speak JA, Frei E, Bernal SD (1985) SQM1 antibody defines a surface membrane antigen in squamous carcinoma of the head and neck. Int J Cancer 36:137–142

Boucher Y and Jain RK (1992) Microvascular pressure is the principal driving force for interstitial hypertension in solid tumors: implications for vascular collapse. Cancer Res 52:5110–5114

Breitz HB, Sullivan K, Nelp WB (1993) Imaging lung cancer with radiolabeled antibodies. Semin Nucl Med 23:127–132

Chang K, Pastan I, Willingham MC (1992) Frequent expression of the tumor antigen CAK1 in squamous-cell carcinomas. Int J Cancer 51:548–554

Cobb LM (1989) Intratumour factors influencing the access of antibody to tumour cells. Cancer Immunol Immunother 28:235–240

Collier BD, Abdel-Nabi H, Doerr RJ, Harwood SJ, Olson J, Kaplan EH, Winzelberg GG, Grossman SJ, Krag DN, Mitchell EP (1992) Immunoscintigraphy performed with In-111-labeled CYT-103 in the management of colorectal cancer. Radiol 185:179–186

De Bree R, Roos JC, Quak JJ, Den Hollander W, Snow GB, Van Dongen GAMS (1994a) Clinical screening of monoclonal antibodies 323/A3, cSF-25, and K928 for suitability of targeting tumors in the upper-aerodigestive and respiratory tract. Nucl Med Commun 15:613–627

De Bree R, Roos JC, Quak JJ, Den Hollander W, Van den Brekel MWM, Van de Wal JE, Snow GB, Van Dongen GAMS (1994b) Clinical imaging of head and neck cancer with $^{99m}$Tc-labeled monoclonal antibody E48 IgG or $F(ab')_2$. J Nucl Med 35:775–783

De Bree R, Roos JC, Quak JJ, Den Hollander W, Snow GB, Van Dongen GAMS (1995) Radioimmunoscintigraphy with $^{99m}$Tc-labeled monoclonal antibody U36 and its biodistribution in patients with head and neck cancer. Clin Cancer Res 1:591–598

Delaloye AB, Delaloye B (1995) Tumor imaging with monoclonal antibodies. Semin Nucl Med 25:144–164

De Rossi G, Maurizi M, Almadori G, Di Giuda D, Paludetti G, Cadoni G, Ottaviani F, Galli J (1997) The contribution of immunoscintigraphy to the diagnosis of head and neck tumors. Bucl Med Commun 18:10–16

Divgi CR, Welt S, Kris M, Real FX, Yeh SDJ, Gralla R, Merchant B, Schweighart S, Unger M, Larson SM, Mendelsohn J (1991) Phase I and imaging trial of Indium-111-labeled anti-epidermal growth factor receptor monoclonal antibody 225 in patients with squamous cell lung carcinoma. J Natl Cancer Inst 83:97–104

Doerr RJ, Abdel-Nabi H, Krag D, Mitchell E (1991) Radiolabeled antibody imaging in the management of colorectal cancer. Results of a multicenter clinical study. Ann Surg 214:118–124

Dominquez JM, Wolff BG, Nelson H, Forstrom LA, Mullan BP (1996) $^{111}$In-CYT-103 scanning in recurrent colorectal cancer – does it affect standard management? Dis Colon Rectum 39:514–519

Hawkins RE, Llewelyn MB, Russell SJ (1992) Adapting antibodies for clinical use. BMJ 305:1348–1352

Hazra DK, Britton KE, Lahiri VL, Gupta AK, Khanna P, Saran S (1995) Immunotechnological trends in radioimmunotargeting: from "magic bullet" to "smart bomb". Nucl Med Commun 16:66–75

Heider K-H, Sproll M, Susani S, Patzelt E, Beaumier P, Ostermann E, Ahorn H, Adolf GR (1996) Characterization of a high-affinity monoclonal antibody specific for CD44v6 as candidate for immunotherapy of squamous cell carcinomas. Cancer Immunol Immunother 43:245–253

Heissler E, Grünert B, Barzen G, Fritsche L, Hell B, Felix R, Bier J (1994) Radioimmunoscintigraphy of squamous cell carcinoma in the head and neck region. Int J Oral Maxillofac Surg 23:149–152

Inoue M, Nakanishi K, Sasagawa T, Tanizawa O, Inoue H, Hakura A (1990) A novel monoclonal antibody against squamous cell carcinoma. Jpn J Cancer Res 81:176–182

Jain RK (1987) Transport of molecules in the tumor interstitium: a review. Cancer Res 47:3039–3051

Jain RK (1988) Determinants of tumor blood flow: a review. Cancer Res 48:2641–2658

Jain RK (1990) Vascular and interstitial barriers to delivery of therapeutic agents in tumors. Cancer Metastasis Rev 9:253–266

Kairemo KJA (1993) Positron emission tomography of monoclonal antibodies Acta Oncol 32:825–830

Kairemo KJA, Hopsu EVM (1990a) Imaging of tumours in the parotid region with Indium-111-labelled monoclonal antibody reacting with carcinoembryonic antigen. Acta Oncol 29:539–543

Kairemo KJA, Hopsu EVM (1990b) Imaging of pharyngeal and laryngeal carcinomas with Indium-111-labeled monoclonal anti-CEA antibodies. Laryngoscope 100:1077–1082

Kimmel KA, Carey TE (1986) Altered expression in squamous cells of an orientation restricted epithelial antigen detected by monoclonal antibody A9. Cancer Res 46:3614–3623

Köhler G, Milstein C (1975) Continuous cultures of fused cells secreting antibody of predefined specificity. Nature 256:495–497

Larson SM, Pentlow KS, Volkow ND, Wolf AP, Finn RD, Lambrecht RM, Graham MC, Di Resta G, Bendriem B, Daghighian F, Yeh SDJ, Wang G-J, Cheung N-KV (1992) PET scanning of Iodine-124-3F9 as an approach to tumor dosimetry during treatment planning for radioimmunotherapy in a child with neuroblastoma. J Nucl Med 33:2020–2023

Maraveyas A, Stafford N, Rowlinson-Busza G, Stewart JSW, Epenetos AA (1995) Pharmacokinetics, biodistribution, and dosimetry of specific and control radiolabeled monoclonal antibodies in patients with primary head and neck squamous cell carcinoma. Cancer Res 55:1060–1069

Mattes MJ, Griffiths GL, Diril H, Goldenberg DM, Ong GL, Shih LB (1994) Processing of antibody-radioisotope conjugates after binding to the surface of tumor cells. Cancer 73:787–793

Meijs WE, Herscheid JDM, Haisma HJ, Wijbrandts R, Van Langevelde F, Van Leuffen PJ, Mooy R, Pinedo HM (1994) Production of highly pure no-carrier-added zirconium-89 for the labelling of antibodies with a positron emitter. Appl Radiat Isot 45:1143–1147

Meijs WE, Haisma HJ, Klok RP, Van Gog FB, Kievit E, Pinedo HM, Herscheid JDM (1997) Zirconium 88/89 labeled monoclonal antibodies: distribution in tumor-bearing nude mice. J Nucl Med 38:112–118

Moffat FL Jr, Pinsky CM, Hammershaimb L, Petrelli NJ, Patt YZ, Whaley FS, Goldenberg DM (1996) Clinical utility of external radioimmunoscintigraphy with the IMMU-4 technetium-99m Fab′ antibody fragment in patients undergoing surgery for carcinoma of the colon and rectum: results of a pivotal, phase III trial. The Immunomedics Study Group. J Clin Oncol 14:2295–2305

Murthy U, Basu A, Rodeck U, Herlyn M, Ross AH, Das M (1987) Binding of an antagonistic monoclonal antibody to an intact and fragmented EGF-receptor polypeptide. Arch Biochem Biophys 252:549–560

Myoken Y, Moroyama T, Miyauchi S, Takada K, Namba M (1987) Monoclonal antibodies against human oral squamous cell carcinoma reacting with keratin proteins. Cancer 60:2927–2937

Parker SL, Tong T, Bolden S, Wingo PA (1996) Cancer statistics 1996. CA Cancer J Clin 65:5–27

Quak JJ, Van Dongen GAMS, Balm AJM, Brakkee JPG, Scheper RJ, Snow GB, Meijer CJLM (1990a) A 22-kDa surface antigen detected by monoclonal antibody E48 is exclusively expressed in stratified squamous and transitional epithelia. Am J Pathol 136:191–197

Quak JJ, Van Dongen GAMS, Gerretsen M, Hayashida D, Balm AJM, Brakkee JPG, Snow GB, Meijer CJLM (1990b) Production of monoclonal antibody (K931) to a squamous cell carcinoma antigen identified as the 17-1A antigen. Hybridoma 9:377–387

Quak JJ, Schrijvers AHGJ, Brakkee JGP, Davis HD, Scheper RJ, Balm AJM, Meijer CJLM, Snow GB, Van Dongen GAMS (1992) Expression and characterization of two differentiation antigens in stratified squamous epithelia and carcinomas. Int J Cancer 50:507–513

Samuel J, Noujaim AA, Willans DJ, Brzezinska GS, Haines DM, Longenecker BM (1989) A novel marker for basal (stem) cells of mammalian stratified squamous epithelia and squamous cell carcinoma. Cancer Res 49:2465–2470

Schrijvers AHGJ, Quak JJ, Uyterlinde AM, Van Walsum M, Meijer CJLM, Snow GB, Van Dongen GAMS (1993) MAb U36, a novel monoclonal antibody successful in immunotargeting of squamous cell carcinoma of the head and neck. Cancer Res 53:4383–4390

Shah JP, Strong E, Vikram B (1981) Neck dissection: current status and future possibilities. Bulletin 11:25–33

Soo KC, Ward M, Roberts KR, Keeling F, Carter RL, McCready VR, Ott RJ, Powell E, Ozanne B, Westwood JH, Gusterson BA (1987) Radioimmunoscintigraphy of squamous carcinomas of the head and neck. Head Neck Surg 9:349–352

Stoldt HS, Aftab F, Chinol M, Paganelli G, Luca F, Testori A, Geraghty JG (1997) Pretargeting strategies for radioimmunoguided tumour localization and therapy. Eur J Cancer 33:186–192

Surwit EA, Childers JM, Krag DN, Katterhagen JG, Gallion HH, Waggoner S, Mann WJ (1993) Clinical assessment of 111In-CYT-103 immunoscintigraphy in ovarian cancer. Gynecol Oncol 48:285–292

Takahashi H, Wilson B, Ozturk M, Motte P, Straus W, Isselbacher KJ, Wands JR (1988) In vivo localization of human colon adenocarcinoma by monoclonal antibody binding to a highly expressed cell surface antigen. Cancer Res 48:6573–6579

Timon CI, McShane D, Hamilton D, Walsh MA (1991) Head and neck cancer localization with Indium labelled carcinoembryonic antigen: a pilot project. J Otolaryngol 20:283–287

Tranter RMD, Fairwheather DS, Bradwell AR, Dykes PW, Watson-James S, Chandler S (1984) The detection of squamous cell tumours of the head and neck using radio-labelled antibodies. J Laryngol Otol 98:71–74

Van den Brekel MWM, Stel HV, Castelijns JA, Nauta JJP, Van der Waal I, Valk J, Golding RP, Meijer CJLM, Snow GB (1990) Cervical lymph node metastases – assessment of radiological criteria. Radiology 177:379–384

Van den Brekel MWM, Castelijns JA, Stel HV, Golding RP, Meijer CJLM, Snow GB (1993) Modern imaging techniques and ultrasound guided aspiration cytology for the assessment of the neck node metastases: a prospective comparative study. Eur Arch Otorhinolaryngol 250:11–17

Verbruggen AM (1990) Radiopharmaceuticals: state of the art. Eur J Nucl Med 17:346–364

Watkinson JC, Johnston D, Jones N, Coady M, Allen S, Hibbert J (1990) The reliability of palpation in the assessment of tumours. Clin Otolaryngol 15:2–9

Wilson CB, Snook DE, Dhokia B, Taylor CV, Watson IA, Lammertsma AA, Lambrecht R, Waxman J, Jones T, Epenetos AA (1991) Quantitative measurement of monoclonal antibody distribution and blood flow using positron emission tomography and 124-iodine in patients with breast cancer. Int J Cancer 47:344–347

Yoshiura M, Murakami H, Tashiro H, Kurisu K (1993) Production of a human monoclonal antibody to normal basal and squamous cell carcinoma-associated antigen. J Oral Pathol Med 22:451–458

Zarbo RJ and Crissman JD (1988) The surgical pathology of head and neck cancer. Semin Oncol 15:10–19

Zuckier LS, DeNardo GL (1997) Trials and tribulations: oncological antibody imaging comes to the fore. Semin Nucl Med 27:10–29

# 12 T2-Weighted Gradient Echo Imaging of the Inner Ear and Inner Auditory Canal

L. Jäger

CONTENTS



MR imaging of the inner ear and the inner auditory canal has become standard clinical procedure in patients with hearing and vestibular problems. Recent advances in MR technology have led to the development of new sequences with in-plane resolutions far below 1 mm, thereby improving the sensitivity and specificity of the diagnosis of pathology in this region. However, only a minority of subjects with sensorineural hearing loss (SNHL) show suggestive MR findings (Casselman et al. 1996). The standard MR investigation of the labyrinth and the cerebellopontine angle consists of a high-resolution T1-weighted spin-echo (SE) sequence before contrast in an axial projection and after the administration of contrast in axial and coronal projections, and in the sagittal projection if needed. The T1-weighted SE sequence is followed by a high-resolution T2-weighted steady state gradient echo sequence, such as the constructive interference in steady state (CISS) sequence. This sequence has proven its significance in delineating inner ear anatomy and pathology and has gained in popularity over the last few years (Arnold et al. 1996; Casselmann et al. 1993a,b, 1994, 1997; Eberhardt et al. 1995; Jäger et al. 1997). In this chapter the basic technical principles and limitations of the CISS sequence and the indications for its application are discussed.

L. Jäger, M.D., Institut für Radiologische Diagnostik, Klinikum Grosshadern, der Ludwig-Maximilians-Universität Munchen, Marchioninistrasse 15, D-81366 München, Germany

## 12.1 Basic Principles of the 3D-CISS Sequence

The 3D CISS sequence is a gradient echo sequence consisting of two true FISP (fast imaging with steady state precession) sequences (Deimling and Laub 1989). All gradients are focused in true FISP sequences (Haacke et al. 1990, 1991). Because the signals of both FISP sequences are summed, fluids, such as endo- and perilymph and cerebrospinal fluid (CSF) appear bright, even when moving fast.

Steady state precession sequences utilize an extra refocusing gradient with an opposite sign to the regular phase-encoding gradient, instead of a spoiler gradient. The steady state is achieved by a short repetition time (TR << T2*). If the TR is much shorter than the T2*, then the persisting transverse magnetization is added to the magnetization regained by T1 relaxation over the TR interval. This enhanced magnetization is finally shifted back into the transversal magnetization by radio frequency (RF) pulses, and tissues with a small T1/T2* ratio (e.g., liquids) appear with high signal intensity. The steady state may be disturbed by moving spins of different velocity along field gradients, because they gather additional phase shifts, which reduce or delete the transverse magnetization. If these flow-induced phase shifts accumulate over several TR intervals, the signal of CSF or of the endo- and perilymph will diminish and finally disappear. This means that motion destroys the residual transverse magnetization and moving fluids will also eventually lose their signal. In order to avoid these phase shifts, a flow compensation for each gradient and each TR interval is needed. If the gradients (Gx, Gy, Gz) are balanced (Patz 1988), as in true FISP sequences, the average value for each gradient will be zero. Therefore, spins moving at a constant velocity will experience no additional shift in phase during the application of gradient pulses. A true FISP sequence involves the refocusing of all three gradients (Haacke et al. 1991), whereas an original FISP sequence (Oppelt et al. 1986) involves the refocusing of only the phase dispersion.

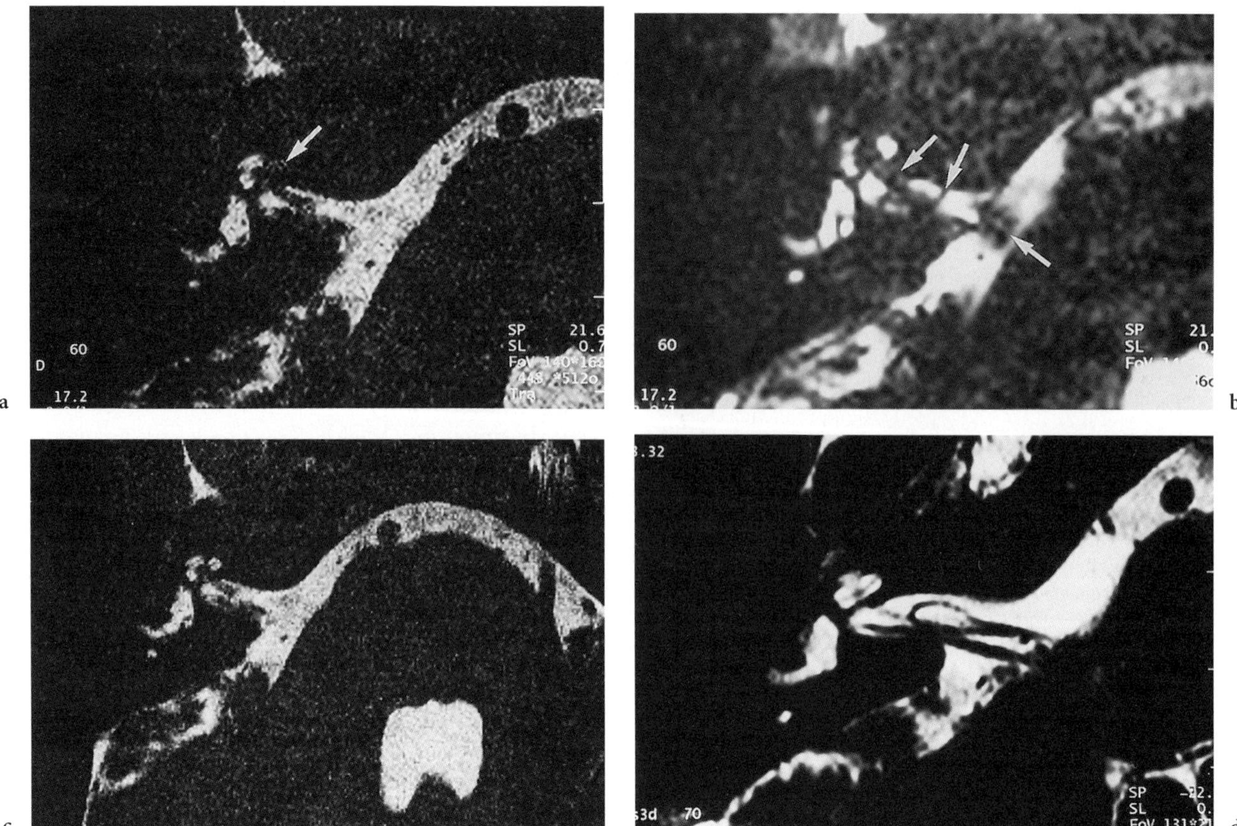


**Fig. 12.1 a.** Axial, T2-weighted 3D CISS images with **a** alternating and **b** nonalternating radio frequency (RF) pulses. Stripes of signal loss (*arrows*) are shifted. **c** These stripes disappeared completely in the calculated postprocessed image. **d** Currently, a 3D CISS sequence is already performing the acquisition of both (alternating and the nonalternating) RF pulses and the final calculation in one step

A major disadvantage of true FISP sequences is their high sensitivity to off-resonance effects, which occur particularly in inhomogenities of magnetic fields. For example, frequency shifts caused by susceptibility changes lead to stripes of signal loss. The black stripes are due to a phase shift of π or an odd multiple of π at a certain location, with a subsequent loss of magnetization. At other locations, the signal of subsequent pulses are in phase because the signal offset is 2π or a multiple of that and the magnetization will be added in stead of cancelled. The phenomenon of stripes of signal loss can be reduced, but not eliminated, by shortening TR. To avoid stripes of signal loss altogether, the acquisition of two true FISP sequences with an alternating and a nonalternating RF pulse is required. This procedure will cause the shift of the signal loss stripes to a location between the data sets of the alternating and nonalternating RF pulses. By taking the maximum value out of two images on a pixel base, an image is obtained without the field inhomogeneity artifacts. Such a combined image is called a CISS image.

Both data acquisitions finally undergo mathematical postprocessing, and the stripes of signal loss disappear in the calculated CISS image (Deimling and Laub 1989) (Fig. 12.1). One drawback of this procedure is that it causes the CISS sequence to be highly susceptible to movements made by the patient during data acquisition.

In order to reduce the artifacts of the T2-weighted steady state gradient echo sequence (e.g., 3D CISS sequence) while still maintaining the high-resolution images, a high-end MR system is needed. To obtain an optimal 3D CISS image, a large excitation angle with an ultrashort TR is needed. This constellation results in a high power deposition. Since the 3D CISS sequence is susceptible to patient movement, the acquisition time should be kept short. Typical imaging protocols for a 1-T and a 1.5-T MR system are given in Tables 12.1 and 12.2. Even with the ultrashort TR and the application of alternating and non-

**Table 12.1.** 3D CISS (three-dimensional constructive interference in steady state) protocols for 1-T (Harmony, Siemens Medical Systems, Erlangen, Germany) and 1.5-T (Vision, Siemens Medical Systems, Erlangen, Germany) MR systems. Currently, a 3D CISS sequence consists of one sequence with two sections. One section has an alternating and the other has a nonalternating radio frequency (RF) pulse

| | 1 T | 1.5 T | 1.5 T |
|---|---|---|---|
| Repetition time (TR) | 17 ms | 12.25 ms | 12.25 ms |
| Echo time (TE) | 8.08 ms | 5.9 ms | 5.9 ms |
| Excitation angle | 70° | 70° | 70° |
| Slab thickness | 41.6 mm | 40 mm | 33.6 mm |
| Effective slice thickness | 0.8 mm | 0.8 mm | 0.51 mm |
| Number of partitions | 52 | 50 | 66 |
| Matrix | 256 × 256 | 320 × 512 | 448 × 512 |
| Field of view (FoV) | 8/8 of 160 mm | 5/8 of 260 mm | 7/8 of 160 mm |
| Pixel size | 0.63 × 0.63 mm | 0.51 × 0.51 mm | 0.31 × 0.31 mm |
| Number of acquisitions | 1 | 1 | 1 |
| Acquisition time | 7 min 34 s | 6 min 33 s | 12 min 56 s |

**Table 12.2.** Recommended imaging planes in relation to anatomical structures

| Projection plane | Region of interest |
|---|---|
| Axial | All structures of the labyrinth, the VIIth and VIIIth cranial nerves, and the cerebellopontine angle |
| Coronal | Internal auditory canal, VIIth and VIIIth cranial nerves, cochlea, vestibule, anterior and lateral semicircular canals, and vascular |
| Sagittal | Loops in the cerebellopontine angle Vestibule, lateral and posterior semicircular canals, the tympanic and mastoid part of the VIIth cranial nerve, endolymphatic duct and sac, andvascular loops in the cerebellopontine angle |

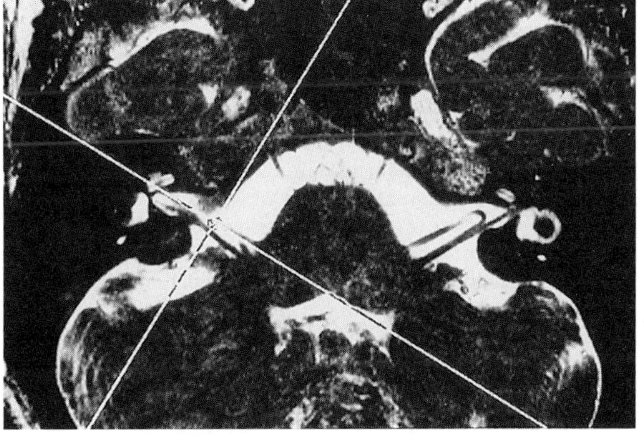

**Fig. 12.2.** Axial, T2-weighted 3D CISS image with both planning axes for the MPR procedure, to achieve reformatted oblique coronal and sagittal images of the right internal auditory canal

alternating RF pulses, there remain slight frequency offsets are areas with strong susceptibility changes and at the borders of the 3D volume slab. When a T2-weighted steady state gradient echo sequence (e.g., the 3D CISS sequence) is used, it is necessary to balance various factors in order to maintain image quality. In other words, it is important to avoid motion artifacts by reducing the acquisition time, while maintaining image quality by utilizing a high signal-to-noise ratio, a high in-plane resolution and diminishing off-resonance effects.

T2-weighted steady state gradient echo imaging is performed in an axial projection. A circular polarized or a phased array head coil is used to image the inner ear and the cerebellopontine angle on both sides simultaneously. Commonly used postimaging reconstruction procedures include the maximum intensity procedure (MIP) and multiplanar reconstruction (MPR). The diagnostic values of 3D MIP and 3D MPR are different. A 3D MIP will result in a clear 3D view of the labyrinth, allowing for the delineation of gross pathology. However, three disadvantages are associated with the MIP procedure: (1) discrete pathology may be missed; (2) it cannot be used to view the internal auditory canal and the cerebellopontine angle; and (3) it is very time consuming. In contrast, MPR is of great value in diagnosis of the pathology of the labyrinth, the internal auditory canal and the cerebellopontine angle. With MPR, oblique projection planes can be easily reconstructed and all three projections (Px, Py, Pz), which are perpendicular to each other, can be visualized simultaneously (Fig. 12.2). The importance of MPR becomes obvious in the evaluation of the semicircular canals and in the detection of a vessel nerve contact in the cerebellopontine angle (Table 12.2).

## 12.2 Anatomy

T2-weighted steady state gradient echo images, depending on the excitation angle and TR, show fluids as a bright signal (Casselman et al. 1993; Jäger et al. 1997; Stillman et al. 1994). Therefore, CSF and the lymph in the lymphatic space of the labyrinth are hyperintense. Differentiation between peri- and endolymph is not possible, however. All other nonliquid structures surrounded by CSF or in the lymphatic space are hypointense, including nerves, vessels, tumors, fibrous tissue and bony structures of the inner ear.

The facial nerve (VIIth cranial nerve) and the vestibulocochlear nerve (VIIIth cranial nerve) run from the brain stem to the internal auditory canal (Fig. 12.3). The facial nerve is rostral to the vestibulocochlear nerve. In the lateral third of the internal auditory canal, the vestibulocochlear nerve is divided into the cochlear nerve and the superior and inferior part of the vestibular nerve. The facial

**Fig. 12.3a–h.** Axial, T2-weighted 3D CISS images. **a,b** The anterior semicircular canal is shown (*arrows*). **c** The posterior semicircular canal (*small arrow*) and a part of the vestibule (*large arrow*) are shown. **d** The facial nerve (*long black arrow*) and the superior part of the vestibular nerve (*short black arrow*) are delineated as a hypointense course in the cerebellopontine angle, surrounded by the hyperintense CSF. The lymph-filled space in the labyrinth is hyperintense: vestibule (*long white arrow*), lateral semicircular canal (*small wide white arrow*), posterior semicircular canal (*short small white arrow*). The ampullary crest of the lateral semicircular canal is hypointense (*curved white arrow*). **e** The lateral part of the first segment of the facial nerve is hypointense (*black arrow*). The cochlear nerve (*long white arrow*) and the inferior part of the vestibular nerve (*short white arrow*) are hypointense and shown in a V-shaped configuration. The osseous modiolus of the cochlea is also hypointense (*small wide white arrow*). **f** The scala vestibuli (*arrowhead*) and the scala tympani (*short arrow*) are hyperintense, separated by the basilar membrane and the osseous spiral lamina (*long arrow*), which are hypointense. The entrance of the vestibular nerve into the vestibule is shown as a hypointense course (*small wide arrow*). The ampullary crest of the lateral semicircular canal is hypointense (*curved white arrow*). **g** The posterior semicircular canal is hyperintense (*long arrow*). The osseous modiolus of the cochlea is hypointense (*small wide arrow*). **h** The hypointense modiolus (*small wide arrow*) is surrounded by the hyperintense scala vestibuli and tympani and the hypointense osseous spiral lamina and the basilar membrane. The helicotrema is shown at the top of the cochlea (*long arrow*). **i,j** Coronal, T2-weighted 3D CISS images reformatted by the multiplanar reconstruction (MPR) procedure. **i** The lymphatic space is hyperintense: anterior semicircular canal (*short white arrow*), vestibule (*long white arrow*), lateral semicircular canal (*short wide white arrow*) and a part of the cochlear canal (*curved white arrow*). The superior part (*black arrowhead*) and the inferior part (*short black arrow*) of the vestibular nerve are hypointense, as is the crista falciformis (*long black arrow*). **j** The facial nerve (*black arrowhead*) and the cochlear nerve (*small black arrow*) are hypointense, surrounded by the hyperintense CSF. In between is a hypointense loop of the anterior infetior cerebellar artery (AICA; *long black arrow*). Modiolus (*short wide white arrow*) and the osseous spiral lamina (*long white arrow*) are also hypointense. The scala vestibuli (*white arrowhead*) and the scala tympani (*short white arrow*) are hyperintense, as they are filled with lymph. **K** Sagittal, T2-weighted 3D-CISS image reformatted by the MPR procedure. The cochlea (*curved white arrow*) and a sagittal cut through the internal auditory canal (*IAC*) are shown. The VIIth and the VIIIth cranial nerves are hypointense, surrounded by the hyperintense CSF. Rostrally in the IAC is the facial nerve (*long white arrow*). Caudal to the facial nerve is the cochlear nerve (*long thin white arrow*). The superior part (*black arrowhead*) and the inferior part (*small white arrow*) of the vestibular nerve are posterior to the facial and cochlear nerve. **l** Sagittal, T2-weighted 3D CISS image reformatted by the MPR procedure. A sagittal slice through the IAC is shown, as is the cochlea. The common crus (*small wide arrow*) and the anterior (*small arrow*) and the posterior (*long white arrow*) semicircular canal can be delineated. **m** Axial, T2-weighted 3D CISS image. The anterior (*curved arrow*) and the posterior (*long arrow*) semicircular canal are shown. The endolymphatic sac (*small wide arrow*) and the endolymphatic duct (*small arrow*) are delineated. **n** Sagittal, T2-weighted 3D-CISS image reformatted by the MPR procedure. The endolymphatic duct (*small arrow*), the common crus (*small thin arrow*), the anterior semicircular canal (*curved arrow*), the lateral semicircular canal (*thin arrows*) and the vestibule (*small wide arrow*) are shown. **o,p** Coronal, T2-weighted 3D CISS images reformatted by the MPR procedure. **o** The cochlea is shown in its apical section (*arrow*). **p** The cochlea is shown in its basal section (*small wide arrow*) as are the vestibule (*small arrow*) and the lateral (*long arrow*) and the superior (*curved arrow*) semicircular canal. **q,r** Cranio-caudal and caudo-cranial view, T2-weighted 3D-CISS image reformatted by the maximum intensity procedure (MIP). **q** The IAC (*small open arrow*), the cochlea (*large open arrow*), the vestibule and the anterior semicircular canal (*small arrow*) and the lateral (*curved arrow*) and the posterior semicircular canal (*small wide arrow*) are shown. **r** The IAC (*small open arrow*), the cochlea (*large open arrow*), the vestibule (*small arrow*), the lateral (*curved arrow*) and the posterior semicircular canal (*small wide arrow*) and the anterior (*long thin arrow*) semicircular canal are shown. **s** Coronal, T2-weighted 3D-CISS image. This patient is suffering from vertigo dependent on the head position. Vestibular tests have suggested pathology of the anterior semicircular canal. On the reformatted coronal projection of the 3D-CISS images the left anterior semicircular canal is easily distinguished. No bony structure can be delineated between the left anterior semicircular canal (*arrow*) and the left middle cranial fossa. This finding argues for vertigo induced by a rise in intracranial pressure, which is transmitted to the vestibular system. **t,** Axial, T2-weighted 3D-CISS images. The ampullary crest of the lateral semicircular canal is hypointense (*arrow*) and surrounded by the lymph in the ampulla

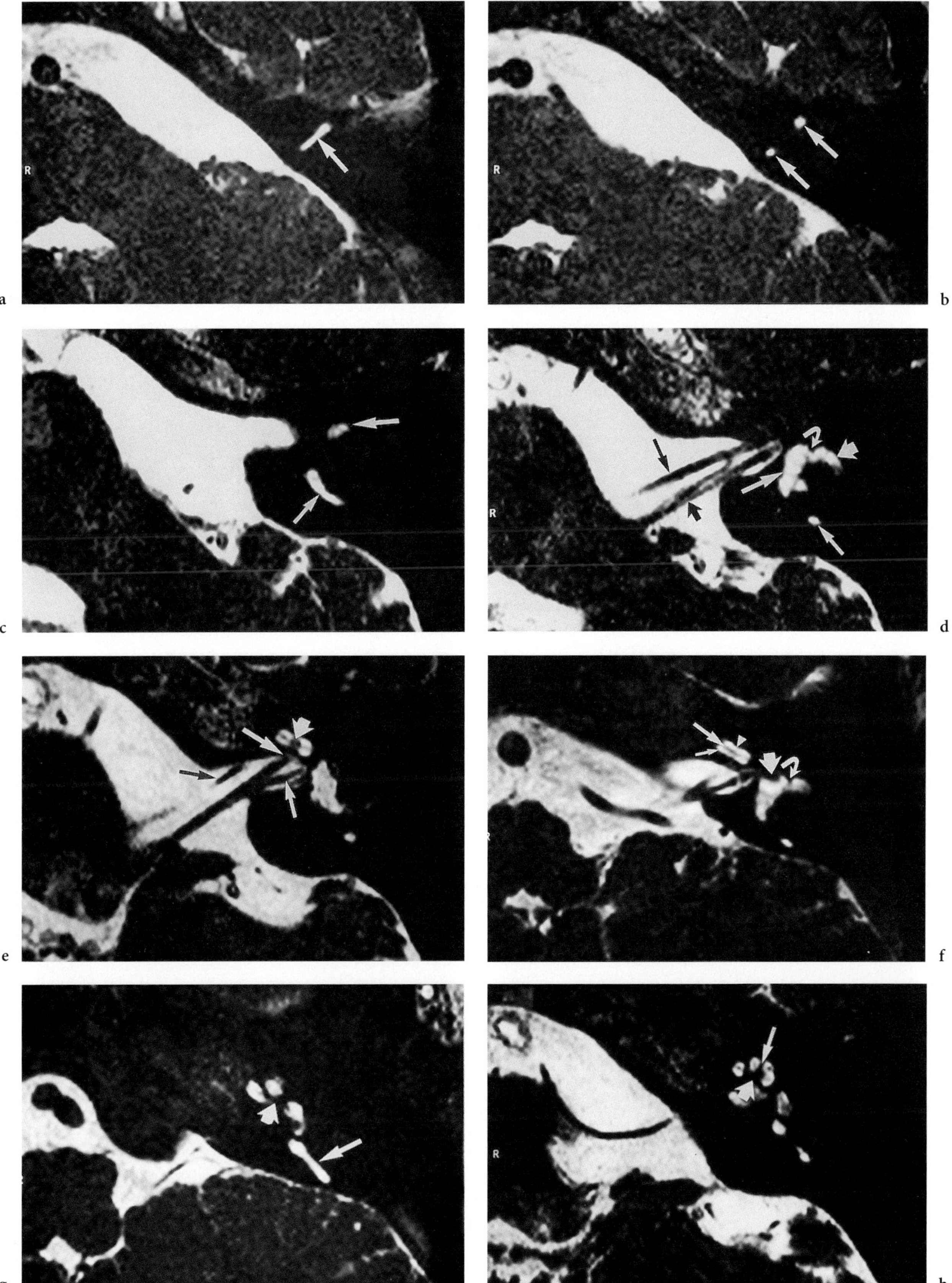


**Fig. 12.3.** *Continued*

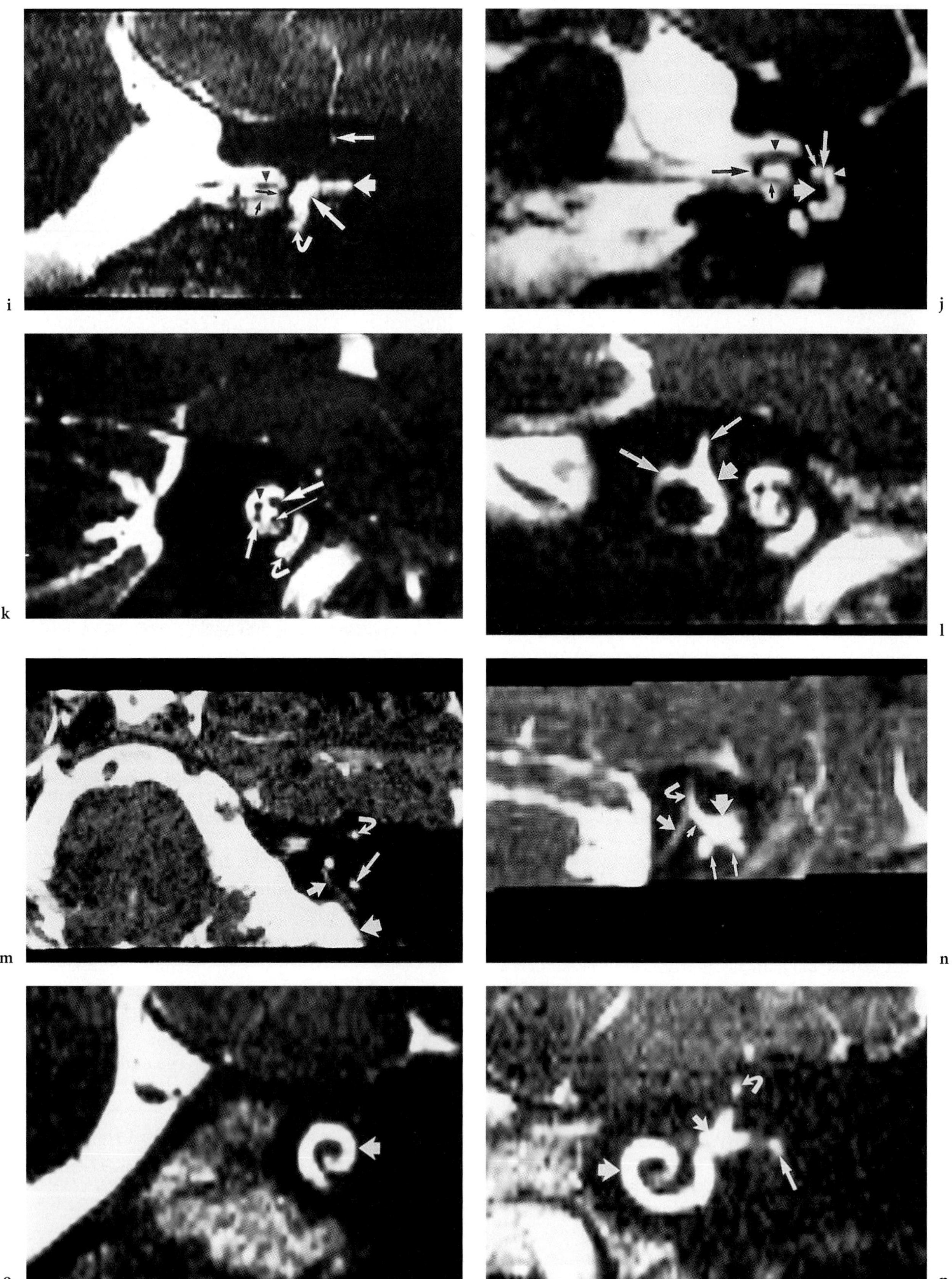


**Fig. 12.3** *Continued*

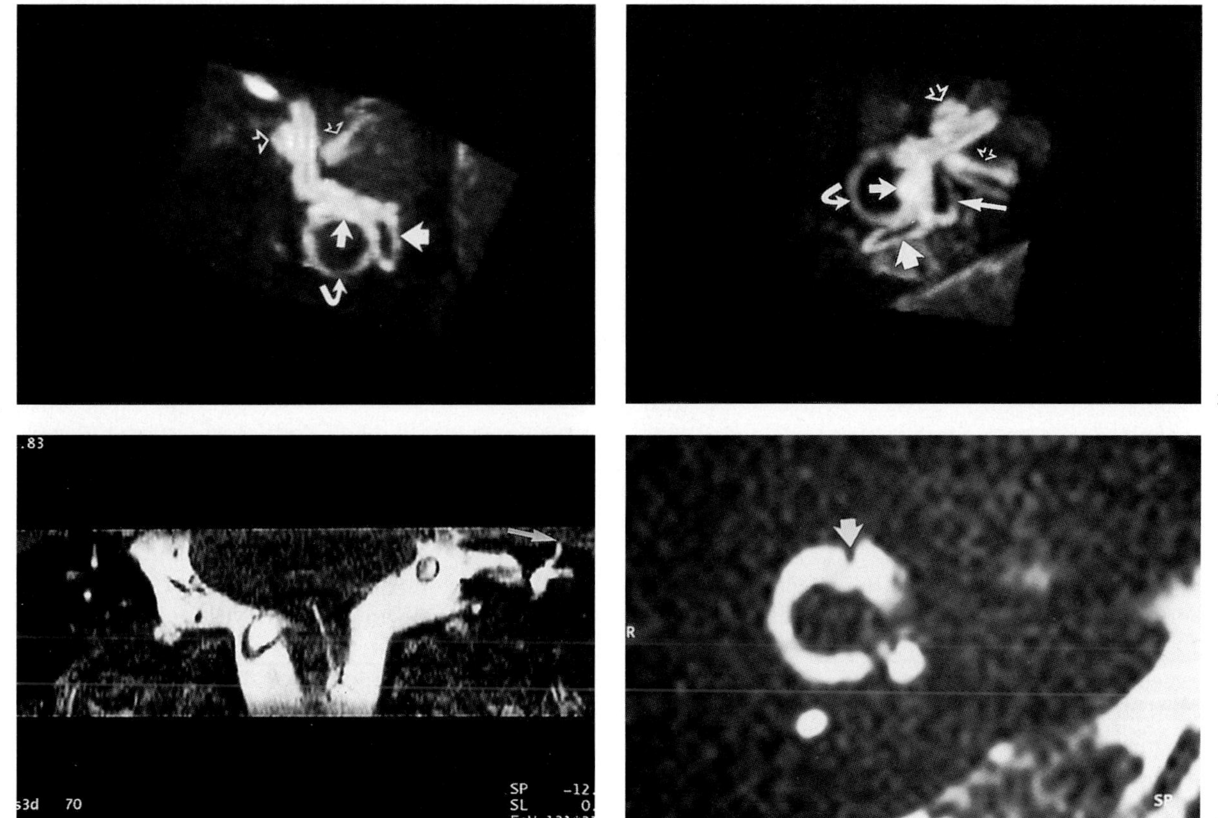


**Fig. 12.3** *Continued*

nerve runs rostrally and parallel to the superior part of the vestibular nerve. The cochlear nerve splits off from the inferior part of the vestibular nerve and runs anterior to the inferior part of the vestibular nerve in a V-shaped configuration and inferior to the facial nerve (Casselman et al. 1993; Rubinstein et al. 1996).

On reformatted coronal MPR images the vertical crest (Bill's bar) and the transverse crest can be delineated. The entrance of the cochlear nerve into the modiolus can also be depicted (Fig. 12.3). The modiolus appears as a hypointense bony structure surrounded by the cochlear duct, which is fluid filled (Fig. 12.3). The osseous spiral lamina and the basilar membrane appear as hypointense structures and separate the scala tympani from the scala vestibuli. The two and a half turns of the lymph-filled cochlear duct are hyperintense, with a hypointense helicotrema at the top. The utricle and the saccule cannot be distinguished with MR; both appear as a single unit, the vestibule. The entrance of the vestibular nerve into the vestibule is detected as a small hypointense dot at its rostral part (Fig. 12.3). The endolymphatic duct runs in an inverted J-configuration from the medial part of the vestibule, first medial to the common crus and then, at the level of the proximal part of the common crus, turning laterally in a dorsocaudal direction (Fig. 12.3). This turning point is called the genu of the endolymphatic duct (Kartush et al. 1986).

The endolymphatic duct enters the endolymphatic sac posterior to the lateral part of the posterior semicircular duct. The distance between the common duct and the endolymphatic duct is about 1.0 mm. The cross-sectional diameter of the endolymphatic duct varies between 0.09 × 0.1 mm and 0.16 × 0.41 mm (Lo et al. 1997). The endolymphatic sac is located intra-and extraosseously at the posterior pyramidal wall. It is close to the sigmoid sinus, and occasionally there is no bony structure separating the endolymphatic sac from the sigmoid sinus. In about 50% of the adult population the extraosseous part is obliterated (Friberg et al. 1988). On T2-weighted steady state gradient echo images it may be difficult to delineate the extraosseous section of the endolymphatic sac, because it has the same signal intensity as the surrounding CSF. The average maximum diameter of the endolymphatic sac is about

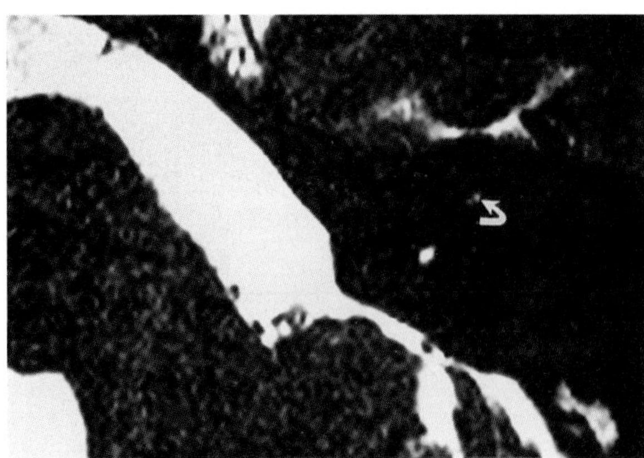

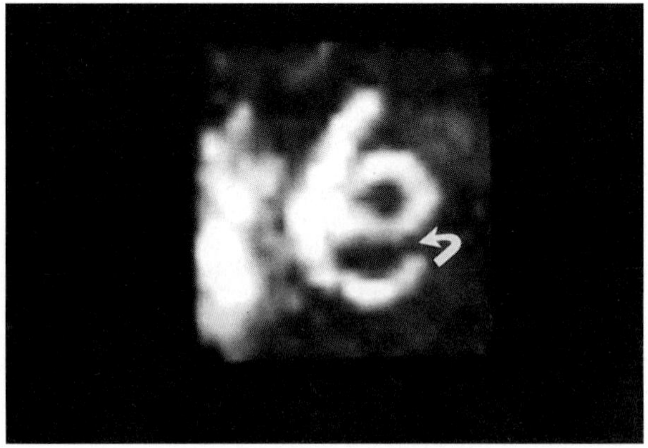

**Fig. 12.4.** **a** Axial, T2-weighted 3D CISS image in a patient with Scheibe syndrome: soft tissue obliteration of a section of the anterior semicircular canal (*curved arrow*). **b** Oblique projection, T2-weighted 3D CISS image reformatted by MIP. Scheibe syndrome, soft tissue obliteration of the posterior semicircular canal (*curved arrow*)

3–15 mm (Lo et al. 1997). The detectability of the endolymphatic duct and sac with high-resolution T2-weighted sequence varies in the literature between 73% (Albers and Casselman 1994) and 95% (Schmalbrock et al. 1996). This range of detectability may be due to the limited number of subjects included in these studies. Because of the small diameter of the endolymphatic duct, which is not far below the in-plane resolution of the MR protocol, detectability may even be below 73% in healthy subjects. Using high-resolution T1-weighted sequences (e.g., 0.51 × 0.51 × 2 mm voxel size), the intraosseous part of the endolymphatic sac and the adjacent part of the endolymphatic duct can easily be delineated. These endolymphatic structures appear as a hyperintense signal in the strongly T2-weighted gradient echo sequence only when they are filled with endolymph. These findings may be explained by the filling of the intraosseous part of the endolymphatic sac with epithelium-lined interconnected tubules surrounded by richly vascular fibroareolar stroma (Linthicum and Galey 1981), which can be imaged more easily with T1-weighted sequences than with T2-weighted steady state gradient echo sequences because these T2-weighted sequences are highly sensitive only to liquid. The evaluation of the endolymphatic system is performed best in axial and sagittal projections. The anterior and posterior semicircular ducts form the common crus before entering the vestibule. The bony covering of the anterior semicircular canal and the middle cranial fossa varies in thickness, and is absent in some cases (Fig. 12.3). Without this bony structure, patients will suffer from vertigo, as changes in CSF pressure or motion are transmitted to the anterior semicircular canal. The ampullae are shown as a widening of the semicircular duct before entering the vestibule. The crista ampullaris can be detected as a hypointense dot at the wall of the ampulla and is surrounded by hyperintense lymph (Fig. 12.3).

## 12.3 Anomalies

Anomalies of the inner ear are caused by disturbed embryogenic maturation. Reasons for this disruption include genetic factors (e.g., Goldenhar syndrome), infections (e.g., rubella) and drug toxins (e.g., thalidomide). Depending on the intensity of these disruptions, membranous dysplasia (Scheibe syndrome) (Fig. 12.4), osseous dysplasia (Mondini syndrome) (Fig. 12.5) and aplastic dysplasia (Michel syndrome) can result. Typical findings include narrowing or widening of the cochlear duct, reduction of the number of cochlear turns, deformity of the cochlea or the labyrinth, narrowing or widening the vestibule, dysplasia or absence of the semicircular ducts and widening of the vestibular aqueduct (Casselman et al. 1996, 1997; Jäger et al. 1997). It is quite common for a narrowing of the internal auditory canal (e.g., thalidomide embryophathy) to be associated with a severe hearing impairment (Fig. 12.6). Widening of the internal auditory canal is often seen in combination with the Mondini syndrome. Narrowing or widening of these various structures can easily be detected with a T2-weighted steady state gradient echo sequence, because either will result in a local defect of the hyperintense intraluminal lymphatic space. Differentiation between

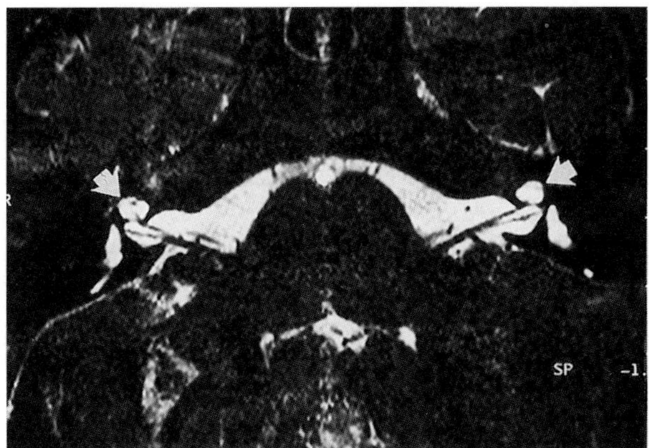


a

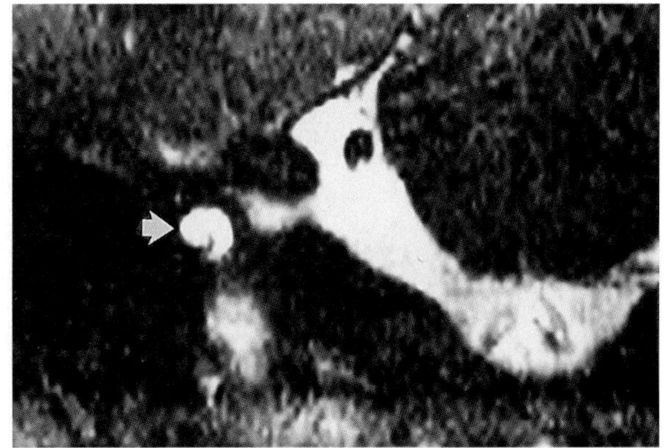

b

**Fig. 12.5.** **a** Axial, T2-weighted 3D CISS image. Mondini syndrome, osseous deformation of the cochlea. **b** Coronal, T2-weighted 3D CISS image reformatted by the MPR procedure. Mondini syndrome, osseous deformation of the cochlea

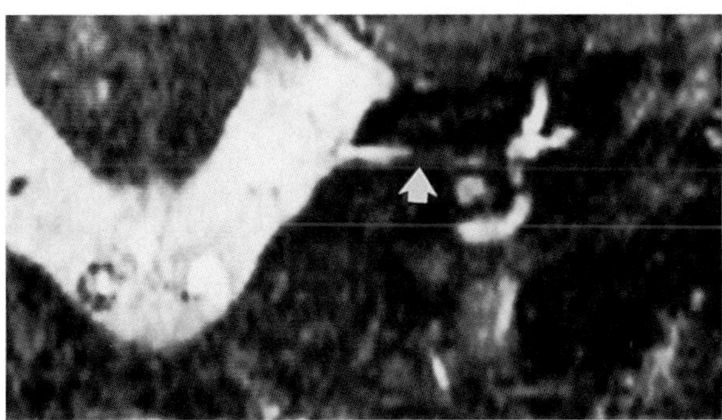

**Fig. 12.6.** Coronal, T2-weighted 3D CISS image reformatted by the MPR procedure. Severe narrowing of the IAC (*arrow*) with hypoplasty of the the VIIIth cranial nerve

an osseous and a fibrous occlusion is easily achieved with CT, but not with a T2-weighted steady state gradient echo sequence. A high-resolution T1-weighted sequence might also be helpful in detecting the soft tissue.

Liquor fistulas, which can be found in combination with anomalies of the inner ear, are classified as direct or indirect. In the latter, liquor finds its way through the perilymph space and passes through the oval window into the middle ear (Jäger et al. 1997). The fistula itself cannot be delineated with MR, but the T2-weighted steady state gradient echo sequence can detect the accumulation of CSF in the middle ear (Mafee et al. 1988; Nurre et al. 1988; Weissman and Curtin 1992). In contrast, direct liquor fistulas run independently from the lymph-filled space of the labyrinth. Because they transport CSF, they may be visualized by the T2-weighted steady state gradient echo sequence. Small intralabyrinthine pneumoceles may also be found (Lipkin et al. 1985), appearing as black dots on the T2-weighted steady state gradient echo sequence. A pre- and postcontrast T1-weighted image may also be helpful. The following liquor paths are possible: along the facial nerve, through a dehiscence at the tegmen tympani, through an eroded cell at the apex of the pyramid, and along the petromastoidal canal.

Another anomaly of the cerebellopontine angle that causes acoustic and vestibular disorders is the presence of arachnoidal cysts (Fig. 12.7). Because they have a layer of choroid plexus on their inner surface, they tend to grow as a result of CSF production. Using the MPR procedure, sagittal and coronal reconstruction of the primary T2-weighted steady state gradient echo sequence (e.g., 3D CISS) will show an arachnoidal cyst in the cerebellopontine angle and the deviation of the VIIth and VIIIth cranial nerves. The CSF inside and outside the cyst has the same signal intensity on the 3D T2-weighted steady state gradient echo images, separated by a hypointense cyst wall. A 3D reconstruction by surface rendering of the arachnoidal cyst in relation to the facial and vestibulocochlear nerve will show the deviation of the nerves affected by the cyst. Symptoms occur depending on head position.

Large vestibular aqueduct syndrome (LVAS) is the most common imaging finding in patients with SNHL between infancy or early childhood. The vestibular aqueduct is considered to be large when the cross-diameter of the duct is more than 1.5 mm at the midpoint between the common crus and the entrance into the endolymphatic sac (Valvassori and Clemis 1978). The term large vestibular aqueduct syndrome is a construct of the CT examination and is not necessarily correlated with MR results. For example, a widening of the vestibular aqueduct may not necessarily correlate with endolymphatic hydrops in the MR, or a T2-weighted T2-weighted steady state gradient echo sequence may detect

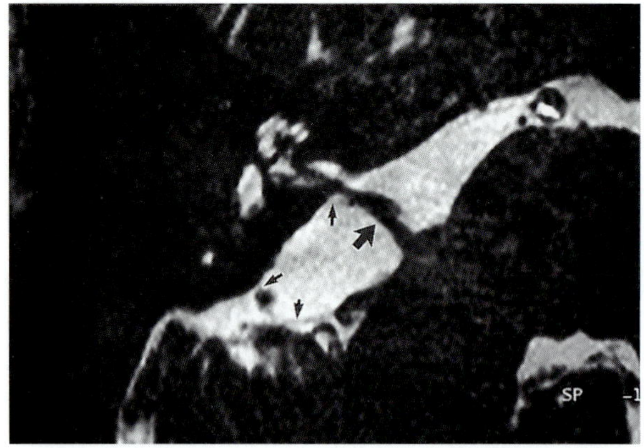


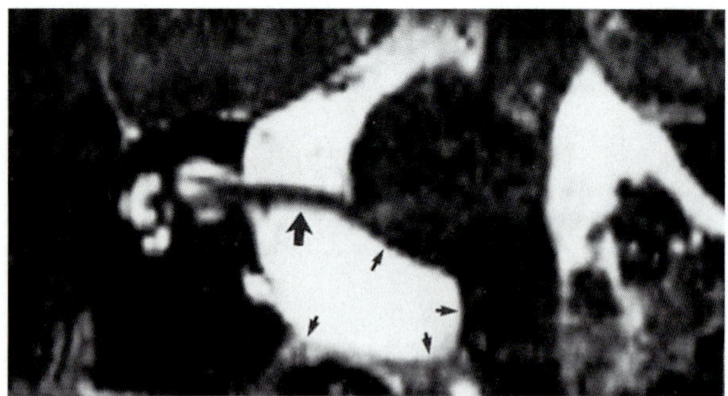

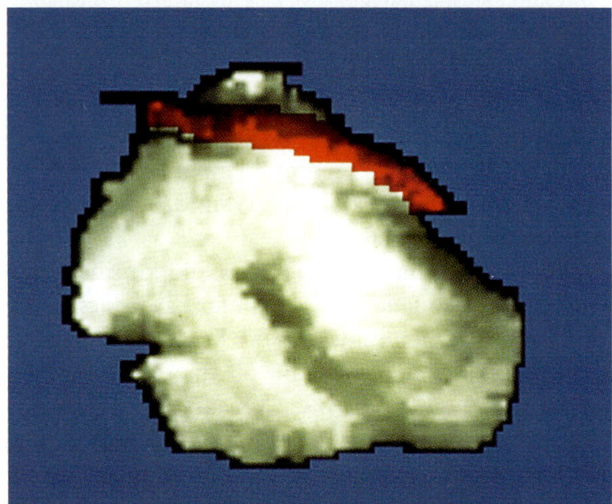

**Fig. 12.7.** **a** Axial, T2-weighted 3D CISS image. An arachnoidal cyst in the cerebellopontine angle causes a deviation of the VIIIth cranial nerve (*large arrow*). The wall of the cyst is shown as a thin course (*small arrows*). **b** Coronal, T2-weighted 3D CISS image reformatted by the MPR procedure. An arachnoidal cyst in the cerebellopontine angle causes a deviation of the VIIIth cranial nerve (*large arrow*). The wall of the cyst in shown as a thin course (*small arrows*). **c** Oblique view. The axial 3D CISS images were segmented and a 3D volume reconstruction was performed. The arachnoidal cyst (*yellow*) is in direct contact with the vestibulocochlear nerve (*red*). The VIIIth cranial nerve shows a cranial deviation

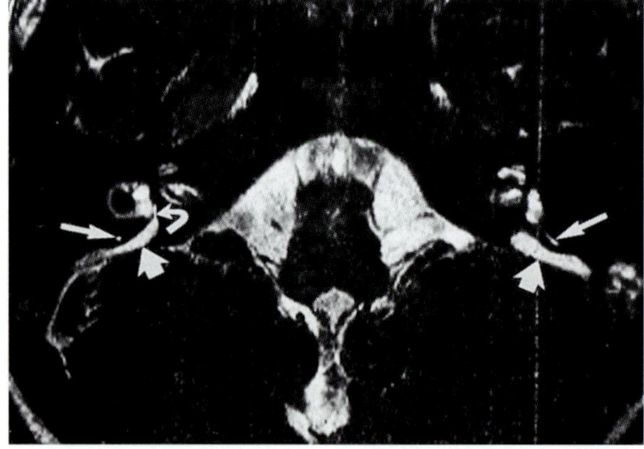

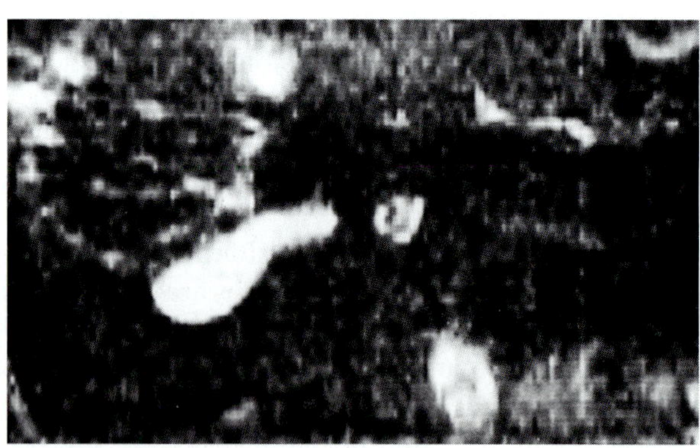

**Fig. 12.8.** **a** Axial, T2-weighted 3D CISS image. An endolymphatic hydrops of the endolymphatic sac is shown on both sides (*small wide arrow*). A stenosis of the endolymphatic duct (*curved arrow*) is delineated on the *right* side. The posterior semicircular canal is imaged (*long arrow*). **b** Sagittal, T2-weighted 3D CISS image reformatted by the MPR procedure. A hydrops of the endolymphatic sac is shown

endolymphatic hydrops (Fig. 12.8), but these findings do not correlate with CT (Dahlen et al. 1997). The appearance of LVAS is usually bilateral. Patients with LVAS suffer from SNHL beginning in early childhood, with deterioration in hearing loss over some years (Valvassori 1983). This gradual loss is associated with minor illness or head trauma. The severity of hearing loss does not correlate with the size of the endolymphatic duct or sac or with the size of the vestibular aqueduct. It is most likely

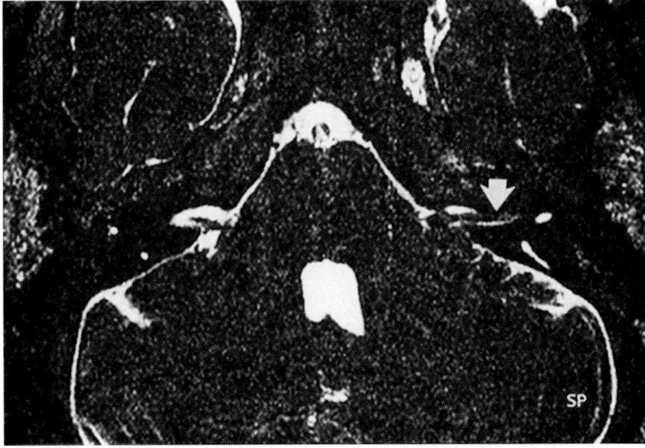


**Fig. 12.9.** Axial, T2-weighted 3D CISS image. A young male patient suffering from osteopetrosis (Albers-Schönberg disease). Severe narrowing of the IAC with compression of the VIIth and VIIIth cranial nerves is seen. The MR diagnosis was confirmed by CT

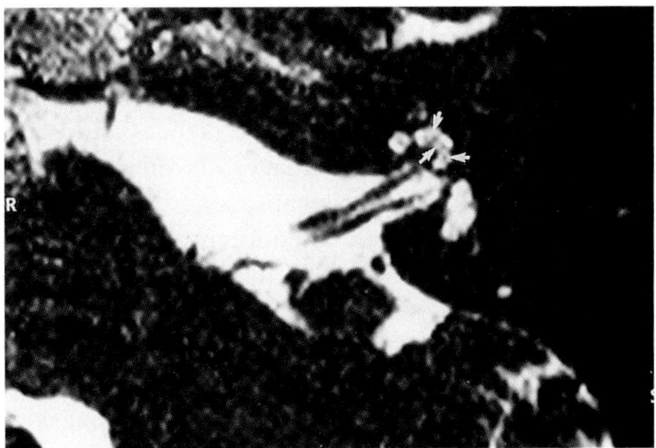


**Fig. 12.10.** Axial, T2-weighted 3D CISS image. A patient suffering from retrofenestral otosclerosis. Areas of signal loss (*arrows*) around the modiolus and the osseous spiral lamina are delineated as a result of osseous plaques, which were confirmed by CT

that LVAS results from an interruption of the differentiation of the endolymphatic duct in the 4th gestational week.

## 12.4 Otodystrophies

The bony changes of otodystrophies (e.g., Paget's disease, fibrous dysplasia, osteopetrosis, osteogenesis imperfecta tarda and otosclerosis) are evaluated best with CT, but narrowing of the internal auditory canal, as well as of the labyrinth, is also seen on T2-weighted steady state gradient echo images (Fig. 12.9). Compression of the VIIth and VIIIth cranial nerves results in symptoms, such as tinnitus and hearing loss, which are often the trigger for an MR examination. A coronal MPR reformation of the images will help in making the diagnosis.

Otosclerosis is the most common otodystrophy consisting of two major types, the fenestral and the retrofenestral type. An immediate diagnosis can be made with CT, but findings are fuller with MR. The fenestral type may result in a thickening of the stapes foot plate and the annular ligament and in the development of plaques in the oval window. If these plaques develop to a certain size they will curve into the cochlear duct and vestibule, which will be detected as a dot of signal loss on the T2-weighted steady state gradient echo images in the axial and coronal projections. A labyrinthine ossification (Fig. 12.10), as a result of a retrofenestral otosclerosis, could result in narrowing of the cochlear duct, which might be difficult to distinguish from labyrinthitis ossificans. The narrowing can be detected best on MR with a T2-weighted steady state gradient echo sequence.

## 12.5 Traumatology

Because the value of MR in the examination of fractures of the temporal bone is limited, CT is the recommended procedure. MR, however, is gaining popularity in cases of SNHL or vertigo that cannot be explained with CT. Fractures of the temporal bone are classified as longitudinal, which rarely affect the labyrinth, and as medial and lateral transverse fractures. Medial transverse fractures cross the internal auditory canal and damage the VIIth and VIIIth cranial nerves. Lateral transverse fractures are those that typically involve the otic capsule and the labyrinth. Liquor or perilymph fistulas may be the consequences. A loss of lymph resulting in pneumolabyrinth can be seen on T2-weighted steady state gradient echo images. The intralabyrinthine pneumoceles are hypointense dots surrounded by the hyperintense lymph. Pre- and postcontrast T1-weighted images can provide further information. CSF otorrhea or a perilymph fistula results in an increasing amount of CSF-like fluid in the middle ear or adjacent cells of the pyramid or mastoid (Mafee et al. 1988; Nurre et al. 1988; Weissman and Curtin 1992). This fluid has the same signal intensity on the T2-weighted steady state gradient echo images as CSF. A disrupture of the VIIth and VIIIth cranial nerve may be detected best on T2-weighted steady state gradient echo sequences and on postcontrast T1-weighted images, as they show an enhancement. A traumatic rupture of the endolymphatic duct will result in an endolymphatic hydrops (SHEA et al. 1995), which is detected best on T2-weighted steady state gradient echo images. A contusio labyrinthi, which results in vertigo and SNHL, may be seen as areas of signal loss on the T2-weighted steady state gradient echo images if hemorrhages are present, but is diagnosed easily with T1-weighted pre- and postcontrast sequences (MARK and FITZGERALD 1993).

## 12.6 Labyrinthitis

Labyrinthitis can be classified as an inflammatory or autoimmune (e.g., Cogan) disease. The inflammatory type is classified further based on the mode of transmission: tympanogenic, meningogenic, hematogenic and posttraumatic. Tympanogenic labyrinthitis is secondary to inflammatory lesions of the middle ear, which are unilateral. Acute otitis media (e.g., scarlet fever) or chronic otitis media (e.g., cholesteatoma) are to blame. Modes of transmission include the oval and round windows, fistulas of the labyrinth, posttraumatic fissure or a dehiscence (e.g., Mondini syndrome). Interestingly, the permeability of the oval and round windows is increased by endo- and exotoxins (e.g., *Pseudomonas* cytotoxin, streptolysin and *Staphylococcus aureus* toxin). Meningogenic labyrinthitis results from meningitis, with the bacterial types (e.g., *Pneumococcus*, *Meningococcus* and *Haemophilus influenzae*) being most common. Modes of transmission include the internal auditory canal and the cochlear aqueduct. Hematogenic labyrinthitis is less common and usually bilateral; the bacterial types are the most frequent (e.g., lues or borelliosis), but viral types are also found (e.g., measles or mumps). Posttraumatic labyrinthitis is commonly the result of a persisting perilymph fistula, which is the mode of transmission for bacterial infection.

T1-weighted pre- and postcontrast sequences are needed to evaluate subacute hemorrhages and the increase of permeability of intralabyrinthine vessel. In acute labyrinthitis, as well as in the residual condition, the signal of the lymph in the labyrinth may be lowered on the T2-weighted steady state gradient echo images (Fig. 12.11). This is probably due to high concentration of proteins. Also, after subacute hemorrhage areas of signal loss may be present on the T2-weighted steady state gradient echo images. Because the signal intensity of a T2-weighted steady state gradient echo sequence is determined by the T1/T2* quotient, by-products of hemoglobin will result in signal loss. Therefore it might be difficult to differentiate between a subacute hemorrhage or a high concentration of proteins and fibrous tissue or a tumor; a high-resolution T1-weighted sequence pre- and postcontrast is recommended for this purpose. However, tumors and fibrous tissue are more likely to be in a discrete area and have more consistent signal behavior than inflammation, which is scattered in the labyrinth and is not as consistent in its appearance. Fibrous occlusions in the labyrinth may occur after labyrinthitis as residual findings (Fig. 12.11). These can be detected on the T2-weighted steady state gradient echo images as areas of signal loss in the intralabyrinthine space surrounded by the hyperin-tense lymph. It is not possible to differentiate between fibrous and bony occlusion with a T2-weighted sequence, but a high-resolution T1-weighted sequence will provide the information needed.

Autoimmune labyrinthitis typically occurs bilaterally. Cogan syndrome is one type of autoimmune labyrinthitis. Because autoimmune labyrinthitis is a chronic disease, periods of acute onset are seen (CASSELMAN et al. 1994; HELMCHEN et al. 1998; JÄGER et al. 1997). These acute onsets can be monitored clinically or with MR and are not associated with a change in labyrinthine antibodies. They result in small hemorrhages, which are scattered in the labyrinth. They are best seen on T1-weighted images. An enhancement is also present, sometimes lasting up to 6 months. Acute onsets are rarely seen with a T2-weighted steady state gradient echo sequence, but residual fibrotic or even bony narrowing or occlusion of the labyrinths can be visualized (Fig. 12.12). Again, for differentiation between fibrous tissue and osseous formations, T1-weighted sequences or CT are very helpful.

Chronic labyrinthitis lasting for several months can lead to labyrinthitis ossificans, with bony narrowing of the labyrinth occurring after several months or years. Such areas of narrowing can be detected with the T2-weighted steady state gradient echo images (Fig. 12.13), but diagnosis is confirmed with CT.

Modern antibiotics have made intracranial abscesses less common, but they are still found in

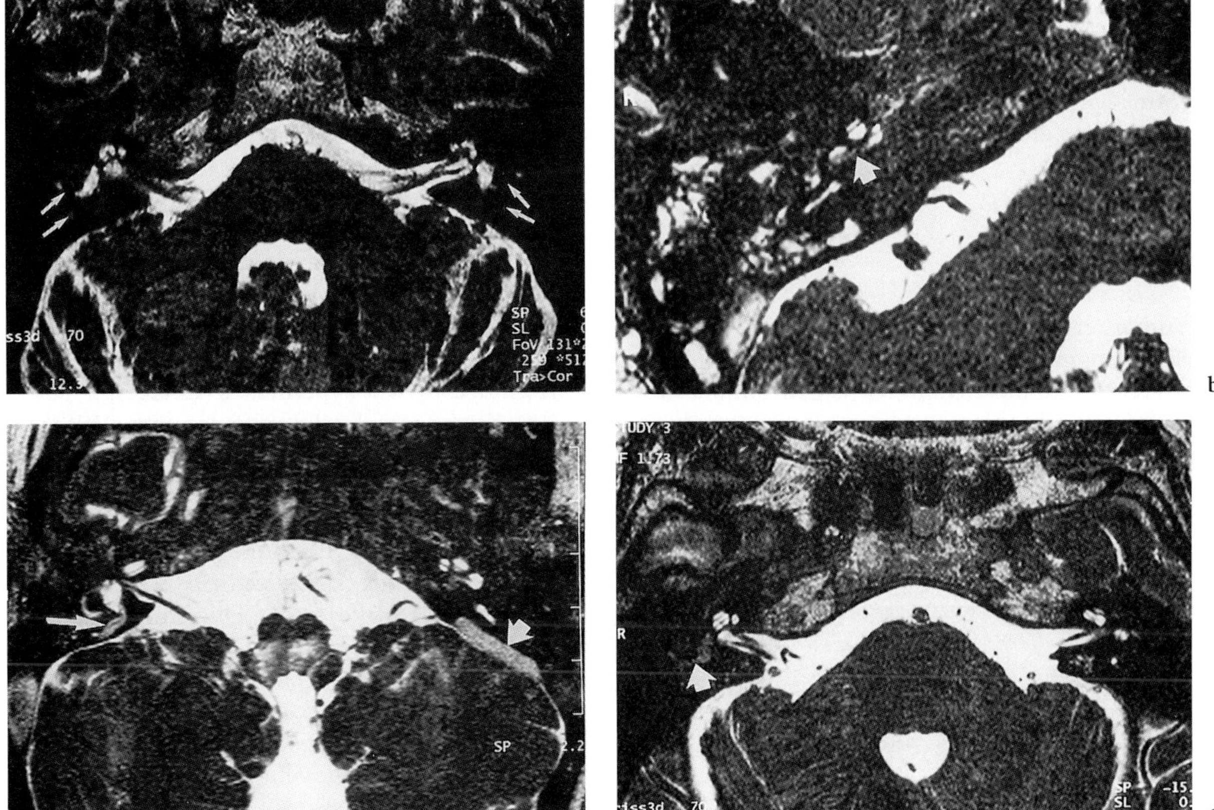

**Fig. 12.11 a–c.** Axial, T2-weighted 3D CISS images. **a** A patient with acute bacterial meningitis and secondary labyrinthitis. As a result of hemorrhage signal loss is found in the semicircular canals on both sides (*arrows*). **b** A patient with an iatrogenic traumatic hemorrhage into the labyrinth during an operation of a fistula at the round window. As a result, a hypointense area (*arrow*) is detected in the scala tympani of the second turn of the right cochlea. **c** A child before a cochlear implant (CI). This young boy had severe bacterial meningitis, which resulted in a hearing disability. A hydrops of the endolymphatic duct (*long arrow*) and the sac (*wide arrow*) are shown. Interestingly, the signal of the endolymphatic space is hypointense compared with the lymph-filled space of the cochlea and the vestibular system. This is most probably due to a high concentration of proteins, which may be the result of labyrinthitis caused by the meningitis. **d** This patient had zoster auricularis of the right side. The right vestibular system shows a signal loss as a result of fibrous tissue obliteration (*wide arrow*).

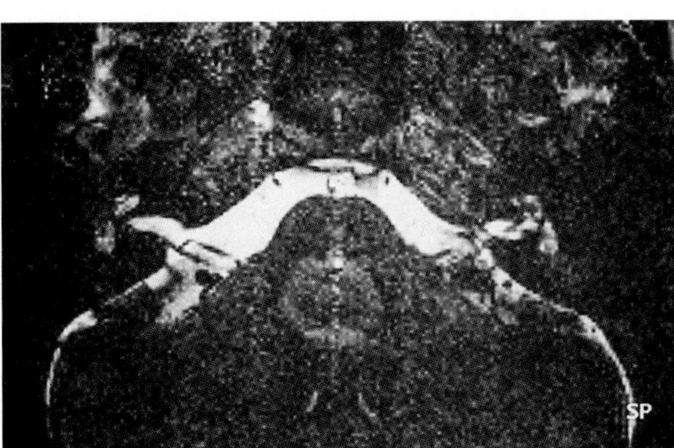

**Fig. 12.12.** Axial, T2-weighted 3D CISS image. Young lady with onset of Cogan syndrome several years ago. The labyrinth shows areas of signal loss as a result of fibrous tissue obliteration.

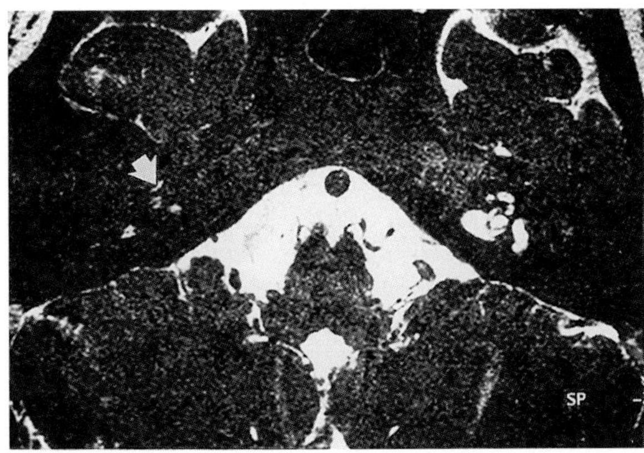

**Fig. 12.13.** Axial, T2-weighted 3D CISS image. This patient has labyrinthitis ossificans on the right side. As a result of subtotal ossification of the cochlea a severe signal loss of the lymphatic space of the cochlea is delineated (*arrow*).

patients with an immune deficit or suppression. Abscesses of the skull base may erode the capsule of the labyrinth and result in a leakage of lymph. Intralabyrinthine areas of signal loss on T2-weighted steady state gradient echo images are the result.

## 12.7 Tumors

Tumors are classified as benign or malignant. Schwannoma of the vestibular, cochlear and facial nerve are the most common benign tumors of the labyrinth and the inner auditory canal. The schwannoma appears as a mass with sharp borders. There is no bone destruction; rather, they extend through the preformed cavity of the labyrinth.

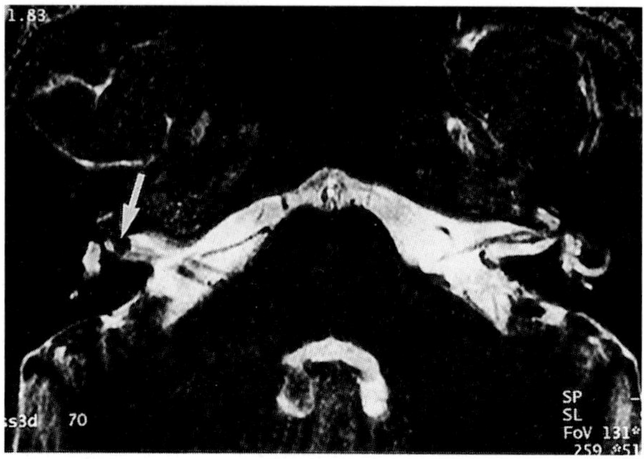

**Fig. 12.14.** Axial, T2-weighted 3D CISS image. An acoustic schwannoma of the cochlear nerve is delineated in the IAC as a hypointense structure with sharp borders (*arrow*)

Schwannomas of the internal auditory canal cause it to widen. Schwannomas of the cerebellopontine angle always extend into the internal auditory canal, but meningiomas rarely do. Whereas schwannomas grow in a more centered manner around the aperture of the internal auditory canal, meningiomas have a more extrinsic growth pattern. The meningeal tail sign on the T1-weighted postcontrast sequences is nonspecific (Bourekas et al. 1995). However, meningiomas and schwannomas appear on T2-weighted steady state gradient echo images as round hypointense tumors in the cerebellopontine angle, surrounded by the hyperintense CSF (Figs. 12.14–12.16). Because small schwannomas of the VIIth and VIIIth cranial nerves appear as dot-like enhancements on the involved cranial nerves, they cannot be differentiated from neuritis on T1-weighted images. The superior in-plane resolution associated with the T2-weighted steady state gradient echo sequence (e.g., 3D CISS) makes it possible to delineate the discrete thickening of the nerve if a schwannoma is present. Neuritis will not change the thickness of the nerve significantly.

Epidermoid and cholesterol cysts of the petrous apex may also erode the internal auditory canal and result in vestibular or auditory symptoms. Epidermoid cysts, also known as congenital cholesteatoma, are congenital lesions of ectodermal inclusions (Hasso and Smith 1989). Symptoms occur in adulthood between the ages of 20 and 50 years. They are the third most common lesion in the cerebellopontine angle, after acoustic schwannoma and meningioma. They are preferably located in the cerebellopontine angle, sellar and parasellar regions, petrous apex and the middle cranial fossa. Epider-

a

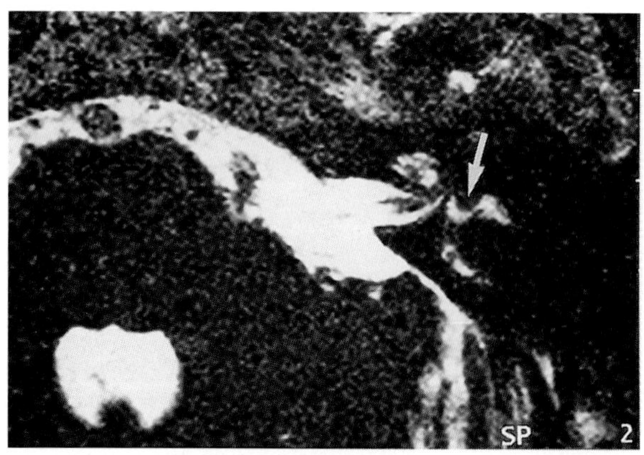

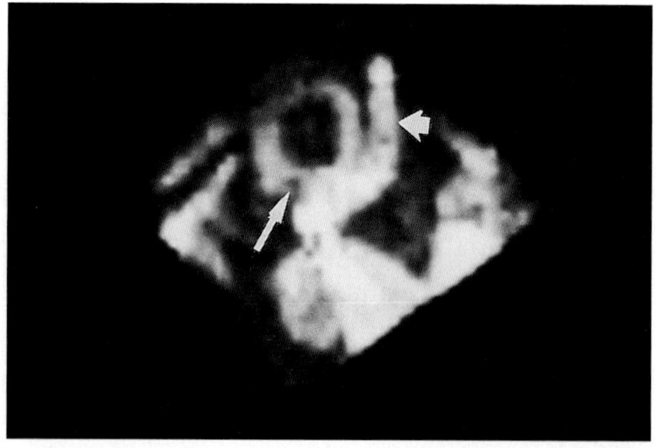

b

**Fig. 12.15.** **a** Axial, T2-weighted 3D CISS image. An acoustic schwannoma of the rostral part of the lateral semicircular canal is imaged as a hypointense structure (*arrow*). **b** Oblique, T2-weighted 3D CISS image reformatted by MIP. The acoustic schwannoma is found as a hypointense structure (*long arrow*) in the lateral semicircular canal. The posterior semicircular canal is also delineated (*wide arrow*)

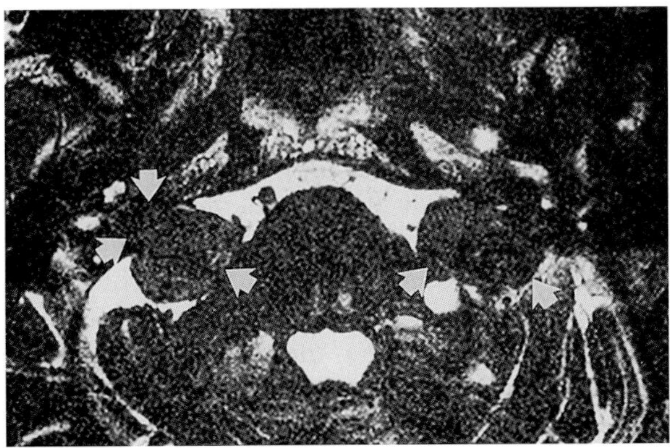

**Fig. 12.16.** Axial, T2-weighted 3D CISS image. A bilateral acoustic schwannoma is shown as a hypointense structure extending from the IAC into the cerebellopontine angle (*arrows*)

moid cysts contain a mixture of keratin debris and cholesterol crystals (Gao et al. 1992; Zimmerman and Bilaniuk 1979), which determines the signal behavior on T1-weighted and on T2-weighted steady state gradient echo images. On T1-, T2- and proton density-weighted images they are isointense or slightly hyperintense relative to CSF (Ikushima et al. 1997; Robert et al. 1995). A discrete rim of enhancement might be present. However, sometimes they are hardly differentiated from arachnoidal cysts. In these cases a T2-weighted steady state gradient echo sequence (e.g., 3D CISS sequence) is very helpful (Ikushima et al. 1997; Sakamoto et al. 1994; Tien et al. 1995), as they appear hypointense to CSF and hyperintense to brain tissue. They have a sharp border and can easily be distinguished from surrounding structures.

Cholesterol cysts are foreign-body granulomas, which occur during an inflammatory reaction to cholesterin crystals, the result of cell death. The cholesterol cysts have cystic compartments in their center. These are surrounded by highly vasculated fibrous tissue with a chronic inflammatory reaction. A hemorrhage into the cyst is common. Other locations of cholesterol cysts are the cerebellopontine angle, the dorsal region of the pyramid and the middle ear. Cholesterol cysts of the middle ear are a result of a chronic ventilation problems. Cholesterol cysts are also found after middle ear surgery, as fibrous tissue might restrict middle ear ventilation. The signal characteristics of cholesterol cysts in MR are determined by the content of cholesterol and the chronical subacute hemorrhage. They have a strong, hyperintense signal relative to CSF to T1- and T2-weighted sequences (Fig. 12.17). This holds true

a

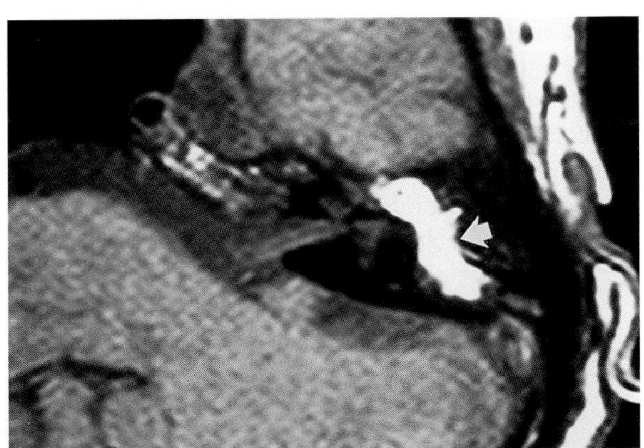

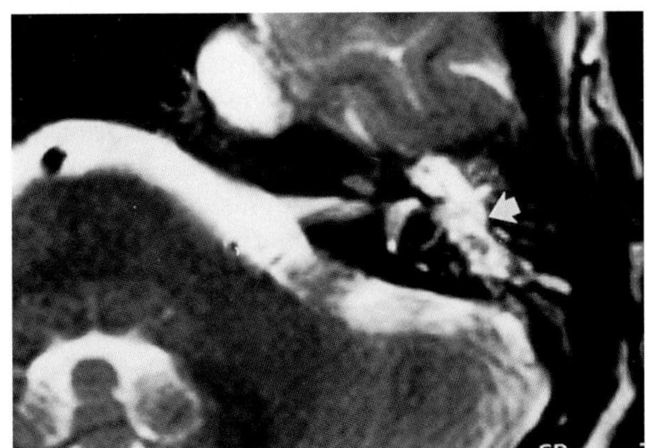

b

c

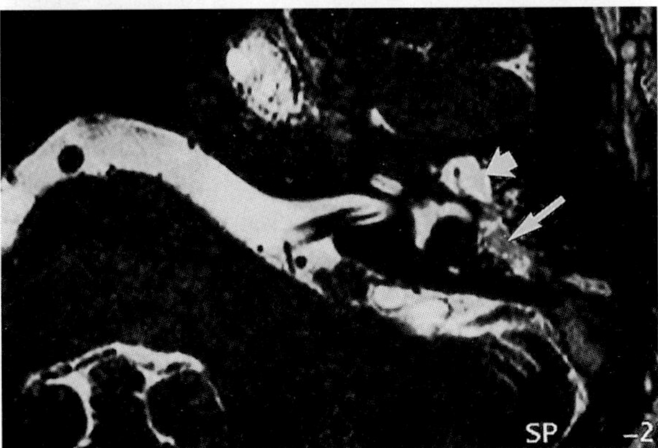


**Fig. 12.17.** **A** Axial, T1-weighted spin echo image. The cholesterol cyst of the middle ear has a hyperintense signal (*wide arrow*). **B** Axial, T2-weighted turbo spin echo image. The cholesterol cyst of the middle ear has a hyperintense signal (*wide arrow*). **C** Axial, T2-weighted 3D CISS image. The cholesterol cyst of the middle ear has a hyperintense signal (*wide arrow*). Hypointense areas are found in the cholesterol cyst (*long arrow*), which are due to hemosiderin.

also for T2-weighted steady state gradient echo sequences (e.g., 3D-CISS; Fig.12.17). Areas of hypointensity on T1- and T2-weighted images are due to hemosiderin deposits.

Malignant tumors (e.g., rhabdomyosarcoma of the middle ear or eustachian tube or metastases) do not respect bony borders and will erode adjacent osseous structures. On T2-weighted images such a tumor can be delineated as a hypointense mass with irregular borders (Fig. 12.18).

## 12.8 Miscellaneous

Cryptogenic vestibular neuritis does not result in changes that are detectable with MR (STRUPP et al. 1998). Benign peripheral paroxysmal vertigo (BPPV) can be evoked by head motion and is caused by canalolithiasis. Traumatic or degenerative inorganic particles that have split away from the otoliths have a higher specific weight than endolymph and move around as a result of gravity. This is seen especially in the posterior semicircular canals. As a result, vertigo and nystagmus occur when the head is laid back. Since canaloliths are smaller than the maximum commonly used in-plane resolution (0.31 × 0.31 × 0.51 mm), they are usually not identified with T2-weighted steady state gradient echo sequences. With a further increase of the in-plane resolution, visualization of these particles may be possible on dedicated MR systems (e.g., head systems) with high field strength and high-power gradients.

Meniere's disease is characterized by vertigo, often lasting for hours, tinnitus, fluctuating and permanent SNHL and the feeling of pressure in the ear. Meniere's disease can occur uni- or bilaterally and can be unisymptomatic or multisymptomatic. Endolymphatic hydrops with periodic ruptures of the membrane between the endo- and perilymph space is believed to be the cause of the onset of symptoms. The diffusion of potassium-rich endolymph into the perilymph space results in potassium-induced depolarization of the vestibulocochlear nerve. It is most likely that endolymphatic hydrops is caused by perisaccular fibrosis or by obliteration of the endolymphatic duct (ARENBERG et al. 1985; IKEDA and SANDO 1984). This results in disturbance of endolymph resorption in the endolymphatic sac and an interruption of the longitudinal endolymph circulation (KIMURA and SCHUKNECHT 1965). This hypothesis is supported by recent MR findings, which suggest narrowing or total invisibility of the endolymphatic duct or sac in 74–80% of the inner ears affected (ALBERS and CASSELMAN 1994; SCHMALBROCK et al. 1996). Endolymphatic hydrops is not found in these patients (TANIOKA et al. 1997). Treatments of Meniere's disease vary. One treatment involves the pharmacological elimination of the peripheral vestibular organ. Gentamicin, a cytotoxic drug, is placed in the middle ear and then diffuses through the oval and round windows into the labyrinth, where it eliminates vestibular function. As a side effect, the SNHL may be worsened, but this effect appears to be dose-dependent. Cytotoxic effects are not detectable with MR during or after treatment with T1-weighted pre- and postcontrast images or with high-resolution T2-weighted steady state gradient echo images.

a 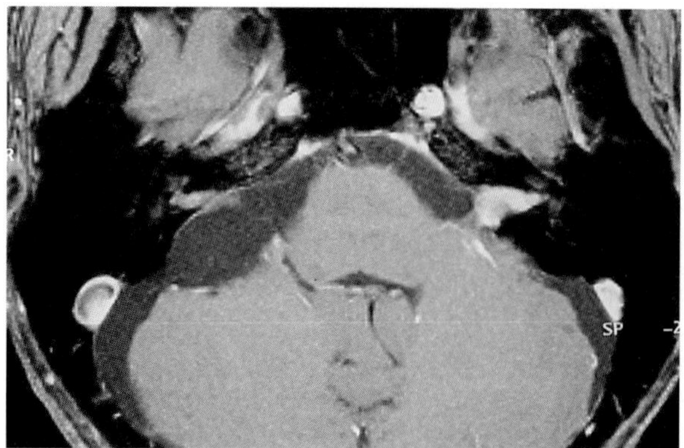


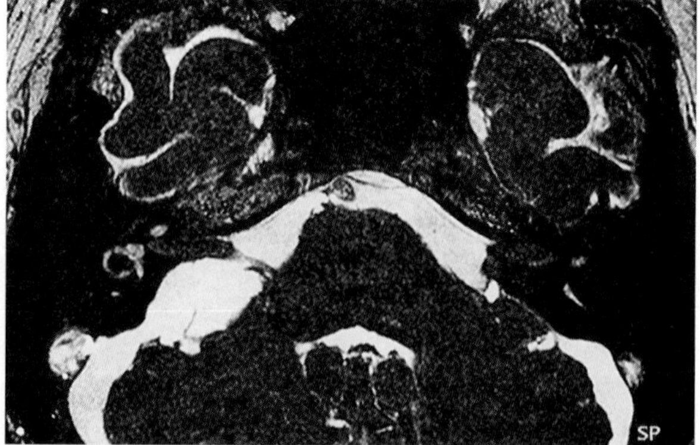 b


**Fig. 12.18.** **a** Axial, T1-weighted postcontrast 2D FLASH (fast low angle shot) and **b** T2-weighted 3D CISS images. Metastases from a bronchial cancer are shown in the IAC bilaterally and in the cerebellopontine angle on the *left* side. The metastases have strong enhancement and are hypointense on the corresponding 3D CISS image. The borders are irregular. The patient had meningitis carcinomatosa

Vestibular paroxysmia is characterized by short onsets of vertigo that are dependent on head position. SNHL and tinnitus occur during the episodic event. Symptoms are improved by carbamazepine. Elongated and dilated arteries in the cerebellopontine angle are thought to evoke demyelinization (oligodendroglia). Thus far, however, it is not possible to detect these areas of demyelinization with high-resolution T1-weighted or T2-weighted sequences, and pathological enhancement is not seen. The trigger for the symptoms are pulsatile nerve compressions and pathological paroxysmal excitations between two adjacent demyelinated axons. MR angiography can detect these arteries easily in the cerebellopontine angle and in the internal auditory canal. But arterial loops in the internal auditory canal are relatively unspecified morphological findings, since they are seen in approximately 40% of the healthy population (Mazzoni 1969). Loops of the anterior and posterior inferior cerebellar arteries (AICA and PICA) are the most common. However, arterial loops close to the exit point of the vestibulocochlear nerve at the brain stem are thought to be the cause of vestibular paroxysmia. The advantage of the MR examination with a high-resolution T2-weighted sequence, such as the 3D-CISS sequence, is the ability to perform an MPR procedure in order to obtain reformatted images in the needed oblique, axial, coronal and sagittal planes (Fig. 12.19). On these images the distance between the arterial loop and the vestibulocochlear nerve can be measured. Contact between the VIIIth cranial nerve and the AICA or PICA are typical findings. An elongated or dilated vertebral or basilar artery in the immediate vicinity is also commonly found.

Cochlear implants (CI) are cutting edge devices used to help deaf individuals process the sound around them. They are implanted in patients who have lost their hearing ability but who have normal function of the retrocochlear part of the acoustic pathway. The CI processor is placed in a retrauricular bony cavity of the mastoid, and the electrodes run from the mastoid through the middle ear to the basal turn of the cochlea, the promontory, to enter the intralabyrinthine cochlear space, the scala tympani. An alternative entrance to the cochlea is from the helicotrema. The purpose of the MR examination is to delineate the intralymphatic space of the cochlea. A lymph-filled cochlea is a prerequisite for a CI. The lymph facilitates the placing of the

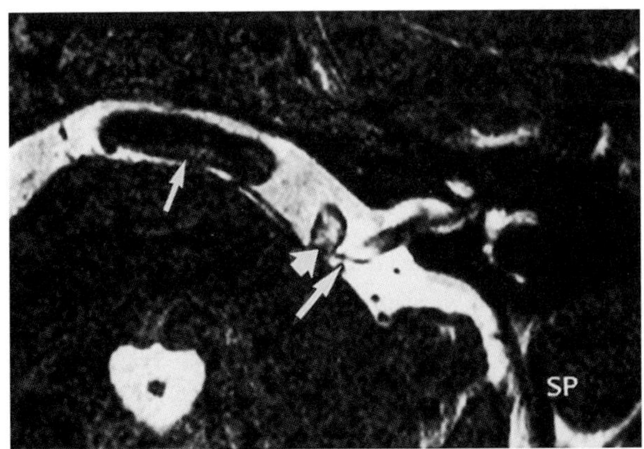


A

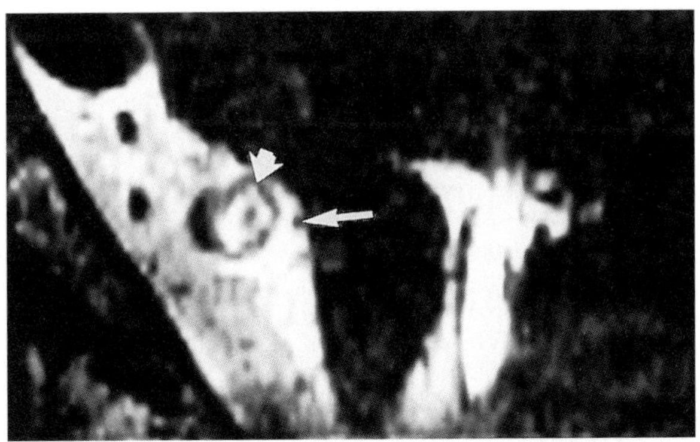

B

C

**Fig. 12.19. A** Axial, T2-weighted 3D CISS image. This is a patient with a vestibular paroxysm. A megadolichobasilar artery (*small arrow*) and a megadolichovertebral artery (*small wide arrow*) are shown in the left cerebellopontine angle. The vertebral artery is in close contact with the VIIIth cranial nerve (*long arrow*). **B** Sagittal, T2-weighted 3D-CISS image reformatted by the MPR procedure. The vertebral artery (*small wide arrow*) and the VIIIth cranial nerve (*long arrow*) are in close proximity to each other, but there is no contact. **C** Sagittal, T2-weighted 3D CISS image reformatted by the MPR procedure. This image is taken medial to that in **B**. The vertebral artery (*small wide* arrow) is in contact with the VIIIth cranial nerve (*long arrow*). The basilar artery is also shown (*small arrow*)

electrode in the cochlear duct. The electrode should be placed helically around the cochlear ganglion in the modiolus. Depending on the consistency and the size of a fibrous obliteration, a bouginage could open the way for the electrode. A bony obliteration of the cochlear duct, on the other hand, would hinder electrode placement. Fibrous and bony obliterations will result in an area of signal loss on the T2-weighted steady state gradient echo images. These areas are surrounded by the bright signal of the lymph. Differentiation between fibrous tissue and osseous structures is not possible with the steady state gradient echo sequence, but high-resolution CT allows easy detection of bony narrowings or occlusions. Since MR can detect lymphatic fluid and intralabyrinthine soft tissue better than CT, whereas CT can detect bony obliterations better than MR, high-resolution T2-weighted steady state gradient echo images in combination with high-resolution CTs are prerequisites in the examination of patients before cochlear impantation.

## References


Albers FWJ, Casselman JW (1994) 3DFT-magnetic resonance imaging of the iner ear in Meniere's disease. In: Filipo R, Barbara M (eds) Menieres disease: perspectives in the 90's. Kugler, Amsterdam, 43–46

Arenberg IK, Norback DH, Shambough GE (1985) Distribution and density of subepithelial collagen in the endolymphatic sac tissue from Meniere's disease patients. Am J Otol 6:449–454

Arnold B, Jäger L, Grevers G et al (1996) Visualisation of inner ear structures by three-dimensional high-resolution MRI. Am J Otol 17:480–485

Bourekas EC, Wildenhain P, Lewin JS et al (1995) The dural tail sign revisited. AJNR 16:1514–1516

Casselman JW, Kuhweide R, Deimling M et al (1993a) Constructive interference in steady state-3DFT MR imaging of the inner ear and cerebellopontine angle. AJNR Am J Neuroradiol 14:47–57

Casselman JW, Kuhweide R, Ampe W et al (1993b) Pathology of the membranous labyrinth: comparison of T1- and T2-weighted and gadolinium-enhanced spin-echo 3DFT-CISS imaging. AJNR Am J Neuroradiol 14:59–69

Casselman JW, Majoor MHJM, Albers FW (1994) MR of the inner ear in patients with Cogan syndrome. AJNR Am J Neuroradiol 15:131–138

Casselman JW, Kuhweide R, Ampe W et al (1996) Inner ear malformations in patients with sensorineural hearing loss: detection with gradient-echo (3DFT-CISS) MRI. Neuroradiology 38:278–286

Casselman JW, Offeciers FE, Govaerts PJ et al (1997) Aplasia and Hypoplasia of the vestibulocochlear nerve: diagnosis with MR Imaging. Radiology 202:773–781

Dahlen RT, Harnsberg HR, Gray SD et al (1997) Overlapping thin section fast spin echo magnetic resonance imaging in the evaluation of the large vestibular aqueduct syndrome: comparison with CT. AJNR 18:67–75

Deimling M, Laub G (1989) Constructive Interference in steady state (CISS) for motion sensitivity reconstruction. In: Book of abstracts: annual meeting of the Society of Magnetic Resonance in Medicine, vol 1, Berkeley, p 842

Eberhardt KEW, Hollenbach HP, Deimling M et al (1995) High-resolution magnetic resonance imaging of the endolymphatic duct and sac. MAGMA 3:77–81

Friberg U, Jansson B, Rask-Andersen H et al (1988) Variations in surgical anatomy of the endolymphatic sac. Arch Otolaryngol Head Neck Surg 114:389–394

Gao PY, Osborn AG, Smirniotopoulos JG et al (1992) Epidermoid tumor of the cerebellopontine angle. AJNR 13: 863–872

Haacke EM, Wielopolski PA, Tkach JA et al (1990) Steady-state free precession imaging in the presence of motion: application for improved visualization of the cerebrospinal fluid. Radiology 175:545–552

Haacke EM, Wielopolski PA, Tkach JA (1991) A comprehensive technical review of short TR, fast magnetic resonance imaging. Rev Mag Res 3:53–170

Hasso AN, Smith DS (1989) The cerebellopontine angle. Semin Ultrasound CT MR 10:280–301

Helmchen C, Jäger L, Büttner U et al (1998) Cogan-syndrome: high-resolution MRI as an indicator of activity. J Vestib Res 8:155–167

Ikeda M, Sando I (1984) Endolymphatic duct an sac in patients with Meniere's disease. Ann Otol Rhinol Laryngol 93: 540–546

Ikushima I, Korogi Y, Hirai T et al (1997) MR of epidermoids with a variety of pulse sequences. AJNR 18: 1359–1363

Jäger L, Strupp M, Brandt T et al (1997) Imaging of the labyrinth and vestibular nerve: clinical relevance for differential diagnosis of vestibular disorders. Nervenarzt 68: 443–458

Kartush JM, Toya S, Shiobara R et al (1986) Anatomic basis for labyrinthine preservation during posterior fossa acoustic tumor surgery. Laryngoscope 96:1024–1028

Kimura RS, Schuknecht HF (1965) Membranous hydrops in the inner ear of the guinea pig after obliteration of the endolymphatic sac. Pract Oto Rhino Larngol 27:343–354

Linthicum FH, Galey FR (1981) Computer-aided reconstruction of the endolymphatic sac. Acta Otolaryngol 91: 423–429

Lipkin AF, Bryan RN, Jenkins HA (1985) Pneumolabyrinth after temporal bone fracture: documentation by high resolution CT. AJNR 6:294–297

Lo WWM, Daniels DL, Chakeres DW et al (1997) The endolymphatic duct and sac. AJNR 18:881–887

Mafee MF, Kumar A, Tahmoressi CN et al (1988) Direct sagittal CT in the evaluation of temporal bone disease. AJNR 8:371–378

Mark AS, Fitzgerald D (1993) Segmental enhancement of the cochlea on contrast-enhanced MR: correlation with the frequency of hearing loss and possible sign of perilymphatic fistula and autoimmune labyrinthitis. AJNR 14:991–996

Mazzoni A (1969) Internal auditory canal arterial relations at the porus acusticus. Ann Otol Rhinol Laryngol 78:797–814

Nurre JG, Neblett CR, Rose JE (1982) Pneumolabyrinth as a late sequela of temporal bone fracture. Am J Otol 9:489–493

Oppelt A, Graumann R, Barfuss H et al (1986) FISP – a new fast MRI sequence. Electromedica 54:15–18

Patz S (1988) Some factors that influence the steady state in the steady-state free precession. Magn Reson Imaging 6:405–413

Robert Y, Carcasset S, Rocourt N et al (1995) Congenital cholesteatoma of the temporal bone: MR findings and comparison with CT. AJNR 16:755–761

Rubinstein D, Sandberg EJ, Cajade-Law AG (1996) Anatomy of the facial and vestibulocochlear nerve in the internal auditory canal. AJNR 17:1099–1105

Sakamoto Y, Takahashi M, Ushio Y et al (1994) Visibility of epidermoid tumors on steady-state free precission images. AJNR 15:1737–1744

Schmalbrock P, Dailiana T, Chakeres DW et al (1996) Submillimeter-resolution MR of the endolymphatic sac in healthy subjects and patients with Meniere disease. AJNR 17:1707–1717

Shea JJ, Ge X, Orchik DJ et al (1995) Traumatic endolymphatic hydrops. Am J Otol 16:235–240

Stillman AE, Remley K, Loes DJ et al (1994) Steady-state free precission imaging of the inner ear. AJNR 15:348–350

Strupp M, Jäger L, Müller-Lisse U et al (1998) High resolution MRI in 60 patients with vestibular neuritis: no contrast enhancement of the labyrinth or vestibular nerve. J Vestib Res (in press)

Tanioka H, Kaga K, Zusho H et al (1997) MR of the endolymphatic duct and sac: findings in Meniere Disease. AJNR 18:45–51

Tien RD, Felsberg GJ, Lirng JF (1995) Variable bandwidth steady-state free-precession MR imaging: a technique for improving characterization of epidermoid tumor and arachnoidal cyst. AJR 164:689–692

Valvassori GE (1983) The large vestibular aqueductand associated anomalies of the inner ear. Otolaryngol Clin North Am 16:95–101

Valvassori GE, Clemis JD (1978) The vestibular aqueduct syndrome. Laryngoscope 88:723–728

Weissman JL, Curtin HD (1992) Pneumolabyrinth: a computed tomographic sign of temporal bone fracture. Am J Otolaryngol 13:113–114

Zimmerman RA, Bilaniuk LT (1979) Cranial computed tomography of epidermoid and congenital fatty tumors of maldevelopmental origin. Comput Tomogr 3:40–50

# 13 3D Visualization of the Extracranial Head and Neck: Explanation of Technique and Review of Clinical Applications

B.M. HEMMINGER and S.K. MUKHERJI

CONTENTS



## 13.1 Introduction

Advances in various imaging modalities have had a significant impact on treatment and management of various skull base lesions over the last 15 years. Technical improvements in CT and MR imaging permit exquisite visualization of bony and soft tissue anatomy, which previously could not be seen. These imaging modalities now permit detailed information of the location and extent of temporal bone and skull base lesions. The presence of bone erosion, perineural spread, tumor margins, and relationship to surrounding neurovascular structures often cannot be determined by clinical examination. Because of their important role in tumor staging, preoperative CT and MR imaging have become an integral component of the preoperative evaluation in patients with temporal bone and skull base tumors (MUKHERJI et al. 1997).

Recent advances in CT and MRI scanners have produced high-quality data suitable for three-dimensional (3D) visualization. Coinciding with progress in image acquisition have been recent developments in computer display technology, which permit viewing CT and MR imaging studies directly as three-dimensional volumes. These advances permit unique ways of visualizing 3D studies that go beyond the standard 2D format. The intent of this chapter is (1) to introduce recent technical advancements in medical image display and (2) to provide an overview of clinical applications of 3D visualization as it pertains to head and neck and skull base imaging.


B.M. HEMMINGER, MS, Department of Radiology, Radiology Research Center, University of North Carolina, Chapel Hill, NC 27599-7515, USA

S.K. MUKHERJI, MD, Departments of Radiology and Surgery, The School of Medicine, and Department of Diagnostic Sciences, University of North Carolina at Chapel Hill, Chapel Hill, NC 27599-7510, USA


## 13.2 Evolution of 3D Visualization Methods Applied to Medical Imaging

Advances in the field of computer graphics have permitted visualization of the human body in ways not previously available. In the 1980s, as computing power increased, developments in the field of computer graphics led to the design of algorithms that would depict 3D anatomical structures on 2D video monitors, so that the human observer would have a sense of the "3D scene" (Fig. 13.1). The appearance of a 3D scene from a static 2D image was accomplished using such visual cues as occlusion, perspective, shading, and stereo (when using a stereo display and stereo glasses). Further, if the observer could manipulate the image on the screen, rotational cues were added, as well as strengthening the previous cues through kinesthetic correspondence. These developments were quickly applied to medical image data that could be acquired as a 3D volume or equivalently, as a stack of 2D slices. The first 3D presentations consisted of a simple 3D visualization of the anatomy from a single viewpoint. This was expanded to multiple 3D static views from different viewpoints, with efforts being made to estimate the ideal viewpoints from a clinical perspective because of the lengthy time required to compute the 3D views. This was followed by the precomputing of a

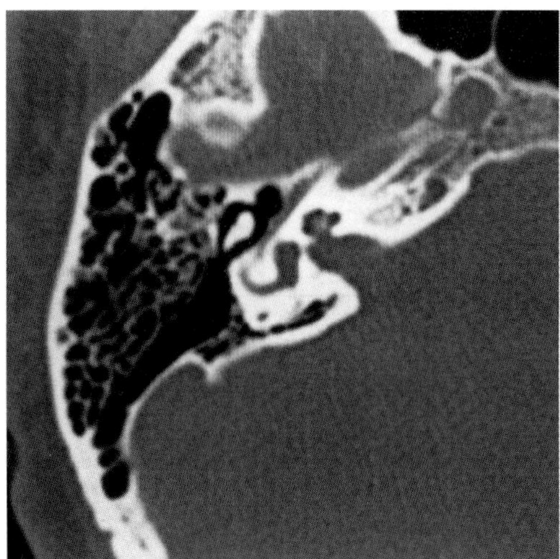
a

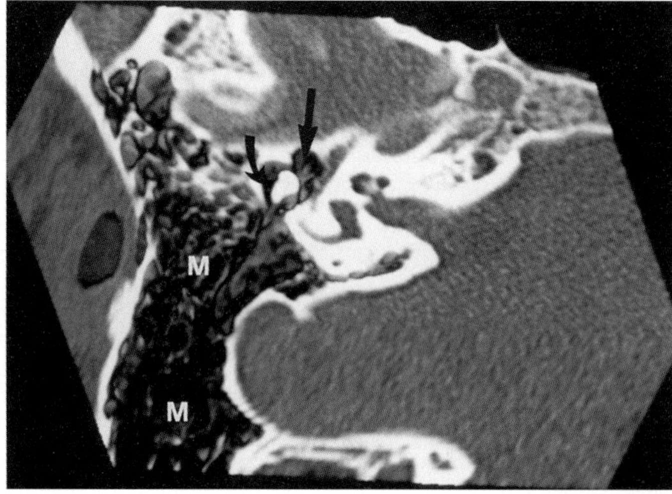

b

**Fig. 13.1.** **a** Axial image of the temporal bone illustrates the standard two-dimensional image routinely obtained for evaluation of the temporal bone. **b** Three-dimensional reconstruction ("3D scene") of the data illustrated in **a**. This visualization provides a better appreciation of the depth and spatial relationships of the ossicles with the epitympanum (*straight arrow*) and fossa incudis (*curved arrow*), and mastoid air cells (*M*)

collection of 3D images about a single axis of rotation of the 3D volume, which could be played back under interactive control as a continuously rotating 3D object. This *cine loop* provided better visual cues, and also provided some kinetic depth effect benefits similar to those of interactive control of the arbitrary rotations. The final step occurred when computers became fast enough to allow for the calculation of the 3D view of the entire data volume in a fraction of a second, so that the 3D presentation could be interactively controlled by the user in real time. Similar to the progression of presentation techniques, the methods for rendering the 3D scene from the 3D volume started with simplified methods (surface rendering), and then advanced to intermediate direct volume rendering methods (Maximum Intensity Projection, MIP) and finally to true direct volume rendering methods. This progression is detailed in the next section.

## 13.3 Techniques of Interactive 3D Visualization

### 13.3.1 Surface Rendering

The initial rendering methods that were developed came from the field of computer graphics and consisted primarily of surface rendering methods that had direct hardware support for surface rendering primitives on the graphics cards in workstations and high-end PCs. The hardware became fast enough to render a large set of 3D surfaces in real time, leading to efforts to describe volumes as surfaces of interest (Fuchs et al. 1997). For the first time, it became practicable to interactively control the display of a clinically realistic 3D surface-rendered visualization, including changing the viewpoint, light sources, and cutting planes. While the addition of real time rendering was a powerful advantage, surface rendering methods have two disadvantages. First, they required the definition of a surface from the volume. This implied time-consuming hand contouring steps and follow-up editing. While image processing techniques could semi-automate this process, high-quality surface generation usually requires the input of highly trained medical personnel. The second disadvantage is that reducing the complexity of the 3D volume by encoding it as surfaces implicitly requires making a binary decision as to where surfaces lie. This can cause sampling artifacts, such as "holes" in surfaces representing continuous portions of anatomy due to thin areas of bone, or voxel averaging. Later, methods like Marching Cubes and its derivatives partially solved this problem by allowing for automated mapping of voxels into polygonal surfaces that more optimally choose surfaces, and reduced sampling artifacts (Lorensen and Cline 1987).

## 13.3.2 Volume Rendering

In the 1990s, as computer power has increased and hardware prices have declined, experimentation with direct rendering of the entire data volume became feasible (Davis et al. 1991; Levoy 1991). This led to rendering the entire volume dataset without the intermediate step of defining surfaces, and is generally referred to as *volume rendering*, or sometimes as *direct volume rendering*. Volume rendering methods model the voxels as objects in space and calculate the interaction of light with these objects as seen from the observer's viewpoint. The treatment of voxels as different types of objects (point samples, blobs, cubes, etc.) with different possible reflectance and scatter characteristics has led to the creation of many different volume rendering techniques. A general discussion of volume rendering can be found in an an article by Drebin et al. (1988), and a recent survey of volume rendering techniques applied to medical imaging has been published by Yoo and Fuchs (1993). The progress of volume rendering towards interactive real time rendering has followed the same sequence of steps as surface rendering with single views, collections of views, single axis cine loops, and finally real time interactive volume rendering.

The first commercially available system capable of real-time volume rendering under interactive user control was the SGI Reality Engine system, released in 1993. A technical description of the SGI Reality Engine is available as a technical report and a paper which describes the application of the Reality Engine to volume rendering (Silicon Graphics 1993; Cabral et al. 1994). Additionally, in-depth discussions of academic realtime volume rendering architectures, such as Pixel Planes, Pixel Flow, and Princeton Engine can be found in computer graphics literature (Fuchs et al. 1992; Kaba et al. 1992; Molnar et al. 1992; Schroeder and Stoll 1992; Taylor et al. 1993). Real-time volume rendering is currently limited to high-end computer graphics systems. However, with the expected increases in computer speeds, interactive volume rendering rates for CT and MRI datasets should be achieved on PCs and low-end workstations by the year 2000.

Several software applications supporting real-time or near real-time volume rendering exist and are used for a variety of applications including pre-surgical planning. The UNC department of Radiology has developed a real-time, interactive 3D visualization tool for medical image data termed "SeeThru" (Hemminger 1994; Hemminger et al. 1994). This technique is highly interactive and permits the user real-time control of view (viewpoint, lighting), data (classification/segmentation) and control of removal (cutting planes, sculpting). This technique is one of the first applications to provide all three of these abilities on commercially available hardware (SGI Reality Engine).

Besides prototype systems (such as SeeThru) developed at academic institutions, there are now several near-real-time 3D visualization software applications for medical imaging available with FDA approval, including those from CT and MRI manufacturers (General Electric and Picker) and independent software companies (Vital Images).

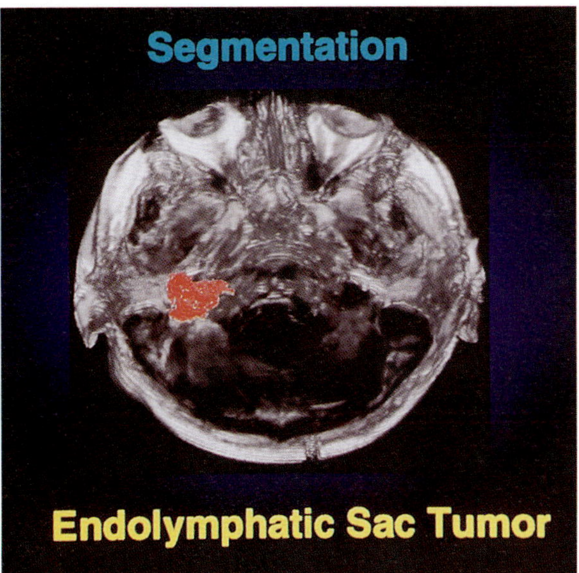


**Fig. 13.2.** Example of segmentation. 3D reconstruction of T1-Weighted MR imaging study performed in a patient with an endolymphatic sac tumor involving the petrous apex. The tumor is defined (segmented) in *red*. This segmentation was performed by manual contouring of the tumor margins

## 13.3.3 Segmentation

An area related to visualization is segmentation. Segmentation is how to segment a 3D volume into different parts, for instance, into separate anatomical structures (Fig. 13.2). Currently, no general-purpose method for segmentation exists. However, for specific problems, and specific image types, some segmentation methods work reasonably well. Methods generally operate by classifying voxels as part of a class by their intensity value, and also by spatial location or other statistical characteristics, such as texture. Segmentation relates to 3D visualization because the process of defining surfaces (for surface rendering) or choosing what set of voxels should have the same opacity and transparency characteristics (for volume rendering) are both segmentation-type problems. Most work in clinical use has evolved from simple image processing techniques, such as thresholding, followed by region growing or shrinking techniques. Newer contour-fitting techniques, such as *snakes*, make use of an expected shape of an object and then shrink wrap to fit the surface of a real object in the volume. As segmentation tools become more powerful and more applicable, we can expect to be able to conveniently and interactively select portions of a volume to highlight them, or make them invisible, in order to improve our perception of the parts of interest in the 3D volume.

### 13.3.4 What Is the Best Presentation Method?

Single, or multiple 2D still images from 3D visualizations are considered the least effective mode of presentation for 3D volume information. As direct volume rendering computation times have decreased to minutes and now seconds, the *cine* presentation has become popular. However, the 2D images representing 3D volumes are even more realistic to the observer if they can be interactively rotated in space via user control due to kinetic depth effect. Since this requires at least 5–10 frames per second update rates to maintain the visual precept of a single object in continuous motion, standard PCs and workstations have not been capable of real-time volume rendering. Ware and Franck (1996) have compared the relative merits of many of the 2D and 3D visual cues available for displaying a 3D volume on a 2D computer video screen. They found that real-time 3D viewing using hand control for rotation of the object was the most accurate, as well as one of the fastest interactions (for accomplishing the tested task). Automatic cine rotations were slightly worse, while a single static 2D image was always the least comprehensible presentation (Ware and Franck 1996). While the best visualization will depend on the clinical task and the dataset, generally for both surface rendering and volume rendering, the most desired presentation method is real-time interactive control of the object and light sources by the user. The other methods (single view, collection of views, cine loops) have all been intermediate steps while waiting for the technology to reach the stage of being able to achieve real-time speeds at affordable prices. Similar benefits to user control of rotation, and also from stereo display, were found by Sollenberg and Milgram (1993).

In most cases, when high-quality volume rendering has been compared to surface rendering it has been considered superior. Further, surface rendering can be considered a subset of volume rendering, since it can be realized by the appropriate choice of volume rendering method (gradient) and parameter (threshold) settings. Again, similar to the progression towards interactive realtime rendering from static views, surface rendering has progressed to volume rendering as computer speeds have become capable of supporting it.

## 13.4 Clinical Applications

In this section we examine published studies that evaluate the clinical applications of 3D visualizations for the extracranial head and neck. The temporal bone and skull base applications will be discussed in more detail in the following chapter.

3D imaging and visualization provides the surgeon with perspectives not available with conventional scans and allows the reconstructed image to be viewed from the expected surgical position. Especially with the ability to observe cutaway and transparency visualizations, the surgeon can reference the procedure to the surface or other landmarks (Andrews et al. 1992).

LaRouere et al. (1990) found that non-real-time surface-rendered 3D offered no significant advantage over 2D for assessing temporal bone anatomy, although it did allow better understanding of the topographic relationship of lesions within the temporal bone (Fig. 13.1). Howard et al. (1990) found no diagnosis was substantially changed by the addition of 3D over 2D for temporal bone studies. However, the 3D did give a direct impression of the lesion and provided spatial relationships not easily appreciated on 2D alone.

The primary advantage of this form of data presentation for temporal bone imaging is the additional information of depth perception, contours, volume, and extent of an abnormality (Darling et al. 1994). 3D display of CT studies of temporal bone and skull base using surface rendering have demonstrated an improvement in surgeons' understanding and planning for temporal bone tumors, middle ear deformities, and cochlear implants. Changing to vol-

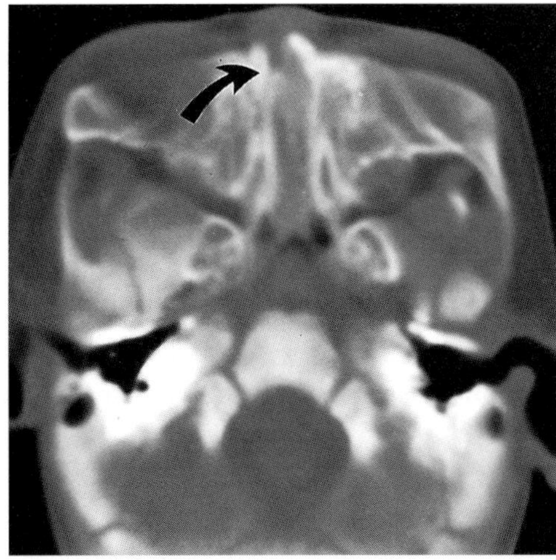

a

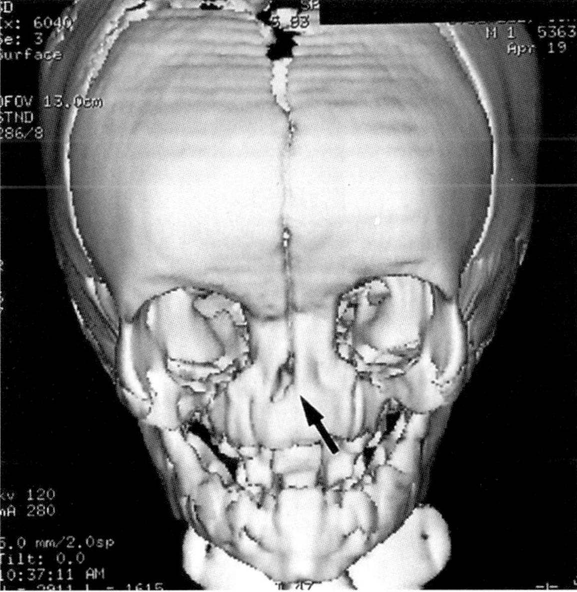

b

**Fig. 13.3.** **a** Axial CT performed at the level of the nasal cavity demonstrates a hypoplastic pyriform aperture and nasal cavity. **b** 3D surface rendering of the CT data of the patient presented in **a** demonstrates the hypoplasia of the pyriform aperture. These reconstructions are performed at our institution for all patients with craniofacial malformations

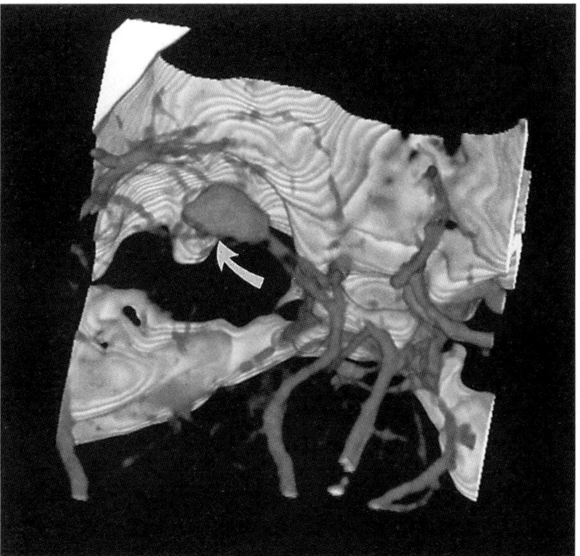

**Fig. 13.4.** 3D volumetric reconstruction of a contrast-enhanced CT (contiguous 1-mm-thick sections) showing an anuerysm of the right middle cerebral artery trifurcation. The neurosurgeon was able to interact with this CT angiogram and used this technique to replicate the expected intraoperative patient position. Because of the excellent visualization of the aneurysm and adjacent vessels on the volume rendered CT angiogram, cerebral angiography was not performed prior to surgery

ume rendered, under real-time control, should further improve surgeon's understanding of the complex anatomy of this region (Schubert et al. 1996). 3D presentation of the study also greatly aids the patients' understanding of the procedure they are about to undergo (Yamamoto et al. 1991).

Mevio et al. (1995) found that 3D CT visualization helped in presenting complex maxillofacial anatomical parts, permitting more specific preoperative analysis and surgical planning. Benson et al. (1996) found that CT with 3D visualization (shaded surface) optimally evaluates the presence and degree of sutural involvement and assesses associated facial and intracranial abnormalities. At our institution, 3D reconstructions are routinely perfomed in patients with congenital craniofacial malformations, craniosynostosis, and complex facial trauma (Fig. 13.3).

3D computed tomography angiography (CTA) has been shown to be useful for evaluating carotid stenosis and detection and evaluation of intracranial aneurysms (Schwartz et al. 1992; Vieco et al. 1995; Fig. 13.4). Recently at our institution, two clinical studies have been completed that attempt to evaluate the clinical utility of real-time interactive 3D visualization. Using the previously described SeeThru 3D visualization and commercially available hardware, significant improvements were demonstrated in diagnostic evaluation and surgery planning for CT cardiothoracic cases and for improving breast cancer staging and evaluation using MR breast studies (Hemmincer et al. 1995; Fig. 13.5).

## 13.5 Summary

In summary, we have attempted to describe the various 3D visualization techniques and provide a per-

a

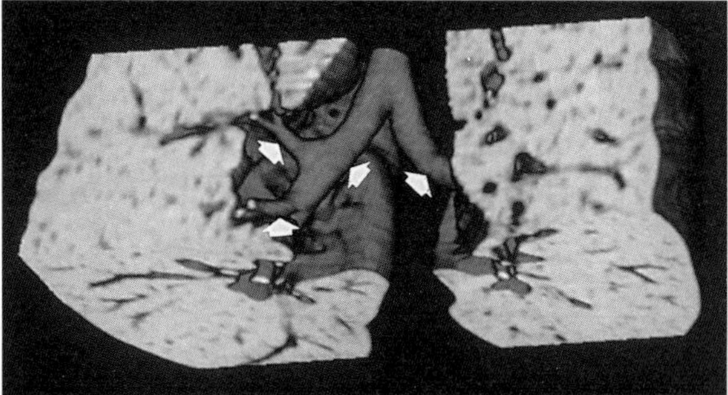

b

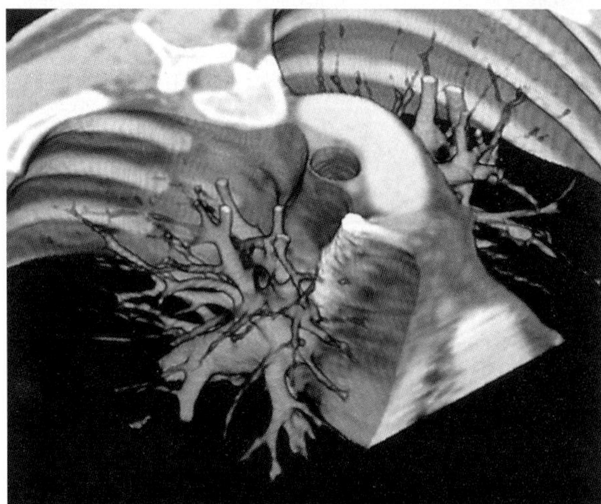

**Fig. 13.5 A,B.** Clinical applications of 3D imaging for preoperative evaluation of living donor lung transplantation. **a** 3D volumetric reconstruction viewed from the front of the patient. The anterior portion of the lungs have been "cut away." This view illustrates the normal bronchial anatomy (*arrows*) in this donor candidate. **b** Superior view of a 3D visualization performed in the same patient as illustrated in **a**. The pretransplant CT examinations are contrast-enhanced studies obtained using a helical (spiral) technique. In this example, the visualization has been interactively changed to remove the lung parenchyma and bronchial anatomy and illustrate the vascular anatomy. The 3D-reconstructed studies are routinely evaluated by the transplant surgeons at our institution to gain a better understanding of the normal bronchial and vascular anatomy in living donor lung candidates

spective on their clinical utility, which can be summarized as follows. First, while 3D alone is generally not better than 2D alone, 3D combined with 2D is as good and generally better than 2D alone. This argues for an integrated 2D plus 3D presentation approach. Secondly, the results of the comparative studies demonstrate that surgeons do benefit from 3D visualization, with the most significant advantages coming in preoperative analysis and surgical plannings. Radiologists, on the other hand, benefited to a lesser extent, mainly being helped in cases with complex or uncommon anatomy where they had less familiarity, and benefited more from the natural presentation of 3D spatial relationships. The third major message is that interactive visualizations (which could be controlled by the user for viewing position, lighting, or parameters to the rendering method, for instance to tune the visualization to show a specific tissue in certain fashion) were always better than noninteractive methods. Fourth and last, high-quality volume rendering was, in general, better than surface renderings or maximum intensity projection methods.

## References


Andrews JC, Yoshimi A, Mankovick NJ, Favilli M, TR, Lubkin RB, Jabour B (1992) Three-dimensional ct scan reconstruction for the assessment of congenital aural atresia. Am J Otol 13:236–240

Benson ML, Oliverio PJ, Yue NC, Zineich SJ (1996) Primary craniosynostosis: imaging features. AMJ Am J Roentgenol 166:697–703

Cabral B, Cam N, Foran F (1994) Accelerated volume rendering and tomographic reconstruction using texture mapping hardware. Proceedings of Symposium on Volume Visualization, Baltimore, October 1994

Darling CF, Byrd SE, Allen ED, Radkowski MA, Wilczynski MA (1994) Three-dimensional computed tomography imaging in the evaluation of craniofacial abnormalities. J Natl Med Assoc 86:676–680

Davis RE, Levoy M, Rosenman JG, Fuchs H, Pizer SM, Skinner A, Pillsburg HC (1991) Three-dimensional high-resolution volume rendering (HRVR) of computed tomography data: applications to otolaryngology-head and neck surgery. Laryngoscope 101:573–582

Drebin RA, Carpenter L, Hanrahan P (1988) Volume rendering. Computer Graphics 22:65–74

Fuchs H, Kedem ZM, Uselton SP (1977) Optimal surface reconstruction for planar contours. Commun Assoc Comput 20:693–702

Fuchs H, Poulton J, Eyles J, Greer T, Goldfeather J, Ellsworth D, Molnar S, Turk G, Tebbs B, Israel L (1992) Pixel-planes 5: a heterogenous multiprocessor graphics system using process enhanced memories. Computer Graphics/Proc Siggraph 1992 26:2231–240

Hemminger BM (1994) Realtime 3D visualization for medical image display. (Technical report TR94-027) Department of Computer Science, University of North Carolina, Chapel Hill

Hemminger BM, Cullip T, North MJ (1994) Interactive visualization of 3D medical image data. In: Boehme JM, Rowberg AH, Wolfman NT (eds) Computer applications to assist radiology. (S/CAR 94) Symposia Foundation, Carlstad, Calib, pp 127–135

Hemminger BM, Molina Pl, Braeuning PM, Detterbeck FC, Egan TM, Pisano ED, Beard DV (1995) Clinical applications of real-time volume rendering. Proceedings of Medical Imaging 1995: Image Display. SPIE 243:165–176

Howard JD, Elster AD, May JS (1990) Temporal bone: three-dimensional CT. I. Normal anatomy, techniques and limitations. Radiology 177:421–425

Kaba J, Matey J, Stoll G, Taylor H, Hanrahan P (1992) Interactive terrain rendering and volume visualization on the Princeton Engine. Proceedings of Visualization 1992, 19–23.10.92. IEEE Computer Society Press, Piscataway, NJ

LaRouere JM, Niparko JK, Gebarski SS, Kemink JL (1990) Three-dimensional x-ray computed tomography of the temporal bone as an aid to surgical planning. Otolaryngol Head Neck Surg 103:740–747

Levoy M (1991) Methods for improving the efficiency and versatility of volume rendering. Prog Clin Biol Res 363:473–488

Lorenson WE, Cline HE (1987) Marching cubes: high resolution 3D surface reconstruction algorithm. Computer graphics Proc Siggraph 1987 21:163–169

Mevio E, Calabro P, Preda L, DiMaggio EM, Caprotti A (1995) Spiral computerized tomography with tridimensional reconstruction (spiral 3d ct) in the study of maxillofacial pathology. Acta Otorhinolaryngol Ital 15:443–448

Molnar S, Eyles J, Poulton J (1992) PixelFlow: high-speed rendering using image composition. Computer Graphics 26:231–240

Mukherji SK, Shelton C, Hemminger BM, Harnsberger HR (1997) Advances in temporal bone imaging. In: Myers EN, Bluestone CD, Brackmann DE, Krause CJ (ed) Advances in otolaryngology-head and neck surgery, vol 11. Mosby Year Book Publishers, St Louis, pp 205–232

Schroeder Stoll G (1992) Data parallel volume rendering through line drawing. Workshop on volume visualization. IEEE Computer Society Press, Piscataway, NJ

Schubert O, Sartor K, Forsting M, Reisser C (1996) Three-dimensional computed display of otosurgical operation sites by spiral CT. Neuroradiology 38:663–668

Schwartz RB, Jones KM, Chernoff DM, Mukherji SK, Khorasni R, Tice HM, Kikinis R, Hooton SM, Steig PE, Polak JF (1992) Common cartoid artery bifurcation: evalution with spiral CT. Radiology 185:513–519

Silicon Graphics (1993) Symmetric multiprocessing systems technical report. Silicon Graphics, San Jose

Sollenberg RL, Milgram P (1993) Effects of stereoscopic and rotational displays in a three-dimensional path tracing task. Human Factors 3:483–499

Taylor HH, Mezrich RS, Shahidi R, Knight S (1993) Real-time interactive volumetric rendering system for medical imaging. Radiology 189P:131

Vieco PT, Shuman WP, Alsofrom FG, et al (1995) Detection of circle of Willis aneurysms in patients with acute subararchnoid hemorrhage: a comparison of CT angiography and digital subtraction angiography. AJR Am J Roentgenol 165:425–430

Ware C, Franck G (1996) Evaluating stereo and motion cues for visualizing information nets in three dimensions. ACM Trans Graphics 15:121–140

Yamamoto E, Mizukami CH, Isono M, Ohmura M, Hirono Y (1991) Observation of the external aperture of the vestibular aqueduct using three-dimensional surface reconstruction imaging. Laryngoscope 101:480–483

Yoo TS, Fuchs H (1993) Three dimensional visualization using medical data: 3D medical visualization from acquisition to application, course 21. Proc Siggraph 1993

# 14 3D Imaging of the Temporal Bone and Skull Base: The Surgeon's Perspective

V. Carrasco

CONTENTS



## 14.1 Introduction

Technologic innovations have varying effects on surgical treatment of disease. But advances in imaging have had a tremendous impact. We can determine much about the pathologic process in a chronically diseased ear with the physical exam and the audiogram. But it is difficult to determine the extent to which a destructive process has progressed within the ear *in full.* This knowledge determines the type of operation performed (tympanoplasty, tympanomastoidectomy, modified radical mastoidectomy, middle ear exploration (MEE) with ossicular reconstruction) and what type of ossicular reconstruction is required (partial or total ossicular replacement prosthesis [PORP, TORP], incus replacement). The addition of computerized tomography (CT) has greatly aided the otologic surgeon by providing a look into the ear preoperatively. Improvements in computerized tomography (CT) and magnetic resonance imaging (MRI) now yield exquisitely detailed images with submillimeter resolution. These improved images, in their typical two-dimensional (2D) presentation format, have served to improve our diagnostic capabilities by providing better visualization of the anatomy. They also improve our understanding of the relationship that pathologic processes have with essential neurovascular structures. These highly detailed images also serve as a data source for advanced image processing and new visualization techniques, furthering their utility to the surgeon. But CT in conjunction with the physical exam does not fully delineate, *preoperatively*, a particular patient's anatomy or fully predict the extent of the pathologic process. Therefore, we continue to search for improvements in technology to achieve these goals. This chapter discusses the development of this technology, the current state of the art and its utility for the otolaryngology head and neck surgeon.

## 14.2 Background

The impact of 3D visualization has been felt for many years in craniofacial surgery and neurosurgery, but has had less of an impact on otolaryngology head and neck surgery because, though impressive to look at, these images lacked the fine detail and interactivity, two elements important for utility. High-resolution studies were needed to show fine anatomic details to be useful for surgical planning. CT scans with a slice thickness in the range of 1.0–1.5 mm produced two-dimensional (2D) images that provide excellent diagnostic data but add little information when formatted into three-dimensional (3D) images, especially with early surface rendering technology.

Recent advances in computer graphics make computerized medical planning possible using these images. These advances are used in disciplines as


V. Carrasco, MD, Division of Otolaryngology Head and Neck Surgery, 610 Burnet Womack, CB #7070, The School of Medicine, University of North Carolina at Chapel Hill, Chapel Hill, NC 27599, USA

diverse as radiation oncology, neurosurgery, orthopedic surgery and craniofacial reconstruction (Rosenman et al. 1989; Smith et al. 1993; Vannier et al. 1994). The advent of 3D treatment-planning systems has made it possible to target with certainty any desired volume within the patient from almost any exterior angle. This ability to localize volumes of internal anatomy is being put to use by neurosurgeons in stereotactically guided surgical systems. Orthopedic and craniofacial surgeons are now making extensive use of 3D computer-generated models for designing various types of prostheses, which are fitted to the patient with better precision than was previously possible (Vannier et al. 1994). This technology is just beginning to appear in the cranial base surgical literature, but has appeared only sporadically in the otolaryngology head and neck surgery literature as a whole (Gandhe et al. 1994).

It was also felt that an interactive computer technology that better organizes these images, permits image processing, and is capable of producing 2D and 3D visualizations could potentially improve surgical planning. The ability to obtain these images is limited by technology and by the nature of certain regions of the body. The more rigid an area is, the easier it is to obtain an accurate reproducible image; the temporal bone, for example, is a good subject. Breathing introduces motion to equation, which can degrade the image. Gating the image acquisition has gone some way toward resolving this problem in certain respects, but has not been perfected in all areas of the body. Another factor that has limited the early use of this technology has been the quality of the images. Initial images that presented a 3D view of the skull proved to be adequate for the craniofacial surgeon, because they were moving relatively large sections of the cranium as part of reconstructive planning. The otologist, for example, needs high-resolution views of the internal anatomy of the temporal bone. Many of the structures that need to be examined are in the millimeter range and until recently were not even seen routinely on 2D CT views. It should be noted at this point that 3D visualizations do not, as a rule, produce *higher* resolution than 2D views. At present, 2D views still provide the most individual details and remain the standard for identification of pathology. But 3D visualizations are catching up and currently provide a valuable contribution by improving the spatial recognition of internal anatomy and pathology.

## 14.3 Hardware

Early computer hardware was capable of producing 3D images that were viewed either statically or with cine loops, a series of sequentially rendered 3D images chained together to provide the illusion of motion in 3D. Advances in hardware with the production of commercially available texture mapped graphic supercomputers made real-time interactivity with multiple large 3D data sets possible. This new hardware spawned the development of new software in the form of volume rendering algorithms, display, image processing and object definition tools (Levoy 1990). It was not until the advent of the SGI Reality Engine, which became available at UNC in 1993, that accelerated volume rendering became available and true real-time interactive 3D imaging was possible (Cullip and Neuman 1993). This allowed the next steps to be taken: taking clinical problems and applying this technology to them, and assessing its usefulness.

## 14.4 Software

Despite these limitations, visualization of axially acquired CT data rendered in three dimensions has aided temporal bone surgeons' approach to the congenital ear. Andrews et al. (1992) and Davis et al. (1991) have shown how a simple "sand-away" approach can be useful for mimicking the actual surgery performed by a temporal bone surgeon. This technology, as more recently applied to the temporal bone using tools developed specifically for the otologic surgeon, has yielded higher resolution 3D images (Carrasco et al. 1995). These images provide fine enough details for reliable preoperative surgical planning for patients with ear disease. Additionally, new software has permitted the application of this technology to skull base surgery, taking and organizing the large amount of image data and putting it into a system that provides 2D and 3D images for use in surgical planning (Carrasco et al. 1995). Other software advances have occurred. Specifically to take advantage of the soft tissue identification characteristics of MR and the bone detail of CT, these images have been fused into a new image with characteristics of both, providing unique information to the skull base surgeon (Carrasco et al. 1995).

The CT scanner, introduced almost 20 years ago, significantly improved the ability of the temporal bone surgeon to plan preoperatively for surgical procedures. It is still considered the study of choice for obtaining bony detail of the middle ear and temporal bone (SHANKAR and MONTANERA 1991). The current state of the art calls for 1-mm CT slices acquired conventionally or spirally. These studies are obtained in axial and coronal planes because fine anatomic details, within the millimeter range, are seen as fragments in each scan plane and can be seen completely only if they happen to lie exactly in the scan plane. These CT data are then displayed as sequential, 2D static panels that may exceed 300 in number. Thus, the spatial relationships of *two* orthogonal CT studies are mentally integrated into a 3D visualization for treatment planning purposes. The ability of individual surgeons to fully assimilate and process this information varies, so that it is frequently difficult for them to fully determine the nature and extent of the disease process confronting them. This ability may also be significantly limited by the current format of image data presentation. Ossicular destruction, cochlear/semicircular canal fenestration, and facial nerve dehiscence are 3D events that are poorly reproduced in a 2D fragmented image format.

## 14.5 Surgical Planning Tool and "SeeThru"

In a multi-departmental collaboration including Otolaryngology, Radiation Oncology, Computer Science and Radiology, a prototype surgical planning tool was developed. High-resolution CT or MR image data sets obtained from the scanners were transferred to the computer workstation. The surgical planning in its early form was composed of a series of visualization programs capable of viewing computerized tomographic image data and magnetic resonance image data simultaneously in a variety of ways. Images were both presented in 2D format and assembled into 3D visualizations. This offered many features, including multiple 3D rendering algorithms, image processing and limited object definition capabilities.

This tool allowed real-time interaction with the data, in a manner making it possible for the surgeon to develop views on the fly. This permitted the surgeon to examine data in a way that personally suited him or her, an extremely important aspect. The addition of motion controlled by the surgeon during evaluation of the image data improved spatial understanding of pathology in three dimensions. GANDHE et al. (1994), in a prospective study, evaluated the value of motion of 3D images using rotational movies sequences of 3D data sets of skull base lesions. We have found that the addition of the individual having control over the data interactively better helps integrate the spatial information. The planning system discussed here also has the added advantage of simultaneous interactive multiple 2D image slice and 3D visualization viewing from CT and MR data (Fig. 14.1). Slices can be enlarged and regions zoomed with very little loss of detail (Fig. 14.2). This system was assembled specifically to satisfy the needs of the otologic surgeon. It was observed that the simultaneous availability of both 2D and 3D images was most beneficial. The 3D images provide information in a "real world" view that simulates clinical circumstances (Figs. 14.3, 14.4).

SeeThru, a real-time interactive 3D visualization tool for medical image data, was developed by the UNC Department of Radiology, also as a part of this multi-departmental collaboration (HEMMINGER 1994; HEMMINGER et al. 1994). It is a visualization tool that makes it possible for a user to view a variety of image modalities, including CT, MR, and CT angiography. It is a highly interactive tool that allows the user real-time control of: viewpoint, "lighting," cut planes (control of removal of data), data classification and segmentation.

## 14.6 Image Fusion

Frequently, the neurotologist/skull base surgeon requires multiple image modalities, CT, and MR in order to diagnose and plan surgical intervention (CARRASCO et al. 1995; MUKHERJI et al. 1996). Specifically in order to take advantages of the soft tissue identification characteristics of MR and the bone detail of CT, these images have been fused into a new image with characteristics of both, providing unique information to the skull base surgeon (MUKHERJI et al. 1996). This requires precise registration of the data sets from each modality. This is performed without the need for internal fiducial markers (Figs. 14.5–14.11).

In the early part of this decade, what was required to perform this task was a Silicon Graphics Onyx and a Reality Engine, as well as the Fusion Tool software

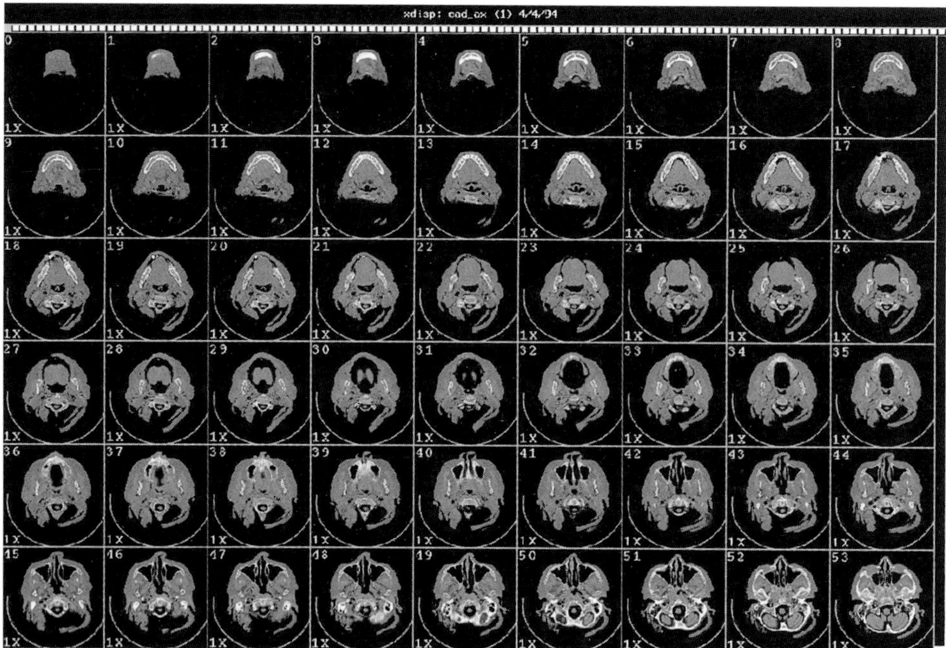

**Fig. 14.1.** Here an entire CT study is displayed side by side in a similar presentation to that we are familiar with. The difference is that slices can be selected individually and enlarged without loss of detail

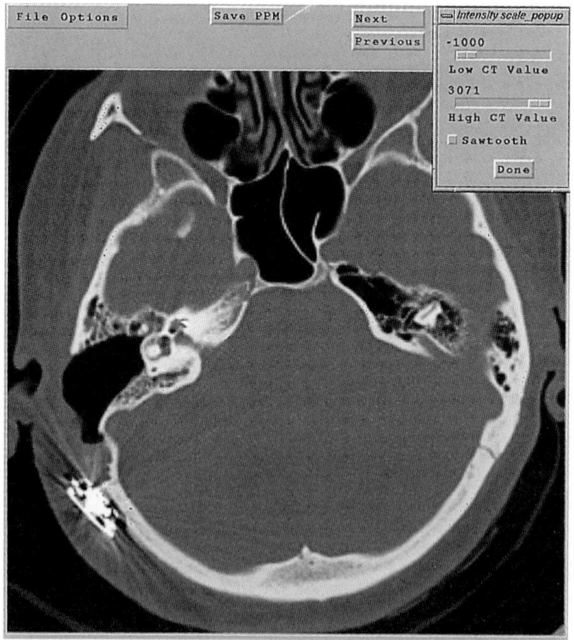


**Fig. 14.2.** This surgical planning module presented individual slices in a large format (18 cm × 18 cm), permitting highly detailed examination of individual slices in 2D. The user could page through the entire study sequentially. Here the CT data set from a patient with a cochlear implant referred for revision is examined

(Soltys et al. 1995). Currently these tasks are performed on a Pentium II-based computer running in excess of 400 mHz. The software has the capability of simultaneous 3D volume rendering of the CT and the MR data sets, and also a "slice view" capacity. The slice view is the modality that enables registration (Figs. 14.5–14.7). The data sets are color labeled for easier identification of the individual studies. White typically represents the CT data set (bone detail), and red typically depicts the MR data set (soft tissue). The volume rendering module is highly interactive, allowing real-time change of viewpoint. Registration is accomplished by real-time manipulation of the data sets, with arbitrary cut plane viewing to verify the registration in multiple planes from multiple viewpoints (Figs. 14.5–14.7). The data sets can be manipulated separately or while "fused." Transverse projection, the viewpoint with the highest resolution, provides the most accurate anatomic registration. Besides being an important presurgical planning tool, this technique is also an integral part of the 3D conformal treatment planning technique used by the Radiation Oncology Department at the University of North Carolina.

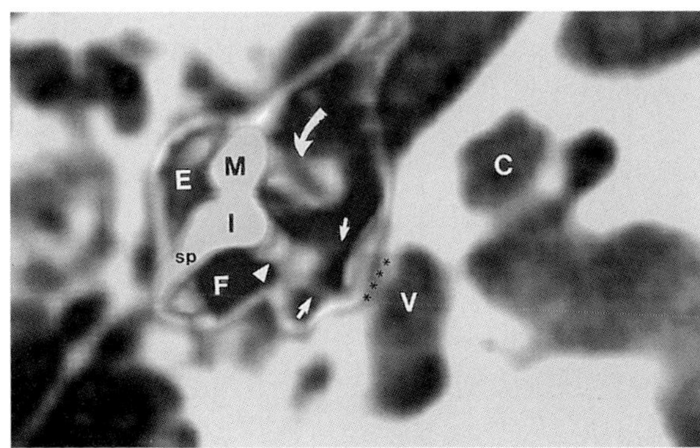


a

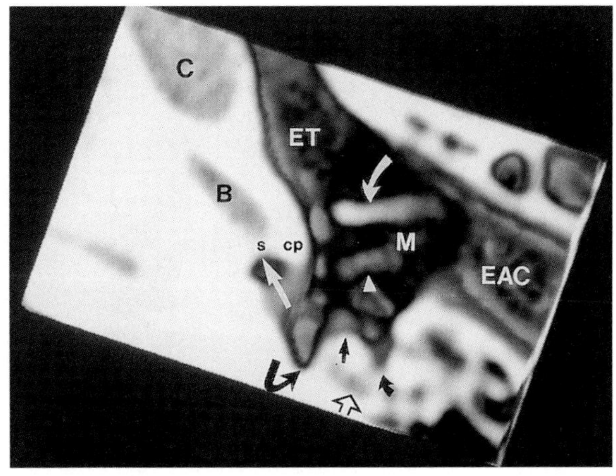


b

**Fig. 14.3 A,B.** 3D volume rendering of the temporal bone. **a** Superior view of the temporal bone illustrates the improvement in understanding of the topographic anatomy and spatial relationships achieved by using 3D reconstruction (*M* malleus, *curved arrow* manubrium of the malleus, *I* incus, *sp* short process of the incus, *arrowhead* long process of the incus, *small arrows* stapes crura, *asterisks* oval window, *V* vestibule, *C* cochlea, *E* lateral epitympanic recess [Prussak's space], *F* fossa incudis). **b** Inferior view of the same region of the middle ear cavity as illustrated in **a** provides a better understanding of the anatomic relationships between the structures of this complex region than is possible with standard axial 2D imaging (*M* middle ear cavity, *curved white arrow* manubrium of the malleus, *arrowhead* long process of the incus, *straight white arrow* round window, *s* subiculum, *B* basal turn of the cochlea, *large curved black arrow* sinus tympani, *straight black arrow* pyramidal eminence, *small curved arrow* facial recess, *open black arrow* descending portion of the facial nerve, *C* petrous portion of the carotid artery, *ET* eustachian tube, *EAC* external auditory canal) (Case courtesy of S. K. Mukherji MD)

## 14.7
## Technique for Acquiring Data from old or Outside Films Where Digital Data Are Not Available (Boxwala and Rosenman 1994)

Digital data are frequently unavailable. To recreate the electronic form of the CT or MR data, the film panels are digitized using a laser scanner. The scanning is done at a resolution of 318 µm (of film) per pixel. The resulting image dimensions are 1120 pixels × 1360 lines for the 14 × 17 inch sheet of CT panels. The spatial distortion introduced by the laser scanner is corrected by a linear transformation. Individual scans are then extracted manually using an interactive program called *xcrop*. Extraction is done so that each CT panel image is registered with respect to the others; the text printed on the CT panels is used as a registration landmark. In other words, the clipping box boundaries of *xcrop* are aligned with the same text in all panels. The scale printed on the CT panels is identified and used to make the correspondence between pixel size and real-world distances. Finally, all the extracted images are concatenated into a single 3D image file and transferred to the treatment planning system. The volume rendered visualizations are not of such high quality as the digitally transferred data sets, but are quite satisfactory.

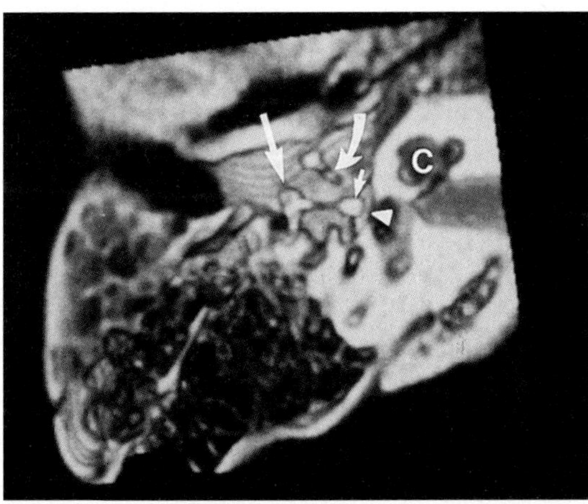


**Fig. 14.4.** Three-dimensional image of a patient who underwent placement of a total ossicular replacement prosthesis (TORP) following ossicular injury sustained in a motor vehicle accident. The study shows the TORP (*large straight arrow*), with the footplate of the prosthesis (*small straight arrow*) adjacent to the oval window *arrowhead*; *C* cochlea, *curved arrow* manubrium of the malleus (Case courtesy of S. K. Mukherji MD)

## 14.8
## Future Development

We believe that the experience and expertise gained at UNC in dealing with computerized medical imaging have contributed significantly to the

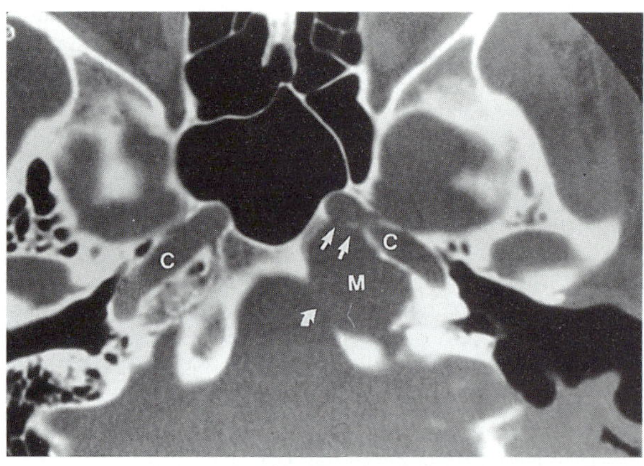


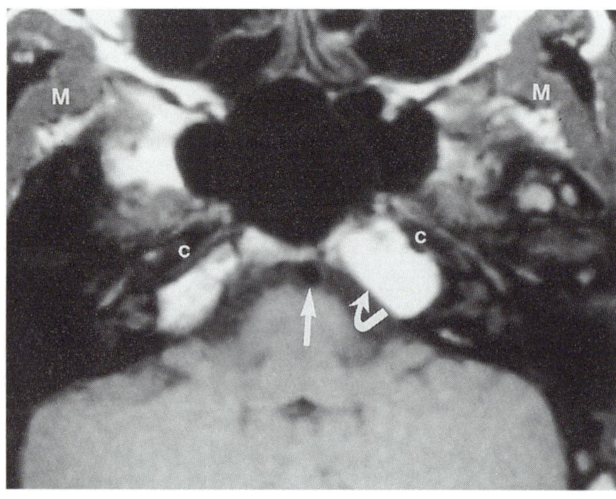


**Fig. 14.5.** **a** Axial CT visualized at bone window settings demonstrates lytic lesion with well-defined margins in left petrous apex (*M*). Note extent of bone erosion involving cortex of the posterior petrous portion of the temporal bone (*curved arrow*) and bony covering (*straight arrows*) of the petrous segment of the internal carotid artery (*C*). **b** Axial T1-weighted non-contrast-enhanced MR imaging performed in same patient as in **a** shows a high-signal-intensity mass located within the left petrous apex (*curved arrow*), which is characteristic of a cholesterol granuloma. Note relationship of the mass to the basilar artery (*straight arrow*). There is excellent visualization of the soft tissues of the brain and masticator spaces (*M*); however, the relationship of the mass to the carotid artery (*c*) and the extent of bone erosion is better seen on CT than on MR imaging. Reprinted, with permission, from Mukherji et al. (1996)

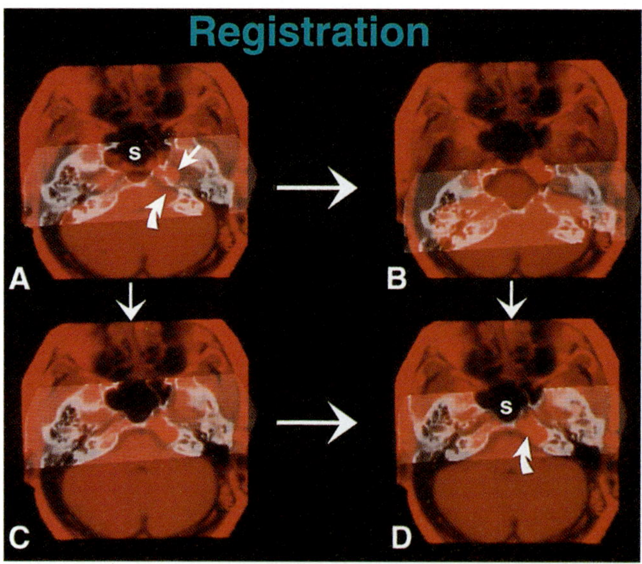


**Fig. 14.6 A–D.** The volumetric data from Fig. 14.5A and B are transferred to •• for image registration; the manual process performed for multimodality image registration. Multiple-slice view projections are presented in the axial plane . The CT data are displayed in *white* and the MR imaging data in *red*. In **A** note the malalignment of the lytic lesion present on CT (*curved arrow*) with the high signal abnormality present on MR imaging (*straight arrow*). Also note the offset of the sphenoid sinuses on CT and MR imaging (*s*). These structures should normally overlie. The data sets are individually manipulated in various patterns (**B, C**) in order to improve their anatomic alignment . Image **D** represents the final alignment. Note the excellent CT and MR imaging alignment of the mass (*arrow*) and the sphenoid sinus (*s*) compared with **A–C.** This data manipulation is also performed in coronal and sagittal slice view projections before a final registration is achieved. Reprinted, with permission, from Mukherji et al. (1996)

development of 3D surgical planning tools for otolaryngology head and neck surgery. Nevertheless, far more could be done with this technology to directly aid the surgeon. These tools could offer sophisticated interaction, ease of use, and a variety of registration modalities, visualizations and object definition instruments useful to our specialty.

This technology will evolve further in several ways. Eventually this system will function not only for treatment planning, but to give continual guidance to the surgeon while operating. However, a complete surgical simulator would have to allow for changes in the 3D model itself. Cut vessels bleed and retract. Pieces of bone and muscles are removed, and cut edges are re-approximated. Changes such as these would have to be calculated on the fly and redisplayed. To ensure that the results of such calculations would lead to realistic changes in the model the computer programs would have to have extensive knowledge of the underlying anatomy and physiology of the model, as well as information

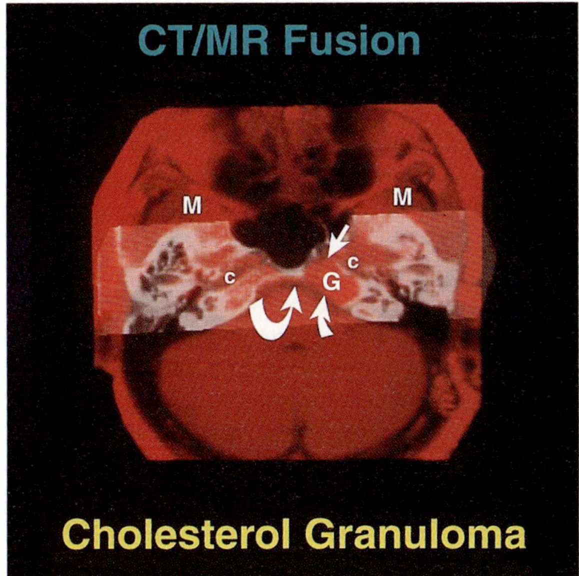


**Fig. 14.7.** Final CT/MR fusion of the patient presented in Fig. 14.5. CT data are presented in *white* and the MR imaging study is displayed in *red*. Co-registered study provides tissue characterization of the cholesterol granuloma (*G*) and excellent soft tissue detail present on the MR imaging study (*M* masticator space, *large curved arrow* basilar artery), along with information regarding the location of the petrous portion of the internal carotid artery (*c*) and the amount and the extent of the bone erosion present on CT (*straight arrow* erosion of bone surrounding the carotid canal, *small curved arrow* erosion of the posterior wall of the petrous portion of the temporal bone). Reprinted, with permission, from MUKHERJI et al. (1996)

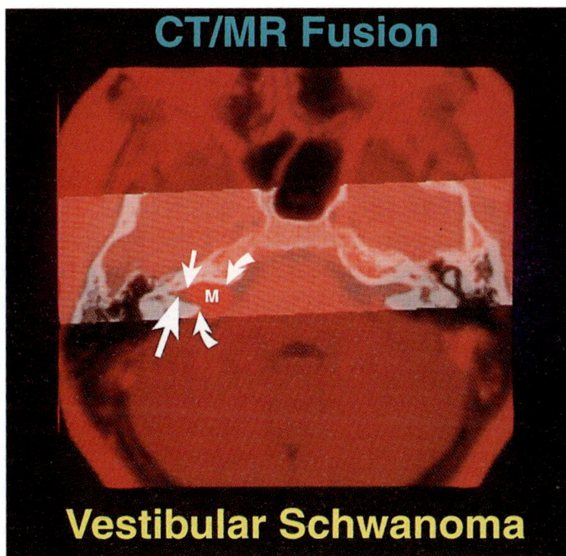


**Fig. 14.8.** CT/MR image fusion of a vestibular schwannoma shows an enhancing mass located within the internal auditory canal (*M*) with enlargement of the porus acusticus (*curved arrows*). Note that the lateral aspect of the schwannoma is proximal (*small arrow*) and does not extend into the fundus of the internal auditor canal (*large arrow*). Reprinted, with permission, from MUKHERJI et al. (1996)

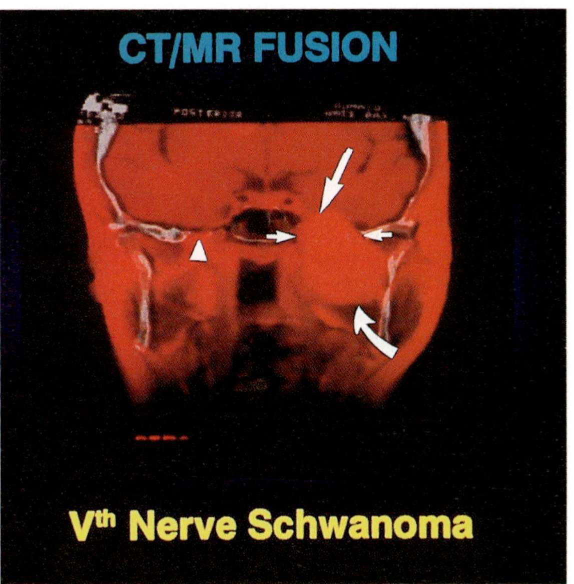


**Fig. 14.9.** CT/MR fusion of a schwannoma involving the mandibular division of the Vth cranial nerve. The mass invloves the masticator space (*curved arrow*) and extends upward into the region of the cavernous sinus (*large straight arrow*). Note the smooth bone expansion of the foramen ovale, which is identified on the CT portion of the fused image (*small straight arrows*). Compare this with the normal appearance of foramen on the contralateral side (*arrowhead*) (Case courtesy of S. K. Mukherji MD)

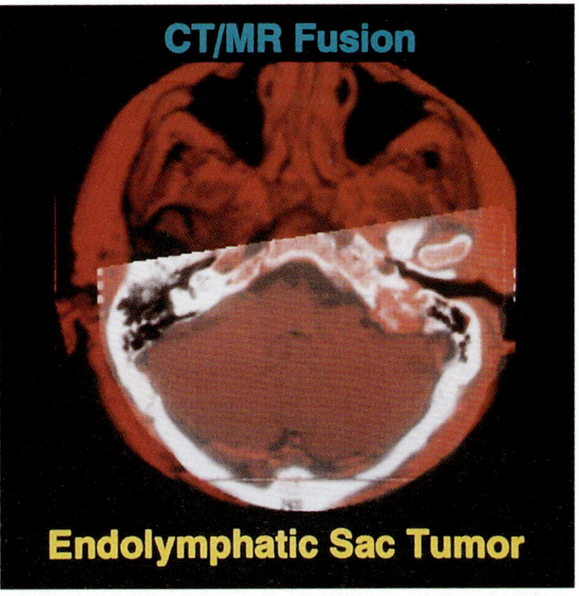


**Fig. 14.10.** CT/MR fusion of an endolymphatic sac tumor involving the left temporal bone. This format allows simultaneous viewing of the CT and MR imaging studies and allows the surgeon to evaluate the extent of the soft tissue abnormality (MR) directly with the degree of bone destruction (CT) (Case courtesy of S. K. Mukherji MD)

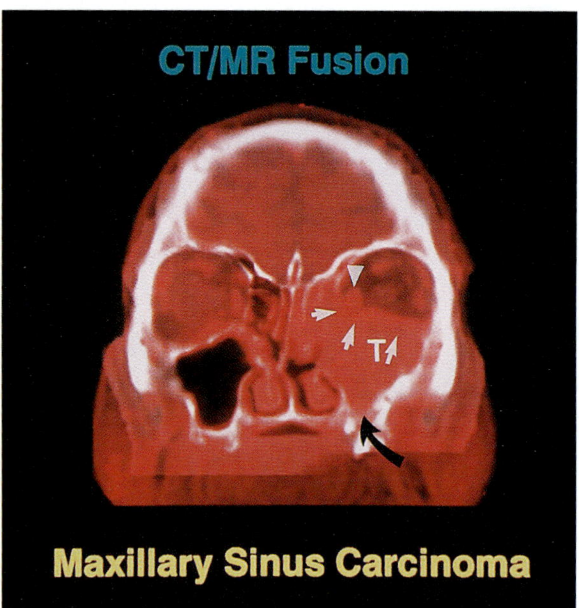


**Fig. 14.11.** CT/MR fusion of a patient with a left maxillary sinus carcinoma (*T*). The co-registered images show that the tumor has spread upward into the orbit and has eroded the floor and medial walls of the orbit (*straight arrows*). The involvement of the orbital floor indicates neoplastic invasion of the maxillary division of the Vth cranial nerve. The tumor has completely encased the inferior rectus muscle and is in close proximity to the medial rectus muscle (*arrowhead*). Note the relative sparing of the alveolar recess of the maxillary sinus (*curved arrow*). Compare the above findings with the normal anatomy seen of the contralateral side (Case courtesy of S. K. Mukherji MD)

pertaining to how the anatomy "reacts" when it is altered. This will require intraoperative real-time updating of image data sets compensating for changes as surgery progresses. Perhaps, based on virtual reality technology, the system of the future will allow the surgeon to practice a procedure, perhaps even using several different approaches, until he or she is comfortable with all the nuances of a particular patient. Our current surgical approach is to establish wide three-dimensional anatomic exposure before attacking the pathology, in order to identify and preserve vital structures. At times, in order to remove the pathology, these structures must be sacrificed. This wide exposure consumes significant operating time. If much of it were eliminated by accurate preoperative identification of the pathology and adjacent vital structures, and guidance intraoperatively past these vital structures with feedback as to when adequate resection had occurred, then surgical exposure, elective sacrifice of and operating time could be reduced. Early forms of this technology currently exist in the form of endoscopic sinus guidance systems. Preoperative CT scan data sets that contain fiducial or landmark information are obtained from the patient at the time of scanning. The CT data sets are registered with the landmark information in the OR in order to provide intraoperative spatial information as to the location of the surgeon's instruments relative to vital structures during the procedure. Future guidance systems may take the form of projecting images of the 3D reconstructed scans that are registered with the patient directly into the eyes of the surgeon. The surgeon could then always keep track of exactly where his or her position is with respect to critical anatomy. True invasive surgery would be developed. Nevertheless, realistic surgical simulators will someday be built. At present, it is more realistic to concentrate on surgical planning tools that can perform tasks well enough to be of practical use.

## 14.9 Conclusion

In order to reach this goal of a true intraoperative computerized surgical guidance system, a number of intervening steps must be achieved. These are: development of higher resolution cross-sectional image studies, higher resolution displays, accurate high-resolution interactive visualizations, image processing, convenient object definition tools, new volume rendering software and an accessible user interface. Many of these have been achieved with recent advances in technology. CT/MR image studies are continually improving, and with the advent of spiral CT and submillimeter CT on the horizon this goal is close to realization for the temporal bone surgeon. Current technology does not support these activities in a useful manner, allowing the surgeon not only to interactively view the image data sets, but to alter them in such a fashion as to simulate procedures. But a reasonable goal at present is a surgical planning system that organizes image data and presents it in an accessible manner to improve anatomic and spatial understanding of underlying pathology. We have discussed here preliminary data on such a system developed at the University of North Carolina. We initially directed our energies to solving some simple problems concerned with determining the most useful methods of displaying image data to the otolaryngologist head and neck surgeon. Next, a series of visualization tools were examined to see whether they provided the optimum views for the surgeon. This addressed the questions, "How does this information need to be presented to the surgeon to obtain optimum planning strategies? What would the surgeon change about these images if he/she had the ability (image processing)?" Obtaining images of adequate quality has been a rate-limiting step in the past for the development of this type of instrumentation for the otolaryngologist. We initially focused our development of a computerized surgical planning tool on the temporal bone, because of the characteristics mentioned above. It is rigid, allowing reproducible accurate scanning with both CT and MR. It also faced us with a formidable problem, in that the anatomy that required visualization, as a rule, was well beyond the current graphics capability of current visualization technology. Future development could yield a set of regionalized (ear, skull base, larynx, sinus and neck) visualization instruments and eventually combine them into a general planning tool. The specific differences between the regionalized tools will be the establishment of preset visualization parameters for specific regions and the specific array of visualization programs that have been determined to be the most useful in these regions. This will serve as the foundation for the future development of surgical simulators and effective intraoperative guidance tools.

## References


Andrews JC, Anzai Y, Mankovich NJ, Favilli M, Lufkin RB, Jabour B (1992) Three-dimensional CT scan reconstruction for the assessment of congenital aural atresia. Am J Otol 13:236–240

Boxwala A, Rosenman JG (1994) Retrospective reconstruction of three dimensional radiotherapy treatment plans from two dimensional planning data. Int J Radiat Oncol Biol Phys 28:1009

Carrasco VN, Murkherji S, Soltys MS, Pizer SM, Rosenman J (1995) A realtime interactive three dimensional visualization system for temporal bone surgical planning. Southern Section of the Triologic Society, Key West, Fla

Carrasco VN, Murhkerji S, Soltys M, Quatrocchi K, Piser S, Rosenman J (1995) Three dimensional surgical planning for resection of skull base tumors using multiple image modalities. North American Skull Base Society, Naples, Fla

Cullip TJ, Neuman U (1993) Accelerating volume construction with 3D texture memory. (Technical report TR93-027) Dept of Computer Science, University of North Carolina, Chapel Hill

Davis RE, Levoy M, Rosenman JG, Fuchs H, Pizer SM, Skinner A, Pillsbury HC (1991) Three-dimensional high-resolution volume rendering (HRVR) of computed tomography data: applications to otolaryngology-head and neck surgery. Laryngoscope 101:573–582

Gandhe AJ, Hill DL, Studhome C, Hawkes DJ, Ruff CL, Cox TC, Gleeson MJ, Strong AJ (1994) Combined and three-dimensional rendered multimodal data for planning cranial base surgery: a prospective evaluation. Neurosurgery 35:463–471

Hemminger RM (1994) Realtime 3D visualization for medical image display. (Technical report TR94-027) Department of Computer Science, University of North Carolina, Chapel Hill

Hemminger BM, Cullip T, North MJ (1994) Interactive visualization of 3D medical image data. In: Boehme JM, Rowberg AH, Wolfman NT (eds) Computer applications to Assist Radiology. (S/CAR 94) Symposia Foundation, Carlsbad, Calif, pp 127–135

Levoy M (1990) Efficient ray tracing of volume data. ACM Trans Graphics 9:245–261

Mukherji SK, Rosenman JG, Soltys M, Boxwala A, Castillo M, Carrasco V, Pizer SM (1996) A new technique for CT/MR image fusion for skull base imaging. Skull Base Surg 6:141–146

Rosenman J, Sherouse GW, Fuchs H, Pizer SM, Skinner AL, Mosher C, Novins K, Tepper JE (1989) Three-dimensional display techniques in radiation therapy treatment planning. Int J Radiat Oncol Biol Phys 61:263–269

Shankar L, Montanera W (1991) Computed tomography versus magnetic resonance imaging and three-dimensional applications. Med Clin North Am 75:1355–1366

Smith GA, Aspden RM, Porter RW (1993) Measurement of vertebral foraminal dimensions using three-dimensional computerized tomography. Spine 18:629–636

Soltys M, Beard D, Carrasco V et al (1995) Fusion: a tool for the registration and visualization of multiple modality 3D medical data. SPIE Med Imaging 24:31

Vannier, MW, Marsh JL, Warren JO (1994) Three-dimensional CT reconstruction images for craniofacial surgical planning and evaluation. Radiology 150:279–284

# 15 Imaging and Interventional Procedures for the Lacrimal Duct System

Alfred G. Janssen

CONTENTS



## 15.1 Anatomy of the Lacrimal Drainage System

### 15.1.1 Anatomy of the Canaliculi

To evaluate the lacrimal drainage system using diagnostic imaging, some knowledge of the anatomy of the lacrimal drainage system is required. The relevant structures are shown in Fig. 15.1a. Figure 15.1b presents a similar image of the lacrimal drainage system obtained by digital subtraction dacryocystography. The lacrimal points are located on the edge of the upper and lower eyelids in the medial corner of the eye. They are turned slightly inward and lie adjacent to the eyeball. The puncta form the entrance to the canaliculi. Initially, the upper and lower canaliculus are almost at right angles with the edge of the eyelid, but after some 2 mm they curve sharply to run more or less parallel with the edge of the eyelid. The total length of the upper canaliculus is about 10 mm, and the lower canaliculus is about 12 mm in length (Cowen and Hurwitz 1996). They merge in the medial corner of the eye to form the common canaliculus, also known as the sinus of Maier, which varies in length from 1 mm to several millimeters and ends in the lacrimal sac. The common canaliculus is not perpendicular to the surface of the lacrimal sac, but enters it at an angle of less than 90°. When an obstruction further down in the lacrimal drainage system causes a pathologic swelling of the lacrimal sac, as may happen with a mucocele or pyocele, for instance, this can cause kinking in the common canaliculus, preventing drainage of the lacrimal sac contents via the canaliculi.

The drainage of tears from the eye via the lacrimal drainage system to the nose is not merely a passive gravitational mechanism. There is also a pump mechanism (Hurwitz 1996a). In the eyelids the canaliculi run between a deep head and a superficial head of the orbicularis muscle. Every blinking movement of the eyelids causes volume changes in the lumen of the canaliculi, which activate a pump mechanism transporting tears via the canaliculi. When the puncta are not adjacent to the eyeball, as in entropion or ectropion, or when there is no blinking of the eyelids, as in facial paresis, the pump mechanism fails, causing epiphora (tearing), despite sufficient patency of the lacrimal drainage system (Tanenbaum and McCord 1993). The passage of tears through the lacrimal sac and the nasolacrimal duct, on the other hand, is mainly a passive process associated with gravity, posture of the head, and the quantity of tears (Hurwitz 1996a).

### 15.1.2 Anatomy of the Lacrimal Sac and Duct

The lacrimal sac is a cylindrical structure with a ball-shaped top extending some millimeters above the

A.G. Janssen, MD, Department of Diagnostic and Interventional Radiology, De Tjongerschans Hospital, Thialfweg 44, Postbus 10500, 8441 PW Heerenveen, The Netherlands

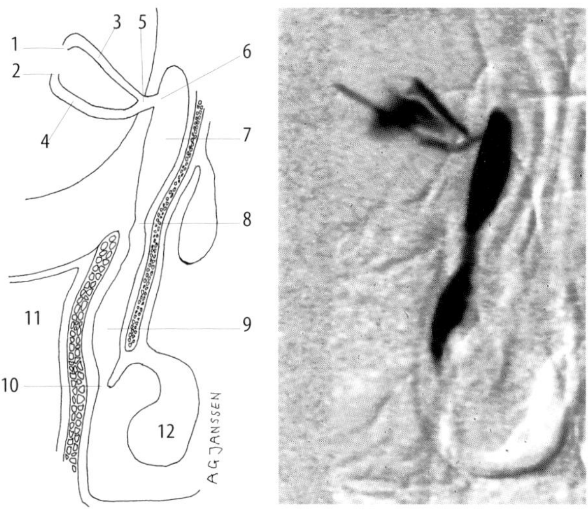


a,b

**Fig. 15.1.** **a** Diagram of the lacrimal excretory passages: *1* superior punctum, *2* inferior punctum, *3* superior canaliculus, *4* inferior canaliculus, *5* common canaliculus or sinus of Maier, *6* valve of Rosenmüller, *7* lacrimal sac, *8* junction between lacrimal sac and duct, also known as valve of Krause, *9* nasolacrimal duct, *10* valve of Hasner, *11* maxillary sinus, *12* inferior turbinate. **b** The lacrimal secretory passages visualized by digital subtraction acryocystography

site where the common canaliculus enters it. The lacrimal sac varies in size and shape. Its length varies from 12 mm to 15 mm, the transverse diameter is 3–5 mm, and the diameter from front to back is 4–8 mm (Cowen and Hurwitz 1996). The lacrimal sac is situated in the medial corner of the eye and is embedded in a skeletal groove, the fossa lacrimalis. The dorsal part of the fossa consists of a part of the lacrimal bone. The medial part of the groove is formed by a part of the maxilla. Further distally the groove deepens and the maxilla closes over the lacrimal duct ventrally, creating a canal in the bone: the lacrimal canal. It runs obliquely backwards and downwards into the maxilla in the bony wall between the nose and the maxillary sinus and ends in the nose underneath the inferior turbinate. The diameter of the bony canal is said to vary between 4 and 6 mm (Duke-Elder 1946), but we have often observed, mainly in patients with low occlusions in the lacrimal drainage system, a slight narrowing of the bony canal to 2.5 mm or 3 mm or less. One should be aware of this when performing interventions in the lacrimal drainage system.

The section of the lacrimal drainage system distal to the lacrimal sac, where the lacrimal drainage system runs through the bony canal, is called the nasolacrimal duct. The length of this tubular structure varies from 15 mm to 18 mm (Cowen and Hurwitz 1996). In the fetal stage the junction of the lacrimal sac and the nasolacrimal duct is initially not very clearly marked, with the entire tract of the lacrimal sac and nasolacrimal duct forming one straight tubular structure. During the embryonic period a distinct waist gradually develops between the lacrimal sac and the nasolacrimal duct. This mucosal fold is also known as the valve of Krause. It is, however, a pseudo-valve. Elsewhere in the lacrimal drainage system valve-like structures are present, consisting of mucosal folds. The most familiar ones are the valve of Rosenmüller, situated at the junction of the common canaliculus and the lacrimal sac, and the valve of Hasner, situated where the nasolacrimal duct ends in the nose. Occasionally, pseudo-valves are found at other sites in the lacrimal drainage system. The mucosa of the lacrimal sac and the nasolacrimal duct consists of columnar epithelium with loose connective tissue underneath. Besides some lymphoid tissue and elastic fibers, it consists of a rich venous plexus, which virtually transforms it into an erectile tissue continuous with the nasal mucosa (Duke-Elder 1946).

### 15.1.3 Congenital Abnormalities

Congenital abnormalities can occur in the lacrimal drainage system. The most common is congenital nasolacrimal duct obstruction, with a complete obstruction at the site of the valve of Hasner owing to a persisting membrane. In 90% of cases the obstruction will disappear spontaneously in the course of the first year of life (Nelson et al. 1985). When the abnormality persists, the ophthalmologist can generally treat it successfully by probing. If probing does not bring the desired result, the interventional radiologist can perform balloon dilatation of the valve of Hasner (Janssen et al. 1998).

Congenital abnormalities in the canaliculi include absent nasolacrimal punctum, punctal reduplication, and accessory canaliculi. Occasionally, a congenital fistula is observed between the lacrimal sac and the overlying skin. Diverticula are frequently found in the lacrimal drainage system. They are generally situated low down lateral to the lacrimal sac, and they vary in size (Figs. 15.2 and 15.3). Rare abnormalities are a severe obstruction of the bony canal or even complete obliteration in cases of craniostenosis, a developmental skull defect. Absence of the common canaliculus is only found in extremely rare cases. Figure 15.4 shows how in these cases the canaliculi end separately in the lacrimal sac.

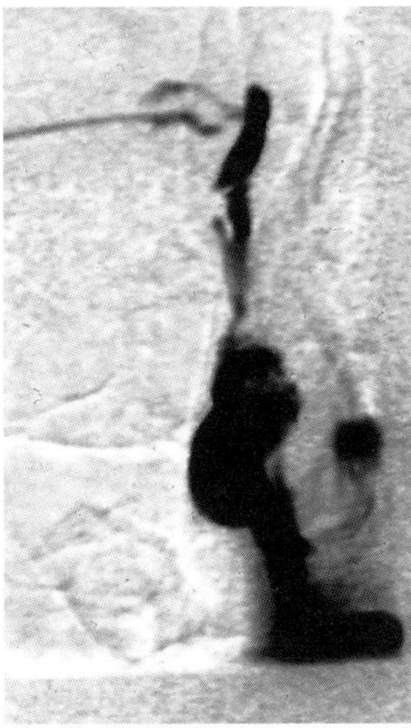

**Fig. 15.2.** Subtraction dacryocystography showing a small diverticulum at the lateral side of the nasolacrimal duct

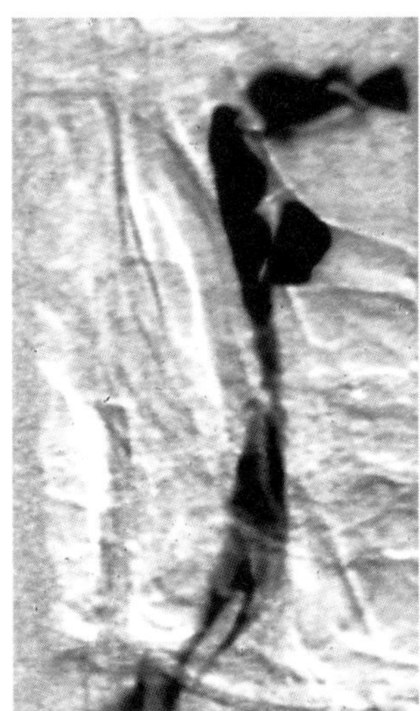

**Fig. 15.3.** Subtraction dacryocystography showing a large diverticulum at the lateral side of the nasolacrimal duct. The patient was found to have a large diverticulum on either side

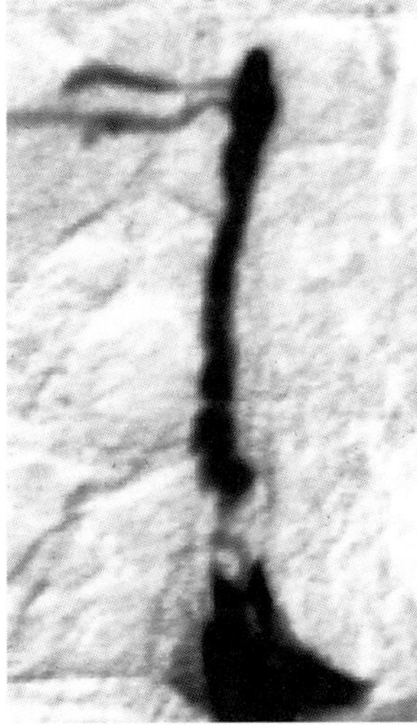

**Fig. 15.4.** Subtraction dacryocystography showing a congenital absence of the common canaliculus. The patient suffers from epiphora owing to a stenosis at the valve of Hasner

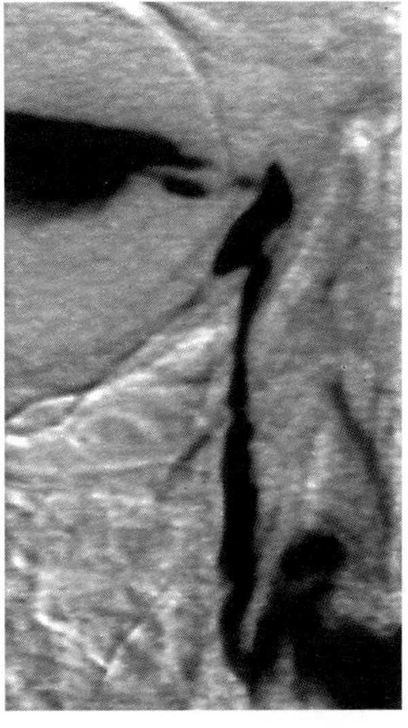

**Fig. 15.5.** Digital subtraction dacryocystography of the right-hand side, showing a common abnormality in the shape of the lacrimal sac: the junction of the lacrimal sac and the nasolacrimal duct is not located at the lowest point of the lacrimal sac

The junction of the larimal sac and the nasolacrimal duct is not always located at the lowest point of the lacrimal sac. Occasionally, the junction is found at the low medial side of the lacrimal sac, some millimeters above the more laterally situated lowest part of the lacrimal sac. This abnormal shape (Fig. 15.5) is quite common, and in such cases it is important to avoid false passage on probing or catheterization of the lacrimal drainage system.

## 15.2 Pathology of the Lacrimal System

### 15.2.1 Diseases of the Canaliculi

It is important that the radiologist should pay attention to pathologic changes in the canaliculi, because there are various ways in which the presence of an obstruction in the canaliculi can affect the success of an intervention in the lacrimal sac or the nasolacrimal duct. If an obstruction in the canaliculi is overlooked when a balloon dilatation is performed in a patient with epiphora or tearing caused by an obstruction of the drainage system in the lacrimal sac or nasolacrimal duct, the chances of successful treatment are very slight indeed. Most abnormalities of the canaliculi involve stenoses or occlusions at one site or over the entire length of the canaliculi. Frequently occurring obstructions are those caused by a bacterial or viral infection. Some drugs can also cause stenoses or occlusions of the canaliculi, such as drugs for glaucoma or chemotherapeutic agents, such as 5-fluorouracil. Tumors of the canaliculi are rare, the most common being papilloma. Occasionally a basal cell carcinoma is observed (Hurwitz 1996b). In some cases where no abnormalities of the canaliculi are detected and patency at irrigation is good, a disorder of the pump mechanism is found. This occurs in particular in abnormalities causing decreased motility and elastic properties of the canaliculi and the immediately surrounding area, such as scleroderma, radiation fibrosis or scar formation in skin burns (Tanenbaum and McCord 1993).

### 15.2.2 Diseases of the Lacrimal Sac and Duct

#### *15.2.2.1 Introduction*

Abnormalities of the lacrimal sac or nasolacrimal duct are another cause of disorders of the drainage system. The patient presents with epiphora, sometimes in combination with an intermittent or permanent infection. Stasis owing to obstructions low down in the lacrimal drainage system is a frequent cause of infection of the lacrimal system. Such an infection is reflected in an increase in tear production, exacerbating the epiphora.

Whereas obstruction of the drainage system in very young patients is nearly always caused by a persisting membrane in the valve of Hasner, as discussed in Section 15.1.3, obstructions of the drainage system in adults are generally attributable to aspecific, gradual atrophy of the lacrimal drainage system. Less frequently, defects are caused by specific disorders, such as acute or chronic inflammation, sarcoidosis, Wegener's granuloma, foreign bodies or stones in the lacrimal sac, and trauma or tumors of the lacrimal system and surrounding area.

#### *15.2.2.2 Primary Acquired Nasolacrimal Duct Obstruction*

In most cases of obstruction of the lacrimal system in adults, no specific cause is found. The most common cause of lacrimal system obstructions is aspecific gradual atrophy of the lacrimal drainage system. Atrophy mainly affects the lacrimal sac and the nasolacrimal duct, causing significant obstructions particularly at sites of physiologic narrowing, i.e. the valve of Rosenmüller, the junction of the sac and duct, and the valve of Hasner, but this is not always the case. Atrophy can affect any site in the lacrimal drainage system and may eventually cause a complete occlusion. The cause of atrophy is not clear. Histologic studies (Linberg and McCormick 1986) have demonstrated that it starts with an obstruction owing to swelling of the mucosa. Infection-induced changes and edema are observed in the wall of the lacrimal drainage system. At a later stage the obstruction increases, mainly owing to increasing fibrosis around the lacrimal drainage system caused by chronic infection. Stasis of cellular debris and mucus occurs in the lacrimal sac and the nasolacrimal duct, not only increasing the infection-induced changes in the walls of the lacrimal drainage system, but also leading to reflex hypersecretion of tears, which in turn exacerbates the epiphora. A bacterial cause of primary acquired nasolacrimal duct obstruction has never been demonstrated. Atrophy of the lacrimal drainage system with increasing age may be primarily attributable to physiologic causes, and it may not always cause symptoms, because of the simultaneous decrease in tear production with increasing age. Ten percent of adults aged 40 years or over have an obstruction of the lacrimal drainage system without any symptoms (Dalgleish 1967). This percentage increases to 35–40% among people aged 90 years or over.

Abnormalities can originate at different sites, but they tend to develop more or less symmetrically. Often, the development of defects on one side lags several years behind that of defects on the other side, with the patient presenting with one-sided epiphora. Figure 15.6 shows an example of multiple stenoses caused by primary acquired nasolacrimal duct obstruction. Figure 15.7 presents an example of the tendency of primary acquired nasolacrimal duct obstruction to develop symmetrically.

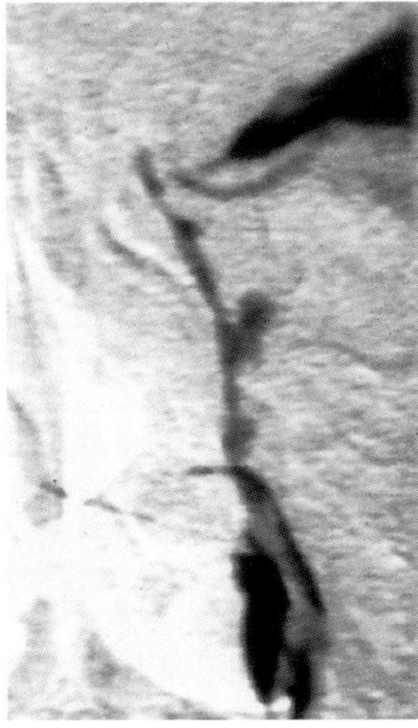

**Fig. 15.6.** Digital subtraction dacryocystography of a 76-year-old woman who has suffered from severe epiphora on the left side for 1 year. Stenosis is found in the entire lacrimal sac and nasolacrimal duct. The common canaliculus is almost completely obstructed. There is a small diverticulum high up at the lateral side of the nasolacrimal duct. The picture is suggestive of primary acquired nasolacrimal duct obstruction

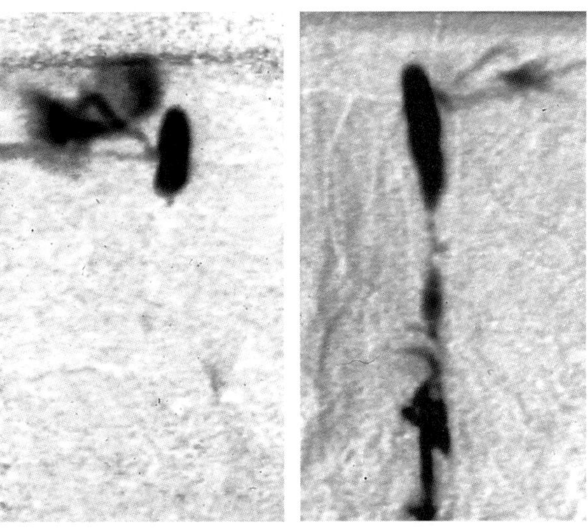

**Fig. 15.7 a,b.** Digital subtraction dacryocystography of a 51-year-old man who has been suffering from severe epiphora on both sides, the right-hand side being more severely affected. **a** On the right side there is a complete obstruction low in the lacrimal sac. **b** On the left side a severe stenosis approximately 1 cm in length can be seen in the nasolacrimal duct. The picture is suggestive of primary acquired nasolacrimal duct obstruction and shows the tendency of the disorder to develop more or less symmetrically

### 15.2.2.3 Acute Dacryocystitis

Acute dacryocystitis presents as a large painful swelling of the lacrimal sac. The overlying skin is red. There may be a preexisting drainage obstruction distal to the lacrimal sac, facilitating the inflammation and preventing distal drainage of pus. The large swelling of the lacrimal sac can cause kinking in the common canaliculus, also preventing the pus from draining via the canaliculi to the eye. In severe cases the inflammation may extend to the area around the eye; it can then even lead to an orbital abscess.

Acute dacryocystitis is treated with systemic antibiotics, if necessary supplemented with dacryocystotomy, which involves making an incision in the skin and the lacrimal sac to relieve the abscess. It is not unthinkable that in the future the interventional radiologist will have a role in the treatment of lacrimal sac abscesses by internal drainage, using a temporary stent in the nasolacrimal duct prior to treatment of an obstruction to avoid a postoperative scar. See also Section 15.5.3.

### 15.2.2.4 Chronic Infections

Chronic infections can be caused by a wide variety of bacteria. Many cases involve infection by *Staphylococcus* spp., *Streptococcus* spp. or *Hemophilus influenzae*, but fungi or viruses are also found. Infections often develop when there is an existing obstruction of the drainage system, and they tend to increase the obstruction by increasing fibrosis in the lacrimal system. Treatment should not be limited to medication to treat the inflammation; if necessary, additional treatment of the stenosis should be performed, either an operation or a radiologic intervention. Figure 15.18 shows an endoscopic image of chronically infected lacrimal sac mucosa.

### 15.2.2.5 Sarcoidosis and Wegener's Granulomatosis

Sarcoidosis is a disease that is pathologically characterized by epithelioid tubercles with inconspicuous necrosis or none at all, affecting any organ or tissue. Wegener's granulomatosis is a rare disorder characterized by acute necrotizing lesions of the respiratory tract, including the nose and upper airways, focal

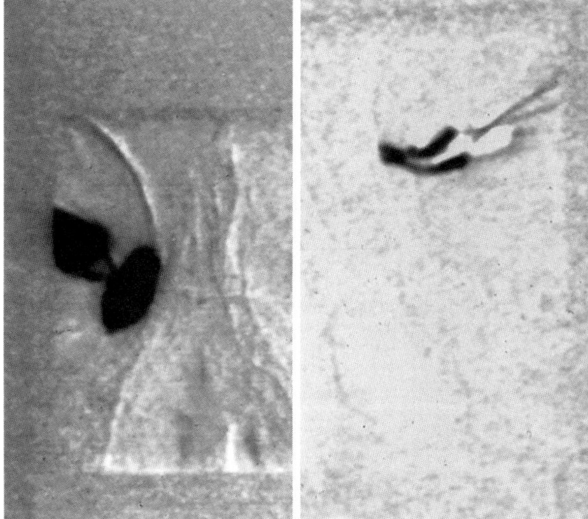

a,b

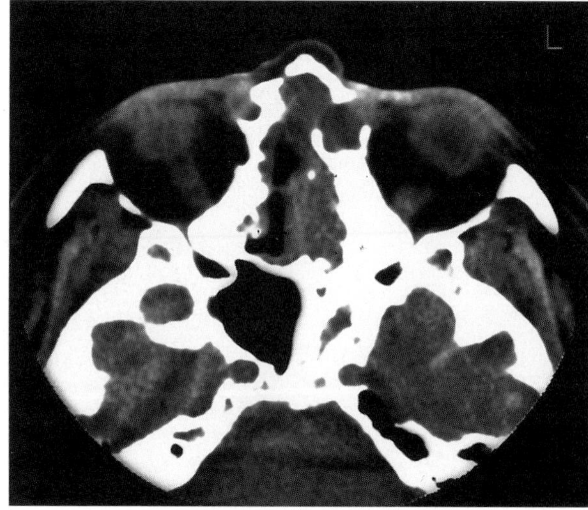

c

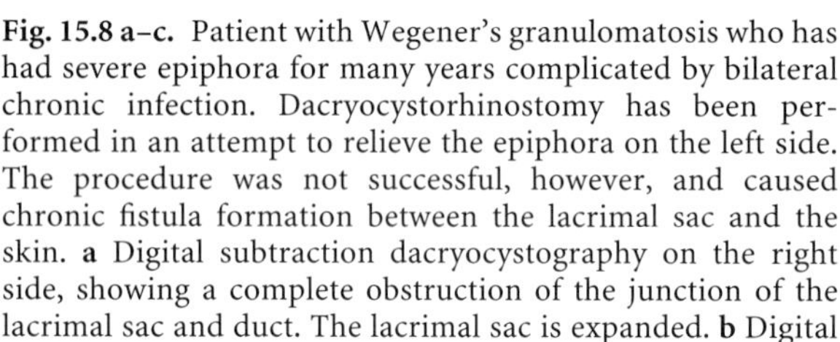

**Fig. 15.8 a–c.** Patient with Wegener's granulomatosis who has had severe epiphora for many years complicated by bilateral chronic infection. Dacryocystorhinostomy has been performed in an attempt to relieve the epiphora on the left side. The procedure was not successful, however, and caused chronic fistula formation between the lacrimal sac and the skin. **a** Digital subtraction dacryocystography on the right side, showing a complete obstruction of the junction of the lacrimal sac and duct. The lacrimal sac is expanded. **b** Digital subtraction dacryocystography on the left side, showing a complete obstruction between the common canaliculus and the lacrimal sac. **c** Conventional axial CT showing an expanded lacrimal sac with a thickened wall in the fossa lacrimalis on the right side and bone destruction in the area of the left lacrimal fossa, which developed partly postoperatively and partly as a result of granuloma formation. There are also granulomas high up in the left nasal cavity

acute necrotizing vasculitis, and renal disease in the form of focal or diffuse glomerulonephritis.

Both sarcoidosis and Wegener's granulomatosis often result in the formation of extensive granulomas and bone destruction in the lacrimal sac and nasolacrimal duct. Figure 15.8a–c shows a patient with Wegener's granulomatosis.

### *15.2.2.6 Foreign Bodies*

Foreign bodies in the lacrimal system can obstruct drainage. In most cases a dacryolith is involved. The stones consist mostly of calcium and phosphate salts (Herzig and Hurwitz 1979). They can be deposited in the lacrimal drainage system de novo or around a core of foreign material, such as rejected epithelial debris, a cilium, or cosmetics that have found their way into the lacrimal sac. Dacryoliths are generally barely radiopaque and they show up on dacryocystography as a gap in the contrast medium. Figure 15.9 shows a large dacryolith in the left lacrimal sac of a 42-year-old woman with intermittent epiphora without complicating infections. The intermittent recurrence of complaints is probably caused by intermittent wedging of the stone in the junction of the lacrimal sac and the nasolacrimal duct.

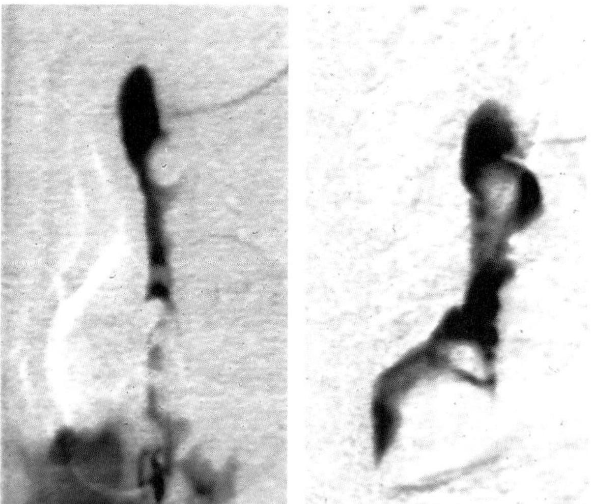

a,b

**Fig. 15.9 a,b.** Digital subtraction dacryocystography showing a large dacryolith in the left lacrimal sac: **a** front view; **b** right anterior oblique view

A foreign body need not always be a dacryolith. Figure 15.10 shows an image of the lacrimal drainage system of a 57-year-old lathe operator. He had been suffering from severe epiphora of the right eye for

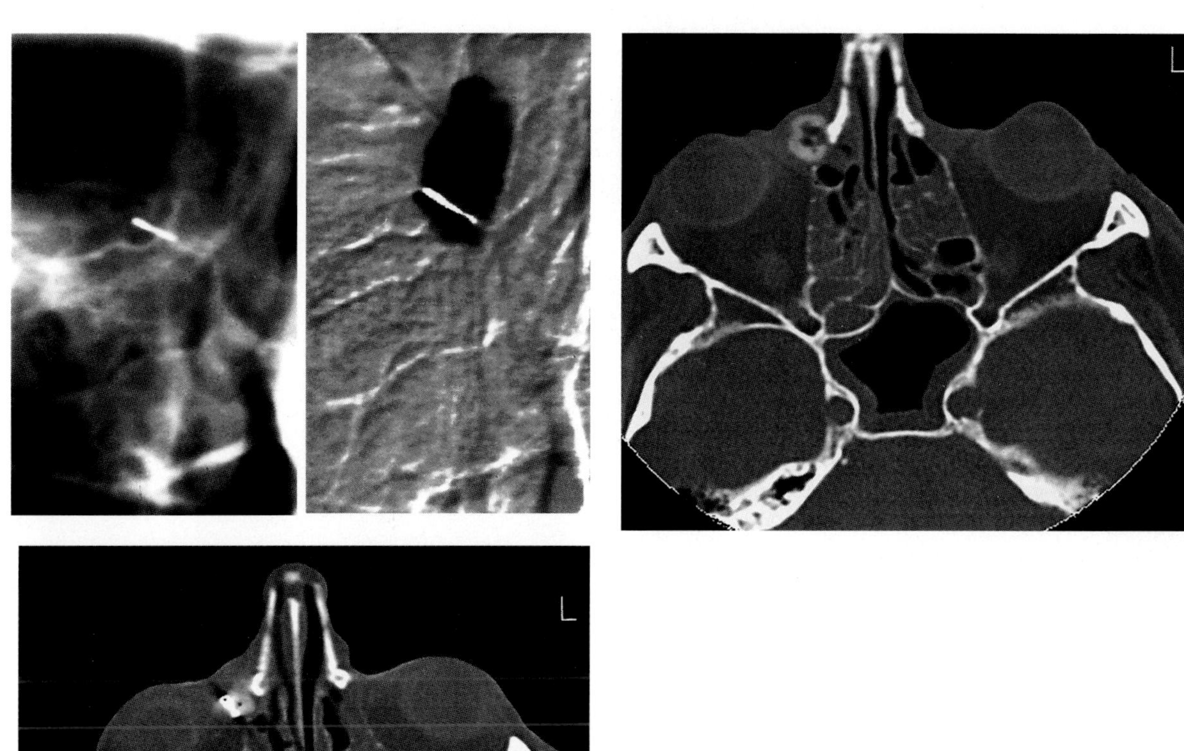

a,b

c

d

Fig. 15.10. **a** Conventional X-ray. A metal splinter is visible in the region of the lacrimal sac. **b** Digital subtraction dacryocystography. The metal splinter is low in the lacrimal sac. **c** Axial CT. On the right side an expanded lacrimal sac with a widened wall is visible. **d** Axial CT. A metal splinter is visible low in the lacrimal sac

4 years though he could not remember any trauma. It turned out that a 5-mm-long steel splinter was lodged in the lacrimal sac, and this was removed surgically.

### 15.2.2.7 Trauma

Traumata can cause obstruction of the drainage system. This occurs mostly with midfacial fractures involving the bony canal, such as Lefort II or Lefort III fractures. Iatrogenic damage to the bone is not uncommon, for example with cosmetic rhinoplasty or a Caldwell-Luc operation. Figure 15.11 shows a complete occlusion high up left in the nasolacrimal duct following a two-sided Caldwell-Luc operation.

### 15.2.2.8 Neoplasms

Tumors of the lacrimal sac and duct are rare. So far, 200 tumors originating in the lacrimal sac have been described (Weber et al. 1996). Some 90% of these were malignant, mainly squamous cell carcinoma, but malignant lymphomas originating in the lymphoid tissue in the wall of the lacrimal sac also occur. Benign tumors include polyps, papillomas, or granulomas. Figure 15.19a,b shows a lacrimal sac polyp in a 60-year-old man who had been suffering from epiphora for several months.

Sometimes an obstruction is not caused by a tumor originating in the lacrimal drainage system, but by a malignancy originating in the surrounding area, such as the nose or the maxillary sinus. Figure 15.12 shows a low obstruction of the lacrimal drain-

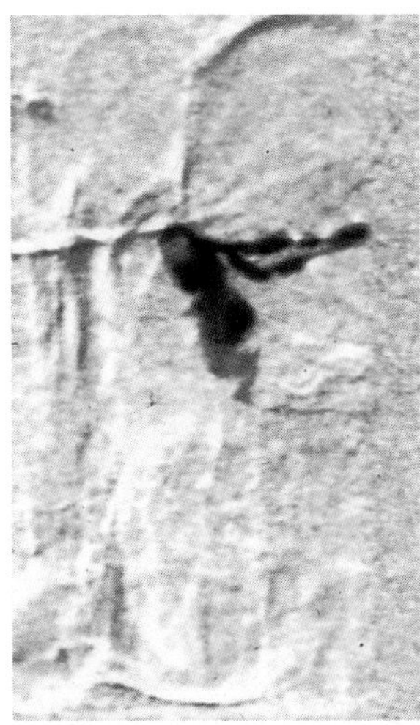

a

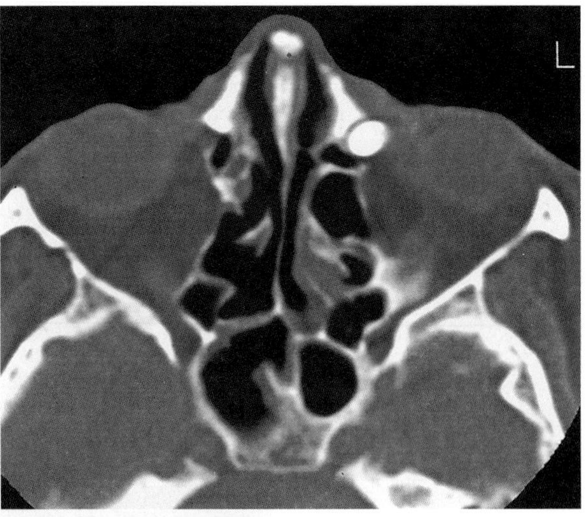

b

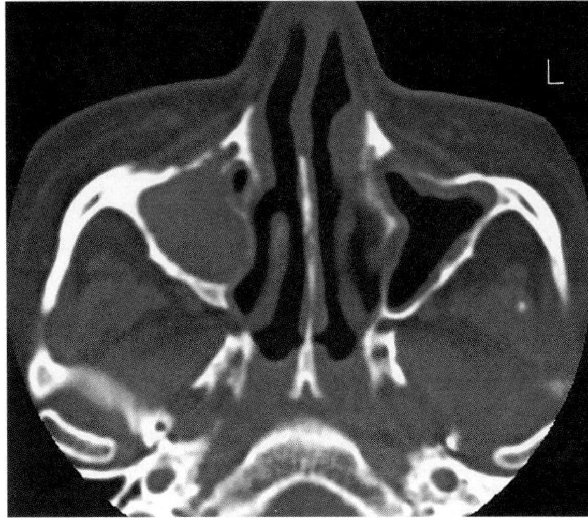

c

**Fig. 15.11 a–c.** A 50-year-old patient suffering from severe epiphora on the left side, following a two-sided Caldwell-Luc operation on the maxillary sinus. **a** Digital subtraction dacryocystography shows a complete obstruction high in the nasolacrimal duct, even after contrast medium has been applied under high pressure. Reflux from the canaliculi was prevented by wedging the second lacrimal punctum with a nonconducting catheter. The lacrimal sac is expanded and contains mucus. **b** CT dacryocystography shows an expanded lacrimal sac on the left side. **c** CT dacryocystography distal to the lacrimal sac shows that cause of the obstruction. When the maxillary sinus was surgically opened, the lacrimal canal on the left side was destroyed, while the bony canal on the right side has remained intact

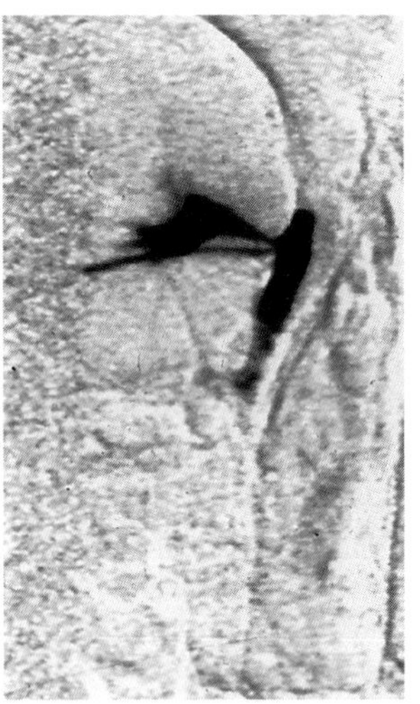

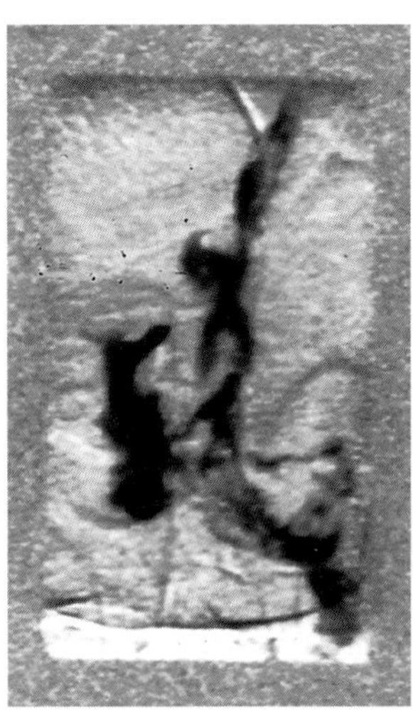

a,b

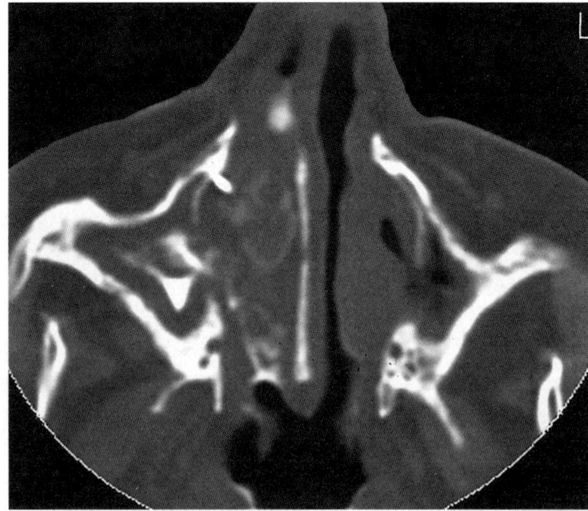

c

**Fig. 15.12 a–c.** An 87-year-old woman who has suffered from severe epiphora on the right side for 1 year. **a** Digital subtraction dacryocystography shows a complete obstruction distal to the lacrimal sac. **b** When a 20-G vascular sheath has been passed over a guidewire low into the lacrimal sac, digital subtraction dacryocystography shows passage of contrast medium to the nose, while simultaneously the lumen in the right maxillary sinus is being filled. Large, irregular filling defects are visible in the nasolacrimal duct. **c** CT dacryocystography performed with the catheter positioned in the lacrimal sac shows a large, irregular tumorous mass low in the right nasal cavity, growing into the inferior turbinate and the wall of the maxillary sinus. The tumor has infiltrated the lacrimal drainage system, where the cathether is visible. Histologic examination demonstrated the presence of a squamous cell carcinoma

age system caused by a carcinoma originating in the right nasal cavity and extending into the nasolacrimal duct.

## 15.3 Radiologic Methods of Examination

### 15.3.1 Dacryocystography

Dacryocystography is the best method of imaging the morphology of the lacrimal drainage system. It involves taking X-rays of the lacrimal drainage system after filling it with contrast medium. In the past, an oil-based contrast medium was used, e.g. lipiodol, but oil-based contrast media have a strong tendency to form drops in a watery environment, preventing adequate coating of the surface of the structures to be imaged. Their use should indeed be considered obsolete, the more so as it can cause granuloma with extravasation (Gulotta and von Denffer 1980). Today, water-soluble contrast media are used, which achieve adequate coating of the mucosa of the lacrimal drainage system. We use iopromide (Ultravist 300 R; Schering, Berlin, Germany), a nonionic contrast medium that does not cause eye irritation.

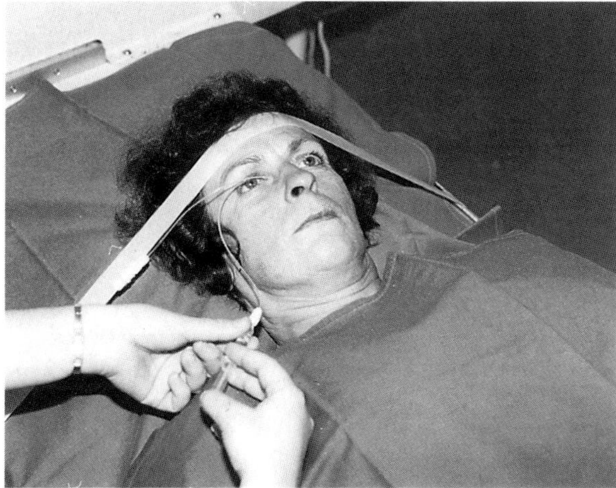

**Fig. 15.13.** Fixation of the patient's head during digital subtraction dacryocystography and administration of contrast medium via a lacrimal catheter in the lower canaliculus while the upper canaliculus is wedged with a second, nonconducting lacrimal catheter to prevent reflux via the upper lacrimal punctum

### 15.3.2 Digital Subtraction Dacryocystography

Digital subtraction dacryocystography can be regarded as the gold standard in lacrimal drainage system imaging.

#### *15.3.2.1 Technique*

In digital subtraction dacryocystography the lacrimal drainage system is imaged with the overprojected facial bone subtracted. Imaging takes place under local anesthesia achieved by applying a few drops of oxybuprocaine 0.4% to the conjunctival sac. The patient is lying prone with the back of the head in a foam fixation pillow and a wide strip of tape running from one side of the X-ray table across the forehead to the other side of the table (Fig. 15.13). The fixation method is similar to that used in cerebral digital subtraction angiography. Good fixation of the head is of the essence for a high-quality examination. Subsequently, one of the puncta is dilated using a lacrimal dilator; the sharp curve of the canaliculus 2 mm distal to the punctum must be borne in mind. Then a flexible lacrimal duct catheter is passed into the canaliculus. We use a sialography catheter (PBN Medicals, Stenlose, Denmark) with the tip cut off obliquely to give an obtuse angle of approximately 30°. The catheter is carefully inserted and at the same time slightly rotated until it is about 1 cm into the canaliculus, the eyelid being slightly drawn away laterally. The patient is asked not to move or swallow, and for a few seconds images are recorded in PA projection direction with a frequency of two images per second, while contrast is simultaneously injected via the catheter into the lacrimal drainage system.

Digital subtraction dacryocystography allows real-time imaging of the lacrimal drainage system. The increasing filling of the lacrimal drainage system with contrast medium can be monitored on screen during injection, so that insufficient filling or overfilling of the lacrimal drainage system can be avoided (Walther et al. 1994). A high-quality examination requires that all the parts of the lacrimal drainage system are well filled with contrast medium during imaging. When there is an excess of mucus in the lacrimal sac this should first be rinsed out with a physiologic saline solution before the series is repeated to obtain better quality images of the lacrimal sac. When the catheter is advanced too far, so that

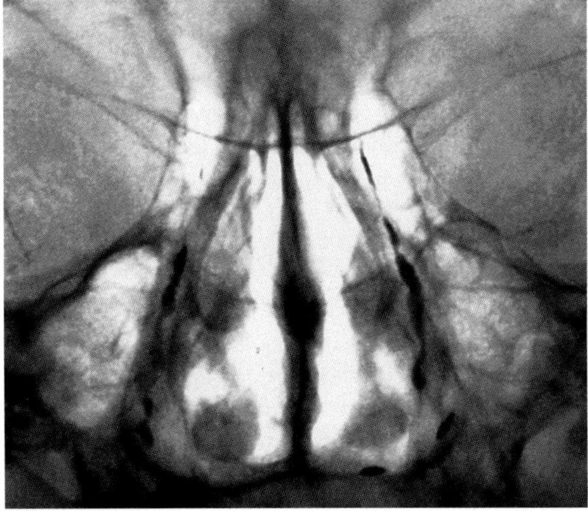
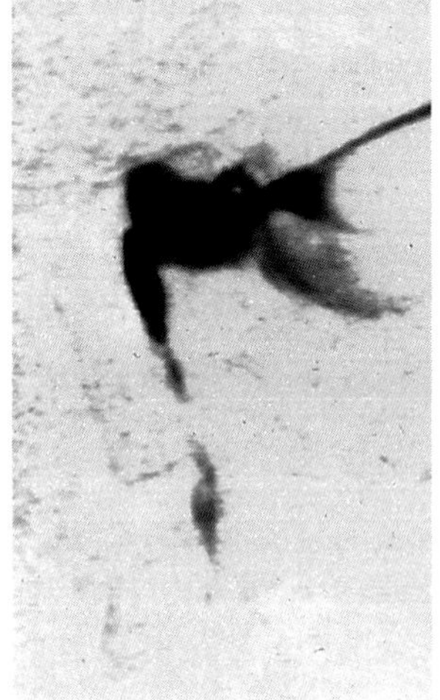
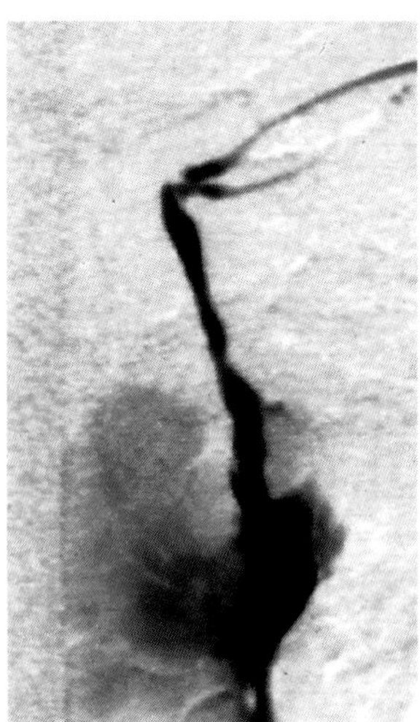

a,b c

**Fig. 15.14. a** Inadequate dacryocystography. The contrast medium was administered on the left- and right-hand sides not during, but prior to, imaging. No contrast medium is present in the canaliculi and only a little is visible in the lacrimal sac. Patency of the lacrimal drainage system was demonstrated on either side. The patient was referred to us for balloon dilatation on both sides for suspected severe stenosis in the lacrimal sac. **b** Digital subtraction dacryocystography of the same patient using one catheter in the lower canaliculus. The lacrimal sac expands well. Owing to substantial reflux of contrast medium via the upper lacrimal punctum the tract of the canaliculi cannot be evaluated. The lack of contrast medium on the distal side suggests the presence of a stenosis in the nasolacrimal duct. This would be a good indication for balloon dilatation. **c** When digital subtraction dacryocystography is performed with the upper lacrimal punctum wedged with a second, nonconducting catheter, the lacrimal drainage system is easy to evaluate. There are no morphologic defects of the lacrimal sac or nasolacrimal duct, but there is a short stenosis in the common canaliculus, implying that balloon dilatation is contraindicated

the tip is inside the lacrimal sac during injection of contrast medium, the canaliculi will not be imaged. In such cases, to avoid missing a stenosis in the canaliculi, the imaging series will have to be repeated after the catheter has been slightly retracted. When there is an excess reflux of contrast medium from the noncatheterized punctum, making evaluation of the tract of the canaliculi and the lacrimal sac impossible owing to overprojection of leaking contrast medium, the best course of action is to repeat the series after wedging the other punctum with a second, nonconducting catheter (Janssen et al. 1994). This method can also be used to evaluate an obstruction in the lacrimal sac or nasolacrimal duct. When an occlusion is detected on digital subtraction dacryocystography using one catheter, the obstruction often turns out to be just patent when the second puncta has been wedged. This may be important should balloon dilatation of the lacrimal drainage system be necessary. In some cases a distal stenosis can only be adequately imaged after a 20-G vascular sheath has been introduced over a guidewire low into the lacrimal sac (Fig. 15.12b). Figure 15.14 shows how inadequate dacryocystography can cause misinterpretation in evaluating the lacrimal drainage system. Digital subtraction dacryocystography is a method of examining the morphology of the lacrimal drainage system, and not a functional examination. When a very severe stenosis is found distal to the lacrimal sac the amount of contrast medium can be increased during digital subtraction dacryocystography. If the lacrimal sac swells up this is often indicative of a significant stenosis.

### *15.3.2.2 Indications*

Digital subtraction dacryocystography is indicated in all cases of epiphora, when ophthalmologic examination has excluded reflex hypersecretion, when there are no anatomic malformations of the eyelids, such as when the puncta are not adjacent to the eyeball due to ectropion or entropion, and when flushing of the lacrimal drainage system during ophthalmologic examination has revealed abnormalities.

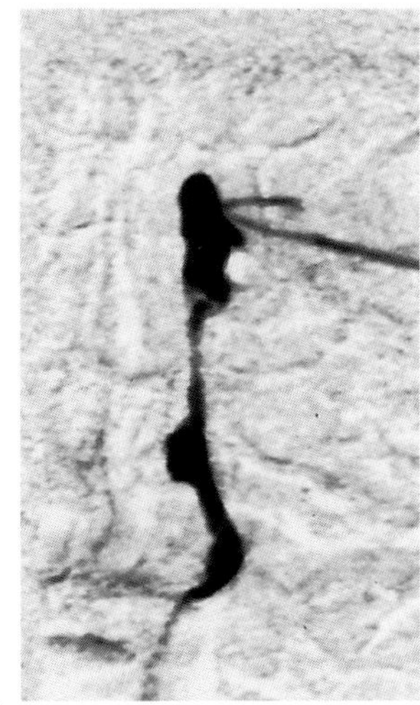

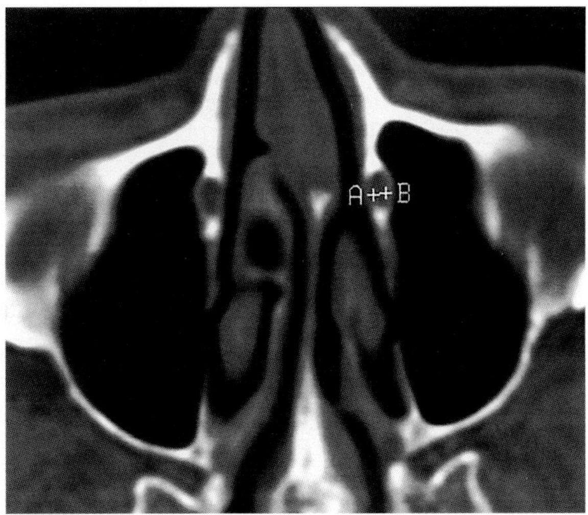


**Fig. 15.15 a,b.** A 43-year-old man who for many years has suffered from severe epiphora associated with a stenosis in the bony canal. **a** Digital subtraction dacryocystography shows dilatation of the lacrimal sac, a substantial short stenosis at the junction, and a long stenosis in the nasolacrimal duct. **b** Conventional, axial CT reveals a stenosis in the bony canal. The diameter across (*A–B*) was at least 1.6 mm

## 15.3.3 CT and CT Dacryocystography

### *15.3.3.1 Computed Tomography*

Computed tomography is a good technique for imaging soft tissues and adjacent bone, including those in the area of the lacrimal drainage system. We use CT mainly to determine the diameter of the bony lacrimal canal. The most common indication for CT of the lacrimal drainage system without contrast medium is a recurrent obstruction in the nasolacrimal duct after balloon dilatation or an extensive stenosis identified in the nasolacrimal duct on digital subtraction dacryocystography prior to balloon dilatation. CT often shows that the diameter of the bony canal is substantially less than 3.5–4 mm. When a balloon dilatation is to be performed in such cases, a balloon with a diameter of 2.0 or 2.5 mm should be considered; alternatively, stent placement might be considered, as discussed in Section 15.5.2, or dacryocystorhinostomy, a surgical procedure during which an opening is made between the lacrimal sac and the nose to bypass the obstruction distal to the lacrimal sac. Figure 15.15 shows such a stenosis in the bony canal.

### *15.3.3.2 CT Dacryocystography*

When more complex pathology is involved, CT dacryocystography can be performed. Zinreich et al. (1990) were the first to combine CT and dacryocystography by performing a CT examination of the lacrimal drainage system after applying contrast medium to the lacrimal drainage system. They did so by inserting some drops of water-soluble contrast medium into the conjunctival sac. Within a few minutes, the contrast medium disperses physiologically into the lacrimal drainage system by capillary action and by the lacrimal pump mechanism that is activated by blinking.

The method was technically further developed with helical CT dacryocystography, which enables multiplanar and even three-dimensional imaging (Moran et al. 1995). Considering the way in which the contrast medium is introduced, the examination is in a sense a functional one. It can show whether contrast medium passes and, if it does, how fast. In this respect it resembles scintigraphy of the lacrimal drainage system, but of course, unlike scintigraphy, it does provide anatomic information about the environment. A disadvantage of this way of introducing contrast medium is that no adequate morphologic information is obtained about the lacrimal drainage system itself owing to slow or incomplete coating of the lacrimal drainage system with the contrast medium.

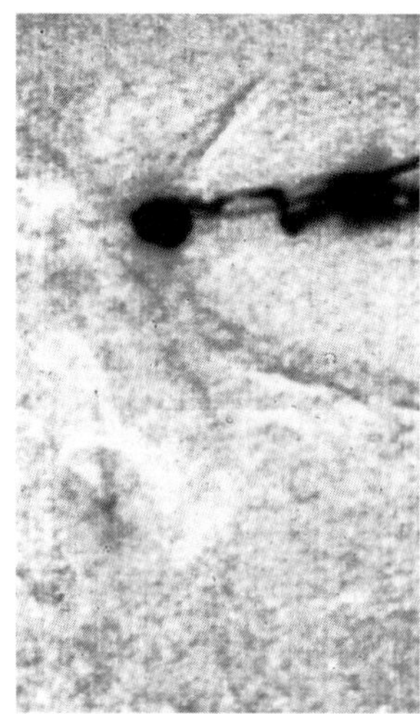

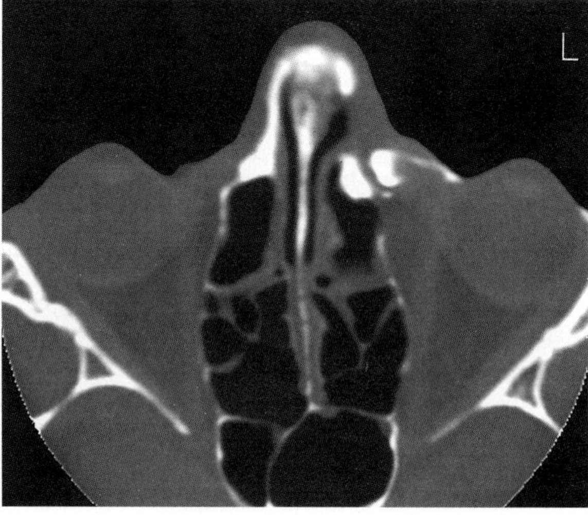


**Fig. 15.16 a,b.** A 31-year-old man with a recurrent obstruction on the left side after dacryocystorhinostomy for a posttraumatic low obstruction. **a** Digital subtraction dacryocystography shows a complete obstruction high up in the lacrimal sac. The canaliculi appear to be normal. **b** CT dacryocystography shows that the opening in the bone made on dacryocystorhinostomy is sufficiently wide and in the right place, but an obstruction has formed in the soft tissue in the area of the operation. Contrast medium is visible in the remainder of the lacrimal sac and one of the canaliculi. At the surface of the lacrimal sac there is minor swelling of the soft tissue caused by scar formation

In our view, the preferred method of examining the morphology of the lacrimal drainage system and its relation to the facial bone and the surrounding soft parts is CT dacryocystography with injection of water-soluble contrast medium via a lacrimal drainage system catheter. This requires local anesthesia, dilatation of a punctum, and catheterization of a canaliculus, but given that the examination is generally performed in combination with digital subtraction dacryocystography this is no problem. The lacrimal catheter inserted for digital subtraction dacryocystography can remain in place when, subsequently, CT dacryocystography is performed. Generally 2-mm contiguous slices in the axial plane suffice when CT dacryocystography is performed immediately after introduction of a few milliliters of diluted contrast medium into the lacrimal drainage system. In evaluating a failed dacryocystorhinostomy, some authors prefer slices in the coronal plane (Glatt et al. 1991). We believe, however, that CT dacryocystography in the axial plane provides the same information when 2-mm contiguous slices are taken (Fig. 15.16). We also prefer the axial plane because imaging takes place with the patient lying prone, a much more comfortable position, particularly for older patients, and because the dimensions of the bony canal are far more reliable in this plane. Figure 15.10 shows how CT dacryocystography can be used in more complex pathology.

#### 15.3.3.3 Indications for CT Dacryocystography

CT dacryocystography has a large number of widely varying indications. It is used in posttraumatic or postoperative obstruction of the lacrimal drainage system. It is recommended after failure of external dacryocystorhinostomy (Waite et al. 1993), after failure of balloon dilatation, and preoperatively before endoscopic transnasal dacryocystorhinostomy. When an obstruction is detected on digital subtraction dacryocystography and cannot be easily passed with a guidewire, CT dacryocystography should be performed prior to any balloon dilatation (Janssen et al. 1997). In some cases pathology can be detected, such as malignant tumors of the lacrimal drainage system or surrounding area, benign tumors of the lacrimal drainage system or nose, and granulomas, such as in Wegener's granulomatosis or sarcoidosis. CT dacryocystography makes an important contribution to diagnosis and directs selection of the treatment.

## 15.3.4 Other Imaging Techniques

### *15.3.4.1 Magnetic Resonance Imaging*

Magnetic resonance imaging is superior to CT in imaging soft tissues. Goldberg et al. (1993) and Rubin et al. (1993) used MRI to examine the lacrimal drainage system in a small group of patients, to assess its advantages over other diagnostic techniques. They used a 1.5-T machine and a 3-in. orbital surface coil. As contrast medium a bolus of gadolinium DTPA was given intravenously (Rubin et al. 1993), diluted gadolinium DTPA was injected into the lacrimal drainage system through a lacrimal catheter (Goldberg et al. 1993), or strongly diluted gadolinium was dripped into the conjunctival sac (Goldberg et al. 1993; Rubin et al. 1993). In the last case the examination becomes a functional one, like scintigraphy of the lacrimal drainage system or CT dacryocystography, which involve contrast medium being dripped into the conjunctival sac.

Advantages of lacrimal system MRI include better assessment of the extent of pathologic processes within the lacrimal drainage system and the fact that ionizing radiation is unnecessary. One of the disadvantages of MRI of the lacrimal drainage system is that MRI does not image the facial bone quite as well as CT does.

We believe that MRI can sometimes offer useful additional information in complex disorders of the lacrimal drainage system, but in most cases it is unlikely to provide any significant more information than digital subtraction dacryocystography and CT dacryocystography.

### *15.3.4.2 Ultrasound of the Lacrimal Sac*

Ultrasound can be used to image the swollen lacrimal sac. In theory, it is possible to use ultrasound to differentiate between a mucocele and a solid tumor in the lacrimal sac. In practice, however, this distinction can be made by using digital subtraction dacryocystography. When it proves impossible to pass the occlusion of the kinked common canaliculus with a guidewire and insert a catheter into the lacrimal sac in cases of a mucocele ultrasound may be considered, although today MRI or CT is more likely to be used. Ultrasound is of hardly any practical value in examination of the lacrimal drainage system.

### *15.3.4.3 Dacryoscintigraphy*

Scintigraphy of the lacrimal drainage system can be valuable when a functional examination is required. The method was introduced by Rossomondo et al. (1972) and involves following the movements of lacrimal fluid from the conjunctival sac, via the lacrimal drainage system to the nose, under almost physiologic conditions (von Denffer et al. 1984). The patient sits in front of a gamma camera with forehead and chin fixed in a holder, after one drop of $^{99m}$Tc-pertechnetate (dosage of less than 4 MBq) has been inserted into the conjunctival sac. Subsequently, images are recorded at fixed time intervals to obtain a good impression of the passage of tracer through the lacrimal drainage system. During the investigation the patient should blink normally to activate the pump mechanism of the lacrimal drainage system. Dacryoscintigraphy is a safe procedure, exposing the lens to a low radiation dose, i.e. 2% of that of an AP skull X-ray (Robertson et al. 1979).

Since lacrimal scintigraphy provides only functional information, it should be regarded as supplementary to methods of examination that provide morphologic information, digital subtraction dacryocystography in particular. Scintigraphy can be used to ascertain whether a minor stenosis identified by digital subtraction dacryocystography is significant or not (Hurwitz and Kirsch 1996). Scintigraphy can also identify a pump dysfunction, for instance in the presence of suspected lid laxity or of facial nerve palsy, when the lacrimal drainage system does not show any morphologic abnormalities on digital subtraction dacryocystography. The presence of pump dysfunction is confirmed when scintigraphy does not reveal any activity in the lacrimal drainage system, but activity remains concentrated in the conjunctival sac. In practice, scintigraphy of the lacrimal drainage system supplementary to flushing the lacrimal drainage system on ophthalmologic examination followed by digital subtraction dacryocystography is hardly ever necessary and is only performed in a limited number of cases.

### *15.3.4.4 Endoscopy of the Lacrimal Drainage System*

In 1990 an endoscope was first used (Hurwitz 1996c) to evaluate the canaliculi. The endoscope had a diameter of barely 1 mm and was rather rigid. In

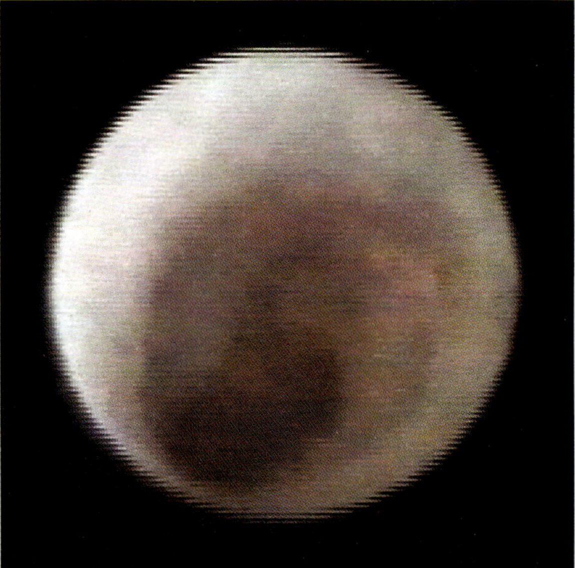

**Fig. 15.17.** Endoscopy of the lacrimal drainage system. The lacrimal sac appears to be normal. The mucosa is smooth and light pink in color

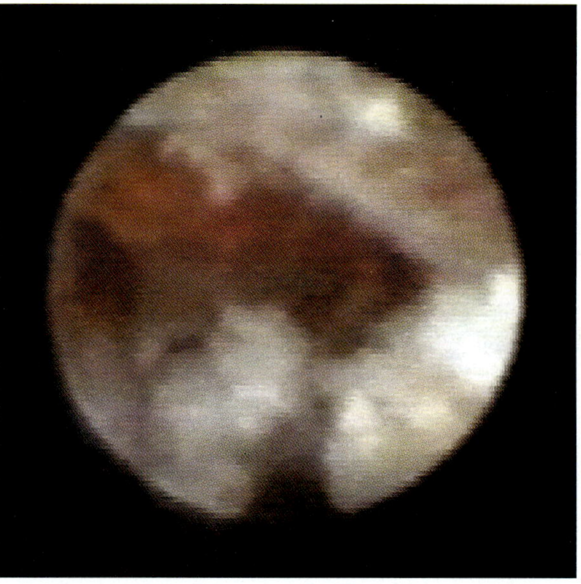

**Fig. 15.18.** Endoscopy of the lacrimal drainage system in chronic infection. There is considerable vascular injection causing the mucosa to color a deep red. The epithelium along the wall of the lacrimal sac appears to be torn, and a large amount of mucus is visible

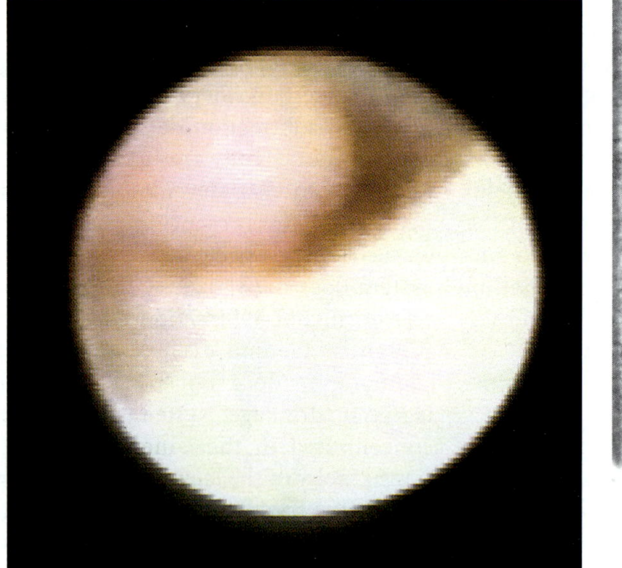

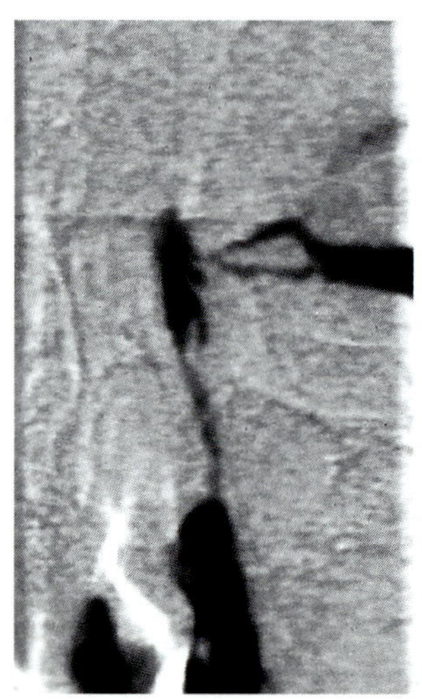

**Fig. 15.19. a** Endoscopy of the lacrimal drainage system. A small polyp is visible in the lacrimal sac. The patient has slight epiphora. **b** Digital subtraction dacryocystography shows a polyp low in the lacrimal sac. The polyp causes a relative obstruction at the junction of the lacrimal sac and the nasolacrimal duct

1996 we used a flexible endoscope with a diameter of approximately 0.5 mm, which made it possible to image the entire length of the lacrimal drainage system (no. 1157/ES Schwind Endognost, Laméris Ootech, Veenendaal, The Netherlands). It proved less than easy to perform an endoscopic examination while simultaneously passing the scope via the lacrimal sac and the nasolacrimal duct to the nose, without damaging the mucosa of the lacrimal drainage system. When, however, a guidewire is first advanced

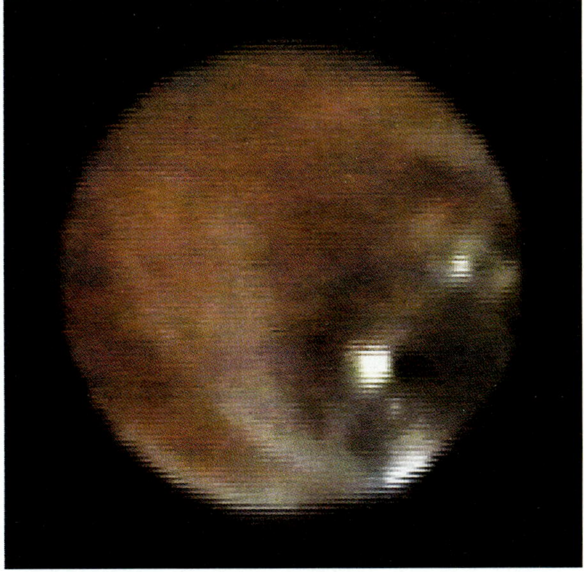

**Fig. 15.20.** Endoscopy of the lacrimal sac during balloon dilatation. The top of the inflated balloon is visible. The tract of the lacrimal sac between the endoscope and the balloon was dilated shortly before. The lacrimal sac expands well on flushing, and no ruptures are visible in the mucosa

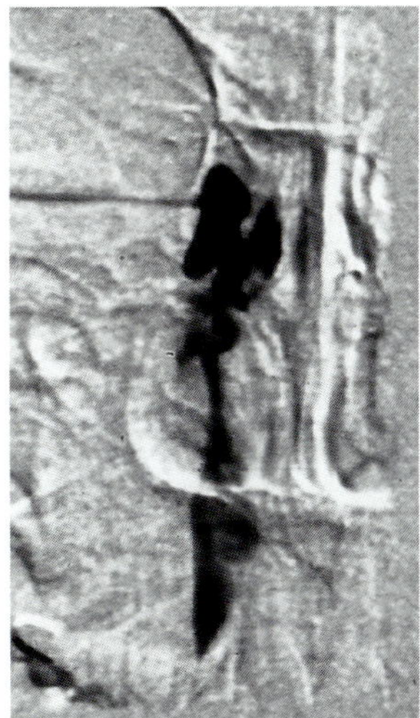

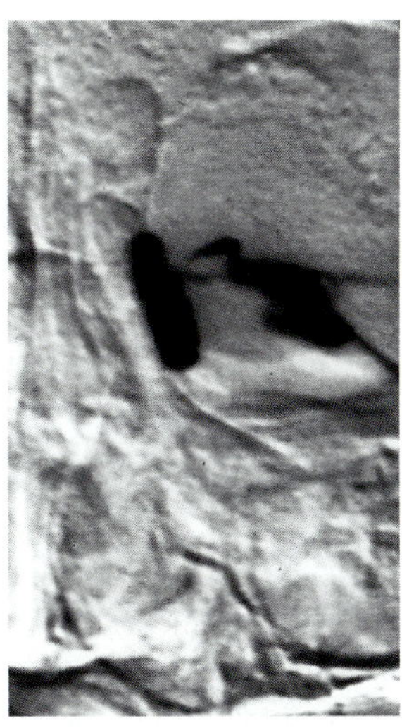

**Fig. 15.21 a,b.** Digital subtraction dacryocystography in a patient who is symptom free after external dacryocystorhinostomy on both sides. **a** On the right side a wide opening is visible between the lacrimal sac and the nose with satisfactory drainage of contrast medium to the nose, which is normal after dacryocystorhinostomy. **b** By contrast, on the left side the surgically created opening between the lacrimal sac and the nose has closed

into the nose via the lacrimal drainage system, followed by a 20-G vascular sheath, the scope can easily be passed into the nose via the sheath and the lacrimal drainage system can then be evaluated while the endoscope is gradually being retracted. In this way we examined the lacrimal drainage system of several volunteers. Figures 15.17–15.19 show endoscopic images of the lacrimal drainage system. Endoscopy of the lacrimal drainage system was also performed during various balloon dilatation procedures (Fig. 15.20). No ruptures of the mucosa were observed after inflation of a 3-mm diameter balloon. At present it remains unclear whether endoscopy of the lacrimal drainage system will have a significant role and will take its place in due course among the range of diagnostic methods used to assess the lacrimal drainage system.

## 15.4 Lacrimal Surgery

Traditionally, acquired obstructions in the nasolacrimal duct or low in the lacrimal sac are treated surgically by dacryocystorhinostomy. This procedure involves removing the bone between the lacrimal sac and the nose, after which the opening is lined with mucosa by suturing the lacrimal sac mucosa to the nasal mucosa. In cases of an obstruction in the common canaliculus, dacryocystorhinostomy can be extended by temporarily placing Silastic tubes in the canaliculi after surgical reduction of the scar tissue surrounding the common canaliculus (canaliculodacryocystorhinostomy). When there is complete occlusion of the canaliculi, conjunctival dacryocystorhinostomy can be performed, which combines dacryocystorhinostomy with a graft between the lacrimal sac and the conjunctiva bypassing the canaliculi (Steinsapir et al. 1990). To ensure a permanent satisfactory result a small glass prosthesis should be worn in this opening. When the glass tube is no longer in place, the opening tends to close rather rapidly. Today, dacrycystorhinostomy is also referred to as external dacryocystorhinostomy, because some years ago a laser-assisted endonasal alternative surgical procedure was developed (Massaro et al. 1990). Currently, it remains unclear whether this endonasal laser dacryocystorhinostomy offers any advantages over conventional external dacryocystorhinostomy. The results of dacryocystorhinostomy are good. When performed by an experienced surgeon the success rate is 90% (Hurwitz and Rutherford 1986). This does not imply, however, that the surgically created opening between the lacrimal sac and the nose remains open in 90% of cases. Occasionally, complete reobstruction of the surgical opening is found in a patient without any or with hardly any symptoms after the operation (Fig. 15.21). In these cases, it could be assumed that dacryocystorhinostomy has succeeded in breaking the vicious circle of obstruction and infection, which we discussed in Section 15.2.2.2.

At present, external dacryocystorhinostomy should be regarded as the gold standard against which all other interventions must be evaluated (Hurwitz 1996d). Indications for external dacryocystorhinostomy include epiphora caused by acquired obstruction within the nasolacrimal sac and duct, mucocele of the lacrimal sac, chronic dacryocystitis due to lacrimal sac obstruction, relief of lacrimal sac infection before intraocular surgery, and congenital nasolacrimal duct obstruction that cannot be cured by probing. Contraindications to dacryocystorhinostomy include acute dacryocystitis and tumor of the lacrimal sac. The following complications of dacryocystorhinostomy are possible: bleeding or infection of the operative area, orbital emphysema and – rarely – CSF leakage via a peroperative fracture in the cribriform plate.

## 15.5 Interventional Procedures

### 15.5.1 Dacryocystoplasty

#### *15.5.1.1 Introduction*

In recent years interventional radiology has made spectacular progress in many areas. Evidence of the interventional radiologist's expanding role in the therapeutic process is also beginning to be seen in the treatment of epiphora, or tearing due to an obstruction in the lacrimal drainage system. In 1978 radiography was first used in passing a probe into the lacrimal drainage system in some patients with a nasolacrimal duct obstruction (Hanafee and Dayton 1978). Fluoroscopy was used to reduce the risk of false passage in probing and thus improve the long-term results of the procedure. Four patients were treated, and the treatment was successful in three. In 1989 a balloon catheter was used for the first time in the lacrimal drainage system (Becker and Berry 1989). A coronary balloon catheter with a 4-mm balloon diameter was used to restore patency of the operative opening in four patients with failed dacryocystorhinostomy as the result of an obstructed nasal ostium. The balloon was passed antegradely over a guidewire via the canaliculus. All four patients demonstrated some improvement during a short follow-up period. In 1990 Munk et al. were the first to describe a method with retrograde passage of an angioplasty catheter via the nose into the lacrimal drainage system over a guidewire that had been advanced antegradely via the canaliculus into the lacrimal drainage system. They used a balloon diameter of 3.0–4.0 mm for dilatation, and they referred to their method as dacryocystoplasty. Eighteen patients with functional or anatomic obstructions were selected to receive this treatment. Technical success of the balloon dilatation was obtained in 16 cases. Over a short follow-up period of 7 weeks to 6 months, 11 of the patients remained free of symptoms.

In the years that followed more and more interventional radiologists performed dacryocystoplasty, and the method developed rapidly, as did the patient selection criteria.

#### *15.5.1.2 Criteria for Patient Selection*

##### 15.5.1.2.1 INCLUSION CRITERIA

Adequate patient selection is important to ensure successful treatment of epiphora by balloon dilatation (Janssen et al. 1998). Selection criteria for dacryocystoplasty after exclusion of reflex hypersecretion by ophthalmologic examination, or presence of anatomic malformations of the eyelids, are demonstration, on digital subtraction dacryocystography, of the presence of a stenosis or occlusion in the lacrimal sac, junction of the lacrimal sac and duct, nasolacrimal duct, or the valve of Hasner, irrespective of the length of the obstruction, the duration of symptoms, and the patient's age. Figure 15.22a–c shows obstructions and stenoses in the lacrimal drainage system that qualify for treatment by dacryocystoplasty. The stenoses and occlusions shown in Figs. 15.4 and 15.7a,b are also suitable for treatment by dacryocystoplasty. A recurrent obstruction after dacryocystorhinostomy can often also be treated by dacryocystoplasty (Fig. 15.16). In these cases it is not the surgically created opening between the nose and lacrimal sac that is dilated, but the original anatomic tract, consisting of the lacrimal sac and nasolacrimal duct.

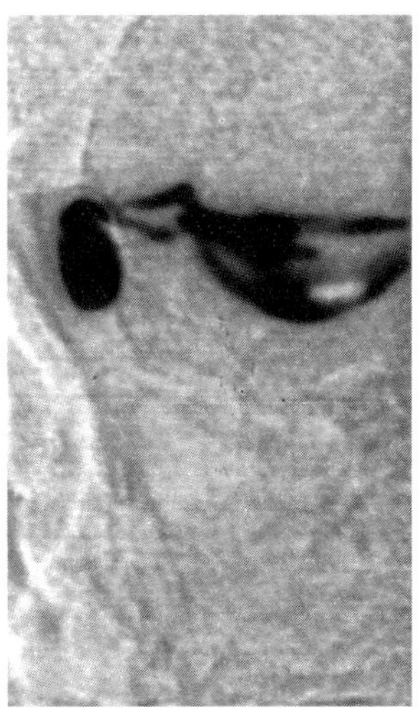
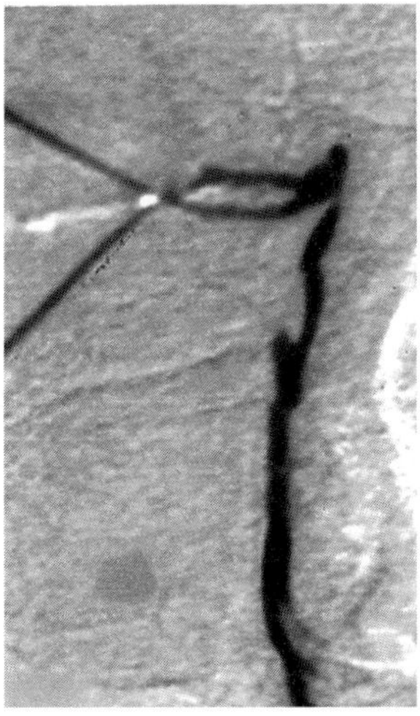
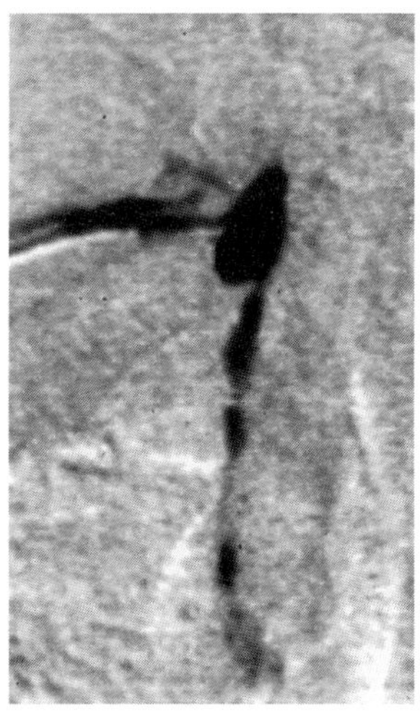

a,b c

**Fig. 15.22 a–c.** Digital subtraction dacryocystography in defects suitable for treatment by dacryocystoplasty. **a** A full obstruction in the junction of the lacrimal sac and the nasolacrimal duct. The lacrimal sac is dilated. **b** A stenosis in the upper half of the lacrimal sac. The common canaliculus expands when contrast medium is injected and, in order to avoid reflux via the upper lacrimal punctum and to pass the large stenosis in the lacrimal sac, it is necessary to wedge the upper canaliculus with a second, nonconducting, catheter. **c** A large stenosis at the junction and two stenoses on the distal side of the nasolacrimal duct. The lacrimal sac is dilated. Reproduced from JANSSEN et al. (1997) with permission from the publisher

15.5.1.2.2
EXCLUSION CRITERIA

Exclusion criteria for dacryocystoplasty are stenoses or occlusions of the canaliculi, acute dacryocystitis, or specific, acquired nasolacrimal sac and duct obstructions, such as posttraumatic obstructions of the bony canal, tumors of the lacrimal drainage system or surrounding area, sarcoidosis of the lacrimal drainage system, or Wegener's granulomatosis. Figure 15.23a,b shows defects that are not suitable for dacryocystoplasty because of their location in the canaliculi. Figures 15.6, 15.8a,b, 15.11 and 15.12 also show defects that should not be treated by dacryocystoplasty.

15.5.1.2.3
QUESTIONABLE INDICATIONS

When there is a long stenosis in the nasolacrimal duct, a narrow bony canal less than 3 mm in diameter is often detected on CT. Further research is needed to determine whether the best results can be achieved with dacryocystorhinostomy, balloon dilatation using a 2-mm balloon diameter, or stent placement. At this moment it is not clear whether commonly occurring stenoses between the common canaliculus and the lacrimal sac should or should not be treated with balloon dilatation. These cases are often accompanied by a hypertrophic appearance of the valve of Rosenmüller (Fig. 15.24). Some authors (ILGIT et al. 1995) have described successful dacryocystoplasty in similar stenoses using a 2-mm balloon. Others (JANSSEN et al. 1994, 1997) take the provisional view that balloon dilatation is contraindicated in cases of a stenosis in the border area be-

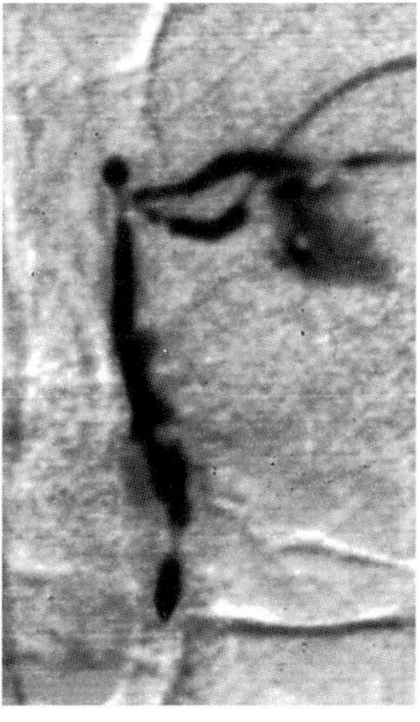
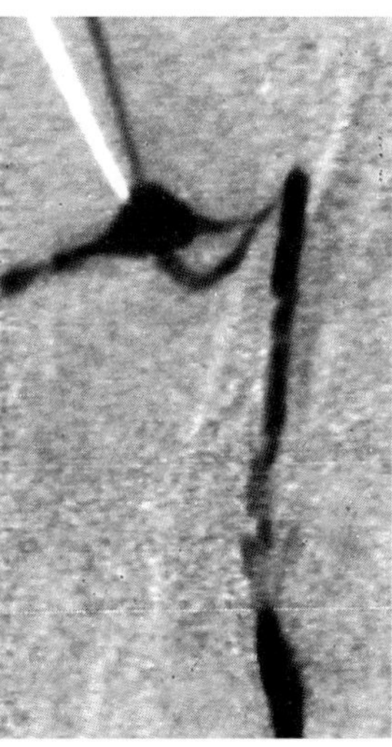

a,b

**Fig. 15.23 a,b.** Digital subtraction dacryocystography of defects for which dacryocystoplasty is not suitable. **a** A stenosis in the upper half of the lacrimal sac, similar to the one in Fig. 14.22b. In this case dacryocystoplasty is contraindicated owing to the presence of an almost complete obstruction in the common canaliculus and multiple stenoses in the lower canaliculus. **b** A stenosis in the common canaliculus. No morphologic defects of the lacrimal sac and nasolacrimal duct are visible. Reproduced from JANSSEN et al. (1997) with permission from the publisher

tween the common canaliculus and the lacrimal sac, to prevent damage to the pump mechanism and the canaliculi.

#### *15.5.1.3 Technique*

Dacryocystoplasty is performed on an outpatient basis after topical anesthesia, usually immediately after digital subtraction dacryocystography. Topical anesthesia is accomplished by applying 0.4% oxybuprocaine hydrochloride (Monofree R; Bournonville-Pharma, Almere, The Netherlands) to the conjunctival sac during digital subtraction dacryocystography. In some cases 1 or 2 additional drops are needed. During digital subtraction dacryocystography anesthetic is applied to the mucosa of the lacrimal drainage system in preparation for dacryocystoplasty, a small amount of 1% lidocaine being mixed with the iopromide. Finally, 10% lidocaine (Xylocaine R spray 10%; Astra, Rijswijk, The Netherlands) is delivered to the nasal mucosa by means of a nebulizer.

On dacryocystoplasty the guidewire is advanced antegradely into the lacrimal drainage system via the lower or upper lacrimal point. When the guidewire extends sufficiently from the nose, the balloon catheter is passed retrogradely over the guidewire via the nose into the lacrimal drainage system.

To pass the lacrimal drainage system, we prefer a shapable 0.025-in. guidewire with hydrophilic coating (Naviguide; Medi-tech/Boston Scientific, Maastricht, The Netherlands), because it is clearly visible under fluoroscopy, easy to push and smooth, because of the hydrophilic coating, and the most distal 4–5 mm of the tip can easily be shaped by hand into a small J-shaped curve (Fig. 15.25). The curve is necessary to enable passage of the sharp curve between the common canaliculus and the lacrimal sac. Guidewires that are supplied with a J-curved tip, such as the 0.025-in. Terumo, are less suitable, because the curve is not at the tip, but 1 cm proximal to the tip.

The guidewire is used in combination with a 20-G plastic vascular sheath (Abbocath; Abbott Ireland, Sligo, Republic of Ireland). Before the procedure, the vascular sheath is also curved at the tip over a wire

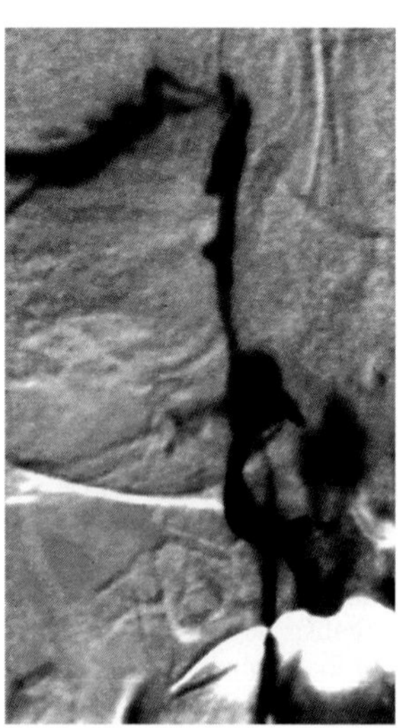

**Fig. 15.24.** Digital subtraction dacryocystography of the lacrimal drainage system on the right side in a patient suffering from epiphora caused by a stenosis between the common canaliculus and the lacrimal sac. The valve of Rosenmüller shows hypertrophy, which is visible as a sickle-shaped gap high on the lateral side of the lacrimal sac. It is questionable whether dacryocystoplasty is indicated in this case.

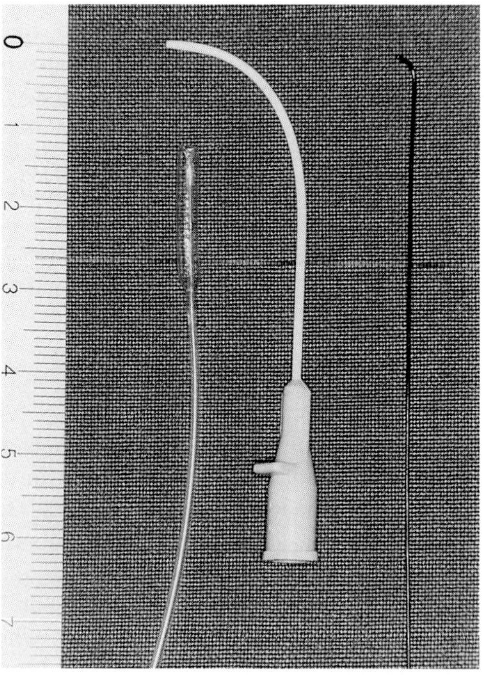


**Fig. 15.25.** The guidewire used in dacryocystoplasty with a J-shaped curve of the most distal 4–5 mm, the 20-G vascular sheath, also with a J-shaped curve at the tip, and the balloon catheter. Note that the catheter has no tip distal to the balloon. The *scale* is in centimeters. Reproduced from Janssen et al. (1997) with permission of the publisher

loop by immersing it in hot water (Fig. 15.26). After cooling of the sheath by immersion in cold water and after removal of the guidewire, the tip has a gradual curved shape (Fig. 15.25).

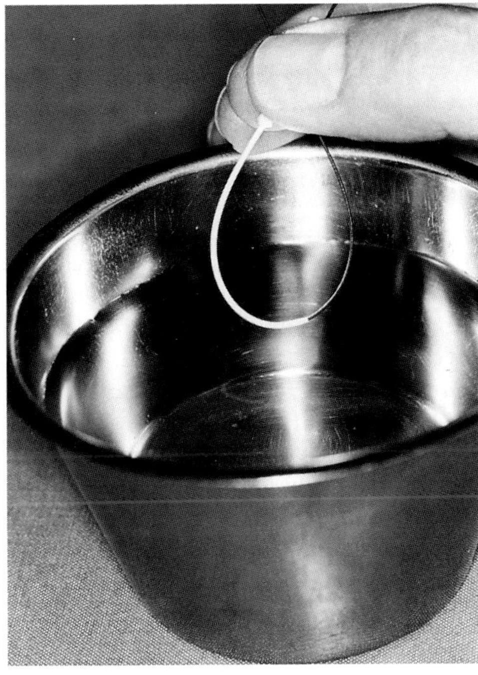

**Fig. 15.26.** The 20-G vascular sheath is curved over a wire loop and immersed in hot water to obtain the desired curve. Reproduced from Janssen et al. (1997) with permission from the publisher

The diagrams in Fig. 15.27a–e show how the guidewire is advanced. One of the lacrimal points is dilated using a lacrimal dilator (Fig. 15.27a). Then the guidewire is advanced via the lacrimal point and the canaliculus until it touches the medial wall of the lacrimal sac. Next the vascular sheath, which is carefully rotated to the left and right, is passed over the guidewire until it has just entered the lacrimal sac (Fig. 15.27b). Subsequently, the vascular sheath is rotated through 180°, causing the sharp curve between the common canaliculus and the lacrimal sac to be straightened (Fig. 15.27c). Under fluoroscopic guidance the guidewire is gently advanced into the lacrimal sac and duct, down to the inferior meatus of the nasal cavity, followed by the sheath (Fig. 15.27a,d,e). The following problems can occur during advancement of the guidewire:

a. The guidewire fails to pass the junction of the common canaliculus and the lacrimal sac. The guidewire cannot be advanced downwards from the common canaliculus. This problem is often associated with slight hypertrophy of the valve of Rosenmüller, creating a small threshold at the bottom of the opening between the common canaliculus and the lacrimal sac. Downward passage should not be forced, because of the risk of false passage from the common canaliculus; rather, the guidewire should be turned through 180° so that the curved tip points towards the

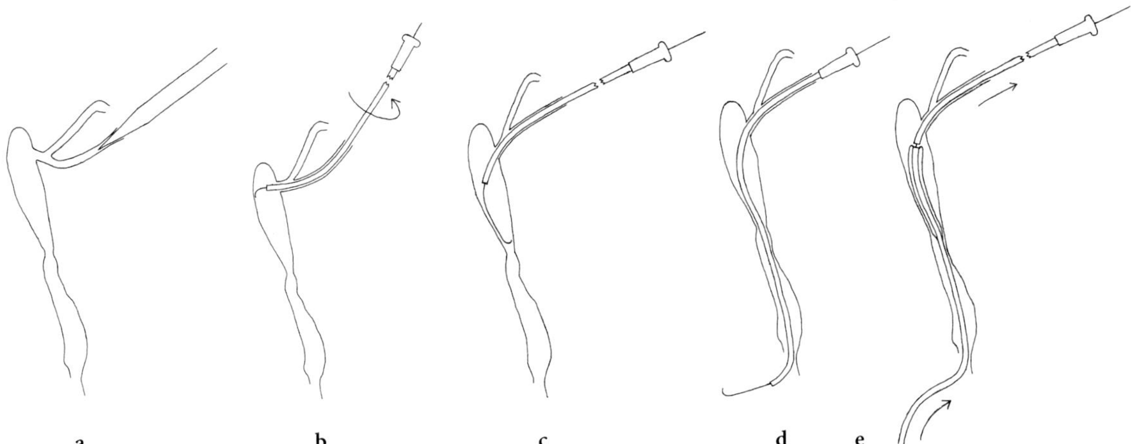


**Fig. 15.27 a–e.** Diagrams illustrating the technique of advancing the guidewire using a curved vascular sheath and positioning the balloon catheter in the lacrimal drainage system. **a** Dilatation of a lacrimal point with a lacrimal dilator. **b** Passage of the vascular sheath over the guidewire until just inside the lacrimal sac, where it is turned through 180°, causing **c** straightening of the sharp curve between the common canaliculus and the lacrimal sac. **d** The guidewire is advanced gently into the lacrimal sac and duct to the inferior meatus of the nasal caurty, followed by the sheath. **e** With fluoroscopic control, the catheter is passed retrogradely into the lacrimal drainage system and positioned at the site of stenosis by pushing the catheter upwards with one hand while pulling the vascular sheath part way out of the canaliculus with the other

cranium and then advanced high into the top of the lacrimal sac. When the guidewire has then again been rotated through 180° the obstruction has been passed.

b. The guidewire cannot pass a stenosis in the lacrimal sac or nasolacrimal duct. Resolution of this problem should be attempted by advancing the guidewire carefully and without pressure and simultaneously rotating it. An attempt should be made to detect the junction of the lacrimal sac and nasolacrimal duct low medial to the lacrimal sac, but in many cases it is not at the lowest point of the lacrimal sac.
c. The guidewire still fails to pass an obstruction in the nasolacrimal duct. First, more extensive pathology of the lacrimal drainage system should be ruled out by CT dacryocystography and the diameter of the bony canal should be determined. When no morphologic abnormalities of the facial bone and soft tissues are found, an attempt can be made to pass the occlusion by applying a little more pressure. To make this possible a 22-G vascular sheath is pushed over a Bowman 4x0 probe. The obstruction is passed by the probe, the probe is removed from the vascular sheath and the guidewire is advanced through the sheath to the nose. Probing can easily be performed by an interventional radiologist experienced in lacrimal drainage system interventions. However, when sufficient experience is lacking, an ophthalmologist should be asked for assistance. Use of a Bowman's probe is only required in 1–2% of dacryocystoplasty procedures. In the majority of cases the obstructions can be passed with the guidewire.
d. The guidewire cannot be advanced far enough to protrude from the nose. It is often possible to advance the guidewire outside the nose under fluoroscopic guidance with lateral projection by turning the curved tip of the vascular sheath forwards. Occasionally, this fails and the guidewire keeps slipping into the epipharynx. A simple solution to this problem is to curve a second guidewire into a loop, which is then inserted into the nose, as close as possible under the inferior turbinate. Under fluoroscopic guidance, the guidewire that points in the direction of the epipharynx can easily be caught with the wire loop and extracted from the nose.
e. It proves impossible to advance the 20-G sheath into the canaliculus despite dilatation of the punctum. Use of a 22-G vascular sheath could be tried, but this has the disadvantage of being slack, in addition to which there is little torque control, so that the curve between the common canaliculus and the lacrimal sac must be passed with the guidewire only.

When the vascular sheath has reached the bottom of the nose with its tip pointing forward, the 0.025-in. wire is replaced by a 0.018-in. wire with a flexible curved tip (Terumo). Changing the wire is necessary because the balloon catheter is adjusted to a 0.018-in. wire. The 0.025-in. wire is used initially, however, because of its excellent shapability, pushability, and visibility under fluoroscopy.

The balloon catheter is passed over the guidewire until its tip touches the tip of the vascular sheath. The guidewire is clipped to either side of the sheath-catheter combination. With fluoroscopic control the balloon catheter is passed retrogradely into the lacrimal drainage system and positioned at the site of the stenosis by pushing the catheter upwards with one hand and pulling the vascular sheath part of the way out of the canaliculus with the other hand (Fig. 15.27e). We prefer a highly flexible 3.4-F balloon catheter with a balloon 3 mm in diameter and 20 mm long (No Tip Bijou 3.0–20; Schneider Europe, Bülach, Switzerland). This catheter has no tip distal to the balloon. Thus, even a stenosis high up in the lacrimal sac can be reached without the catheter tip damaging the common canaliculus.

Dilatation of the lacrimal drainage system can be achieved by inflating the balloon once or twice for 30 s, just long enough to tear the fibrotic component of the obstruction. Other authors (Ilgit et al. 1995; Lee et al. 1994; Song et al. 1993a) recommend a longer inflation time, but this does not improve results (Janssen et al. 1997). Patients tolerate the treatment well under local anesthesia. Occasionally, they experience some pain during balloon inflation. At the end of the procedure the guidewire is removed from the sheath and the balloon catheter is removed via the nose.

#### 15.5.1.4
#### *Postprocedure Treatment*

At the end of the procedure the lacrimal drainage system is flushed with physiologic saline through the vascular sheath that is still in place. This is followed by irrigation of the lacrimal ducts with 0.5 ml (2 mg) dexamethasone (Formulary Dutch Pharmacists). Simultaneously, the vascular sheath is pulled out of the canaliculus. After the procedure, eyedrops [1 mg/ml dexamethasone and 3 mg/ml gentamicin sulfate (Dexamytrex R; Tramedico, Weesp, The Netherlands)] are prescribed: one drop in the affected eye, six times daily for 1 week.

### 15.5.1.5 Complications

Few complications of balloon dilatation of the lacrimal drainage system have been described. When a smooth guidewire with a floppy tip and hydrophilic coating is used no false passage is caused. When a balloon with a diameter of 3 mm is used no significant bleeding is caused. Occasionally, bleeding does occur when a balloon 4 or 5 mm in diameter is used (Lee et al. 1994). In contrast to dacryocystorhinostomy, dacryocystoplasty does not lead to infection in the lacrimal drainage system or the orbita.

### 15.5.1.6 Results

In recent years different authors have published papers on dacryocystoplasty, often reporting differing results in small patient groups with limited follow-up. The series vary widely in patient selection and technique used for the procedure, which makes it difficult to compare the results. Only three fairly large series with longer follow-up periods have been published.

In 1994 Lee et al. published the results of dacryocystoplasty in 81 eyes, with a maximum follow-up of 30 months. They reported a cumulative patency rate of 23%. This series also included stenoses in the canaliculi, and there were many instances of slight bleeding from the lacrimal drainage system, probably owing to the use of a large balloon (4–5 mm in diameter). These disappointing results induced this group of authors to develop an additional treatment involving stent placement.

Ilgit et al. published the results of dacryocystoplasty in 80 eyes, with a follow-up of 6–8 months, in 1995. The results of dacryocystoplasty for stenoses in this series were very good (100%), including the results observed during follow-up, but in the case of occlusions the initial success rate (after 2 months of follow-up) was only 59%, and in the course of continued follow-up another 26% restenoses occurred. Dilatation was performed using a 4 mm balloon. Some of the patients in this series had obstructions in the canaliculi and restenoses after dacryocystorhinostomy, for which the surgically created opening between the lacrimal sac and the nose was dilated.

In 1997, Janssen et al. reported the results of dacryocystoplasty in 100 eyes with 5–48 months follow-up. In this series the long-term cumulative primary patency rate was 70 ± 7% SE. Restenosis occurred in 22 cases during follow-up. These patients were offered repeat dacryocystoplasty, and 11 of them underwent repeat dacryocystoplasty, which was successful in 10 cases. The resulting long-term cumulative secondary patency rate was 81 ± 7% SE. The higher success rate in this series may be explained by stricter selection criteria: patients with stenoses in the canaliculi were excluded, and CT dacryocystography was performed to assess obstructions in the lacrimal sac and nasolacrimal duct that were difficult to pass, before the patients were offered dacryocystoplasty. Another potentially decisive factor is the use of a 3-mm balloon. The difference between the initial and long-term success rates after dacryocystoplasty for an incomplete vs a complete obstruction was statistically significant, with higher success rates for incomplete obstructions. Surprisingly, there was no statistically significant association between success and either the length of the obstruction or the duration of symptoms before dacryocystoplasty.

Dacryocystoplasty is a safe and simple procedure that could replace surgical treatment by dacryocystorhinostomy as the treatment of choice for epiphora caused by a stenosis or occlusion of the lacrimal sac or the nasolacrimal duct. Further research is required into the criteria for optimum patient selection. After a restenosis repeat dacryocystoplasty can be performed and is often successful, but dacryocystorhinostomy or stent placement could also be considered. Dacryocystoplasty does not lead to increased complaints and there are no contraindications to repeat dacryocystoplasty. It never precludes a future dacryocystorhinostomy (Lee et al. 1994; Ilgit et al. 1995; Janssen et al. 1997).

### 15.5.1.7 The Underlying Mechanism of Dacryocystoplasty

Although balloon dilatation of the lacrimal drainage system is increasingly being performed to treat epiphora caused by an obstruction in the lacrimal drainage system, little is known about the mechanism of the procedure. The success of vascular balloon dilatation depends on long-term patency of the stenosis afterwards. The same does not necessarily apply in the case of balloon dilatation of the lacrimal drainage system, because in the course of their lives many people develop obstructions in the lacrimal drainage system without any symptoms (Dalgleish 1967). There are also reports of people who are symptom free after dacryocystorhinostomy, even though they have a re-obstruction of the surgically created opening between the lacrimal sac and the nose (Fig. 15.21). The important factor is the balance between tear production on the one hand and drainage capacity on the other. Studies of the patency of the lacrimal drainage system in persons who have had no symptoms for several years after dacryocystoplasty are likely to reveal some obstructions of the lacrimal drainage system in this group. It is indeed likely that part of the success of dacryocytoplasty is attributable to an interruption of the vicious circle of obstruction, stasis, infection and swelling of the mucosa in the lacrimal drainage system (Janssen et al. 1997). Another factor contributing to this vicious circle, which was also mentioned by Linberg and McCormick (1986), could be reflex hypersecretion of tears when a chronic infection flares up. This might explain why flushing the lacrimal drainage system with physiologic saline and dexamethasone after balloon dilatation followed by further treatment with eyedrops containing dexamethasone and gentamicin could be an important aspect of the treatment (Janssen et al. 1997).

### 15.5.2 Lacrimal Stenting

Encouraged by the poor results of dacryocystoplasty in their series, especially in complete obstructions, Song and coworkers (1993b) focused on alternative treatment methods. Initially, they believed they had found a good alternative in the form of a metallic stent. They developed a self-expandable, "Gianturco-style" stent 4 mm in diameter and 2 cm in length, which was placed in seven patients. During a short follow-up period one stent became obstructed while the others remained patent. A disadvantage of these metallic stents was that they were inflexible, which made placement rather difficult. In addition, a dysfunctional stent, once in place, could only be removed surgically.

Subsequently, Song and coworkers (1994) developed a plastic stent to overcome the limitations of the metallic ones. They developed a stent approximately 5 cm in length, which was made from the tip of a 5-F nylon angiography catheter. To keep the stent in place in the lacrimal drainage system, the outside diameter at the tip of the stent was increased in a way making it similar to the tip of a Malecot catheter, by making incisions lengthways and curving the stent in hot water. Prior to retrograde stent placement via a 6-F sheath, the lacrimal drainage system was dilated using a 3-mm balloon.

In 1996 Song et al. published long-term results obtained in a large series. The stent, which by then was commercially available (Song nasolacrimal duct stent R; Cook Australia, Queensland, Australia) was placed in 283 patients. Follow-up varied from 12 to 30 months. One week after stent placement 87% of patients were symptom free, but approximately 31% of the patients in this group developed a restenosis. Restenosis occurred shortly after stent placement, after a mean period of 16 weeks. Patency could be restored in some stents by flushing the lacrimal drainage system with physiologic saline, but the majority of the obstructed stents had to be removed. Restenosis was often caused by ingrowing granulation tissue, combined with mucus plugging. In 27% of the patients in the group requiring stent removal, restenosis of the lacrimal drainage system occurred immediately after removal. In 73% patency of the lacrimal drainage system after removal was good, but in two thirds of this group restenosis occurred after a mean period of 1 year. The chance of permanent patency after stent removal appears to be slim. Song and coworkers estimated patency rates after stent placement of 46%, 74%, and 85% for obstructions at the site of the lacrimal sac, the site of the junction of the lacrimal sac and duct, and in the nasolacrimal duct, respectively. They conclude that primary stent placement can be a valuable treatment for obstructions in the nasolacrimal duct.

When the long-term results of stent placement (Song et al. 1996) are compared with those of balloon dilatation (Janssen et al. 1998), primary and secondary patency rates after dacryocystoplasty without stent placement are demonstrated to be slightly higher than those for primary stent placement.

Not only can a polyurethane stent become obstructed; it can also sustain a subclinical chronic infection because of bacterial overgrowth, which probably contributes to the vicious circle of infection, swelling of the mucosa, increased obstruction, and stasis. Removal of a dysfunctional stent is followed by rapid restenosis in the lacrimal drainage system in the majority of cases. Because of this and because of the risk of the formation of granulation tissue, stent placement in the lacrimal drainage system might have a negative effect on a dacryocystorhinostomy that may be necessary in the future. Balloon dilatation without stent placement, on the other hand, never precludes future dacryocystorhinostomy. Given that the results of primary stent placement are not superior to those of dacryocystoplasty when the right technique is used in carefully selected patients, that stent placement is more expensive than dacryocystoplasty, and that stents can sustain an infection and frequently cause granulation tissue to develop, there appears to be no indication for primary stent placement in the treatment of an obstruction of the lacrimal drainage system. Therefore, dacryocystoplasty should be the treatment of choice. Further research should identify indications for stent placement. Stent placement may be considered, together with dacryocystorhinostomy, as a treatment for restenosis after dacryocystoplasty and repeat dacryocystoplasty, and it should not be ruled out as a valuable treatment in the case of a lacrimal sac abscess that does not respond favorably to treatment with antibiotics.

### 15.5.3 Drainage of a Lacrimal Sac Abscess

When there is an obstruction distal to the lacrimal sac, the lacrimal sac may swell up and extend laterally, forming a palpable mass in the lacrimal fossa. In some cases careful compression suffices to empty the contents of the lacrimal sac via the canaliculi. However, further swelling of the lacrimal sac may cause kinking of the common canaliculus, thus preventing emptying of the lacrimal sac via the canaliculus. Clear mucus in the lacrimal sac is indicative of a mucocele. When the contents of the lacrimal sac become infected a lacrimal sac abscess develops. A lacrimal sac abscess is extremely painful, and spontaneous rupture via the skin is possible. When a fistula between the lacrimal sac and the skin has developed in this way it will tend to close rather slowly, because tears continue to flow from the lacrimal sac via the fistula. A serious complication of a lacrimal sac abscess can involve spread of the infection to the orbits, which may eventually cause an orbital abscess. A acute lacrimal sac abscess is treated by systemic antibiotics, and possibly additional stab incision of the skin and the lacrimal sac when there is a danger of fistula formation. At a later stage, after the infection has been overcome, the obstruction should be dealt with.

When a lacrimal sac abscess does not respond well to antibiotics and becames chronic and the infection is limited to the lacrimal sac, the interventional radiologist can drain the abscess. The same guidewire and vascular sheath are used as in dacryocystoplasty. By moving the guidewire with great care the kinking of the common canaliculus can be removed. When the guidewire has been advanced into the lacrimal sac and the sheath is passed over the guidewire, the abscess can drain via the sheath after removal of the guidewire. The abscess can be carefully irrigated via the sheath. This treatment is supported by systemic antibiotics. When, after irrigation of the abscess and aspiration of the content of the lacrimal sac as far as possible, the guidewire can be advanced with relative ease via the nasolacrimal duct to the nose, balloon dilatation of the stenosis can be performed and a stent can be left in the lacrimal drainage system for 2–4 weeks. This allows natural drainage of the abscess. A good, cheap stent can be made from a 6-F polyurethane enteral feeding tube (Flocare R; Nutricia Nederland BV, Zoetermeer, The Netherlands). Before use the tube is shortened to 4.5 cm so that the stent remains just visible below the inferior turbinate after placement, allowing easy removal by tweezers after several weeks. The stent is inserted retrogradely into the lacrimal drainage system over a guidewire, using part of the remainder of the enteral feeding tube as a pusher. When the valve of Hasner cannot be passed, the stent can be placed via a 6-F sheath, which is first advanced into the lacrimal drainage system together with a well-tapered dilator. Figure 15.28a–c shows images of such an abscess drainage, which has been successfully performed in some patients; admittedly follow-up is limited to 2–4 months so far.

## 15.6 Conclusions

Epiphora or tearing due to an obstruction in the lacrimal drainage system can be surgically treated by dacryocystorhinostomy. When the operation is performed by an experienced surgeon the success rate is 90%. Recently, an alternative treatment has been developed, i.e., balloon dilatation of the lacrimal drainage system. With careful patient selection and the right technique the results of balloon dilatation are encouraging, and a long-term cumulative secondary

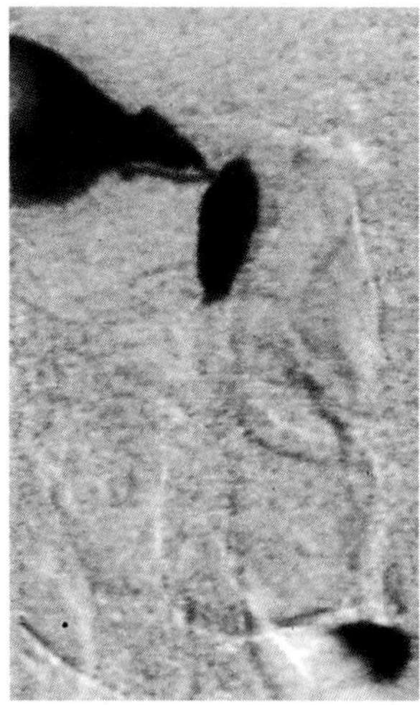
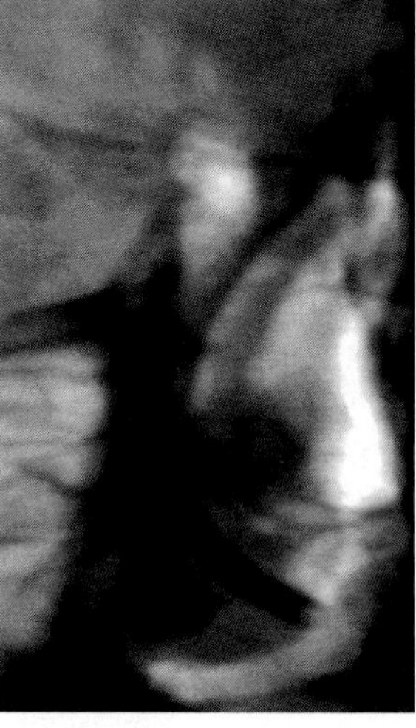
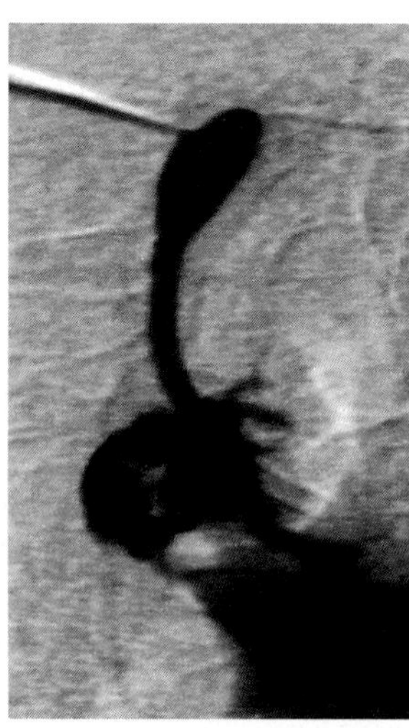

a,b c

**Fig. 15.28.** **a** Digital subtraction dacryocystography of a patient suffering from a lacrimal sac abscess not extending to the surrounding area, which did not respond sufficiently to systemic antibiotics. After flushing of the abscess via the vascular sheath passed into the lacrimal sac over a guidewire, digital subtraction dacryocystography reveals a complete obstruction at the junction of the lacrimal sac and the nasolacrimal duct. **b** X-ray showing the temporary stent, which allowed drainage of the abscess. **c** Digital subtraction dacryocystography showing a well-placed and well-functioning stent. The stent was removed after 4 weeks

patency rate of 81 ± 7% (SE) has been reported. Dacryocystoplasty appears to be a simple, safe procedure performed with local anesthesia as outpatient surgery. Compared with dacryocystorhinostomy, dacryocystoplasty is a less invasive and a less costly procedure. Dacryocystoplasty may become the treatment of choice for epiphora caused by obstruction of the nasolacrimal duct system at the saccular or subsaccular level. Placement of a stent in the lacrimal duct system does not appear to be suitable as primary treatment, because stents often become obstructed by mucus plugging and ingrowing granulation tissue and may cause chronic infection and fibrotic reactions in the long run, leading to restenosis of the lacrimal duct system after removal of a dysfunctional stent. Further research is needed to determine when stent placement is indicated and whether permanent or temporary stent placement should be used in the lacrimal duct system. Indications for stents might include restenosis after dacrycystoplasty and repeat dacryocystoplasty, a relatively narrow bony canal (2.5 or 3 mm), and drainage of a lacrimal abscess that fails to respond adequately to treatment with systemic antibiotics.

*Acknowledgments.* I thank Mereke L.B. Gorsira for translating and correcting the manuscript and Ad J. Petersen for his help with the photographs.

## References

Becker BB, Berry FD (1989) Balloon catheter dilatation in lacrimal surgery. Ophthalmic Surg 20:193–198

Cowen D, Hurwitz JJ (1996) Anatomy of the lacrimal drainage system. In: Hurwitz JJ (ed) The lacrimal system. Lippincott-Raven, Philadelphia, pp 18–21

Dalgleish R (1967) Idiopathic acquired lacrimal drainage obstruction. Br J Ophthalmol 51:463–468

Duke-Elder S (1946) The development, form and function of the visual apparatus. In: Duke Elder S (ed) Text-book of ophthalmology, vol I. Kimpton, London, pp 235–239

Glatt HJ, Chan AC, Barrett L (1991) Evaluation of dacryocystorhinostomy failure with computed tomography and computed tomographic dacryocystography. Am J Ophthalmol 112:431–436

Goldberg RA, Heinz GW, Chiu L (1993) Gadolinium magnetic resonance imaging dacryocystography. Am J Ophthalmol 115:738–741

Gulotta U, Von Denffer H (1980) Dacryocystography: an atlas and textbook. Thieme, Stuttgart

Hanafee WN, Dayton GO (1978) Dilatation of the nasolacrimal duct under radiographic control. Radiology 127:813–815

Herzig S, Hurwitz JJ (1979) Lacrimal sac calculi. Can J Ophthalmol 14:17–20

Hurwitz JJ (1996a) Physiology of the lacrimal drainage system. In: Hurwitz JJ (ed) The lacrimal system. Lippincott-Raven, Philadelphia, pp 23–27

Hurwitz JJ (1996b) Canalicular diseases. In: Hurwitz JJ (ed) The lacrimal system. Lippincott-Raven, Philadelphia, pp 139–141

Hurwitz JJ (1996c) Endoscopy canaliculus. In: Hurwitz JJ (ed) The lacrimal system. Lippincott-Raven, Philadelphia, pp 103–104

Hurwitz JJ (1996d) Dacryocystorhinostomy. In: Hurwitz JJ (ed) The lacrimal system. Lippincott-Raven, Philadelphia, p 261

Hurwitz JJ, Kirsch J (1996) Nuclear lacrimal scanning. In: Hurwitz JJ (ed) The lacrimal system. Lippincott-Raven, Philadelphia, pp 73–81

Hurwitz JJ, Rutherford S (1986) Computerized survey of lacrimal surgery patients. Ophthalmology 93:14–19

Ilgit ET, Yüksel D, Unal M, Akpak S, Isik S, Hasanreisoglu B (1995) Transluminal balloon dilatation of the lacrimal drainage system for the treatment of epiphora. AJR 165:1517–1524

Janssen AG, Mansour K, Krabbe GJ, Van Veen S, Helder AH (1994) Dacryocystoplasty: treatment of epiphora by means of balloon dilatation of the obstructed nasolacrimal duct system. Radiology 193:453–456

Janssen AG, Mansour K, Bos JJ (1997) Obstructed nasolacrimal duct system in epiphora: long-term results of dacryocystoplasty by means of balloon dilatation. Radiology 205:791–796

Lee JM, Song HY, Han YM et al (1994) Balloon dacryocystoplasty: results in the treatment of complete and partial obstructions of the nasolacrimal system. Radiology 192:503–508

Linberg JV, McCormick SA (1986) Primary acquired nasolacrimal duct obstruction: a clinicopathologic report and biopsy technique. Ophthalmology 93:1055–1063

Massaro BM, Gonnering RS, Harris GJ (1990) Endonasal laser dacryocystorhinostomy. A new approach to nasolacrimal duct obstruction. Arch Ophthalmol 108: 1172–1176

Moran CC, Buckwalter K, Caldemeyer KS, Smith RR (1995) Helical CT with topical water-soluble contrast media for imaging of the lacrimal drainage apparatus. AJR 164:995–996

Munk PL, Lin DTC, Morris DC (1990) Epiphora: treatment by means of dacryocystoplasty with balloon dilatation of the nasolacrimal drainage apparatus. Radiology 177:687–690

Nelson LB, Calhoun JH, Menduke H (1985) Medical management of congenital nasolacrimal duct obstruction. Ophthalmol 92:1187–1190

Robertson JS, Brown ML, Colvard DM (1979) Radiation absorbed dose to the lens in dacryoscintigraphy with $^{99m}$Tc $0_4$. Radiology 133:747–750

Rossomondo RM, Carlton W, Trueblood JH, Thomas RP (1972) A new method of evaluating lacrimal drainage. Arch Ophthalmol 88:523–525

Rubin PAD, Bilyk JR, Shore JW, Sutula FC, Cheng HM (1993) Magnetic resonance imaging of the lacrimal drainage system. Ophthalmology 101:235–243

Song HY, Ahn HS, Park CK et al (1993a) Complete obstruction of the nasolacrimal system. Part I. Treatment with balloon dilation. Radiology 186:367–371

Song HY, Ahn HS, Park CK et al (1993b) Complete obstruction of the nasolacrimal system. Part II. Treatment with expandable metallic stents. Radiology 186: 372–376

Song HY, Jin YH, Kim JH et al (1994) Nasolacrimal duct obstruction treated nonsurgically with use of plastic stents. Radiology 190:535–539

Song HY, Jin YH, Kim JH et al (1996) Nonsurgical placement of a nasolacrimal polyurethane stent: long-term effectiveness. Radiology 200:759–763

Steinsapir KD, Glatt HJ, Putterman AM (1990) A 16-year study of conjunctival dacryocystorhinostomy. Am J Ophthalmol 109:387–393

Tanenbaum M, McCord CD (1993) The lacrimal drainage system. In: Tasman W (ed) Duane's clinical ophthalmology, vol IV, chap 13. Lippincott, Philadelphia, p 12

Von Denffer H, Dressler J, Pabst HW (1984) Lacrimal dacryoscintigraphy. Semin Nucl Med 14:8–15

Waite DW, Whittet HB, Shun-Shin GA (1993) Technical note: computed tomographic dacryocystography. Br J Radiol 66:711–713

Walther EK, Herberhold C, Lippel R (1994) Digitale Subtraktions-dakryozystographie (DS-DCG) und Ergebnisbilanz endonasaler Tränenwegschirurgie. Laryngorhinootologie 73:609–613

Weber AL, Rodriquez-DeVelasquez A, Lucarelli MJ, Cheng HM (1996) Normal anatomy and lesions of the lacrimal sac and duct. In: Weber AL (ed) Imaging of the globe, orbit and visual pathway, neuroimaging clinics of North America February 1996. Saunders, Philadelphia, p 200

Zinreich SJ, Miller NR, Freeman LN, Gloriose LW, Rosenbaum AD (1990) Computed tomographic dacryocystography using topical contrast media for lacrimal system visualisation. Orbit 9:79–87

# Subject Index

# List of Contributors

B. Biswal, PhD
Department of Biophysics
Medical College of Wisconsin
Froedtert Memorial Lutheran Hospital
9200 West Wisconsin Avenue
Milwaukee, WI 53226
USA

Vincent Carrasco, MD
Division of Otolaryngology
Head and Neck Surgery
610 Burnet Womack, CB #7070
and Department of Radiology
The School of Medicine
University of North Carolina at Chapel Hill
Chapel Hill, NC 27599
USA

J. A. Castelijns, MD
Academic Hospital
Vrije Universiteit
Department of Radiology
Postbus 7057
1007 MB Amsterdam
The Netherlands

Mauricio Castillo, MD
Departments of Radiology
The School of Medicine
University of North Carolina at Chapel Hill
Chapel Hill, NC 27599-7510
USA

Vincent Chong, MD
Department of Diagnostic Radiology
Singapore General Hospital
Outsam Road
Singapore

D. L. Daniels, MD
Department of Radiology
Medical College of Wisconsin
Froedtert Memorial Lutheran Hospital
9200 West Wisconsin Avenue
Milwaukee, WI 53226
USA

R. De Bree, MD
Department of Otolaryngology/
Head and Neck Surgery
Free University Hospital
De Boelelaan 1117
1081 HV Amsterdam
The Netherlands

Jeffrey L. Duerk, PhD
Department of Radiology
University Hospitals of Cleveland
Case Western Reserve University
11100 Euclid Avenue
Cleveland, OH 44106
USA

Markus Gapany, MD
Division of Otolaryngology
Veterans Affairs Medical Center
One Veterans Drive
Minneapolis, MN 55417
USA

Frank M. Grund, MD
Department of Nuclear Medicine
Veterans Affairs Medical Center
One Veterans Drive
Minneapolis, MN 55417
USA

Bradley M. Hemminger, MS
Department of Radiology
Radiology Research Center
University of North Carolina
Chapel Hill, NC 27599-7515
USA

R. Hermans, MD
Catholic University Leuven
Department of Radiology
University Hospitals
UZ Gasthuisberg
Herestraat 49
B-3000 Leuven
Belgium

Lorenz Jäger, MD
Institut für Radiologische Diagnostik
Klinikum Großhadern
der Ludwig-Maximilians-Universität
München
Marchioninistrasse 15
D-81366 München
Germany

Alfred G. Janssen, MD
Department of Diagnostic and
Interventional Radiology
De Tjongerschans Hospital
Thialfweg 44
Postbus 10500
8441 PW Heerenveen
The Netherlands

Maria Lapela, MD
Department of Oncology and Radiotherapy
and Turku PET Centre
Turku University Central Hospital
PL 52
FIN-20521 Turku
Finland

Sirkku Leskinen, MD
Department of Oncology and Radiotherapy
and Turku PET Centre
Turku University Central Hospital
PL 52
FIN-20521 Turku
Finland

Jonathan S. Lewin, MD
Department of Radiology
University Hospitals of Cleveland
Case Western Reserve University
11100 Euclid Avenue
Cleveland, OH 44106
USA

Paula Lindholm, MD, PhD
Department of Oncology and Radiotherapy
and Turku PET Centre
Turku University Central Hospital
PL 52
FIN-20521 Turku
Finland

Martin G. Mack, MD
Virchow-Klinikum
Humboldt University of Berlin
Strahlenklinik und Poliklinik
Augustenburger Platz 1
D-13353 Berlin
Germany

L. P. Mark, MD
Department of Radiology
Medical College of Wisconsin
Froedtert Memorial Lutheran Hospital
9200 West Wisconsin Avenue
Milwaukee, WI 53226
USA

Elmar M. Merkle, MD
Department of Radiology
University Hospitals of Cleveland
Case Western Reserve University
11100 Euclid Avenue
Cleveland, OH 44106
USA

Heikki Minn, MD
Department of Oncology and Radiotherapy
and Turku PET Centre
Turku University Central Hospital
PL 52
FIN-20521 Turku
Finland

Kristine Mosier, DMD, PhD
Division of OMF Radiology and
Department of Oral Pathology and
Diagnostic Sciences
New Jersey Dental School and
Department of Radiology
University Hospital, University of Medicine and
Dentistry of New Jersey RmC-829
110 Bergen Street
Newark, NJ 07103-2400
USA

Suresh K. Mukherji, MD
Departments of Radiology and Surgery
The School of Medicine and
Department of Diagnostic Sciences and
The School of Dentistry
610 Burnet Womack CB # 7070
University of North Carolina at Chapel Hill
Chapel Hill, NC 27599-7510
USA

J. J. Quak, MD
Department of Otolaryngology/
Head and Neck Surgery
Free University Hospital
De Boelelaan 1117
1081 HV Amsterdam
The Netherlands

J. C. Roos, MD
Department of Nuclear Medicine
Free University Hospital
De Boelelaan 1117
1081 HV Amsterdam
The Netherlands

G.B. Snow, MD
Department of Otolaryngology/
Head and Neck Surgery
Free University Hospital
De Boelelaan 1117
1081 HV Amsterdam
The Netherlands

John L. Ulmer, MD
Department of Radiology
Medical College of Wisconsin
Froedtert Memorial Lutheran Hospital
9200 West Wisconsin Avenue
Milwaukee, WI 53226
USA

M.W.M. van den Brekel, MD
Department of Otolaryngology
Free University Hospital Amsterdam
P.O. Box 7057
1007 MB Amsterdam
The Netherlands

G.A.M.S. van Dongen, PhD
Department of Otolaryngology/
Head and Neck Surgery
Free University Hospital
De Boelelaan 1117
1081 HV Amsterdam
The Netherlands

Thomas J. Vogl, MD
Virchow-Klinikum
Humboldt University of Berlin
Strahlenklinik und Poliklinik
Augustenburger Platz 1
D-13353 Berlin
Germany

David M. Yousem, MD
Departments of Radiology and
Otorhinolaryngology: Head and Neck Surgery
University of Pennsylvania Medical Center
3400 Spruce Street
Philadelphia, PA 19104
USA

Printing and binding: Druckerei Triltsch, Würzburg

# Medical Radiology

## Diagnostic Imaging and Radiation Oncology

*Titles in the series already published*

### Diagnostic Imaging

**Innovations in Diagnostic Imaging**
Edited by J.H. Anderson

**Radiology of the Upper Urinary Tract**
Edited by E.K. Lang

**The Thymus - Diagnostic Imaging, Functions, and Pathologic Anatomy**
Edited by E. Walter, E. Willich, and W.R. Webb

**Interventional Neuroradiology**
Edited by A. Valavanis

**Radiology of the Pancreas**
Edited by A.L. Baert, co-edited by G. Delorme

**Radiology of the Lower Urinary Tract**
Edited by E.K. Lang

**Magnetic Resonance Angiography**
Edited by I.P. Arlart, G.M. Bongartz, and G. Marchal

**Contrast-Enhanced MRI of the Breast**
S. Heywang-Köbrunner and R. Beck

**Spiral CT of the Chest**
Edited by M. Rémy-Jardin and J. Rémy

**Radiological Diagnosis of Breast Diseases**
Edited by M. Friedrich and E.A. Sickles

**Radiology of the Trauma**
Edited by M. Heller and A. Fink

**Biliary Tract Radiology**
Edited by P. Rossi

**Radiological Imaging of Sports Injuries**
Edited by C. Masciocchi

**Modern Imaging of the Alimentary Tube**
Edited by A. R. Margulis

**Diagnosis and Therapy of Spinal Tumors**
Edited by P. R. Algra, J. Valk, and J. J. Heimans

**Interventional Magnetic Resonance Imaging**
Edited by J. F. Debatin and G. Adam

**Abdominal and Pelvic MRI**
Edited by A. Heuck and M. Reiser

**Orthopedic Imaging**
Edited by A.M. Davies and H. Pettersson

**Radiology of the Female Pelvic Organs**
Edited by E.K.Lang

**Magnetic Resonance of the Heart and Great Vessels**
Clinical Applications
Edited by J. Bogaert, A. J. Duerinckx, and F. E. Rademakers

**Modern Head and Neck Imaging**
Edited by S. K. Mukherji and J. A. Castelijns

### Radiation Oncology

**Lung Cancer**
Edited by C.W. Scarantino

**Innovations in Radiation Oncology**
Edited by H.R. Withers and L.J. Peters

**Radiation Therapy of Head and Neck Cancer**
Edited by G.E. Laramore

**Gastrointestinal Cancer – Radiation Therapy**
Edited by R.R. Dobelbower, Jr.

**Radiation Exposure and Occupational Risks**
Edited by E. Scherer, C. Streffer, and K.-R. Trott

**Radiation Therapy of Benign Diseases - A Clinical Guide**
S.E. Order and S.S. Donaldson

# MEDICAL RADIOLOGY
## Diagnostic Imaging and Radiation Oncology

*Titles in the series already published*

### RADIATION ONCOLOGY

**Interventional Radiation Therapy Techniques - Brachytherapy**
Edited by R. Sauer

**Radiopathology of Organs and Tissues**
Edited by E. Scherer, C. Streffer, and K.-R. Trott

**Concomitant Continuous Infusion Chemotherapy and Radiation**
Edited by M. Rotman and C.J. Rosenthal

**Intraoperative Radiotherapy – Clinical Experiences and Results**
Edited by F.A. Calvo, M. Santos, and L.W. Brady

**Radiotherapy of Intraocular and Orbital Tumors**
Edited by W.E. Alberti and R.H. Sagerman

**Interstitial and Intracavitary Thermoradiotherapy**
Edited by M.H. Seegenschmiedt and R. Sauer

**Non-Disseminated Breast Cancer**
Controversial Issues in Management
Edited by G.H. Fletcher and S.H. Levitt

**Current Topics in Clinical Radiobiology of Tumors**
Edited by H.-P. Beck-Bornholdt

**Practical Approaches to Cancer Invasion and Metastases**
A Compendium of Radiation Oncologists' Responses to 40 Histories
Edited by A.R. Kagan with the Assistance of R.J. Steckel

**Radiation Therapy in Pediatric Oncology**
Edited by J.R. Cassady

**Radiation Therapy Physics**
Edited by A.R. Smith

**Late Sequelae in Oncology**
Edited by J. Dunst and R. Sauer

**Mediastinal Tumors. Update 1995**
Edited by D.E. Wood and C.R. Thomas, Jr.

**Thermoradiotherapy and Thermochemotherapy**
Volume 1:
Biology, Physiology, and Physics
Volume 2:
Clinical Applications
Edited by M.H. Seegenschmiedt, P. Fessenden, and C.C. Vernon

**Carcinoma of the Prostate**
Innovations in Management
Edited by Z. Petrovich, L. Baert, and L.W. Brady

**Radiation Oncology of Gynecological Cancers**
Edited by H.W. Vahrson

**Carcinoma of the Bladder**
Innovations in Management
Edited by Z. Petrovich, L. Baert, and L.W. Brady

**Blood Perfusion and Microenvironment of Human Tumors**
Implications for Clinical Radiooncology
Edited by M. Molls and P. Vaupel

**Radiation Therapy of Benign Diseases. A Clinical Guide**
2nd revised edition
S.E. Order and S.S. Donaldson

**Carcinoma of the Kidney and Testis, and Rare Urologic Malignancies**
Innovations in Management
Edited by Z. Petrovich, L. Baert, and L.W. Brady